PRACTICAL PHYSIOLOGY

PRACTICAL PHYSIOLOGY

As per the Competency-based Medical Education Curriculum (NMC)

SECOND EDITION

N Geetha MBBS MD (Physiology)
Principal
Government Medical College
Manjeri, Kerala, India

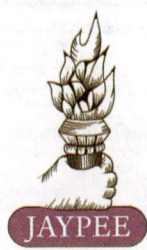

JAYPEE BROTHERS MEDICAL PUBLISHERS
The Health Sciences Publisher
New Delhi | London

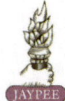
Jaypee Brothers Medical Publishers (P) Ltd

Headquarters
Jaypee Brothers Medical Publishers (P) Ltd
EMCA House, 23/23-B
Ansari Road, Daryaganj
New Delhi 110 002, India
Landline: +91-11-23272143, +91-11-23272703
+91-11-23282021, +91-11-23245672
Email: jaypee@jaypeebrothers.com

Corporate Office
Jaypee Brothers Medical Publishers (P) Ltd
4838/24, Ansari Road, Daryaganj
New Delhi 110 002, India
Phone: +91-11-43574357
Fax: +91-11-43574314
Email: jaypee@jaypeebrothers.com

Overseas Office
J.P. Medical Ltd
83 Victoria Street, London
SW1H 0HW (UK)
Phone: +44 20 3170 8910
Fax: +44 (0)20 3008 6180
Email: info@jpmedpub.com

Website: www.jaypeebrothers.com
Website: www.jaypeedigital.com

© 2025, Jaypee Brothers Medical Publishers

The views and opinions expressed in this book are solely those of the original contributor(s)/author(s) and do not necessarily represent those of editor(s) and publisher of the book.

All rights reserved. No part of this publication may be reproduced, stored or transmitted in any form or by any means, electronic, mechanical, photocopying, recording or otherwise, without the prior permission in writing of the publishers.

All brand names and product names used in this book are trade names, service marks, trademarks or registered trademarks of their respective owners. The publisher is not associated with any product or vendor mentioned in this book.

Medical knowledge and practice change constantly. This book is designed to provide accurate, authoritative information about the subject matter in question. However, readers are advised to check the most current information available on procedures included and check information from the manufacturer of each product to be administered, to verify the recommended dose, formula, method and duration of administration, adverse effects and contraindications. It is the responsibility of the practitioner to take all appropriate safety precautions. Neither the publisher nor the author(s)/editor(s) assume any liability for any injury and/or damage to persons or property arising from or related to use of material in this book.

This book is sold on the understanding that the publisher is not engaged in providing professional medical services. If such advice or services are required, the services of a competent medical professional should be sought.

Every effort has been made where necessary to contact holders of copyright to obtain permission to reproduce copyright material. If any have been inadvertently overlooked, the publisher will be pleased to make the necessary arrangements at the first opportunity.

Inquiries for bulk sales may be solicited at: jaypee@jaypeebrothers.com

Practical Physiology

First Edition: 2017
Second Edition: **2025**
ISBN: 978-93-5696-933-9

Printed in India at Sterling Graphics Pvt. Ltd.

Dedicated to

My parents
K Saraladevi who was and still is my pillar of strength and
N Natarajan who told me never to settle for good but
to chase perfection.

Preface to the Second Edition

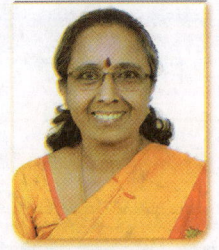

The book was originally structured strictly with the then latest curriculum in mind. But as we progress, what was new then becomes old now. The revised book aims to maintain the simplicity of the previous version while updating its applied aspects. The viva questions and model answers have also been updated to reflect recent trends.

I am still extremely obliged to Dr Diveen Sengeeth, for his help.

I am also indebted to Shri Jitendar P Vij (Group Chairman), Mr Ankit Vij (Managing Director), Mr MS Mani (Group President), Dr Madhu Choudhary (Director–Educational Publishing), Ms Pooja Bhandari [Director–Production (Books and Journals)], Mr Ajay Kumar Sharma [Deputy General Manager (Books and Journals)], Ms Sunita Katla (Executive Assistant to Group Chairman and Publishing Manager), Ms Samina Khan (Executive Assistant to Director–Educational Publishing), Dr Aditya Tayal (Editorial Manager–Content Strategy), Ms Jitika Royal (Content Strategist–Nursing), Mr Rajesh Sharma (Production Coordinator), Ms Seema Dogra (Cover Visualizer), Ms Neha Verma (Graphic Designer–Cover), Mr Laxmidhar Padhiary (Quality Controller), Mr Kulwant Singh (Typesetter), and Mr Radhey Shyam Singh (Graphic Designer) of M/s Jaypee Brothers Medical Publishers (P) Ltd, New Delhi, India, and their team for the sincere work in bringing out this book.

God bless.

N Geetha

Preface to the First Edition

As an aspiring doctor, every medical student should have a clear and unambiguous understanding of the field. As you know, second chances are very rare in our field and a mistake can even cost a life. To further your understanding of this vast arena, I have endeavored to bring out this edition of *Practical Physiology*. The book has been structured keeping the requirements of the present day curriculum in mind. It is constructed in a simple manner and includes the basic principles of physiology and its applied aspects. The viva questions and model answers given at the end of each chapter will help the students in preparing for their examination.

For ease of use, the book is divided into five main sections: Hematology, Clinical Examination, Amphibian, Biophysics and Mammalian Experiments. In the sixth section, the normal hematological and biochemical values are given. In the seventh section, the model of practical examination and sample questions with model answers are provided.

I extend my sincere thanks to Dr Diveen Sengeeth for his help in taking photographs and editing them. I also express my gratitude to my teachers and my dear students who are both the motivation and encouragement for this book.

I am indebted to Shri Jitendar P Vij (Group Chairman) and Ms Chetna Malhotra Vohra (Associate Director–Content Strategy) of Jaypee Brothers Medical Publishers and their team for the sincere work in bringing out this book.

I thank Almighty for giving me health and strength in completing the book.

N Geetha

Contents

Section 1: Hematology

Chapter 1: Compound Microscope   3
- Light Microscopes   3

Chapter 2: Microscopic Examination of Blood   10
- Aim   10
- Apparatus   10
- Examination of Fresh Blood Under the Microscope   10
- Examination of Blood in Isotonic Solution   11
- Blood in Hypotonic Saline   11
- Blood in Hypertonic Saline   11

Chapter 3: Collection of Blood Sample   13
- Collection of Blood   14

Chapter 4: Erythrocyte Sedimentation Rate   17
- Principle   17
- Methods   17
- Result   19

Chapter 5: Packed Cell Volume or Hematocrit   23
- Principle   23
- Methods   23

Chapter 6: Estimation of Hemoglobin (Hemoglobinometry)   28
- Colorimetric Estimation of Hemoglobin   28
- Other Methods of Estimation of Hemoglobin   31

Chapter 7: Hemocytometer and Red Blood Cell Count   34
- Hemocytometry   34
- Hemocytometer   34
- Red Blood Cell Count   36
- Result   39
- Discussion   39
- Normal RBC Count   39

Chapter 8: Red Blood Cell Indices—MCV, MCH and MCHC   44
- Mean Corpuscular Volume or MCV   44
- Mean Corpuscular Hemoglobin or MCH   44
- Mean Corpuscular Hemoglobin Concentration or MCHC   45

Chapter 9: Determination of Specific Gravity of Blood   47
- Principle   47

Chapter 10: Determination of Osmotic Fragility of Red Blood Cells   50
- Principle   50
- Apparatus   50
- Procedure   50
- Observations   50
- Result   51

Chapter 11: White Blood Cell Count or Total Leukocyte Count   54
- Principle   54
- Apparatus   54
- WBC Pipette   54
- WBC Diluting Fluid (Turk's Fluid)   54

Chapter 12: Differential Leukocyte Count   58
- Principle   58
- Apparatus   58
- Methods of Making a Blood Smear   59

Chapter 13: Absolute Eosinophil Count by Hemocytometry   71
- Principle   71
- Apparatus   71

Chapter 14: Reticulocyte Count   74
- Principle   74
- Procedure   74

Chapter 15: Platelet Count   77
- Apparatus   77
- Automated Analyzer   78

Chapter 16: Determination of Bleeding Time and Clotting Time   80
- Bleeding Time   80
- Clotting Time   81

Chapter 17: Determination of Blood Group   85
- Principle   85
- Apparatus   85
- Procedure   85
- Observations   86

Section 2: Clinical Examination

Chapter 18: General Examination   93

Chapter 19: Physical Examination   99
- Inspection   99
- Palpation   99
- Percussion   100
- Auscultation   101

Chapter 20: Determination of Arterial Blood Pressure   103
- Aim *103*
- Principle of Manual Blood Pressure Measurement *103*
- Methods of Sphygmomanometry *104*
- Recording of Blood Pressure in Different Postures and After Exercise *105*
- Sample Report Pattern *106*

Chapter 21: Examination of the Respiratory System   109
- Inspection *109*
- Palpation *110*
- Percussion *112*
- Auscultation *113*
- Report Pattern *114*
- General Examination *114*
- Respiratory System Examination *114*

Chapter 22: Examination of Cardiovascular System   116
- Examination of Arterial Pulse *116*
- Measurement of Arterial Blood Pressure *118*
- Jugular Venous Pressure *118*
- Examination of Precordium *119*
- Report Pattern *123*

Chapter 23: Recording of Arterial Pulse   126
- Aim *126*
- Apparatus: Physiograph *126*
- Procedure *126*
- Discussion *127*
- Abnormalities of Arterial Pulse *127*

Chapter 24: Examination of Abdomen   129
- Aim *129*
- Requirements *129*
- Procedure *129*
- Abdominal Examination *129*
- Inspection *129*
- Palpation *130*
- Percussion *133*
- Auscultation *133*
- Report Pattern *134*
- Impression *134*

Chapter 25: Examination of Nervous System   135
- Examination of Higher Functions *135*
- Mental State *135*
- Memory *136*
- Speech *136*
- Posture and Gait *136*

Chapter 26: Examination of the Sensory System   138
- Requirements *138*
- Method *138*
- Touch Sensation *138*
- Pain Sensation *139*
- Vibration Sense *139*
- Temperature *140*
- Stereognosis *140*
- Appreciation of Passive Movement and Sense of Position (Proprioception) *140*
- Graphesthesia *141*
- Double Simultaneous Stimulation *141*
- Test the Sensory Cranial Nerves (I, II, VIII) and the Sensory Parts of Mixed Nerves *141*
- Report Pattern of a Normal Subject *141*
- Impression *142*

Chapter 27: Examination of Motor System   145
- Inspection *145*
- Bulk of Muscle *145*
- Muscle Tone *146*
- Coordination of Movement *147*
- Muscle Power or Strength of the Muscles *150*
- Muscles of Upper Limb *151*
- Muscles of Shoulder *153*
- Muscles of Neck, Abdomen and Back *154*
- Muscles of Lower Limb *155*
- Grading of Power of Muscles *155*
- Motor Cranial Nerves *155*
- Gait *156*
- Abnormal Movements *156*
- Report Pattern *156*

Chapter 28: Examination of the Cranial Nerves   159
- Olfactory Nerve *159*
- Optic Nerve *160*
- Oculomotor, Trochlear and Abducent Nerves (III, IV, VI) *163*
- Trigeminal Nerve *165*
- Facial Nerve *166*
- Vestibulocochlear (Acoustic) Nerve *168*
- Vestibular Part *169*
- Glossopharyngeal Nerve *170*
- Vagus Nerve *170*
- Accessory Nerve *171*
- Hypoglossal Nerve *172*
- Examination of Cranial Nerves *172*
- Olfactory Nerve *172*
- Optic Nerve *172*
- Oculomotor, Trochlear and Abducent Nerve *172*
- Trigeminal Nerve *172*
- Facial Nerve *172*
- Vestibulocochlear Nerve *173*
- Glossopharyngeal Nerve *173*
- Vagus Nerve *173*
- Spinal Accessory Nerve *173*
- Hypoglossal Nerve *173*

Chapter 29:	Examination of Reflexes	176

- Deep Reflexes or Muscle Stretch Reflexes (Tendon Jerks) *177*
- Superficial Reflexes *180*
- Corneal and the Conjunctival Reflexes (V and VII Cranial Nerve) *180*
- Pharyngeal and Palatal Reflexes (IX and X Cranial Nerves) *180*
- Pupillary Reflexes (II and III Cranial Nerves) *180*
- Abdominal Reflex (T6 to T12 Spinal Segments) *180*
- Cremasteric Reflex (L1, 2) *181*
- Plantar Reflex (L4, 5, S1, 2) *181*
- Anal Reflex (Pudendal Nerve; S3, 4, 5) *182*
- Visceral Reflexes or Organic Reflexes *182*

Section 3: Experimental Physiology (Amphibian Experiments)

Chapter 30:	Common Appliances Used in the Experimental Physiology Laboratory	187

- Study of Instruments Used *187*
- Electrical Equipments *187*
- Mechanical Equipments *190*

Chapter 31:	Pithing of Frog and Dissection of Muscle Nerve Preparation	194

- Pithing of Frog *194*
- Dissection of the Nerve-Muscle Preparation *195*

Chapter 32:	Mounting the Muscle-Nerve Preparation	197

- Procedure *197*

Chapter 33:	Simple Muscle Twitch	199

- Materials *199*
- Observation *200*

Chapter 34:	Effects of Two Successive Stimuli on Muscle Contraction	202

- Requirements *202*
- Method *202*
- Observations *203*

Chapter 35:	Genesis of Tetanus	205

- Apparatus *205*
- Procedure *205*
- Observation *205*

Chapter 36:	Effect of Afterload and Freeload in Skeletal Muscle Contraction	208

- Principle *208*
- Requirements *208*

Chapter 37:	Effect of Continuous Stimulation of a Muscle (Study of Fatigue and Recovery)	211

- Principle *211*
- Requirements *211*
- Electrical Connections *211*
- Procedure *211*
- Observations *212*
- Precautions *212*

Chapter 38:	Effects of Temperature on Muscle Contraction	213

- Principle *213*
- Requirements *213*
- Procedure *213*
- Precautions *214*
- Observation *214*

Chapter 39:	Velocity of Nerve Impulses	216

- Principle *216*
- Requirements *216*
- Calculations *217*

Chapter 40:	Normal Cardiogram of Frog	218

- Anatomy of the Frog's Heart *218*
- Requirements *219*
- Recording of the Normal Cardiogram *219*
- Observation *219*
- Precautions *219*

Chapter 41:	Effect of Temperature on Frog's Heart	221

- Requirements *221*
- Procedure *221*
- Observation *221*

Chapter 42:	Stannius Ligatures	223

- Requirements *223*
- Procedure *223*
- Observation *224*

Chapter 43:	Extrasystole and Compensatory Pause	225
Chapter 44:	Effect of Vagal Stimulation on Frog's Heart	227
Chapter 45:	Effect of Drugs and Ions on Isolated Frog's Heart	230

- Principle *230*
- Requirements *230*
- Procedure *230*
- Precautions *231*

Section 4: Biophysics Experiments

Chapter 46:	Cathode Ray Oscilloscope	235
Chapter 47:	Electrocardiography	237

- Electrocardiograph *237*
- Method *239*

Chapter 48:	Spirometry	247

- Spirometer *247*

Chapter 49:	Stethography	251

- Aim *251*

- ❖ Apparatus *251*
- ❖ Procedure *252*
- ❖ Observation *252*
- ❖ Precautions *253*

Chapter 50: Perimetry *255*
- ❖ Perimeter *255*
- ❖ Apparatus *256*
- ❖ Procedure *256*
- ❖ Observations and Inferences *257*
- ❖ Precautions *257*

Chapter 51: Electromyography *259*
- ❖ Principle *259*
- ❖ Apparatus *259*
- ❖ Electrodes *259*

Chapter 52: Audiometry *261*
- ❖ Apparatus *261*
- ❖ Procedure *262*
- ❖ Observation *262*

Chapter 53: Ergography *264*
- ❖ Procedure *264*

Chapter 54: Peak Expiratory Flow Rate *266*
- ❖ Aim *266*
- ❖ Apparatus *266*
- ❖ Procedure *266*

Chapter 55: Ophthalmoscopy *268*
- ❖ Aim *268*
- ❖ Apparatus *268*
- ❖ Principle *268*
- ❖ Procedure *268*
- ❖ Discussion *269*

Chapter 56: Harvard Step Test *271*
- ❖ Aim *271*
- ❖ Equipment Required *271*
- ❖ Principle *271*
- ❖ Procedure *271*

Chapter 57: Cardiovascular Autonomic Function Tests *274*
- ❖ Aim *274*
- ❖ Cardiovascular Response to Standing (30:15 R-R Ratio) *274*
- ❖ Heart Rate and Blood Pressure Response to Passive Tilting *275*
- ❖ Valsalva Ratio *275*
- ❖ Heart Rate Variation with Deep Breathing (Sinus Arrhythmia) *277*
- ❖ Isometric Exercise (Sustained Hand Grip Test) *277*

Section 5: Mammalian (Rabbit) Experiments

Chapter 58: Perfusion of Isolated Rabbit's Heart and the Effects of Drugs and Ions *281*
- ❖ Principle *281*
- ❖ Requirements *281*
- ❖ Procedure *281*
- ❖ Precautions *282*
- ❖ Observation *282*

Chapter 59: Recording of Rabbit's Normal Intestinal Movements and the Effects of Drugs *285*
- ❖ Principle *285*
- ❖ Requirements *285*
- ❖ Procedure *285*

Section 6: Normal Values

Chapter 60: Hematologic Values and Fluids Used in the Laboratory *291*
- ❖ Normal Values *291*
- ❖ Composition of Different Fluids Used in the Laboratory *292*

Section 7: Model of Practical Examination

Chapter 61: Sample Questions *295*
- ❖ Pattern of Practical Examination *295*
- ❖ Mark Distribution for I MBBS Physiology Practical Examination *310*

Index *313*

Competency Table

Number	Competency: The student should be able to	Core (Y/N)	Chapter number	Page number
PY 2.8	Describe the physiological basis of hemostasis and, anticoagulants. Describe bleeding and clotting disorders (hemophilia, purpura)	Y	16	80
PY 2.9	Describe different blood groups and discuss the clinical importance of blood grouping, blood banking and transfusion	Y	17	85
PY 2.11	Estimate Hb, RBC, TLC, RBC indices, DLC, blood groups, BT/CT	Y	6, 7, 8, 11, 12, 16, 17	28, 34, 44, 54, 58, 80, 85
PY 2.12	Describe test for ESR, osmotic fragility, hematocrit. Note the findings and interpret the test results, etc.	Y	4, 5, 10	17, 23, 50
PY 2.13	Describe steps for reticulocyte and platelet count	Y	14, 15	74, 77
PY 3.15	Demonstrate effect of mild, moderate and severe exercise and record changes in cardiorespiratory parameters	Y	56	271
PY 3.18	Observe with computer-assisted learning: (i) amphibian nerve-muscle experiments, (ii) amphibian cardiac experiments	Y	30, 31, 32, 33, 34, 35, 36, 37, 38, 39, 40, 41, 42, 43, 44, 45	187, 194, 197, 199, 202, 205, 208, 211, 213, 216, 218, 221, 223, 225, 227, 230
PY 4.10	Demonstrate the correct clinical examination of the abdomen in a normal volunteer or simulated environment	Y	24	129
PY 5.12	Record blood pressure and pulse at rest and in different grades of exercise and postures in a volunteer or simulated environment	Y	20	103
PY 5.13	Record and interpret normal ECG in a volunteer or simulated environment	Y	47	237
PY 5.14	Observe cardiovascular autonomic function tests in a volunteer or simulated environment	N	57	274
PY 5.15	Demonstrate the correct clinical examination of the cardiovascular system in a normal volunteer or simulated environment	Y	22	116
PY 5.16	Record arterial pulse tracing using finger plethysmography in a volunteer or simulated environment	N	23	126
PY 6.8	Demonstrate the correct technique to perform and interpret spirometry	Y	48, 54	247, 266
PY 6.9	Demonstrate the correct clinical examination of the respiratory system in a normal volunteer or simulated environment	Y	21	109

Number	Competency: The student should be able to	Core (Y/N)	Chapter number	Page number
PY 10.11	Demonstrate the correct clinical examination of the nervous system: Higher functions, sensory system, motor system, reflexes, cranial nerves in a normal volunteer or simulated environment	Y	26, 27, 28, 29	138, 145, 159, 176
PY 10.17	Describe and discuss functional anatomy of eye, physiology of image formation, physiology of vision including color vision, refractive errors, color blindness, physiology of pupil and light reflex	Y	55	268
PY 10.20	Demonstrate: (i) testing of visual acuity, color and field of vision and (ii) hearing, (iii) testing for smell and (iv) taste sensation in volunteer/simulated environment	Y	50, 52	255, 261
PY 11.13	Obtain history and perform general examination in the volunteer/simulated environment	Y	18	93

Section 1

Hematology

1. Compound Microscope
2. Microscopic Examination of Blood
3. Collection of Blood Sample
4. Erythrocyte Sedimentation Rate
5. Packed Cell Volume or Hematocrit
6. Estimation of Hemoglobin (Hemoglobinometry)
7. Hemocytometer and Red Blood Cell Count
8. Red Blood Cell Indices—MCV, MCH and MCHC
9. Determination of Specific Gravity of Blood
10. Determination of Osmotic Fragility of Red Blood Cells
11. White Blood Cell Count or Total Leukocyte Count
12. Differential Leukocyte Count
13. Absolute Eosinophil Count by Hemocytometry
14. Reticulocyte Count
15. Platelet Count
16. Determination of Bleeding Time and Clotting Time
17. Determination of Blood Group

Chapter 1

Compound Microscope

LEARNING OBJECTIVES

- Describe the uses of the different parts of the compound microscope
- Adjustment of microscope for viewing object under low-power, high-power and oil immersion objective
- Enumerate the precautions to be taken while handling and while using the microscope
- Define resolution, magnification, working distance and numerical aperture of microscope
- Describe other types of microscopy and their principles

INTRODUCTION

Fine structural organization of tissues can be appreciated only by the use of microscopes. **Hooke** made the first compound microscope in 1695. It has been made perfect by others. Microscopy works on the principles of optics.

Microscopy is of two types—**light microscopy and electron microscopy**. Light microscopy involves the use of either artificial light or natural sunlight. Electron microscopy involves the use of a beam of electrons, which, by virtue of refraction/diffraction or absorbance through a series of converging/diverging electrostatic plate lenses or magnets, renders the view of the object enlarged.

LIGHT MICROSCOPES

Light microscopes include simple microscope and compound microscope.

Simple microscope works on the principle of simple biconvex lens. The image formed is virtual and erect. The magnification in simple microscope ranges from 2 to 20 times. They do not give a three-dimensional appreciation of the object. They are used in preliminary screening examination of the object.

Compound microscopes are called so because they are combinations of a double set of lenses referred to as objective lens that lies in proximity to the object and eyepiece lens which lies near the observer's eye. The eyepiece and objective lenses have different magnification. Compound microscopes include monocular compound

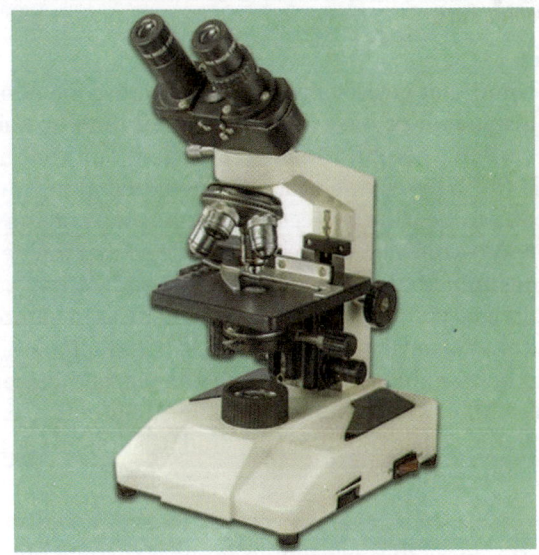

Fig. 1.1: Binocular microscope.

microscope having single eyepiece, binocular compound microscope that has two eyepieces **(Fig. 1.1)**, phase contrast microscope, polarizing microscope, fluorescence microscope, etc. Monocular compound microscope is discussed in detail.

Parts of the Compound Microscope

Compound microscope consists of:
- Mechanical parts
- Optical parts

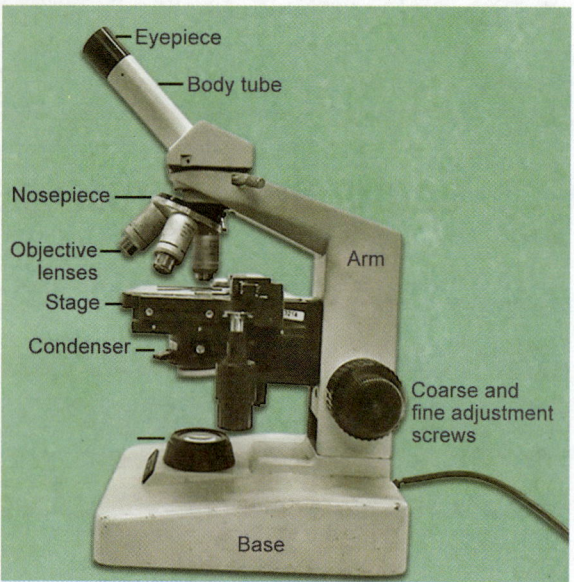

Fig. 1.2: Compound microscope (monocular).

The mechanical parts consist of the stand and the arm. The optical parts consist of eyepiece and the nosepiece that carries the objectives **(Fig. 1.2)**.

Mechanical Parts

Stand
The stand that gives stability to the microscope consists of a heavy **foot or base and a C-shaped limb or handle** that contain the optical parts. A hinged joint that helps to tilt the microscope to any angle convenient for the observer to view the object connects the limb and the foot. The microscope can be inclined a little so that the person looking into the microscope need not bend. This is useful if prolonged continuous work is to be done as in pathology departments to view histology slides. If fluid preparations are to be examined the stage must be placed horizontal. For example, while doing RBC count, WBC count, etc., if the microscope is kept tilted the fluid will drain away from the counting chamber.

Arm
The arm carries the body tube in its upper part and the stage and the sub-stage in its lower part.

- **Body tube:** Body tube is fitted at the upper end of the handle. The optical parts are held in position by the body tube that can be moved up and down by means of **coarse and fine adjustment screws** one pair on either side. The coarse adjustment screw is identified by the bigger size of the knob while fine adjustment has a smaller knob. When one coarse or fine adjustment screw is turned, the one on the other side also rotates at the same time. Coarse adjustment moves the tube rapidly through a large distance when the adjusting screw is rotated. The fine adjustment works in a similar way but several rotations of the screw head are required to move the tube through a very small distance, i.e., one rotation is equal to 0.01 mm or less. Thus the height of the tube can be adjusted so that the objective lens can be kept at its optimal working distance from the object. (The body of the microscope may be of two types. In one type, the stage is fixed and the body tube can be moved up or down; while in the other type, the body tube is fixed and the stage is moved up and down.)

  The body tube is 16–17 cm in length and is called the **tube length**. It is the distance between the upper end of the objective and the upper-end of the eyepiece. The distance between the lower focal point of the objective and the upper focal point of the eyepiece is called the **optical tube length**, which is about 25 cm. Increase in the tube length increases the magnification but this may result in loss of clarity of the image. It is through the body tube that light passes to the eyepiece.

- **Stage:** Stage is a rigid platform on which the slide containing the specimen to be examined or, the counting chamber is kept. It consists of a fixed stage and a mechanical stage. The **fixed stage** is a square platform with an aperture in its center to permit light to reach the object. **Mechanical stage** is a calibrated mechanical frame located on the right edge of the fixed stage. It consists of a **slide holder** that keeps the slide in position. There are two screws for moving the slide forwards, backwards, and from side to side.

- **Sub-stage:** The sub-stage lies below the stage. It carries the condenser and the iris diaphragm fitted in a short cylinder. Sub-stage can be lowered and raised with the help of a screw.

The **sub-stage condenser** consists of two lenses that are corrected for spherical and chromatic aberration and it is used to focus light on the object to be viewed. It can be raised or lowered and thus the focus of light can be changed. It also helps in resolving the image. The full resolving power of the objective is possible only by the use of a proper condenser system. An ideal condenser system is an optically inverted objective. It is constructed in such a way that it gives a solid cone of rays that reaches the object in a perpendicular direction.

The **numerical aperture (NA)** of a lens is the ratio of its diameter to its focal length. As the numerical aperture increases, the resolving power of the lens also increases. The condenser has a fixed NA for a particular amount of light passing through the lens. Decreasing the amount of light passing through the lens can decrease the numerical aperture. Therefore, the illumination has to be increased as the objectives are changed from low power, to high power, or to oil immersion. Raising or lowering the condenser can vary its numerical aperture. While viewing under a particular objective, the NA of condenser and the objective should be the same.

All the light passing through the condenser is collected by the objective and helps in maximum clarity of the object viewed. So the position of the condenser must be changed with each objective to get the light focused and to increase the resolving power of the microscope. The proper use of the condenser is necessary for obtaining the maximum resolution of an image.

The **iris diaphragm** is seen below the condenser and is attached to it. Function is to control the amount of light reaching the object. It can be opened or closed with the help of a lever on its side. By narrowing the aperture of iris diaphragm, the numerical aperture of the condenser can be decreased.

Illumination System

Below the condenser a double-sided reflecting mirror is attached which is plane on one side and concave on the other side. It can be tilted in all directions. A microscope can function optimally only if proper illumination is there. All the light reaching the eye of the observer should come from the object. In the microscope, proper illumination is provided by the position of the condenser, mirror, and the size of the iris diaphragm. The source of illumination can be sunlight that is collected by the mirror, or it can be an inbuilt electric microscope lamp for all powers of the objectives. A frosted tungsten lamp provides uniform white light. If the light source is inbuilt, there is no need of the mirror. Here the intensity of light can be adjusted with a knob provided at the base in front.

Optical Magnifying Parts

Eyepiece

Eyepiece is fitted at the top of the body tube. The height of the eyepiece varies—5X is the tallest and 15X is the shortest one. 5X and 10X eyepieces are commonly used (× denotes the magnification, i.e., 5X means the image reaching the eye piece is magnified 5 times). 6X, 8X, and 15X eyepieces are also available. Each eyepiece has two planoconvex lenses, one at the top and the other fitted at the bottom. The lower lens called the **field lens** collects the divergent rays of the image magnified by the objective and passes them to the **eye lens** that further magnifies the image. A pointer eyepiece has a small pin mounted in it. It is used to point out a specific object in a field. A demonstration eyepiece has two separate eyepieces mounted on a horizontal barrel. Two people can simultaneously observe the mounted object.

Nosepiece

Nosepiece is fitted at the lower-end of the body tube. It has two parts, **fixed nosepiece and revolving nosepiece**. The revolving nosepiece carries three objectives lenses whose magnification power is 10X, 40X, and 100X, respectively which is imprinted on the objective. Oil immersion objective also has a black rim around its lower end. The desired objective can be rotated into position and the correct position is indicated by a click sound. The aperture of the low power lens is the largest and it has the maximum focal length. The oil immersion lens has only a pinhole aperture. The oil immersion lens has a very short focal length and if the aperture is large, spherical, and chromatic aberration will distort the image.

Image Formation by the Microscope

Image is formed with the help of two convex lenses, the objective lens and the eyepiece lens. The objective lens forms a real inverted and magnified image of the object, which is further magnified by the eyepiece lens. The function of the field lens of the eyepiece is to collect the diverging rays of the primary image formed by the objective lens and pass it to the eye lens of the eyepiece. A virtual magnified image of the object is seen through the eyepiece. The image appears to be at a distance of 25 cm in front of the eyes.

Working Distance

The working distance is the distance between the objective and the slide under study. The distance decreases with increasing magnification. An objective operates at a distance from the object that is roughly equal to its focal length. Focal length is maximal for low power lens and minimum for oil immersion lens. The working distance is 10–13 mm for low power, 1–3 mm for high power, and less than 0.5 mm for oil immersion lens, respectively.

Magnification of the Microscope

Magnification power of the microscope is the degree of image enlargement. The magnification produced by the microscope is obtained by multiplying the objective magnification by the eyepiece magnification. For example, if the eyepiece used is 5X, and the objective is 10X, then the total magnification is $5 \times 10 = 50$. That is, the image of the object is magnified 50 times. The maximum magnification in compound microscope is obtained with an oil immersion objective that gives a total magnification of 1,000 times. The maximum resolution of the magnified image, by the most powerful light microscope, is limited by the wavelength of the light source used. Further magnification, therefore, can be obtained only by reducing the wavelength of the light source.

Resolving Power

Resolving power of the eye indicates the capacity of the eye to differentiate between two points kept close to each other as separate and distinct from each other. The resolving power of unaided human eye is between 0.15 mm and 0.25 mm. The resolving power of lens depends on its NA as well as the wavelength of incidental light (λ). The resolving power of a microscope is expressed in terms of **limit of resolution (LR) or the minimum separable distance**. If the distance between two points is less than LR, the two points appear as one. The limit of resolution of a standard light microscope is around 200 nm. The electron microscope gives very high magnification and has a resolving power of 0.5 nm.

$$\text{Resolving power (R)} = \frac{0.61\lambda}{NA}$$

Taking into consideration the resolving power of the eye, only a magnification capable of separating 1/100th of an inch would be useful. Further magnification will cause strain to the eye.

Adjustments of the Microscope

Low Power Adjustments

- The low power objective in which is labeled 10X is brought in line with the eyepiece lens.
- The condenser is lowered.
- Iris diaphragm is half opened so that a narrow rim of light rays at the periphery is cut-off.
- If mirror is used, concave mirror is turned toward the source of light.
- Look at the lower end of the objective by bending by the side of the microscope and by coarse adjustment bring down the low power objective near the slide, but take care that the objective does not touch the slide.
- Then look into the microscope through the eyepiece and slowly raise the objective by using the coarse adjustment screw till the object can be clearly seen.
- The cells and their components are three-dimensional structures and lie at different levels. So under any magnification, the focus should not be kept fixed but continuously use the fine adjustment screw to see the details of the object. This process of continuously adjusting the fine adjustment screw to bring the various structures into view clearly into and out of focus alternately is called **racking the microscope**.

High Power Adjustments

- High power objective, which is marked 40X or 45X, is brought into position and confirmed by the click sound.
- Condenser is half raised.
- Plane mirror is turned toward the source of light if mirror is present or switch on the light.
- Iris diaphragm is 3/4th opened.
- As for low power adjustment, raise the body tube very slowly till the object is clearly seen. While viewing under high power, the working distance is very little. So it is better to do the adjustments using the fine adjustment screw.
- While looking through the eyepiece, the objective should never be brought down with coarse adjustment screw. This may lead to damage of the costly objective lens.

Adjustments for Oil Immersion

- Oil immersion objective, which is labeled 100X, is brought in line with the eyepiece lens.
- Condenser is raised fully.
- Iris diaphragm is fully opened.
- Plane mirror is used.
- After keeping the slide on the stage, put a drop of cedar wood oil on the slide over the area to be observed.
- Looking through the side of the microscope, bring down slowly the oil immersion objective till it just touches the oil.
- Look through the eyepiece and by fine adjustment focus the image accurately.

Precautions

- While changing the objective, make sure that the objective clicks into its proper position.
- Position of the condenser and the aperture of the iris should be checked while using each objective.
- Before placing the slide on the stage make sure that the microscopic adjustments are correct.
- While focusing the object, lower the objective close to the slide by looking directly at the objective so that it does not touch the object. Then by looking through the eye piece, focus the object by very slowly raising the objective.
- Never bring down the objective with the coarse adjustment screw while looking through the eyepiece.
- Always examine the slide under low power first and then observe under high power and oil immersion objective. This is to make sure that the prepared slide satisfies the criteria for a good one.

Care of Microscope

- Always keep the microscope in its case when not in use in order to protect it from moisture and dust.
- Place it on the table in a stable position. Take care of the eyepiece when it is removed from the tube.
- Always keep the microscope clean and free from dust.
- Clean the eye piece frequently since it comes in contact with the observer's eye.
- Cedar wood oil should be removed from the oil immersion lens immediately after completing the experiment. Otherwise it may seep into the body of the objective and damage the lens. The oil should be removed first with a dry soft cloth or with clean tissue lens paper and then with a little of xylol on it. Use of organic solvents like xylene or ethanol frequently should be avoided. It loosens the cement material in which the objective is fixed.

- The surface of the objectives and the eyepieces should be cleaned with soft linen or polishing cloth. Always take care not to touch the glass with fingers and not to blow on them to remove dust.
- While lifting the microscope, one hand should be placed under the base and the other hand should hold the handle.
- Each microscope should be thoroughly checked by a mechanic at least once a year.
- *Never bring the objective down using the coarse adjustment screw while looking into the microscope. It may hit the slide and cause damage to the lens, which is costly.*

Other Microscopes

Phase Contrast Microscope

Phase contrast microscope uses principles of light refraction and it helps to identify structures that cannot be seen with ordinary light microscope. It works on the principle of interference. Unstained wet preparations can be studied. In this microscope, a special plate is inserted into the condenser, which can retard the speed of some light waves. Since the different cells have different refractive indices, this microscope uses these differences to produce an image with good contrast of light and shade.

Electron Microscope

Electron microscope is used to study the ultra-structural details of tissues and cells. In an electron microscope the electron beam of much lesser wavelength replaces the light source. Electromagnetic fields are used in place of glass lenses. A series of electromagnets are used for converging or diverging the beam of electrons. This renders the view of the object as enlarged one. The electron microscope gives very high magnification and can separate dots that are about 0.2 nm apart. There are two types of electron microscopy:

a. Transmission electron microscopy (TEM) gives a two-dimensional image of the object. It uses a beam of electrons instead of light and electromagnetic field instead of glass lens. Magnification is about 100,000 times.

b. Scanning electron microscopy (SEM) gives a three-dimensional image. The image is produced in a cathode ray oscilloscope and it can be magnified.

Fluorescence Microscope

A fluorescent dye is used to stain tissues or microorganisms like *Mycobacterium tuberculosis*; lipids, and elastic fibers, etc., which are then studied under this microscope. Ultraviolet light is used for illumination.

Dark-Field Microscope

To view a specimen in dark field, an opaque disk is placed underneath the condensor lens, so that light that is scattered by objects on the slide can reach the eye. Instead of coming up through the specimen, the light is reflected by particles on the slide. The condensor system is modified so that the specimen is not illuminated directly. The field in view looks dark since light does not pass from the condensor to the objective. The object under study, appears light against a dark background. Living specimens can be observed more readily with dark-field than with bright-field microscopy. Dark-field is used for the demonstration of *Treponema pallidum*, the motility of flagellated bacteria and protozoa, and is also used to study mounted cells and tissues.

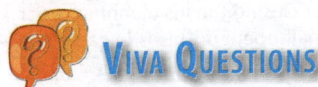

Viva Questions

1. **Who invented microscope?**
   Robert Hooke.
2. **What are the adjustments of microscope for low power, high power, and oil immersion?**
   Refer page 6.
3. **What is meant by resolution?**
   Refer page 5 and 6.
4. **What does the term numerical aperture mean?**
   Refer page 4.
5. **Why oil is used while viewing under oil immersion objective?**
   Cedar wood oil is used in oil immersion to avoid the thin layer of air between the slide and the objective so that the glass slide and the objective lens become a continuous column. This avoids refraction of light rays coming from the condenser and allows enough light to enter the objective. When light rays pass from a denser medium (glass slide) to a rarer medium (air) the rays get refracted away from the aperture of the objective. The oil immersion lens has only a pinhole aperture. Any factor that reduces the amount of rays falling on the objective impairs the quality of the image and the image will be faint. Oil removes the layer of air and prevents refraction of light.
6. **Why cedar wood oil is used specifically in oil immersion?**
   Cedar wood oil is used because it has the same refractive index as that of glass (1.515) and least refraction of light rays occur. Liquid paraffin and glycerin can also be used but cedar wood oil gives best result.

7. **What are the precautions you should take while using the microscope?**
   Refer page 6.

8. **Why the oil immersion objective has only a pinhole aperture?**
   The focal length of oil immersion lens is very short. So if it has a large aperture, more light will enter through the periphery of the lens leading to spherical and chromatic aberration, which will distort the image. Since the aperture is small, it allows only the central cone of light to pass through and form the image which will be very clear.

9. **What is the magnification for low power, high power, and oil immersion when a 10X eyepiece is used?**
   Magnification power of the microscope is the degree of image enlargement. The magnification produced by the microscope is obtained by multiplying the objective magnification by the eyepiece magnification.
   Low power—100 times (objective 10X)
   High power—400 times (objective 40X)
   Oil immersion—1,000 times (objective 100X)

10. **What does working distance mean? Give its value for different magnifications.**
    The distance between the object and the objective lens in the microscope at which the object is sharply focused is called working distance. The objective working distance decreases as the magnification and numerical aperture increase. It is maximal for low power 10X (5–8 mm), less for high power 40X (0.5 mm), and least for oil immersion 100X (0.13 mm).

11. **What are the functions of the condenser and iris diaphragm?**
    Condenser condenses the light rays and focuses them on the object. All the light passing through the condenser is collected by the objective and helps in maximum clarity of the object viewed. So the position of the condenser must be changed with each objective to get the light focused and to increase the resolving power of the microscope. If the condenser is raised too high maximum light reaches the objective lens. The aperture of the low power lens is largest and it will allow large amount of light to pass through. So if the condenser is raised to the maximum while viewing under low power the clarity of the image will be lost due to excessive brightness. So the condenser should be lowered while using low power objective to avoid glare. The rays passing through the condenser system when collected by the objective now suffer from minimum diffraction. The oil immersion objective lens has only a pinhole aperture and so for maximum clarity the condenser should be raised. The proper use of the condenser is necessary for obtaining the maximum resolution of an image. Adjusting the iris diaphragm that is placed immediately below the condenser can control light reaching the condenser.

12. **What is meant by 'racking the microscope'?**
    While viewing an object under the microscope, using the fine adjustment screw the structures in the slide can be brought into clear focus by turning it very slowly. The focus should be continuously changed to see all the structures. This is because, the cells and their organelles are three-dimensional and lie at different levels. So, instead of viewing the object under a fixed focus the microscope can be continuously racked using the fine adjustment screw so that different structures come into focus at different times and all structures can be clearly viewed.

13. **Why is this microscope called compound microscope?**
    In a simple microscope, only a single convex lens is required to view the object. But details of the object cannot be studied. In the compound microscope, there are two lens systems. One is the objective lens and other is the eye piece lens. Since two lenses take part in image formation this is called a compound microscope. A real, inverted and magnified image is produced by the objective lens which is called the primary image. The image seen by our eye is a virtual, inverted and magnified image produced by the eye piece from the image produced by the objective lens.

14. **What is the significance of changing the illumination while using different objectives?**
    Illumination in the microscope can be changed by raising or lowering the condensor and opening or closing the iris diaphragm. For example, while using low power objective, the condensor should be lowered and iris diaphragm half opened. This is because the clarity of the image depends on an optimal amount of light reaching the object. Greater illumination is required while viewing under oil immersion lens.

OBJECTIVE STRUCTURED PRACTICAL EXAMINATION

I. Make microscopic adjustments for viewing an object under low power objective
1. Adjust concave mirror if adjustable mirror is present, otherwise switch on the light
2. Open the iris diaphragm 1/2
3. Adjust the low power objective till a click sound is heard
4. Lower the condenser to the maximum
5. Raise the body tube and place the slide on the stage
6. Look from the side while lowering the body tube
7. Make coarse adjustments to focus the image
8. Then use the fine adjustment screw for final focusing

II. Make microscopic adjustments for focusing an object under high power
1. Use plane mirror or switch on the light
2. Open the iris diaphragm 3/4th
3. Condensor to be half raised
4. After raising the body tube place the slide on the stage
5. Look from the side while lowering the body tube
6. First view the object under low power objective to see whether the staining is perfect
7. Then bring the high power objective into position
8. Make coarse adjustments to focus the image
9. Then use fine adjustment screw for final focusing

III. Make microscopic adjustments to focus an object under oil immersion objective
1. Adjust plane mirror or put on the light
2. Open the iris diaphragm fully
3. Condensor should be fully raised
4. Place a drop of cedar wood oil in the center of the slide
5. Place the slide on the stage
6. First view the object under low power and then under high power and if it is perfect
7. Bring the oil immersion objective into position
8. Adjust the slide on the stage so that the oil immersion objective just touches the oil
9. Make coarse adjustments to focus the image
10. Then use the fine adjustment screw to view the image clearly

Chapter 2

Microscopic Examination of Blood

LEARNING OBJECTIVES

- Normal appearance of fresh blood under the microscope
- Identify the morphology of red blood cells and rouleaux formation
- Appreciate the change in the morphology of red cells in hypotonic and hypertonic solutions
- Identify abnormal size, color and shape of red cells in disease conditions like anemia

AIM

To study the appearance of red blood cells (RBCs) in whole blood and to study the morphological changes in RBCs when suspended in isotonic saline, hypotonic saline, and in hypertonic saline. The students can be trained to use the microscope properly using this experiment.

APPARATUS

Compound microscope, glass slides, cotton, spirit, isotonic, hypotonic and hypertonic saline, sterile lancet or needle.

EXAMINATION OF FRESH BLOOD UNDER THE MICROSCOPE

Examining whole blood under the microscope is an extremely useful method for studying the color, size, and shape of red cells; the white blood cells (WBCs), etc. Fresh blood can be examined as a wet mount. Prick the fingertip using a sterile needle and place a drop of blood on a clean glass slide. Put a cover slip over it and seal the edges of the coverslip with paraffin wax to prevent drying. Examine it under the high power of the microscope. Wet mounts are used to detect sickling of red cells, spherocytes and parasites within erythrocytes. Their typical movement in the field can detect some organisms such as spirochetes and trypanosomes. In the physiology laboratory, students can study the normal biconcave shape of RBCs, formation of rouleaux, presence of anisocytosis, poikilocytosis, etc.

Observation

The RBCs are seen singly and in groups. Single red cells have biconcave shape and pink color with a central pallor. Size varies between 7.2 and 7.5 μm. Nucleus is absent. When present in groups, they are seen attached to one another at their broad surfaces like a pile of coins. This is referred to as rouleaux formation **(Fig. 2.1)**. It is a peculiar phenomenon observed in the whole blood when it is allowed to stand. The number of cells in each pile varies between 2 and 16. Most of the piles have 10–12 cells. In circulation as the blood is constantly moving, no piling can occur. Formation of these piles or rouleaux depends upon the presence of globulins and fibrinogen in the plasma.

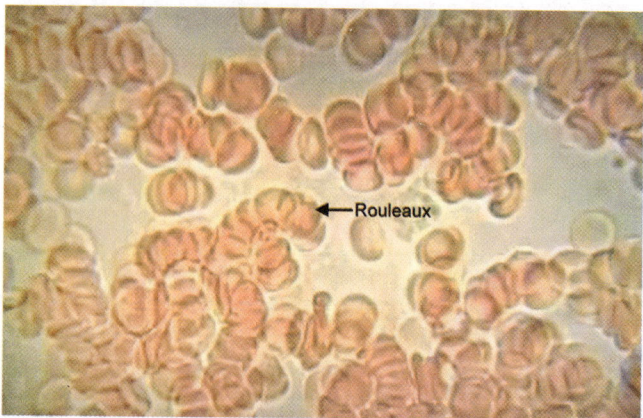

Fig. 2.1: Fresh blood under the microscope (note the biconcave shape of erythrocytes and rouleaux formation).

Different types of white blood cells are also seen. Many white cells show motility, some have irregular shapes due to the formation of pseudopodia. Formation of the fibrin fibers may also be seen after some time.

EXAMINATION OF BLOOD IN ISOTONIC SOLUTION

A drop of isotonic solution or normal saline (0.9% sodium chloride solution) is taken in a glass slide. To this add one drop of fresh blood obtained by the finger prick. Cover it with the cover slip and observe under the microscope. The red cells are seen with normal morphology having normal size (7.2–7.5 µm diameter) and shape (dumb-bell shape). Rouleaux formation is usually not seen due to dilution.

BLOOD IN HYPOTONIC SALINE

A drop of hypotonic saline is taken on the glass slide and to this add one drop of fresh blood. Cover with the cover slip and observe under the high power. The RBCs are found to be swollen and spherical in shape. Pores appear in the stretched RBC membrane through which hemoglobin escapes out and the remaining cell is called ghost cell **(Fig. 2.2)**. Most of the RBCs are ruptured and the remnants of the cell membrane seen are also called ghost cells. When suspended in hypotonic saline, water enters the red cells by endosmosis since the osmotic pressure inside the RBC is more when compared to the fluid outside. This causes swelling of the RBCs and finally they rupture which is referred to as **hemolysis**.

BLOOD IN HYPERTONIC SALINE

Blood is mixed with hypertonic saline and observed under the microscope. The red cells are seen to be shrunken and

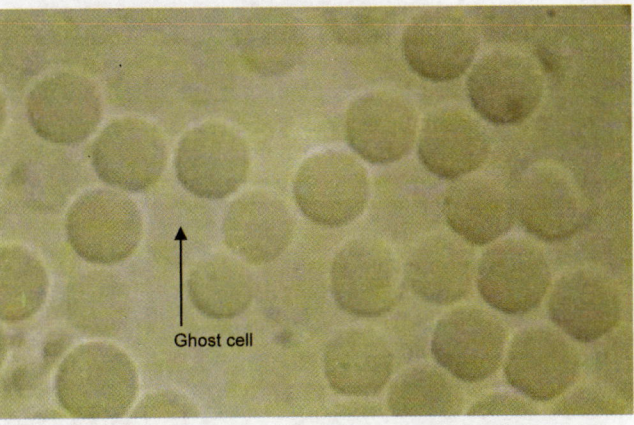

Fig. 2.2: Blood in hypotonic saline (note the swollen erythrocytes and cell membrane remnants referred to as ghost cell).

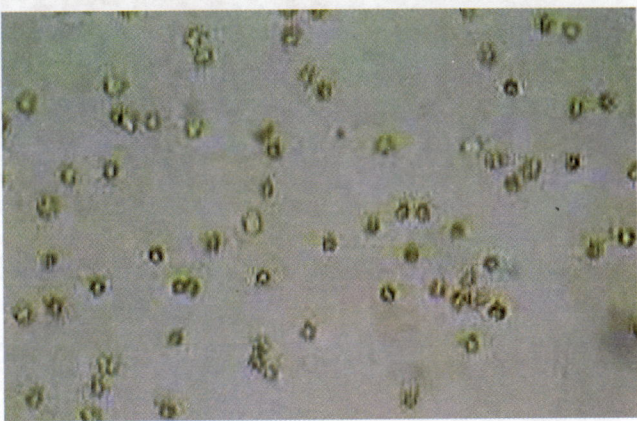

Fig. 2.3: Blood in hypertonic saline (note the crenated or star shaped erythrocytes).

crenated (star shaped) due to exosmosis **(Fig. 2.3)**. Water moves from inside the cell to the outside since the amount of osmotically active particles is more outside.

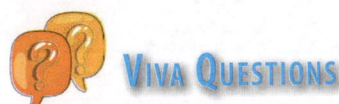

Viva Questions

1. **What is the normal appearance of RBCs under the microscope?**
   Red blood cells are biconcave shaped, red in color with a central pallor.
2. **What is rouleaux?**
   When fresh blood is examined under the microscope, the RBCs are seen attached to their broad surfaces as a pile of coins. This is called rouleaux. This is a reversible phenomenon.
3. **Why rouleaux formation does not occur in the body during life?**
   » Blood is in constant motion.
   » Negative charges on the RBC membrane repel them.
4. **What are ghost cells?**
   When blood is mixed with hypotonic solution, the RBCs swell up due to endosmosis and become spherical. When the volume increases the cells break and the contents go out. The remnants of the cell membrane appear as ghost cells when viewed under a microscope.
5. **What is the difference between isotonic and iso-osmotic solutions?**
   Isotonic solution has the same salt concentration as blood and cells of the human body. Isosmotic solutions have the same number of solutes. The difference between isosmotic and isotonic solutions is that isotonic solutions contain only nonpenetrating solutes and they can be termed as solutions having same osmotic pressure as the cells they surround. They are neither absorbed nor do they absorb anything from the cell. On the other hand, isosmotic solutions contain both penetrating as well as nonpenetrating solutes. They have

the same osmotic pressure as the cell they surround. Penetrating solutes are solutes that can pass through the membrane of the cell and increase the osmotic pressure in the cell. This forces the cell to absorb more water to equalize the difference in pressure. This may lead to bursting of the cell when too much water is absorbed.

6. **What is meant by exosmosis and endosmosis?**
   Movement of water molecules from the cell to the outside across the cell membrane (semipermeable membrane) when the cell is suspended in hypertonic solution is called exosmosis. Movement of water molecules from the outside to the interior of the cell across the cell membrane when it is suspended in hypotonic solution is called endosmosis. The cell swells up in endosmosis and it shrinks and become crenated in exosmosis.

7. **What is anisopoikilocytosis?**
   Presence of different sized and different shaped RBCs in the smear is called anisopoikilocytosis. Difference in shape of erythrocytes is anisocytosis and difference in the shape is referred to as poikilocytosis **(Fig. 2.4)**.

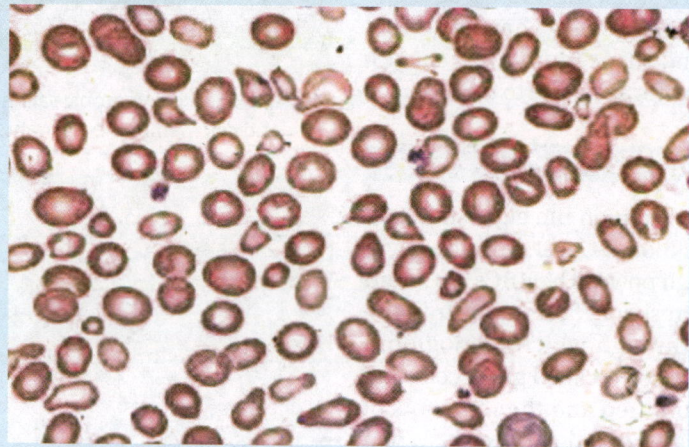

Fig. 2.4: Peripheral smear showing anisopoikilocytosis.

Chapter 3

Collection of Blood Sample

LEARNING OBJECTIVES

- Different methods of collection of blood samples
- List the precautions to be taken while collecting blood
- Should be able to collect blood by finger prick method
- Technique of collecting venous blood from a peripheral vein
- Explain the mechanism of action of anticoagulants used in the laboratory
- Methods to separate serum and plasma from whole blood

INTRODUCTION

Before taking a blood sample, the skin at the puncture site should be thoroughly sterilized. This is because skin surface contains a number of bacteria that may enter the body tissues if strict aseptic (the condition free from bacteria) precautions are not taken while pricking the skin. Not only the skin but also all the instruments coming in contact with the puncture site should be sterile. As far as possible, use the sterile lancet or the pricking needle only once.

The site of puncture should be cleaned with a sterile swab of cotton or wool soaked in methylated spirit or 70% alcohol. After wiping the area, the spirit should be allowed to dry by evaporation or the area can be wiped with a piece of sterile cotton. If the skin is wet with spirit, the blood will spread over the finger and a well-defined drop is not obtained which is very essential for the blood test. Mixing of blood with spirit also interferes with the result. The excess alcohol will also enter the puncture wound and cause pain. The sterilized site should not be touched to prevent contamination.

Blood is usually taken from a capillary or from a vein depending on the purpose for which blood is drawn. Venous blood is preferred for most hematological examinations. Rarely arterial blood is taken for blood gas analysis.

After taking the blood sample, the site of puncture should be cleaned to remove the blood sticking over the area. The swab should then be pressed upon the puncture for some time, i.e., till the oozing of blood stops.

If venous blood is taken it should be transferred into a container containing appropriate anticoagulant. If serum is required for the investigation, then there is no need to add anticoagulant.

Anticoagulants: The anticoagulants commonly used are:

1. **Trisodium citrate:** 3.8% solution of trisodium citrate is isotonic with blood. It acts as anticoagulant by forming calcium sodium citrate, thus removing calcium ions from blood. Ca^{2+} is necessary for all steps in coagulation except activation of factor XII, factor XI, and conversion of fibrinogen to fibrin monomer. One part of this solution is mixed with 4 parts of blood for determination of erythrocyte sedimentation rate (ESR) by Westergren's method or Esrite method. It is also used for determining prothrombin time and for other plasma coagulation tests.

2. **Ethylenediaminetetraacetic acid (EDTA):** 1.2 mg of EDTA per milliliter of blood is used. It is the anticoagulant of choice since it preserves the cellular components of blood for adequate time and it is the most powerful calcium-chelating agent used as anticoagulant. It acts by chelating calcium ions and can be used for hemocytometry and ESR. EDTA also inhibits platelet clumping and so it is also used for doing platelet count. It should not be used for estimating prothrombin time.

3. **Double oxalate mixture (Wintrobe's mixture):** Contains ammonium oxalate and potassium oxalate in the ratio 3:2. The two are used together because if ammonium oxalate alone is used, it causes swelling of blood cells and if potassium oxalate alone is used, it causes shrinking of cells. To balance the swelling effect of ammonium oxalate and the shrinking effect of

potassium oxalate these two are combined in a mixture with a ratio of 3 parts of ammonium oxalate to 2 parts of potassium oxalate. Ten milligram of double oxalate is mixed with 10 mL of blood. It acts as anticoagulant by chelating calcium ions. It is used for determining packed cell volume (PCV) or hematocrit, Hb estimation, ESR, total RBC and WBC count. Oxalated blood is not used for studying the WBC morphology in blood smears and for platelet count. WBC morphology is distorted when this anticoagulant is used because the calcium oxalate formed is insoluble and precipitates out. The neutrophils phagocytose the precipitated oxalate.

4. **Heparin:** Heparin was first isolated from liver and hence the name. It can be used as anticoagulant in the laboratory but it is costly. One unit is added to 10 mL of blood. It cannot be used for doing leukocyte count because heparin causes clumping of leukocytes. Heparinized blood should not be used for making blood films as its highly acidic reaction gives a faint blue coloration to the background when the films are stained by Romanowsky stains. It acts as an anticoagulant by inactivating clotting factors IX, X, XI, and XII. It also forms a complex with antithrombin III in the plasma and prevents thrombin formation. Heparin is used for the biochemical testing of electrolytes and blood gases and also during open-heart surgery.

5. **Sodium fluoride:** It is the anticoagulant of choice for blood sugar estimation. It combines with calcium to form calcium fluoride. It also prevents glycolysis by blocking phosphorylase enzymes in red cells thus preventing loss of glucose.

6. **Acid-citrate-dextrose (ACD) and citrate-phosphate-dextrose-adenine (CPD-A)** are anticoagulants used for storing blood in blood bank. CPD-A is superior to ACD because it preserves 2,3-BPG (2,3-bisphosphoglycerate) better.

In Vivo Anticoagulants

In vivo anticoagulants are used in patients who are prone to develop thromboembolism, to prevent blood clotting in patients who are bed ridden, etc. Commonly used in vivo anticoagulants are **heparin and coumarin** derivatives like dicoumarol and warfarin sodium. Coumarin derivatives are vitamin K antagonists. They prevent the synthesis of vitamin K dependent factors like factor II, VII, IX, and X, and protein C and protein S in the liver. Protein C and protein S are not clotting factors; they come under fibrinolytic system.

Heparin is used during open-heart surgery and during hemodialysis.

COLLECTION OF BLOOD

Capillary Blood

The ring finger or the middle finger of the left hand is used for puncturing. Clean the fingertip with cotton swab dipped in methylated spirit. Allow it to dry because blood will not form a drop on a wet finger. It will spread out. Spirit may also cause hemolysis of blood and pain. A sterile needle or lancet is used for pricking. Before collecting blood, wear sterile gloves to prevent subject's blood from coming in contact with your hand. This precaution is taken to prevent the risk of transmission of serious diseases like hepatitis, AIDS, etc.

Procedure

Hold the finger to be punctured in the left hand and make a deep prick on the ball of the finger with the right hand. The prick should be deep enough (2–3 mm) so that there is free flow of blood **(Fig. 3.1)**. If the finger is squeezed for obtaining blood, it will contain more of tissue fluid and the cell counts become inaccurate. The first small drop of blood that comes out should be wiped off with sterile swab since it contains more tissue fluid that may dilute the blood. Then allow a large drop of blood to be formed and it can be pipetted at once or can be used for making blood smear. The blood should be used for the experiment immediately, otherwise it will clot and become useless. After collecting blood, apply a sterile cotton swab and ask the subject to press on the puncture site until bleeding stops. If the finger appears pale, before pricking, the hand can be dipped in warm water at about 40°C for 3–4 minutes and this will allow free flow of blood.

In infants, capillary blood is collected by a deep puncture of the plantar surface of the heel. It must be restricted to the outer medial or lateral portions of the plantar surface of the foot. Otherwise it will injure the underlying tarsal bones. The ball of the big toe can also be used for pricking.

Precautions to be taken by students in the laboratory
- Keep all equipments ready before giving a prick
- Students should use their own lancets. Sharing of lancets may lead to sharing of diseases.
- The site should be sterilized
- The prick should be deep enough to get free flowing blood

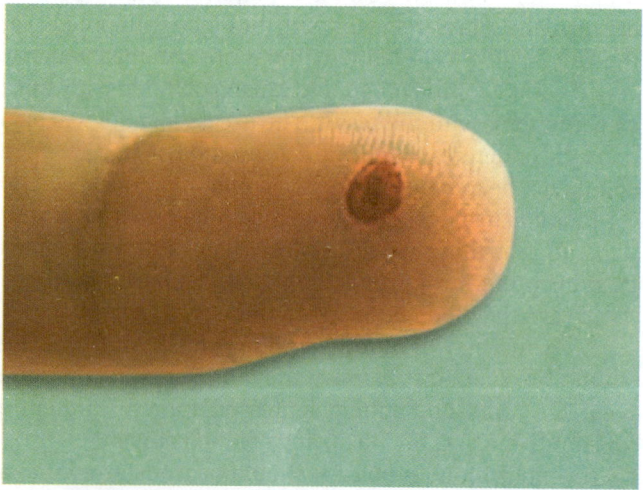

Fig. 3.1: Collection of capillary blood by finger prick.

- Wipe off the first drop of blood since it contains more of tissue fluid.
- Do not squeeze the finger tip for obtaining blood
- If blood is not coming freely, give a second prick

Collection of Venous Blood

Venous blood sample is obtained by venipuncture. It is usually done when more blood is required for the investigation. A superficial suitable vein is selected in the arm usually one in the cubital fossa preferably on the left side. A vein on the dorsum of the hand can also be selected if the veins in the elbow are not suitable. The selected vein should be straight for at least 2 cm and should be sufficiently large to introduce the needle. A vein that is connected by two other veins is more suitable since it is immovable and it will be easy to introduce the needle in such a vein. The subject is asked to sit down on a chair and keep his arm on the armrest or he can be made to lie down on a bed.

Procedure

Tie a tourniquet around the upper arm in such a way that it can be easily removed by one hand immediately after collecting blood in the syringe. The tourniquet should never be left in place for more than 2 minutes. The tourniquet should not be too tight because the pressure may compress the arteries and decrease arterial blood flow to the lower arm and the area suffers from ischemia, which is very painful. (Instead of tourniquet, a sphygmomanometer cuff can be applied to the upper arm and it can be inflated approximately to the diastolic pressure.) Ask the subject to open and close the fist a few times and the veins below the tourniquet become prominent due to increased venous flow from the hand. A dry sterile syringe with a wide bored (19G or 21G for adults and 23G for children) sharp needle is selected. If very fine needles are used, it causes hemolysis.

Clean the skin over the selected vein with methylated spirit and allow it to dry. While puncturing the vein, the bevel of the needle should face the person who is collecting blood. When the vein is punctured, blood will appear in the syringe and slowly withdraw the piston and blood starts entering the syringe **(Fig. 3.2)**. During this time ask the subject to open and close his fist repeatedly so that the vein gets engorged. When sufficient amount of blood is withdrawn, remove the tourniquet and place a sterile cotton swab on the puncture site with the left hand and press lightly. Withdraw the needle with the syringe and press the swab firmly on the puncture. Instruct the subject to press the swab and to fold the arm. It is better to cover the puncture site with medicated adhesive tape.

The whole procedure should be completed within 2 minutes. Otherwise stagnation of blood in the vein for more time will affect the composition of blood. The cell count usually increases.

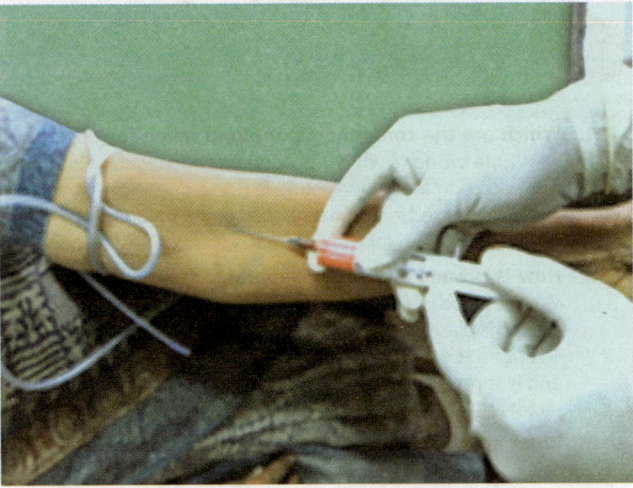

Fig. 3.2: Collection of blood from the anterior cubital vein.

Hold the syringe vertically with the needle directed upwards and remove the needle carefully. To obtain plasma, transfer the blood into a container that contains the proper anticoagulant by slowly pushing down the piston. Hold the tube between the palms of the hands and rotate it gently to mix the anticoagulant thoroughly with blood. The movement should not be too vigorous since it causes hemolysis. Close the tube and label it. To obtain serum, transfer the blood into a container without anticoagulant. *Destroy the syringe and needle if it is disposable* so that reuse can be prevented. Many diseases having high mortality like hepatitis, AIDS, etc., are transmitted through contaminated syringe and needle.

Collection of Arterial Blood

Arterial blood is needed for tests like blood gas analysis, estimation of blood pH, etc. An artery such as radial artery or femoral artery is punctured using a syringe and needle. This procedure requires expertise. Not a routine procedure.

Collection of Blood from Heart Chambers

Blood from the chambers of heart is collected by cardiac catheterization.

Transport of Blood to Laboratory

The collected blood should be transferred into suitable containers from the syringe. The needle should be removed before transferring blood from the syringe into the container. Otherwise blood cells may lyse. Clean and dry collection bottles are used. To send a sample of whole blood or plasma, blood is collected in a container containing suitable anticoagulant. This prevents clotting of blood.

To get a sample of serum, blood is collected in a container with no anticoagulant. The blood is allowed to clot in the container and serum is collected.

Section 1: Hematology

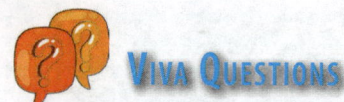
VIVA QUESTIONS

1. **Which are the components of blood taken for different analysis?**
   » **Whole blood** to which appropriate anticoagulant is added is taken for the analysis of glucose, urea, pH estimation, etc. It is also used to do complete blood count, ESR, etc.
   » **Serum** is used for estimating total protein, albumin, globulin, bilirubin, cholesterol, creatinine, uric acid, and phosphate, SGOT, SGPT, etc.
   » **Plasma** is used for the estimation of chloride, fibrinogen, bicarbonate, etc.

2. **How is plasma and serum separated from whole blood? What is the difference between plasma and serum?**
   Venous blood is taken and mixed with proper anticoagulant. Centrifuge this blood for 20–30 minutes at 2,500 rpm. The clear fluid formed at the top is plasma. It is pipetted and transferred to another container. It contains all the components of blood except the formed elements. To obtain serum, blood is transferred to a container with no anticoagulant. Keep it undisturbed for an hour or two. A clot will be formed and it shrinks and expresses out a clear fluid, which is serum. Serum differs from plasma in that serum does not contain the clotting factors I, II, V, VIII, and XIII.

3. **What are the changes that occur in the blood on keeping it for some time?**
   » Change in the RBC morphology (swelling or crenation of RBC may occur)
   » Autolysis and disintegration of WBC
   » Decrease in ESR
   » Increase in the osmotic fragility of RBC
   » Prolongation of prothrombin time and other plasma coagulation times
   » Loss of CO_2 since it diffuses to air
   » K^+ enters the cells leading to decrease in plasma K^+ level
   » Conversion of glucose to lactic acid by glycolysis
   » Conversion of pyruvate to lactic acid
   » Formation of NH_3 from nitrogenous substances like urea
   » Increase in plasma inorganic phosphates.

4. **What are the precautions to be taken while collecting blood?**
   » The subject should be in a comfortable position
   » Sterilize the puncture site thoroughly and never touch the sterilized area before collecting blood
   » Spirit should not be present at the puncture site before puncturing
   » While collecting blood from a subject wear sterile gloves, glasses to protect the eyes, and mask
   » Never squeeze the fingertip to obtain capillary blood
   » The tourniquet should not be tied too tightly and remove it immediately after drawing venous blood
   » Remove the needle from the syringe before transferring the blood into the container
   » After collecting blood, apply a sterile cotton swab and ask the subject to press on the puncture site until bleeding stops
   » Destroy the disposable syringe and needle immediately after use.

5. **What is the reason for not pricking the thumb and little finger for obtaining capillary blood?**
   The palmar fascia of the thumb and little finger extends to the forearm. While pricking these fingers if this fascia is injured, it may lead to spread of infection to the forearm.

6. **Why is it not advisable to squeeze the fingertip to obtain blood?**
   If the fingertip is squeezed, more tissue fluid comes out which dilutes the blood and gives false low values for the test.

7. **Why should the prick be given only after drying the area to be pricked?**
   If the pricking area is wet the blood drop spreads over the skin and a definite drop of blood will not be obtained. If the part is wet with spirit, it causes lysis of the blood cells. Spirit also increases the pain in the area after the prick. Sterilization with alcohol will be complete only if the area dries by evaporation.

8. **Name the sites for collecting capillary blood.**
   In adults, capillary blood can be collected from finger tips and ear lobes. Finger tip is the ideal site. In infants, blood is collected from the heel or from the plantar surface of big toe.

9. **Why is median cubital vein chosen for venipuncture?**
   This vein is larger than the veins in the wrist, forearm or ankle. It does not slip beneath the skin.

10. **What are the differences in the complete blood count when capillary and venous blood samples are used?**
    Venous blood and capillary blood are not quite the same. The packed cell volume, red cell count, and hemoglobin content of capillary blood are slightly greater than in venous blood. The total leukocyte and neutrophil counts are higher by 8% and monocyte count by 12% in capillary blood. Conversely, the platelet count appears to be higher in venous blood than in capillary blood by about 9–32%. This may be due to adhesion of platelets at the site of skin puncture.

11. **What is the mechanism of action of various anticoagulants?**
    Refer page 13 and 14.

12. **How to collect capillary blood if the finger is cold and pale?**
    Immerse the finger in warm water for 2–3 minutes before pricking.

Chapter 4

Erythrocyte Sedimentation Rate

LEARNING OBJECTIVES

- Fill the ESR tube with blood accurately
- List the different methods of determination of ESR
- Define ESR and explain the factors affecting ESR
- List the normal value of ESR in different age groups and in male and female
- State the conditions which alters ESR
- State the precautions and the sources of error while determining ESR

PY2.12: Describe test for ESR, osmotic fragility, hematocrit; note the findings and interpret the test results.

PRINCIPLE

Anticoagulated blood is taken in a graduated glass tube with narrow bore and is mounted vertically on a stand. The specific gravity of red blood cells (1.095) is more than that of plasma (1.032) and the cells settle down gradually towards the bottom of the tube. As the cells settle down, the upper layer of plasma gets cleared of the red cells. The height in mm of plasma cleared of the cells at the end of first hour is recorded.

METHODS

- Westergren's method
- Wintrobe's method
- Esrite method
- Micro-erythrocyte sedimentation rate (ESR) method

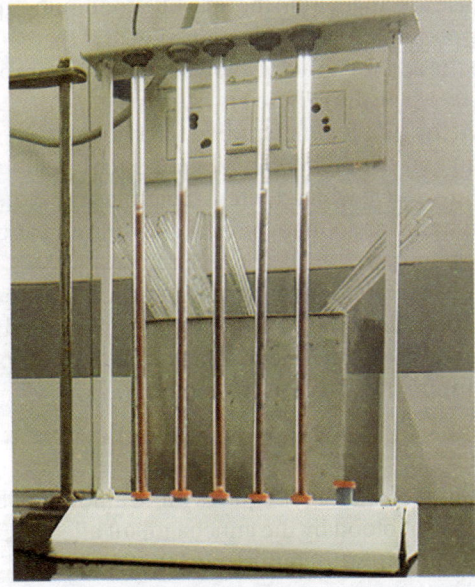

Fig. 4.1: Westergren's pipettes mounted on the Westergren's stand.

Westergren's Method

Apparatus

Westergren's pipette, stand, centrifuge, 3.8% sodium citrate, lancet, cotton and spirit. Westergren's pipette has an internal bore diameter of 2.5 mm and a length of about 300 mm. It is open at both the ends and is calibrated from 0–200 mm from top to bottom along the lower 2/3rd of its length. The Westergren's stand can accommodate three pipettes at a time **(Fig. 4.1)**. There is a rubber cushion at the base of the stand on which the lower end of the Westergren's pipette is made to rest. At the upper end is a screw cap that fits upon the pipette. It can be screwed down to exert sufficient pressure on the pipette. This prevents any leakage of blood from the bottom of the tube. The stand allows the pipettes to remain exactly in a vertical position.

- Procedure
- A sample of blood is obtained with all precautions by venepuncture.
- The blood is mixed with 3.8% trisodium citrate ($Na_3C_6H_5O_7.2H_2O$) solution in proportion of 4 parts of blood to 1 part of citrate solution. Minimum amount of blood required is 1.6 mL mixed with 0.4 mL of citrate solution. Citrate acts as an anticoagulant and the concentration taken here is isotonic with blood.
- Mix the blood by rotating the sample gently between the palms.
- Suck the blood into the Westergren's pipette slowly up to the zero mark without air bubbles. Because of the risk of diseases like AIDS, hepatitis, etc., filling of blood by mouth pipetting should be strictly discouraged. Instead of sucking, blood can be filled with the help of a rubber teat by vacuum filling.
- If it rises above the zero mark, allow it to drain slowly so that the upper level of blood is exactly at the zero mark.
- Close the upper end of the pipette with the finger tightly to prevent outflow of blood. Carefully press the lower end of the pipette on the rubber cushion of the Westergren's stand taking care that no blood escapes.
- Release the finger from the tip while continuing applying the pressure on the rubber cushion and fix the pipette with the screw cap at the top. The pipette must be fitted exactly vertically **(Fig. 4.1)**.
- Leave the pipette undisturbed for 1 hour.
- At the end of one hour, read the upper level of the red column above which there is clear plasma. Note down the reading as so many mm of clear plasma at the end of first hour.
- In cases of extreme anemia or where the ESR is very high, the upper level of the red column is not clearly seen. In such cases, take the reading at the highest point of maximum density of the red column.

Disadvantages

- Westergren's method requires more amount of blood.
- Dilution of blood by the anticoagulant affects ESR.
- Mouth pipetting increases the risk of spread of diseases like AIDS.

Wintrobe's Method

Apparatus

Wintrobe's hematocrit tube and stand (description of Wintrobe's tube is given in Chapter 5).

Procedure

- Keep the Wintrobe's stand on the table in the horizontal plane.
- Add 1 mL of venous blood into the tube or bottle containing double oxalate powder (2 mg of potassium oxalate and 3 mg of ammonium oxalate) and mix it gently. Do not shake.
- Rotate the tube containing the oxalated blood to mix the cells and the plasma well just before taking the blood in the pipette.
- Fill the Wintrobe's tube with anticoagulated blood with the long narrow pipette (Pasteur pipette) up to the '0' mark.
- Place the tube on the stand perfectly in the vertical position.
- Note the time.
- Take the reading at the end of first hour by placing the tube at the level of the eyes.

Advantages

- Wintrobe's method has the additional advantage that, after noting down the erythrocyte sedimentation rate (ESR) the same tube can be used for determining the packed cell volume (PCV).
- The amount of blood required is also less in this method. This is significant in small children and in conditions like anemia.
- There is no dilution with anticoagulant.
- Filling of the tube with Pasteur pipette eliminates chance of infection due to handling of blood.

Disadvantages

- The disadvantage is that if the ESR is more than 100 mm, it cannot be measured.
- Blood should be used within 2 hours.

Esrite Method

Apparatus

Esrite glass Westergren's tube, filling vials, Esrite stand and scale, spirit, etc. Esrite tube is a glass pipette with no markings. The tip of Esrite tube is cylindrical in shape and the diameter is just adequate to fit into the vial containing the blood sample to form a leak proof seal. The stand can hold the Esrite tubes in their vials in an exactly vertical position. Behind the row of tubes, the stand provides a permanently marked millimeter scale. The filling vials are made of chemically inert plastic with a cylindrical internal bore which makes a leak proof seal with the Esrite tube.

Procedure

Take trisodium citrate in the vial up to the groove marked. Add about 1 mL of venous blood into the vial and close it. Mix the contents well. Place the vial on the Esrite stand and open it. Introduce the conical tip of the Esrite tube vertically into the vial containing the blood sample and gently push the tube down till blood rises in the tube up to the zero mark

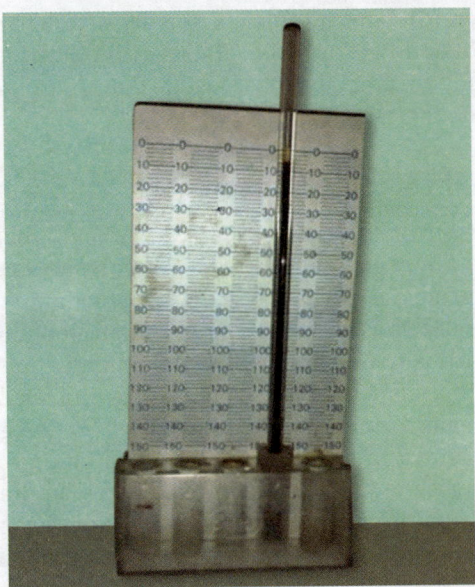

Fig. 4.2: Normal ESR reading by Esrite method (6 mm in the first hour).

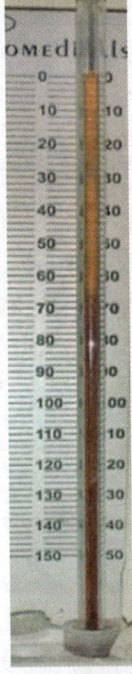

Fig. 4.3: ESR reading in anemia (70 mm in the first hour). Since the plasma is tinted red, this can be a case of hemolytic anemia.

on the scale provided at the back **(Figs. 4.2 and 4.3)**. Note the time. After 1 hour, measure the height of clear plasma formed at the top of the column of blood. Record it as so many millimeters in the first hour.

Precautions While Doing ESR

- Blood should be collected preferably in the fasting state. Fasting is not mandatory.
- Even a small clot in the blood leads to a reduction in the fibrinogen content and the ESR decreases. Such samples should be discarded. Hemolyzed blood also should be discarded.
- Anticoagulants used do affect the ESR either by acting on the plasma or on the cell size. Standard anticoagulants should therefore be used for getting reliable results. Excess anticoagulant should not be used.
- Proper anticoagulant should be used for each method. If 3.8% sodium citrate is used in Wintrobe's method, the blood will be too much diluted and this will give false high values for ESR.
- The test should be done within 2 hours of collecting the blood sample.
- Seasonal variations in the room temperature can produce errors in the readings taken at different times.
- If the tube in which the ESR is measured is kept in an inclined position, an increase in the rate of sedimentation of RBCs is observed.
- The bore of the tubing should have a diameter between 2.5 and 3 mm. Small diameter tubing retards the rate and large diameter one requires large quantities of blood.
- The reading should be taken exactly after the end of one hour after mounting the blood vertically. This is because the method has been standardized for one hour. Moreover, 95–98% of red cells settle down by the end of one hour.

Micro-ESR Kit

Micro-ESR kit is used for pediatric cases and adults suffering from severe burns, eczema, etc., where it is difficult to obtain venous blood. Micro-capillary ESR provides results, which may be correlated and standardized with reference to conventional ESR. In this method, a capillary tube 160 mm long with an internal bore diameter of 1 mm is used. It is graduated 1 mm apart for 50 mm, with two red lines on it.

Citrate solution is taken up to the first red mark in the micro-capillary tube provided in the kit. Blood is taken from a finger prick up to the second red mark. Rotate the capillary or invert it several times to mix the contents and seal the capillary end with wax. Insert the capillary in the non-corroding plastic stand to hold it vertically. Record the readings after one hour as that for Westergren's method.

RESULT

The result is expressed in mm of clear plasma formed at the top of the column of blood at the end of first hour.

DISCUSSION

During acute inflammatory conditions and during the active phases of chronic inflammation, there will be alteration in the concentration of plasma proteins. There will be a rise in fibrinogen and C-reactive protein (CRP) and a fall in albumin. Estimation of ESR, fibrinogen and CRP help to measure the extent of inflammation.

In Wintrobe's method: The normal range is 0 to 7 mm in males at the end of first hour and in females 0 to 15 mm at the end of first hour. The same values are obtained after two hours by Westergren's method.

Blood is a suspension of the red blood cells in plasma. The red blood cells are heavier than the plasma (specific gravity of red cells is 1090 and that of plasma is 1030). In the body, the blood is circulating and the cells and plasma are mixed up. When the blood is taken out and is allowed to stand in a tube, the cells tend to settle down at the bottom. Physical factors like specific gravity of the cells and the plasma, the temperature and the viscosity of plasma determine the rate of settling down. The single important factor affecting the rate of sedimentation is rouleaux formation.

Rouleaux Formation

- The red blood cells are negatively charged, as they remain suspended in the plasma. These charges tend to keep them separate from one another due to their mutual repulsion in the circulating blood. This repulsion force is known as **zeta potential**.
- Protein molecules in plasma especially fibrinogen and globulin make the red cells sticky. It overcomes the repulsion caused by the negative charge when blood is taken in the tube. When the cells strike each other because of the random thermodynamic movements they tend to stick to each other and get piled over one another to form a rouleaux. Each rouleau consists of 8–12 cells.
- When RBCs form rouleaux, the density increases and it sinks down quickly. Thus sedimentation rate is mostly governed by those factors that control rouleaux formation.

Factors Affecting Rouleaux Formation

- Different molecules in plasma, e.g., proteins, cholesterol, etc., affect the rate of rouleaux formation. Larger molecules usually increase the rate of sedimentation of red cells. Thus fibrinogen is better than globulin, which in turn is better than albumin. Not only the size but also the shape and the structure of the molecule affect rouleaux formation. In various diseases, the globulin concentration and also its pattern change. These changes are responsible for the change in the rate of rouleaux formation and the sedimentation. For example, in collagen disorders like systemic lupus erythematosus (SLE), there is increase in globulin content which in turn increases ESR. Fibrinogen and globulin concentrations are increased in both acute and chronic infections.
- Cell size, shape and composition: biconcave shape of RBCs favors rouleaux formation. An increase in the MCV, a decrease in the MCH, and spherocytosis, all retard the rate of rouleaux formation. In certain clinical conditions, many of these changes occur simultaneously and cause a decrease in the ESR.
- Increase in body temperature increases rouleaux formation.
- An increase in the viscosity of blood decreases ESR. For example, in hyperproteinemia, polycythemia, etc., there is decrease in ESR.

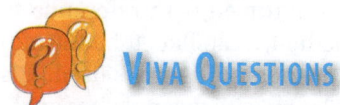

Viva Questions

1. **Define ESR. Give its normal value.**
   Depth in millimeters of clear plasma formed at the top of a vertical column of anticoagulated blood kept undisturbed for one hour in a tube of standard dimensions is called ESR or suspension stability of RBC. It is expressed in mm at the end of the first hour.
   The normal range of ESR in Westergren's method is:
   Males: 3–5 mm at the end of 1st hour
   Females: 4–7 mm at the end of 1st hour

2. **Will the value of ESR double after the 2nd hour?**
   No, this is because at the end of 1st hour, 95–98% of cells have settled down. The value taken at the end of 1st hour is the most accurate reading.

3. **What is the proportion of blood and anticoagulant for doing ESR?**
   The blood is mixed with 3.8% trisodium citrate solution in proportion of 4 parts of blood to 1 part of citrate solution. Minimum amount of blood required is 1.6 mL mixed with 0.4 mL of citrate solution.

4. **What are the three stages of ESR?**
   » Rouleaux formation or **stage of aggregation** which takes about 10 minutes.
   » Rapid settling or **stage of sedimentation** or stage of fall of the aggregates that takes place at a constant speed. This stage lasts for 40 minutes.
   » **Stage of packing** takes about 10 minutes during which aggregated cells pack at the bottom of the tube.

5. **What are the advantages of Esrite method over Westergren's method?**
   » Esrite method eliminates the risk of infection from patients due to mouth pipetting.
   » Filling of the tube is easy and the blood level can be maintained without repeated sucking while fitting the pipette on the stand.
   » Only 1 mL of blood is needed to fill the tube.
   » Blood taken from the vein can be directly transferred into the sample vial containing anticoagulant which, when closed, is leak proof.
   » Aluminium screen with permanent scale helps to easily get the reading of sedimentation rate.

6. **What is the significance of doing ESR routinely?**
   » ESR is an index of inflammatory activity in the body. It is increased in infective and non-infective inflammatory conditions. So it is not a specific test.
   » An increase in the ESR indicates quick rouleaux formation caused by alteration in the concentration of plasma proteins. This pattern indicates the presence of inflammatory diseases associated with increased production of acute phase proteins like fibrinogen and C-reactive protein. It does not indicate the nature of the disease.
   » It helps to assess the progress of a disease which affects ESR.
   » Increase in the ESR in two or more consecutive tests carried out at definite intervals indicates the continuation or increased activity of the disease process.
   » A decrease in ESR in consecutive tests is the sign of arrest of the process and improvement.
   » Change in the ESR in consecutive tests is of more significance than the initial value observed.
   » ESR estimation helps to distinguish between benign and malignant tumors. In malignancy, ESR will be significantly increased.
   » It also helps to assess the prognosis of a disease, i.e., to assess whether the patient is responding to the specific treatment. If the ESR goes on decreasing, it means that the patient is responding to treatment, i.e., his condition is becoming better.
   » A reading of 8 mm in the first hour for males and 15 mm for females in the first hour is not considered as a significant increase in ESR.

7. **Enumerate the physiological and pathological conditions that cause increase and decrease in ESR values.**
   Physiological increase is seen in females in the reproductive age group due to the effect of estrogen, during pregnancy (due to hemodilution), parturition, menstruation (due to increase in fibrinogen) and in old age.
   Physiological decrease is seen in males and newborn babies due to high RBC count. ESR is decreased in stored blood.
   Pathological Increase
   (ESR is said to be increased only if it is more than 15 mm in females and 20 mm in males less than 50 years of age)
   » Acute and chronic infections (globulin, fibrinogen and products of tissue destruction increase rouleaux formation). ESR is very high in septicemia and tuberculosis.
   » Collagen disorders, like systemic lupus erythematosus (SLE), rheumatoid arthritis, etc. (due to immune reactions and increase in globulin).
   » Malignancy (due to products of tissue destruction and increased fibrinogen).
   » Renal diseases decrease erythropoiesis due to decreased erythropoietin secretion leading to reduction in RBC count. There is also increased loss of albumin in urine leading to hypoproteinemia and decrease in the viscosity of blood.
   » Anemia especially iron deficiency anemia (Exception: in sickle cell anemia and spherocytic anemia, ESR is decreased because of defective rouleaux formation).
   Pathological Decrease
   » Severe allergic reactions
   » Polycythemia
   » Sickle cell anemia and spherocytic anemia
   » Hypofibrinogenemia

8. **What are the factors affecting ESR?**
   » All factors that affect rouleaux formation affect ESR. When the rate of rouleaux formation increases, there will be an increase in ESR and vice versa. Plasma proteins fibrinogen and globulin increase rouleaux and albumin decrease rouleaux formation.
   » Increase in viscosity decreases ESR and vice versa.
   » Liquid anticoagulants dilute blood and hence increase ESR.
   » RBC count: ESR is decreased in polycythemia and increased in anemia.
   » Size and shape of RBCs: increased size leads to increase in ESR. Macrocytes settle more quickly and increase ESR. Spherocytes retard rouleaux formation and decrease ESR.
   » ESR increases when the temperature increases within physiological limits. Increase in temperature decreases blood viscosity.
   » Increase in plasma cholesterol increases ESR and lecithin decreases ESR.

9. **What is rouleaux? Give its cause. Why is it not being formed in circulation during life?**
   Piling of RBCs one above the other along their broad surfaces when blood is taken out of the body is called rouleaux. Protein molecules in plasma especially fibrinogen and globulin make the red cells sticky when blood is taken out of the body. It overcomes the repulsion of RBCs caused by the negative charge on their surface. When the cells strike each other because of the random thermodynamic movements, they tend to stick to each other and get piled over one another along their flat surface to form rouleaux.
   Rouleaux formation does not occur in the body due to the following reasons:
   » Blood is in constant motion.
   » RBC membrane is negatively charged and so they get repelled from each other preventing rouleaux formation.

Section 1: Hematology

10. **Name the anticoagulant used for doing ESR in Westergren's method. What is its mechanism of action?**
    3.8% sodium citrate is the anticoagulant. It removes ionic calcium by forming calcium citrate. Ionic calcium is necessary for almost all steps in coagulation except for the conversion of inactive clotting factors XII and XI to their active forms and conversion of fibrinogen to fibrin monomer.

11. **Can 3.8% sodium citrate be used for determining ESR by Wintrobe's method?**
    No, sodium citrate cannot be used in Wintrobe's method because the length of the tube is less and the blood will be too much diluted as compared to the length of the tube. This will give false high value for ESR.

12. **What is the reason for increase in ESR in malignancy?**
    Certain proteins like fibrinogen, C-reactive protein, etc., that decrease the negativity of RBC membrane increases clumping of RBC and increase their sedimentation rate. Such proteins are released in excess amounts by the malignant tissues that lead to an increase in ESR.

13. **Why is blood collected on an empty stomach for determining ESR?**
    After a meal, ESR is found to be increased slightly. Since there is no significant difference, it is not mandatory to do ESR on a fasting blood sample.

14. **Give five differences between Westergren's pipette and Wintrobe's hematocrit tube.**

Westergren's pipette	*Wintrobe's tube*
300 mm in length	110 mm in length
2.5 mm bore diameter	3 mm
Both ends are open	Lower end is closed
Graduated from 0 to 200 from top to bottom	Marked 0 to 10 on one side and 10 to zero on the opposite side of the tube
Used for finding ESR	Used for finding PCV and ESR, and demonstration of LE cells

# **OBJECTIVE STRUCTURED PRACTICAL EXAMINATION**

I. Load the Westergren pipette for doing ESR with the blood sample provided
1. Take a clean dry Westergren pipette (Y/N)
2. Gently mix the blood (Y/N)
3. Pipette blood to the zero mark carefully to avoid air bubbles in the blood column (Y/N)
4. Immediately close the upper end of the pipette with finger tip
5. Make sure that the upper end of blood column is exactly at the zero mark (Y/N)
6. Place the pipette on the rubber pad of the stand and fix it vertically with the metal screw or the metal clip provided at the top (Y/N)
7. Note the time

II. Load the Esrite tube with the blood provided for doing ESR
1. Take a clean dry Esrite tube (Y/N)
2. Add about 1 mL of anticoagulated venous blood into the vial (Y/N)
3. Place the vial on the Esrite stand and introduce the conical tip of the Esrite tube vertically into the vial containing the blood sample (Y/N)
4. Gently push the tube down till blood rises in the tube up to the zero mark on the scale provided at the back (Y/N)
5. Note the time (Y/N)

Chapter 5

Packed Cell Volume or Hematocrit

LEARNING OBJECTIVES

- List the methods of determination of hematocrit
- Differentiate between Wintrobe's tube and Westergren's pipette
- Fill the Wintrobe's tube with the blood provided and determine the PCV
- State the significance of buffy coat layer and plasma column
- Precautions to be taken while filling the tube
- List the conditions where there is variation in PCV

PY2.12: Describe test for ESR, osmotic fragility, hematocrit; note the findings and interpret the test results.

Measurement of the packed cell volume (PCV) or the hematocrit value of blood is the most accurate and simplest of all the methods for determining the presence or absence of anemia or polycythemia and measuring their degrees.

PRINCIPLE

The red blood cells are heavier than plasma. When blood is placed in a long tube and is centrifuged, the cells settle down and pack themselves because of the centrifugal force. The volume occupied by the cells is measured and its ratio with the volume of the whole blood in the tube is calculated. This ratio gives the packed cell volume.

METHODS

- Wintrobe's method
- Microhematocrit method

Wintrobe's Method

Apparatus

Wintrobe's hematocrit tube, Pasteur pipette, which is a long glass capillary pipette (150 mm long) with a rubber teat **(Fig. 5.1B)**, sterile syringe and needle, anticoagulant preferably double oxalate (EDTA or heparin can also be used), cotton swab, methylated spirit and a centrifuge, which can create the necessary force are required.

Wintrobe's hematocrit tube is a thick cylindrical tube of uniform bore and a closed bottom. It is 110 mm long and has an internal bore diameter of 2.5 mm. It is graduated on both sides: on the left hand side, from the top to bottom of the tube as 0 to 10 and on the right hand side as 10 to 0 **(Fig. 5.1A)**. It is graduated in this manner in order to do PCV

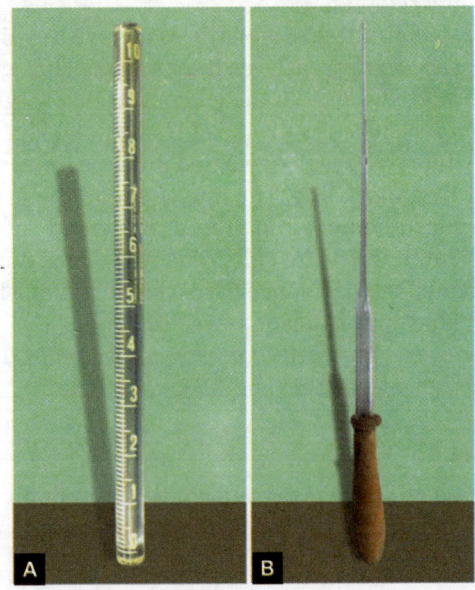

Figs. 5.1A and B: (A) Wintrobe's hematocrit tube; (B) Pasteur pipette.

and ESR with the same tube. Each main division represents 1 cm and each smaller one represents 1 mm. To convert the reading to percentage when the tube has been filled up to zero, multiply the reading (in centimeters) by ten.

Procedure

- 1 mL of blood is collected by a venipuncture.
- It is transferred into a container containing correct amount of anticoagulant, preferably double oxalate mixture (ammonium oxalate and potassium oxalate in the ratio 3:2).
- Take the blood in the dry long capillary stem of the Pasteur pipette after mixing the blood well by rotating the container between the palms. There should not be any air bubble in the capillary stem.
- Now insert the tip of the Pasteur pipette into the bottom of the Wintrobe's tube.
- By gentle pressure on the rubber teat, fill the hematocrit tube by slowly withdrawing the pipette and release the pressure when blood reaches the upper zero mark.
- If more blood is accidentally added remove the excess blood.
- If blood added is less, bring the volume to zero level.
- Centrifuge the tube for 30 minutes at a speed of 3,000 revolutions per minute. If the centrifugal force to which the blood is subjected is not adequate, the cells do not pack to the minimum value. The pack cell volume obtained then will be high.
- Take out the tube and read the upper level of the cell layer and it gives the PCV.

Observations

- The tube shows an uppermost layer of plasma. It is pale and straw colored.
- Just beneath the plasma layer is a greyish-white thin layer called buffy coat layer. It consists of platelets above (thin white layer) and the leucocytes below (greyish-pink layer). It is usually 0.5–1 mm thick **(Fig. 5.2)**.
- The white cell layer is separated from the lower red cell layer by a black line. The line is due to the presence of reduced hemoglobin present in the red cells lying adjacent to the white cells. The white cells during its metabolic activity reduce the oxyhemoglobin. This line marks the upper limit of the red cell layer.
- The height of red cells corresponds to the PCV and it varies between 4.2 cm and 4.7 cm normally.

Calculations

The packed cell volume percent is given by multiplying the reading obtained by 10. Thus if the red cell layer is 4.2 cm, then PCV = 4.2 × 10 = 42%.

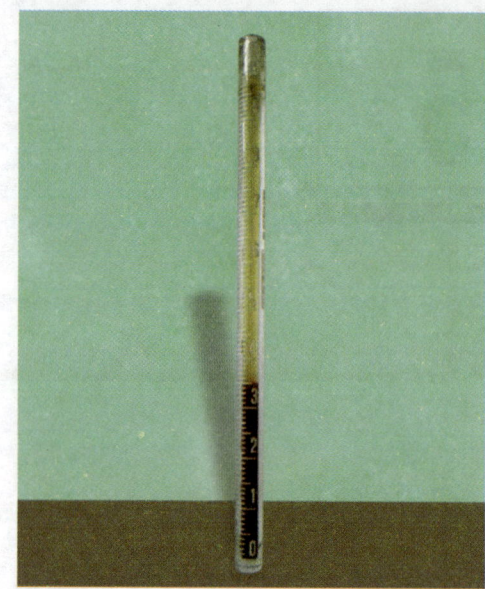

Fig. 5.2: Hematocrit reading (PCV—35%; plasma volume—65%; note the normal straw colored plasma).

Even under standard conditions the packed cell volume contains some 'trapped plasma'. To obtain the actual red cell volume, the packed cell volume obtained should be multiplied by a correction factor of 0.97–0.99 depending upon the centrifugal force of the machine used.

Microhematocrit Method (Micro-PCV)

- A heparinized capillary tube 70 mm long with an internal bore diameter of 1 mm is used in this method. Capillary blood is taken into the tube by capillary action up to 60 mm. Heparin mixes with the blood and prevents coagulation.
- Seal the empty end of the tube with a small plug of plasticine.
- Centrifuge it in a microhematocrit centrifuge at 12,000 rpm for 5 minutes with the sealed end away from the center **(Fig. 5.3)**.
- The red cell column is measured using a reading device incorporated in the centrifuge. PCV can be read from the chart directly without any calculation.

Advantages

- The amount of blood required is very small and can be easily obtained from a finger prick.
- The time required for centrifugation is much less.
- Some of the automated blood cell counters are designed to calculate the PCV from the number of RBC and mean cell volume.

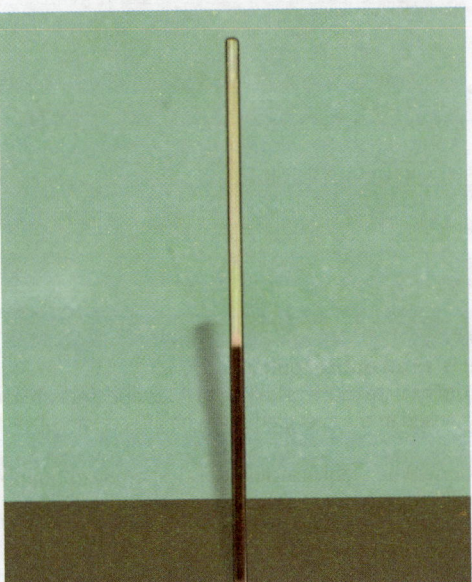

Fig. 5.3: Determination of PCV by microhematocrit method.

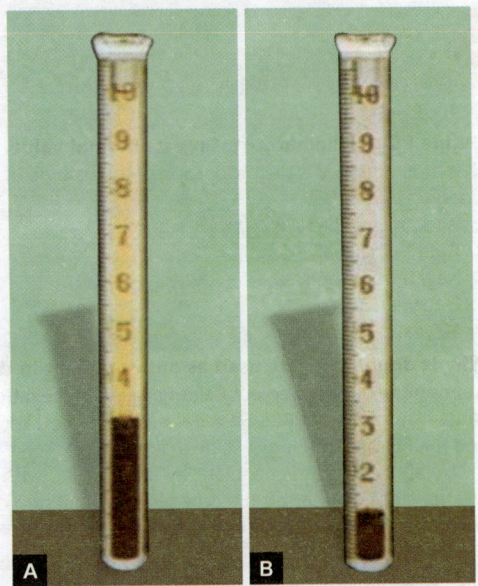

Figs. 5.4A and B: Hematocrit findings: (A) Mild anemia (PCV—30%), (B) Severe anemia (PCV—13%). In tube 'B', see that the color of plasma is very pale which is typical of severe anemia.

DISCUSSION

- Normally plasma is straw colored **(Fig. 5.2)**. By noting the color of plasma some pathological conditions can be suspected.
- Red color of plasma indicates hemolysis **(Fig. 5.5)**. It may occur due to some disease in the body as in hemolytic anemia. If the blood is vigorously shaken with the anticoagulant, it may cause hemolysis.
- If the plasma layer is deep yellow it suggests increase in bilirubin content in blood.
- If it is cloudy and milky it indicates hyperlipidemia (normally seen after a heavy fatty meal due to the presence of chylomicrons).
- In iron deficiency anemia, plasma layer is very much increased and it will be very pale **(Figs. 5.4A and B)**.
- If the buffy coat layer is exceedingly thin it indicates leucopenia. If it is thicker than normal, it indicates leukocytosis or thrombocytosis.
- Normal buffy coat layer is about 1 mm in thickness. 0.1 mm of buffy coat layer is equivalent to 1,000 leukocytes/mm^3. Thus by noting the thickness of buffy coat layer the total leukocyte count can be assessed roughly. For example, if it is 0.5 mm thick then the blood contains 5,000 leukocytes/mm^3 of blood. Leukocytosis and marked increase in the number of platelets may cause an increase in the thickness of buffy coat. In leukemia the buffy coat layer will be very thick.

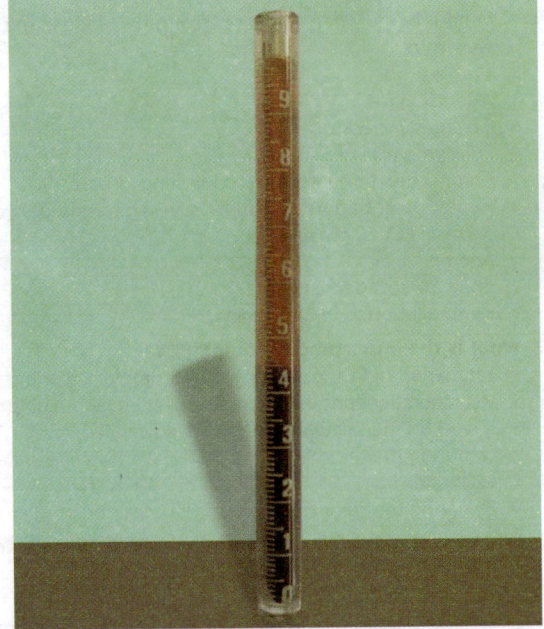

Fig. 5.5: Hematocrit reading (PCV—45%, plasma volume—55%; plasma is tinted red due to hemolysis of RBCs) (normally plasma is straw colored; *see* **Fig. 5.2**).

- If PCV is more than normal, it indicates increase in the number of red blood cells (polycythemia). If it is less it indicates anemia.

Section 1: Hematology

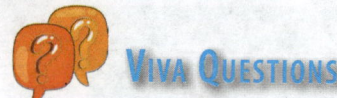
VIVA QUESTIONS

1. **Define PCV or hematocrit. Give its normal value.**
   Hematocrit or PCV is the proportion of the volume of a blood sample that is occupied by red cells.
   Normal range of PCV
   » Adult male: 40–55%
   » Adult female: 35–45%
   » New born: 53–68%
   » One year: 35%
   » 10 years: 38%

2. **Why is double oxalate used as anticoagulant in doing PCV? How it acts as an anticoagulant?**
   Ammonium oxalate and potassium oxalate in the ratio 3:2 is used. Ammonium oxalate causes swelling of RBCs and potassium oxalate causes shrinking of RBCs. So they cannot be used separately. When both are used in the specified ratio the effects cancel each other and the RBC morphology will be maintained.

   Oxalate acts as anticoagulant by forming salt with ionic calcium (chelation). When ionic calcium (Ca^{2+}) is removed from blood, it will not clot because calcium is necessary for all steps of coagulation except for the activation of inactive factors XII and XI and for the conversion of fibrinogen to fibrin monomer.

3. **Comment on the three layers seen in the PCV tube after centrifugation of blood.**
   Refer page 24.

4. **What is the reason for the difference in PCV in arterial and venous blood?**
   PCV in venous blood is 3% greater than that of arterial blood. This is because of the increased size of RBCs in venous blood due to the phenomenon of chloride shift or Hamburger phenomenon. Another reason is that some amount of plasma filtered from the arterial capillaries instead of entering the venous blood, will be returned to circulation via the lymphatics.

5. **Enumerate the conditions where PCV is increased and decreased.**
   Physiological increase
   » Venous blood when compared to arterial blood in the same individual
   » Newborn
   » High altitude
   » After exercise
   Pathological increase
   » Polycythemia
   » Chronic heart disease and chronic lung disease
   » Hemoconcentration as in burns, severe diarrhea, dehydration due to increased sweating.
   Decrease in PCV is seen in
   » Anemia
   » Bone marrow depression
   » Hemodilution as in pregnancy.

6. **What is the importance of doing PCV?**
   » Estimation of PCV can be used as a simple screening test for anemia. Hematocrit will be decreased in anemia and the extent of reduction depends on the degree of anemia. The plasma layer will be very pale in severe anemia.
   » It helps in the calculation of blood indices like MCHC.
   » By noting the thickness of the buffy coat layer we get an idea about the total leukocyte count and conditions like leukemia can be excluded.
   » By noting the color of the plasma layer, conditions like hemolysis, hyperbilirubinemia (jaundice), lipemia etc., can be assessed.

7. **What are the disadvantages of doing PCV? What is true hematocrit?**
   a. Reading error is more.
   b. Hematocrit value gives only the concentration of red cells, i.e., the red cells present in a particular volume of blood. It does not give an idea of the total red cell mass. For example, in hypovolemic shock due to hemorrhage, the PCV will be normal but the total red cell mass is drastically reduced.
   c. About 2% of plasma remains trapped in between the red cells after centrifugation. This will be more if the red cells are of abnormal shape as in spherocytosis. The true hematocrit value can be found out by using a correction factor.
      True hematocrit = obtained hematocrit multiplied by 0.98 (correction factor)
   d. If the blood provided is not mixed properly there will be error in the reading of PCV
   e. Improper reading of PCV. If buffy coat layer is also included while taking the reading, PCV will be high
   f. If centrifugation is not adequate, there will be a reduction in the PCV value

8. **What is the importance of the buffy coat layer?**
   » The thickness of buffy coat gives a rough estimation of total WBC count. 0.1 mm of buffy coat corresponds to 1,000 WBCs.
   » A smear of the buffy coat layer can be prepared to study the morphology of WBCs in conditions like leukemia, multiple myeloma, etc. Blasts cells are seen in leukemia and plasma cells are seen in multiple myeloma.
   » The thickness of buffy coat layer is increased in leukocytosis, leukemia and in thrombocytosis and it is decreased in leukopenia and thrombocytopenia. Platelets occupy the upper most part of the buffy coat.

9. **What is the effect of increased PCV in circulation?**
   Increase in PCV increases the viscosity of blood, which in turn increases resistance to the flow of blood (peripheral resistance). This leads to increase in diastolic blood pressure.

10. **Hematocrit value in microcirculation is lower than that in large vessels. Give reason.**
    Hematocrit value of blood in microcirculation (arterioles, metarterioles and capillaries) is lower because of the effect of **plasma skimming**. In the blood vessel with laminar flow, the red cells move in the center of the blood stream (axial flow) and the blood along the sides of the vessel has less number of RBCs. Branches arising at right angles to the vessel may receive cell-poor blood. This is known as plasma skimming and is marked in the capillaries. Hence hematocrit of capillary blood will be 25% lower than the venous blood.

11. **Why is PCV value less in females when compared to males?**
    In males, the red blood cell count is more because testosterone stimulates erythropoiesis. So PCV will be a little higher in males when compared to females.

OBJECTIVE STRUCTURED PRACTICAL EXAMINATION

I. Fill the Wintrobe's tube with the blood provided for the estimation of hematocrit
   1. Take a clean and dry Wintrobe's tube (Y/N)
   2. Mix the blood provided gently (Y/N)
   3. Take blood in the Pasteur pipette
   4. Bring the tip of the Pasteur pipette to the bottom of the tube (Y/N)
   5. Fill the tube with blood by gradually withdrawing the tube upwards while compressing the teat gently making sure that bubbles are not being formed in the blood in the tube (Y/N)
   6. Stop filling when the blood column reaches exactly the zero mark in the tube (Y/N)
   7. If the tube is overfilled remove the extra blood using a dropper

Chapter 6

Estimation of Hemoglobin (Hemoglobinometry)

LEARNING OBJECTIVES

- List the different methods of estimation of hemoglobin
- Estimate hemoglobin content of your blood by Sahli's acid hematin method
- Advantages and disadvantages of Sahli's method
- Principle of Sahli's method
- Mention the normal values of hemoglobin concentration in infants, adult and old age
- Why is hemoglobin content more in males
- Name the conditions where there is variation in the hemoglobin content of blood
- Define anemia and mention the types of anemia depending on hemoglobin content
- Describe the steps in the synthesis of hemoglobin
- List the derivatives of hemoglobin
- Describe different types of anemia

PY2.11: Estimate hemoglobin, red blood cell count, total leukocyte count, RBC indices, differential leukocyte count, blood groups, BT/CT.

COLORIMETRIC ESTIMATION OF HEMOGLOBIN

Different colorimetric methods are:
- Sahli's method
- Tallquist's method
- Haldane's method
- Cyanmethemoglobin method (most accurate method)
- Gasometric method

Principle

The hemoglobin present in a measured sample of blood is converted into a derivative having a definite tinge of color. In Sahli's method acid hematin is prepared. In Tallquist's method the color of oxyhemoglobin is compared. In Haldane's method, carboxyhemoglobin is prepared. Cyanmethemoglobin derivative is also used to give accurate results. The density of this color is compared with a standard solution of the same derivative. Iron estimation or spectrophotometry is used while deciding the strength and the color of the standard.

Such a standard solution of the derivative cannot be prepared every time. They do not maintain their color for long. There is always a difficulty in obtaining a known sample of blood for its preparation.

So, artificially tinted glass rods matching exactly with the color of the standard solution are used as the standard color. These rods maintain their color for long time.

For comparing the color, first a concentrated solution is prepared. This solution is then diluted till its color density matches with that of the standard. The degree of dilution gives a measure of the amount of hemoglobin (as derivative) present in the sample. The tube in which the blood is diluted is calibrated to give a direct reading of hemoglobin in grams.

Sahli's Method

Principle

Sahli's method is the commonly employed method for hemoglobin estimation. The hemoglobin present in a particular volume of blood is converted to acid hematin by treating it with N/10 HCl. Acid hematin is brown in color and the solution is diluted with distilled water till the color matches with the standard color. The standard color is prepared by treating a sample of blood containing 14.5 g of hemoglobin per 100 mL of blood with N/10 HCl and diluting it 100 times. So 100% reading in the diluting tube corresponds to 14.5 g% of hemoglobin.

Apparatus

Sahli's hemoglobinometer set **(Fig. 6.1)** contains the following:

- A rectangular plastic box with two color standards on either side with a central provision for keeping the diluting tube. The color standard is made of nonfading, standardized, golden brown glass rods **(Fig. 6.2)**.
- Specially graduated diluting tube is square or round in shape. It is graduated in percentage (20–140%) on one side and in gm per deciliter (2–24 g%) on the opposite side.
- A glass rod with flat tip to stir the contents.
- Hemoglobin pipette with a 20 mm^3 mark and rubber tubing with a mouthpiece to suck the blood. There is no bulb in the hemoglobin pipette and the 20 mm^3 mark indicates a definite measured volume and not an arbitrary volume as in the case of RBC and WBC pipette.
- Needle or lancet.
- Bottle containing distilled water and a dropper with teat.
- Bottle containing N/10 hydrochloric acid, which is prepared by mixing 3 mL of concentrated HCl and 997 mL of distilled water.
- Brush to clean the tube.

Procedure

- See that the hemoglobin pipette is clean and dry.
- Place the graduated tube between the standards in the plastic box.
- Fill it with N/10 HCl up to the lowest mark.
- Prick the tip of the finger to get a large drop of blood.
- Hold the pipette in the right hand with the graduation in front.
- Place the mouthpiece between the lips.
- Hold the pipette at an angle of 45° above the horizontal and touch the tip of the pipette to one side of the drop.
- Suck the blood till the blood reaches the 20 mm^3 mark (if any air bubble enters the pipette, repeat with a new dry one).
- Remove the pipette and clean the outer surface with a cotton swab by wiping it towards the tip to remove any blood that is present on the outer surface of the pipette. Do not touch the open end while wiping because blood will come out of the pipette due to capillary action.
- If the blood has slightly crossed the mark, take the excess blood out by touching the tip of the pipette on the palm of the hand for a couple of times and the blood will recede back in the pipette. Make sure that you are wearing gloves if blood is taken from another person.
- Do not use a swab or a filter paper to remove the excess blood. It will absorb a very large quantity of blood.
- While transferring the blood to the HCl in the diluting tube, blow down slowly.
- Dip its tip in the acid and blow out gently to transfer all the blood into the tube.
- Suck the superficial acid and rinse the pipette repeatedly till all the blood in the pipette is transferred into the diluting tube.
- Mix the blood and the acid with the glass rod provided.
- Note the time. Wait for 10 minutes to allow the brown color of acid hematin to develop. The color does not develop immediately. Its intensity changes with time. 95% of the color is reached by the end of 10 minutes.

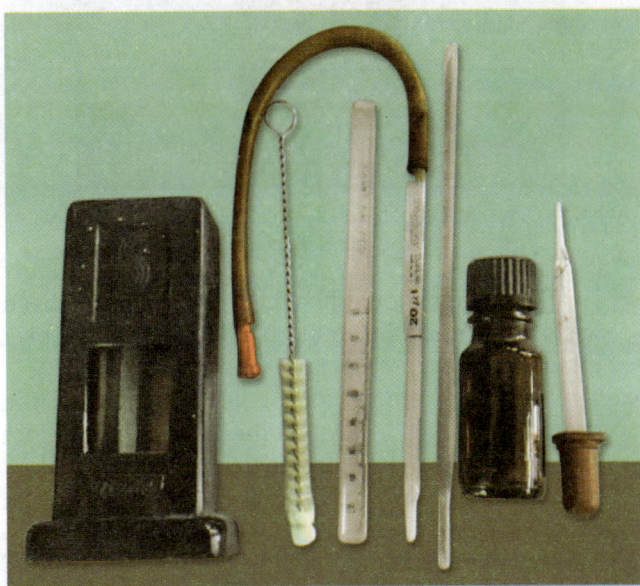

Fig. 6.1: Sahli's hemoglobinometer showing the box with standard color, brush, diluting tube, pipette, glass rod, N/10 HCl and dropper.

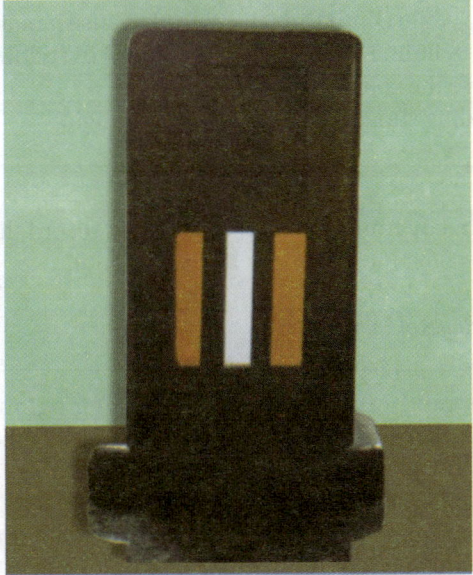

Fig. 6.2: Sahli's hemoglobinometer showing the color standards.

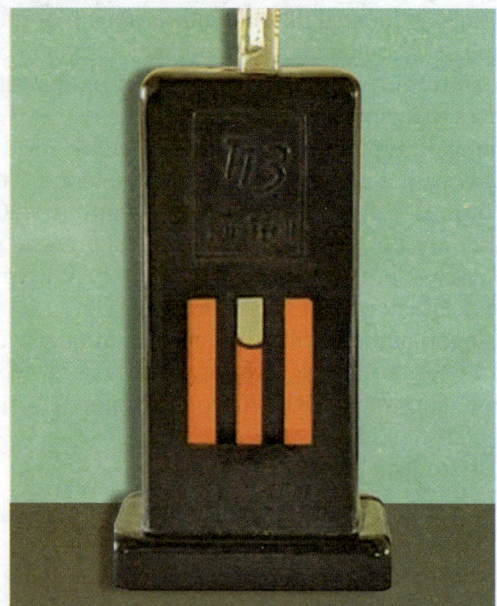

Fig. 6.3: Correct matching of sample with standard color.

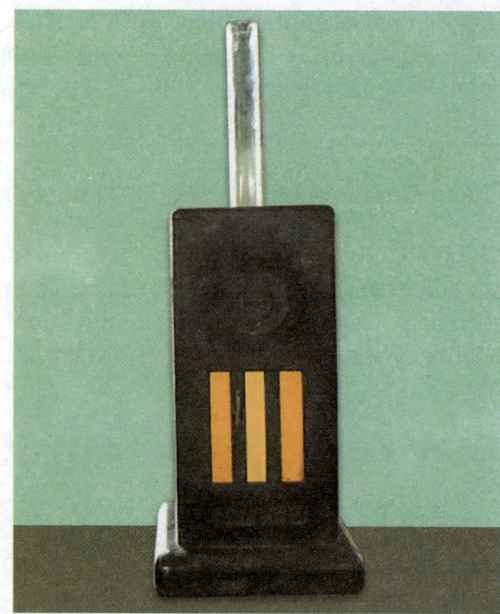

Fig. 6.4: Overdilution of blood sample, color not matching with the standard color.

- Add distilled water drop by drop mixing the solution with the glass rod after the addition of each drop.
- After adding two or three drops of water and mixing, compare the color of the solution with the standard color of the glass block. While comparing, lift the stirrer above the level of the solution but it should not be completely taken out of the tube. If comparison is done with the glass rod in the solution, the solution will appear lighter. While comparing the color, avoid viewing through the markings on the tube and hold the apparatus against natural light.
- Add water drop by drop, mix and compare each time after every addition.
- Continue till the colors match **(Fig. 6.3)**.
- Raise the glass rod and take the reading in g/dL.
- Read the lower meniscus. Since the solution is transparent the lower meniscus is clearly seen even though it is colored.

Precautions

- The color of the standard should be examined from time to time to exclude any fading or change in color.
- After pricking, the finger should not be squeezed to obtain blood. This may give a false low value for hemoglobin since the blood gets diluted with tissue fluid. A free flowing drop should be obtained.
- There should not be any air bubble in the blood column in the pipette.
- Blood from the pipette should be immediately transferred into the tube containing N/10 HCl. Otherwise blood may clot.

- Distilled water should be added dropbydrop, mixed well and compared with the standard. Otherwise over dilution may occur **(Fig. 6.4).**
- The diluting tube should be kept in between the standards in such a way that the graduations are not interfering with the comparison.
- Take the reading without delay because on keeping, the color will deepen.
- Matching and reading should be taken after lifting the glass rod from the solution. If it is left in the solution while comparing the color, the solution will appear lighter.
- The glass rod should not be removed from the diluting tube while comparing the color, because it may lead to loss of fluid. Hold it against the side of the diluting tube above the solution.
- Reading should be taken in good daylight.

Result

Read directly from the diluting tube and record the result in grams of hemoglobin per 100 mL of blood.

Disadvantages of Sahli's Method

- There can be visual error.
- This method estimates only oxyhemoglobin and reduced hemoglobin. Carboxy, met and sulfhemoglobin cannot be converted to acid hematin.
- The color of the standard fades over time.
- If the reading is not taken immediately, the color of acid hematin changes.

Cyanmethemoglobin Method

Principle

The basis of this method is dilution of blood in a diluent called Drabkin cyanide–ferricyanide solution. Ferrous ion of hemoglobin is converted to ferric ion by ferricyanide and methemoglobin so produced is combined with potassium ferricyanide to produce cyanmethemoglobin which is red colored. All hemoglobin derivatives of blood except sulfhemoglobin are measured by this technique. But sulfhemoglobin is rarely present in significant amounts in blood. *Cyanmethemoglobin method is one of the most reliable and the most accurate method and is the WHO'S recommended method for determining the hemoglobin concentration of blood.* The color of cyanmethemoglobin in the unknown blood is compared with the standard solution of cyanmethemoglobin.

Procedure

To 5 mL of Drabkin solution add 20 μL of blood. Mix well and after 5 minutes read the absorbance in a spectrometer at 540 nm or in a photoelectric colorimeter with a yellow-green filter. Drabkin solution consists of dihydrogen potassium phosphate (140 mg), potassium ferricyanide (200 mg), potassium cyanide (50 mg) and distilled water to 1,000 mL. The oxy, carboxy and methemoglobin are all converted into cyanmethemoglobin and there is development of pink color. The color intensity is proportional to the concentration of hemoglobin in the blood sample. The color is compared with that of a standard cyanmethemoglobin solution.

Tallquist's Method

A drop of blood is placed on an absorbent paper and is then matched against a series of lithographed color supposed to represent hemoglobin values in grades of 10–100%. Though quick, this method is inaccurate and is only used in mass surveys for anemia.

Haldane's Method or Carboxyhemoglobin Method

Blood is treated with ammonia solution and is then saturated with CO. The carboxyhemoglobin formed is compared with a glass tube containing carboxyhemoglobin as the standard.

Gasometric Method

It is also called van Slyke's oxygen capacity method. It estimates the amount of hemoglobin from the amount of O_2 it absorbs.

OTHER METHODS OF ESTIMATION OF HEMOGLOBIN

Estimation of Iron

The amount of iron present in a known volume of blood can be accurately measured by chemical methods. Normally, 1 g of hemoglobin contains 3.35 mg of iron. By finding out the amount of iron present in the blood sample the amount of hemoglobin can be calculated. This method is time consuming.

Spectrophotometry

This method is based on the ability of hemoglobin to refract definite wavelengths of light giving typical absorption bands. If light is passed through a solution of hemoglobin, definite wave lengths of light are absorbed by hemoglobin. By using suitable wavelengths of light, the con centration of hemoglobin can be measured by a photoelectric colorimeter.

Oxygen Carrying Capacity Determination

The maximum amount of oxygen the sample of blood is capable of carrying is called the oxygen carrying capacity of the blood. The amount of oxygen present in the blood can be measured very accurately with the Van Slyke's apparatus. A sample of blood is exposed to the atmosphere. The partial pressure of oxygen in the atmospheric air is about 150 mm Hg. At this partial pressure the hemoglobin gets completely saturated with oxygen. This oxygenated sample of blood is treated with ferricyanide and exposed to vacuum in the Van Slyke's apparatus when all the oxygen present is evolved out and it is measured. One gram of hemoglobin combines with 1.34 mL of oxygen at normal temperature and pressure. By measuring the amount of O_2 evolved, the amount of hemoglobin in the given blood sample can be calculated.

The above three methods cannot be used for routine estimation of hemoglobin since it is time consuming and requires sophisticated equipment.

DISCUSSION

Hemoglobin is the red coloring pigment and the O_2 binding protein of RBC. It forms 95% of the dry weight of RBC. The function of hemoglobin is to carry O_2 as oxyhemoglobin and CO_2 as carbaminohemoglobin. The iron atoms are in their reduced state, i.e., ferrous state in the hemoglobin molecule and in this state each iron atom can combine with one molecule of O_2. When the iron atoms get oxidized to their ferric state then it is called methemoglobin. Methemoglobin has no ability to carry O_2.

Section 1: Hematology

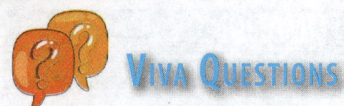
Viva Questions

1. **Give the normal hemoglobin content.**
   » At birth: 23–25 g%
   » Adult male: 14–16 g%
   » Adult female: 12–15 g%

2. **Mention the variations in hemoglobin content.**
   » Increase in hemoglobin content is seen in newborn, at high altitude, after exercise, hemoconcentration, polycythemia vera, etc.
   » Technical error like increase in the amount of blood taken in the pipette (>20 µL) gives a higher value.
   » Decrease in hemoglobin content is anemia. All conditions producing anemia will result in decrease in hemoglobin content.
   » In hemodilution as in pregnancy, Hb concentration will be less than normal.
   » Technical errors like less amount of blood taken in the pipette and blood sample obtained by squeezing the fingertip will give a lower value. When the fingertip is squeezed, the fluid coming will contain more of tissue fluid and less number of RBCs. Failure to wait for 10 minutes after mixing blood with N/10 HCl will give a low hemoglobin value. If the amount of N/10 HCl taken is not adequate, all the hemoglobin present in the sample will not be converted to acid hematin and a low value will be obtained.

3. **What happens if hemoglobin is found in plasma as the free hemoglobin?**
   If Hb is present dissolved in plasma and not confined within the RBC, it leads to the following problems:
   » It increases the viscosity of blood leading to an increase in the blood pressure.
   » Increase in the osmotic pressure of blood.
   » Free hemoglobin will be filtered and excreted by the kidneys leading to hemoglobinuria and precipitation of hemoglobin in the renal tubules leading to renal failure and anemia.
   » Free hemoglobin will be rapidly destroyed by the reticuloendothelial cells leading to increase in the bilirubin content of blood.

4. **What is the reason for increase in hemoglobin content in the newborn?**
   During fetal life the type of hemoglobin in blood is HbF (fetal hemoglobin). It contains two α and two γ chains. The γ chain does not combine with 2, 3bisphosphoglycerate (2, 3 BPG) and so HbF has greater affinity for oxygen. It releases less O_2 at the tissue level and tissues suffer from hypoxia, which is the most potent stimulant for erythropoietin secretion. Since erythropoiesis is increased there is increase in hemoglobin content in newborn.

5. **What is physiological jaundice?**
   Yellowish discoloration of skin and mucous membrane seen in newborn is called physiological jaundice. It disappears in 2 weeks. After birth fetal hemoglobin is replaced by adult hemoglobin. There is increased destruction of red blood cells after birth in order to bring the RBC count to normal level. This leads to increase in the level of bilirubin in blood leading to jaundice.

6. **What is the principle behind Sahli's method of hemoglobin estimation?**
   Refer page 28.

7. **How is the standard color in Sahli's method obtained?**
   The standard color is prepared by treating 20 mm^3 of blood containing 14.5 g of hemoglobin per 100 mL with N/10 HCl and diluting it 100 times.

8. **What is the reason for waiting for 10 min after adding blood into the diluting tube?**
   This much time is needed for the complete hemolysis of RBCs and for the conversion of all the hemoglobin present to form acid hematin.

9. **What are the functions of hemoglobin?**
   » It helps in the transport of O_2 from lungs to tissues by forming oxyhemoglobin.
   » Helps in the transport of CO_2 from tissues to lungs by forming carbaminohemoglobin.
   » It acts as a buffer to maintain the normal pH of blood. Hemoglobin being a protein is responsible for 70% of the buffering capacity of whole blood.
   » The β-chain F hemoglobin has an additional nitric oxide (NO) binding site. The affinity of hemoglobin for NO is increased by O_2. So hemoglobin binds with NO in the lungs and releases it in the tissues where it promotes vasodilatation.

10. **What are the various forms of hemoglobin present in blood?**
    » Oxyhemoglobin (HbO_2)—Hb in combination with O_2.
    » Carbaminohemoglobin (HbNHCOOH)—Hb combined with CO_2.
    » Carboxy hemoglobin (HbCO)—Hb in combination with CO.
    » Sulfhemoglobin (SHb)—in combination with sulfur containing compounds.
    » Methemoglobin—when the ferrous form of iron is oxidized to the ferric form.
    » Adult hemoglobin are HbA ($α_2β_2$) and HbA_2 ($α_2δ_2$).
    » Fetal hemoglobin or HbF ($α_2γ_2$).

11. **What is anemia? How is it graded?**
    Reduction in the hemoglobin content of blood or RBC count or both below the normal range for that age and sex is called anemia. When the RBC count is less than 4 million/mm^3 of blood or hemoglobin content less than 12 g/dL in an adult the condition is anemia. Severity of anemia can be graded depending on the hemoglobin content as follows:
    Mild anemia where the hemoglobin content is 10–11 g%. **Moderate anemia** where the hemoglobin content is 7–9 g%. **Severe anemia** when the hemoglobin content falls below 6 g%.

12. **What is the etiological classification of anemia?**
    » Anemia due to increased destruction of RBC (hemolytic anemia).
    » Anemia due to defective formation of RBC (deficiency anemia and anemia due to bone marrow depression).
    » Posthemorrhagic anemia (acute and chronic blood loss).
13. **What are the disadvantages of Sahli's method?**
    » This method estimates only oxyhemoglobin and reduced hemoglobin. Other forms such as carboxyhemoglobin and met hemoglobin are not estimated.
    » The color of the standard may fade and become lighter after a few years and this will give a wrong result.
14. **Which is the most accurate method for estimating hemoglobin content? Why?**
    Cyanmethemoglobin method. All hemoglobin derivatives of blood except sulfhemoglobin are measured by this technique. But sulfhemoglobin is rarely present in significant amounts in blood.
15. **What is oxygen carrying capacity of blood?**
    The amount of oxygen present in 100 mL of blood, when all the hemoglobin present in it is completely saturated with O_2 is the oxygen carrying capacity. Normally it is about 21 mL/100 mL of blood. One gram of hemoglobin can combine with 1.35 mL of O_2.
16. **At what stage of erythropoiesis does hemoglobin appear in red cells?**
    Hemoglobin appears in the early normoblast stage and maximum level is reached in the late normoblast stage.
17. **Which is the most common cause of anemia in India?**
    Worm infestation especially hook worm infestation is the most common cause. It produces iron deficiency anemia.

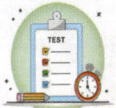

OBJECTIVE STRUCTURED PRACTICAL EXAMINATION

I. Suck blood in the hemoglobin pipette for estimating your hemoglobin concentration
   1. Take a clean and dry hemoglobin pipette
   2. Sterilize the finger tip
   3. Give a deep prick using a sterile lancet (do not squeeze the finger tip for obtaining blood)
   4. Wipe off the first drop using sterile cotton
   5. Apply gentle pressure so that a drop of blood appears on the finger tip
   6. Suck blood into the pipette exactly up to the 20 mm³ mark on the pipette
   7. Wipe the tip of the pipette
   8. Press the finger tip with clean cotton

II. Do the hemoglobin estimation with the blood taken in the hemoglobin pipette
   1. Take a clean diluting tube
   2. Take N/10 HCl up to the lower mark in the tube
   3. Blow the blood in the pipette into the acid solution in the diluting tube.
   4. Rinse the pipette in the acid solution 2 more times and blow out into the diluting tube so that whole of blood remaining in the pipette is transferred to the diluting tube
   5. Place the diluting tube between the standard colors
   6. Note the time and wait for 10 minutes for the formation of acid hematin
   7. Add distilled water drop by drop mixing the solution with the glass rod after the addition of each drop.
   8. After adding two or three drops of water and mixing, compare the color of the solution with the standard color of the glass block. While comparing, lift the stirrer above the level of the solution but it should not be completely taken out of the tube.
   9. Add water drop by drop, mix and compare each time after every addition.
   10. Continue till the colors match.
   11. Raise the glass rod and take the reading in g/dL.
   12. Read the lower meniscus.

Hemocytometer and Red Blood Cell Count

LEARNING OBJECTIVES

- Mention the differences between RBC and WBC pipettes
- Focus the ruled area of the counting chamber under low power and high power of the microscope and identify the WBC and RBC counting areas
- Dilute the blood in the RBC pipette up to the correct mark for doing RBC count
- Charge the counting chamber precisely
- Mention the precautions to be taken while charging
- Write the calculations stepwise for finding out the RBC count

PY2.11: Estimate hemoglobin, red blood cell count, total leukocyte count, RBC indices, differential leukocyte count, blood groups, BT/CT.

HEMOCYTOMETRY

Hemocytometry is the technique of counting the different blood cells. The red blood cells (RBCs), white blood cells (WBCs) and platelets are counted separately.

Since manual methods for counting the blood cells have proven to be very inaccurate, automated counters provide a much more accurate reflection of the various blood cell counts like RBC count, WBC count, platelet count, etc.

HEMOCYTOMETER

Hemocytometer is a box containing the following: RBC pipette, WBC pipette, improved Neubauer counting chamber, special cover glass, RBC diluting fluid, WBC diluting fluid, spirit, etc.

RBC Pipette

The **RBC pipette** or Thoma glass pipette has a capillary stem of uniform bore with a conical tip. Just above the stem is a large bulb that contains a small red glass bead **(Fig. 7.1)**. The pipette is so constructed that the capacity of the bulb is 100 times that of the stem. The junction between the stem and the bulb is prominently marked as '1'. The capillary stem is divided into ten equal parts from the tip

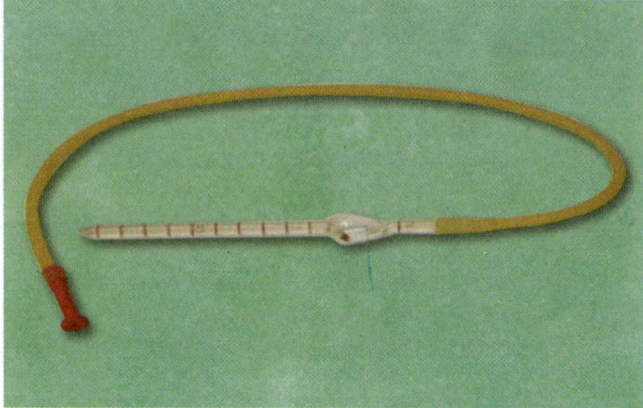

Fig. 7.1: RBC pipette showing red bead in the bulb.

to the mark '1' and the fifth division is again prominently marked as 0.5. Smaller calibrations in between allow greater dilutions if needed. There is another line just above the bulb that is marked '101'. The markings have no units and it only represents relative volumes. The bulb narrows proximally into a glass capillary tube to which a long narrow soft rubber tube bearing a mouthpiece is attached. The rubber tube must have a length of 30–40 cm so that when the mouthpiece is held between the lips, the markings in the pipette could be easily seen while it is being filled with blood. The pipette has a white glossy surface opposite the graduation marks. This helps to see the markings in the pipette distinctly.

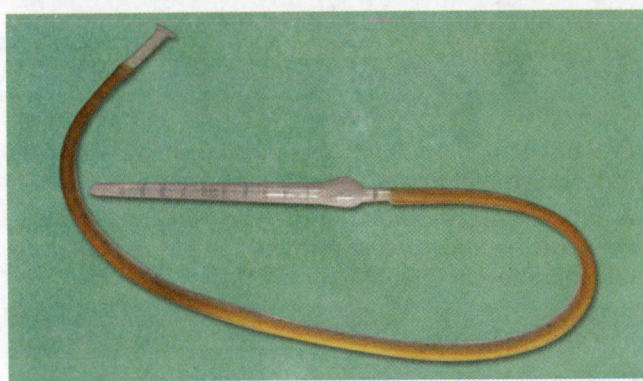

Fig. 7.2: WBC pipette.

WBC Pipette

The bulb of the WBC pipette is smaller than that of RBC pipette and has a capacity only 10 times that of its stem. It is marked with the number 11 at its top. In the middle of the stem, there is a 0.5 mark and just below the bulb it is marked 1. The bulb of the pipette contains a **white bead** to identify the pipette and also to mix the blood and diluting fluid thoroughly **(Fig. 7.2)**.

The Hemocytometer or Neubauer Counting Chamber

The counting chamber is a thick glass slide with a central depressed platform separated on either side from the remaining platform by deep moats **(Fig. 7.3)**.

The surface level of this platform is exactly 0.1 mm lower than the general surface on which the cover glass rests. That is, when the cover slip is laid across between the two ridges there is exactly 0.1 mm distance between the surface of the depressed platform and the under surface of the cover slip **(Fig. 7.4)**. This depressed platform is accurately ruled in squares. The length and breadth of the smallest square on it is always 1/20 mm each, i.e., each of the smallest squares has an area of 1/400 sq. mm. These squares are grouped in various ways in different types of chambers.

The improved **Neubauer double counting chamber** (called so because it has two counting areas in a single slide and it is used for counting RBCs and WBCs) has an H-shaped depression in the center called moat. The central depressed platform is divided into two parts by a lengthwise moat and from the surrounding slide by two breadthwise moats. On either side of the transverse depression, there are ruled areas of squares that are used for counting red blood cells and white blood cells. The chamber is called improved double counting chamber because the ruling in the counting chamber is done using diamond and, therefore, the lines will never fade away. The lines are coated with silver to make it more prominent under the microscope.

Each ruled area is square-shaped with the side measuring 3 mm. The total area of the square is 9 mm². The squares are divided into 9 equal parts by means of 4 vertical and 4 horizontal triple lines. The side of each of these large squares is 1 mm. The four corner squares are used for counting WBCs. Each of the corner squares is again divided into 16 smaller squares by single lines **(Fig. 7.5)**.

The central square in the ruled area of the counting chamber measuring 1 mm × 1 mm is used for counting red blood cells **(Fig. 7.6)**. This square is divided into 25 medium-sized squares by means of triple lines so that the side of one small square is 1/5 mm. This small square is

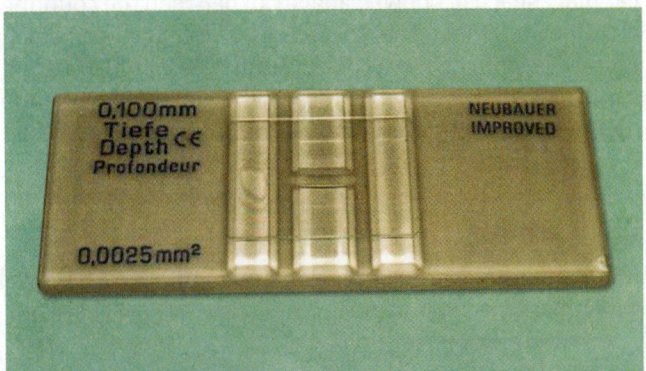

Fig. 7.3: Neubauer double counting chamber.

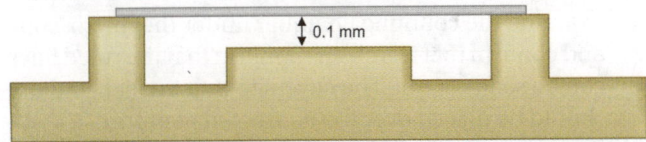

Fig. 7.4: The moats of the counting chamber as viewed from the side.

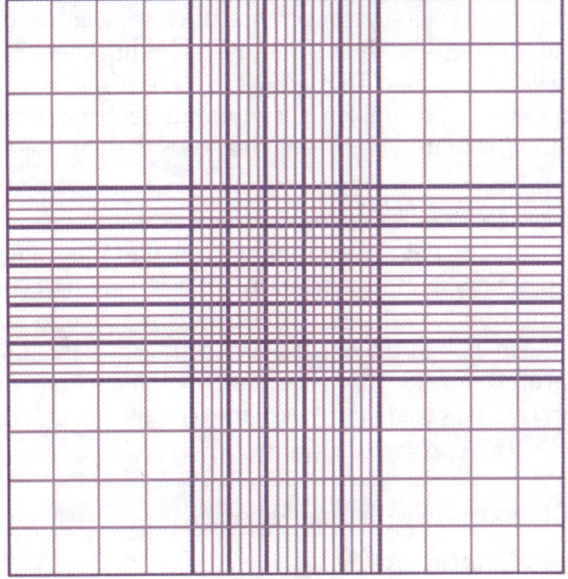

Fig. 7.5: Ruled area of the counting chamber (the four corner squares each divided into 16 smaller squares are the WBC counting areas and the central large square divided into 25 smaller squares is the RBC counting area, each small square is again divided into 16 smallest squares in the RBC counting area).

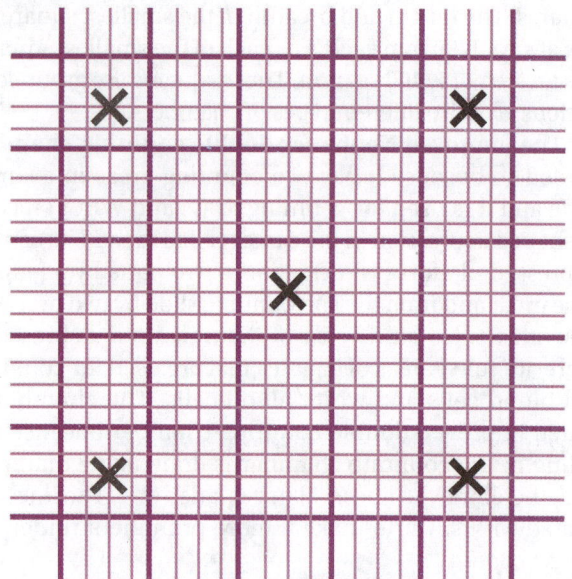

Fig. 7.6: RBC counting area in the counting chamber. The squares marked 'X' are used for counting RBCs.

again divided into 16 smaller squares by single lines so that the side of the smallest square in the RBC counting area is $1/5 \times 1/4 = 1/20$ mm. The area of the smallest square is $1/20 \times 1/20$ mm = $1/400$ mm². *The four, corner squares and the central one in the RBC counting area (a total of $16 \times 5 = 80$ smallest squares) are used for counting RBCs.*

Special Cover Glass

A special coverslip is used along with the counting chamber, which is thicker and stronger than the cover slips used for mounting on slides. 0.3, 0.4 and 0.5 mm thickness cover glasses are available. They are of two sizes, 16 mm × 22 mm and 22 mm × 22 mm. For the improved Neubauer double counting chamber, the larger cover glass must be used.

WBC Diluting Fluid (Turk's Fluid)

WBC diluting fluid is not isotonic as that of RBC diluting fluid. It contains **glacial acetic acid 0.2 mL, gentian violet 1% solution 0.1 mL** and distilled water is added to make the volume up to 100 mL. Glacial acetic acid is the purest form of acetic acid. This very dilute hypotonic acid solution quickly causes complete lysis of the red cells so that WBCs can be distinctly seen.

RBC Diluting Fluid (Hayem's Fluid)

Composition of Hayem's Fluid

NaCl—0.5 gram, Na_2SO_4—2.5 grams, mercuric perchloride—0.25 gram and distilled water to be added to make up the volume to 100 mL.

Dissolve the chemicals in distilled water and filter several times through filter paper. In this fluid, NaCl and Na_2SO_4 make the solution isotonic with plasma, Na_2SO_4 acts as a fixative to preserve the shape of the cells and it also prevents clumping of RBCs; mercuric perchloride acts as a preservative and prevents growth of any organism.

But in many diseased conditions, this fluid tends to clump the red cells. 0.01 gram of gelatin per 100 mL of the fluid may prevent this clumping.

Other RBC Diluting Fluids

❖ **Dacie's fluid**
   Composition:
   Trisodium citrate : 3.13 g
   37% formalin: 1 mL
   Distilled water up to 100 mL
   The advantages of Dacie's fluid is that (i) it is easy to prepare; (ii) no preservatives needed; (iii) RBC count can be performed even after several hours of dilution of blood
❖ **Isotonic saline**
   In emergencies, isotonic saline can be used as diluting fluid. But the count should be performed immediately after dilution. Otherwise, the red cells will aggregate.

RED BLOOD CELL COUNT

Principle

The number of red cells in the blood is too many and the size of the cells is too small. It is therefore not possible to count the cells even under high power. This difficulty is partially overcome by diluting the blood with Hayem's fluid to a known degree. The diluted blood is placed in a capillary space of known capacity in between the counting chamber and the special cover glass. The cells spread out in a single layer in this space. The number of cells in the small capillary space of known volume is then counted under the high power of a microscope. The result is reported as the number of cells per cubic mm of blood.

Requirements

RBC pipette, Hayem's fluid, Neubauer counting chamber, watch glass, compound microscope, clean absorbable cloth, lancet and spirit.

Procedure

❖ Examine the counting chamber under the microscope and confirm that it is clean. Confirm that the ruled lines can be seen clearly. The coverslip that is clean and dry should be placed over the depressed platform.
❖ Pour about 2 mL of Hayem's fluid in the watch glass.

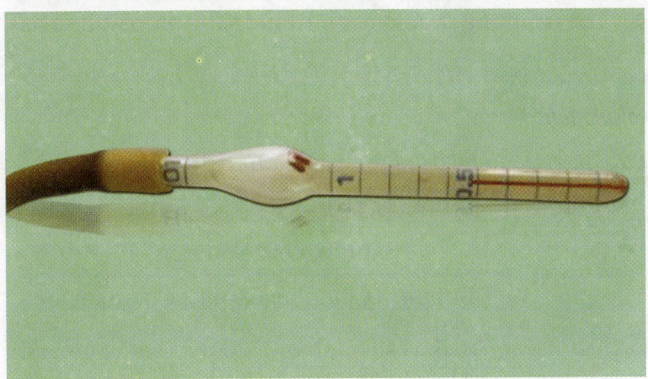

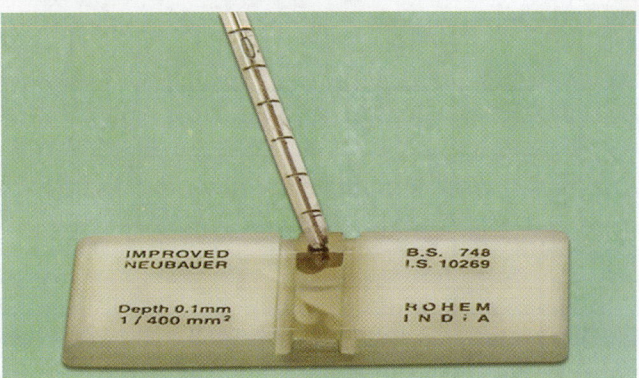

Fig. 7.7: Blood taken up to the 0.5 mark in the RBC pipette for doing RBC count.

Fig. 7.8: Charging the counting chamber.

- Hold the mouthpiece of the RBC pipette between the lips and allow the pipette to hang down.
- The blood is obtained by a deep finger prick with a sterile lancet (stored venous sample can also be used).
- Suck blood into the pipette accurately up to the 0.5 mark **(Fig. 7.7)**. If any air bubble enters the pipette discard it and repeat with a fresh, clean and dry pipette.
- Wipe off the blood sticking to the sides of the tip of the pipette.
- Dip the tip of the pipette in the diluting fluid in the watch glass and suck the fluid accurately up to the 101 mark. If fluid goes beyond the mark, or if air bubble enters by accident, repeat the procedure with fresh sample and fresh pipette. Dilution of the blood must be done quickly otherwise blood may clot in the stem.
- Hold the pipette horizontally and roll it between the palms to ensure thorough mixing.
- This mixture can be kept for up to a maximum of four hours before counting. But before charging, the contents should be properly mixed.

Charging the Counting Chamber

- Place the counting chamber on a plane horizontal surface.
- Roll the pipette once more between the palms to ensure complete mixing of the cells in the fluid immediately before charging.
- Discard at least three drops of fluid from the pipette.
- Hold the pipette at an angle of about 45° and touch its tip on the platform adjacent to the edge of the coverslip **(Fig. 7.8)**.
- Allow a small drop of fluid to form at the tip of the pipette. As the drop formed touch the junction of the counting chamber and the cover glass, because of the capillary action, the fluid will spread under the coverslip. If the drop is too big, it will flow into the moat and over the cover glass. In such a case, the procedure will have to be repeated after cleaning the chamber and the cover glass.
- The capillary space should be completely filled up without leaving any air bubbles in the fluid. Air bubbles are formed if the slide is unclean or moist.
- If the fluid runs down in the moat or if any air bubble is seen, remove the cover glass, clean the slide and the cover glass, and replace it and charge again.
- Before recharging, rotate the pipette to mix the cells and the fluid; remove two drops so that the fluid and the cells settled in the capillary stem are washed out.
- After charging the chamber correctly, allow the RBCs to settle for a period of three minutes on the stage of microscope, before counting. Counting cannot be undertaken when cells are moving and changing their positions due to currents in the fluid.

Counting the Cells

- Fix the slide on the stage with clips.
- Focus the central 1 mm^2 ruled area (RBC squares) under the low power (10X objective) and see whether the cells are uniformly distributed.
- Change over to high power, focus and adjust the light till the cells and the rulings are seen clearly.
- Check whether the cells are uniformly distributed in the chamber.
- The four corner squares and the central square in the RBC counting area is used.
- Move the slide carefully till the left upper corner block of 16 small squares are brought into the field.
- Confirm that the cells have settled down and there is no movement of cells.
- Start counting the cells in the upper and left small square **(Fig. 7.9)**. Leukocytes should not be counted. They appear grayish and granular. One WBC is seen in 750 red cells except in disease conditions like leukemia.
- Obey the 'rules of counting'. The cells lying across the upper horizontal and the left vertical border line should

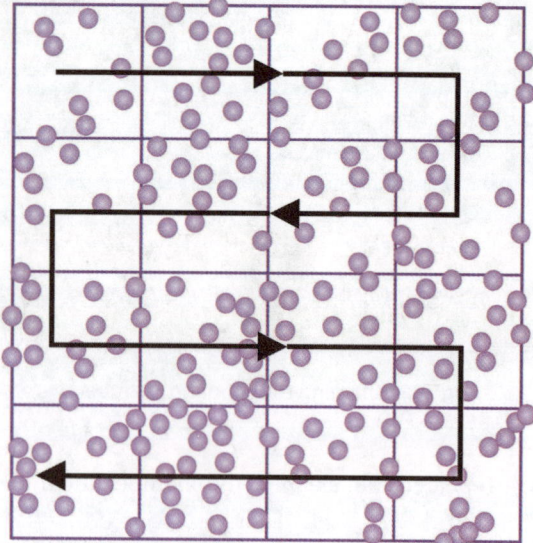

Fig. 7.9: Method of counting RBCs.

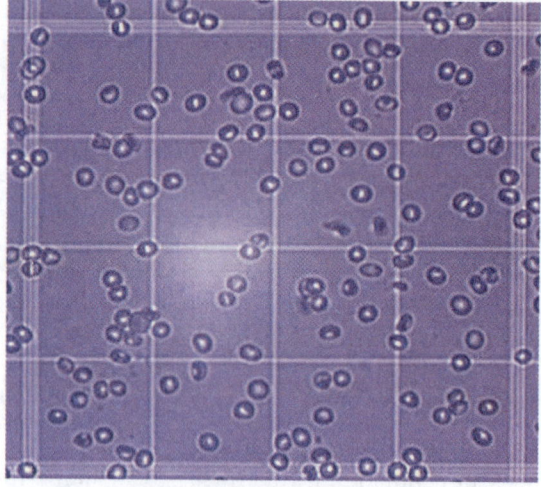

Fig. 7.10: RBCs focused under high power for counting.

be counted in the square under consideration; while those lying across the lower horizontal and the right vertical border line should be counted in the adjacent squares **(Fig. 7.10)**.

- Count the cells in all the sixteen small squares. Note down the reading. Repeat the counting two more times and find out the mean.
- Move the slide carefully toward the left till the upper right big block comes under view.
- Count the cells as previously in this big block 3 times and take the mean.
- Similarly count the cells in the lower right, lower left and the central big square in this order.
- Note down the readings.
- The number of cells in the five different squares should not differ widely from each other. The difference should not be more than 10–20 cells. If the difference is more, it means that the distribution of cells is not very even.
- The counting should not be done if the preparation has dried.

Calculations

The formula to be used for calculation is as follows:

Number of cells/mm^3 of blood

$$= \frac{\text{Number of cells counted}}{\text{Dilution} \times \text{Chamber depth} \times \text{Chamber area}}$$

Each small square has a length of 1/20 mm and a breadth of 1/20 mm and a height of 1/10 mm between the cover slip and the chamber.

The volume of the smallest square is 1/20 × 1/20 × 1/10 = 1/4000 cubic mm. The five big squares counted contain 80 such small squares.

The volume of 80 small square spaces is 1/4000 × 80 = 1/50 cubic mm.

If 'N' is the number of cells counted in the 80 small squares, 1/50 cubic mm contains N cells. So, 1 cubic mm will contain 50 × N cells.

These cells are present in the diluted blood. Blood is taken up to the 0.5 mark and drawn fluid up to the 101 mark. The blood was diluted from 0.5 volumes to 100 volumes, i.e., 1 in 200. The volume of fluid up to the 1 mark in the capillary stem of the pipette did not mix with the blood and this volume was discarded before counting.

The number of cells in the blood must, therefore, be 200 times the one in the diluted. The number of cells in 1 cubic mm of diluted blood sample is $N \times 50$.

The number of cells in 1 cubic mm of undiluted blood will be $N \times 50 \times 200$ or $N \times 10,000$.

Precautions

- The fingertip should not be squeezed because blood gets diluted with tissue fluid and a false low count will be obtained.
- Blood should be drawn exactly up to the 0.5 mark without air bubbles.
- Wipe away the blood on the outside of the tip of the pipette taking care not to touch the tip. Otherwise falsely high counts will be obtained.
- As soon as blood is drawn into the pipette, it should be immediately diluted with the diluting fluid to prevent clotting. Diluting fluid should be drawn exactly up to the 101 mark.
- Mix the blood and the diluting fluid thoroughly by rolling the pipette between the palms.
- Discard three drops from the pipette before charging the chamber.
- Overcharging should not be done, i.e., the fluid should not run over into the gutters and there should be no air bubbles under the cover slip.

- After charging, give time for RBCs to settle.
- Do not keep the microscope tilted.
- Counting should be done under high power after adjusting the microscope.
- 'Rules of counting' should be followed to avoid counting the same cells again.
- Drying of the fluid in the counting chamber should be prevented.
- There should be no errors in calculation.
- The pipette should be thoroughly washed with distilled water, and then rinsed with alcohol. To remove the alcohol, it is rinsed with acetone and dried.

RESULT

The RBC count of the subject is ...... million cells/mm^3 of blood.

DISCUSSION

Estimation of red cell count in blood is mainly done for calculating the blood indices like mean corpuscular volume (MCV) and mean corpuscular hemoglobin (MCH). Otherwise estimation of packed cell volume and hemoglobin estimation is superior to RBC count to get sufficient information about the RBC status. This is because the red cell count varies in different parts of the body. For example, RBC count is more in venous and capillary blood than in arterial blood and it is increased after exercise and meals. So, it is not that reliable. A variation of 10% can occur due to technical error and repeated counts should be done on repeated charging for accuracy.

NORMAL RBC COUNT

- **Newborn:** 6–7 million/mm^3 of blood
- **Males:** 5–6 million cells/mm^3 of blood
- **Female:** 4.5–5.5 million cells/mm^3 of blood

Variations in RBC Count

Physiological Variations in the Red Blood Cell Count

- 5 millions of red cells are present per cubic mm of blood in healthy adult male while 4.5 million in the female. This difference is attributed mainly to the menstrual loss of blood in females. Moreover in males, testosterone stimulates erythropoiesis and this accounts for the increase in RBC count in males when compared to females. The difference does not appear until puberty in man.
- In the newborn, very high counts are obtained. Count is less in children from 4 weeks to about 14 years of age when compared to that of normal adults.
- RBC count is decreased in old age.
- During pregnancy, there is an increase in the plasma volume and hence definite but apparent decreases in the cell count results.
- Exercise and dehydration will tend to increase the count while ingestion of large quantities of water will tend to decrease the count. In exercise, more of stored red cells will be released into circulation especially from spleen which contracts during exercise. In dehydration there is hemoconcentration and there is relative increase in RBC count.
- Emotional polycythemia or stress erythrocytosis is known to occur in many individuals and is due to redistribution of the cells in the vascular system (caused by splenic contraction).
- Athletes undergoing training in strenuous exercise tend to show higher counts that can possibly be attributed to the hypoxic stimulus.
- People staying at high altitudes (12,000 feet and above) show increase in the red cell count even up to 8 million per cubic mm of blood which is due to the hypoxia at the high altitude.
- There is a diurnal variation of about 5%, the count is least during sleep and maximum during evening.

Pathological Variation in Red Cell Count

There are pathological reasons for variation in red cell count. Increase in RBC count is known as polycythemia and decrease in count is called anemia.

Polycythemia

An increase in the number of the red cells above normal is called **polycythemia**. An increase in the amount of the hemoglobin without an increase in the number of red cells cannot occur as the red cells in healthy individuals are completely saturated with hemoglobin.

Types of Polycythemia

1. **Polycythemia vera** is a *malignant condition of red bone marrow*. It is always associated with increase in leukocyte count. RBC count will be more than 14 million/mm^3 of blood.
2. **Secondary polycythemia** is secondary to other pathological conditions that produce a state of chronic hypoxia. Secondary polycythemia is seen in:
   - Chronic lung diseases
   - Congenital cyanotic heart disease
   - Carbon monoxide poisoning
   - Repeated small hemorrhages that stimulates erythropoiesis
   - Phosphorus and arsenic poisoning
   - Endocrine disorders like Cushing syndrome, hyperthyroidism, etc.
   - **Relative polycythemia** is seen in conditions that produce hemoconcentration like burns, diarrhea, vomiting, excessive sweating, etc.

Anemia: Decrease in RBC count below the normal value is anemia.

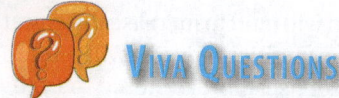
VIVA QUESTIONS

1. **What are the uses of Newbauer's counting chamber?**
   » It is used for finding out RBC count, WBC count and platelet count.
   » It is also used for counting the cells in cerebrospinal fluid, peritoneal and pleural fluid.
   » Used for doing sperm count.

2. **What are the functions of the red bead inside the bulb of RBC pipette?**
   The red bead in the bulb helps in mixing the blood with the diluting fluid and also allows easy identification of the RBC pipette at a distance. The bead also helps to verify whether the pipette is dry. If it is dry, the bead will move freely inside the bulb. If the bulb is wet, the bead will stick to one side of the bulb. The volume of the bead will not decrease the dilution because the volume of the bead is taken into consideration during its manufacture.

3. **What is a fixative?**
   After removal from the body, the tissues start decomposing due to the action of autolytic enzymes and putrefaction by bacteria. Fixative is a substance that preserves cells and tissues in life-like conditions as far as possible. Examples include 100% methyl alcohol, 95% ethyl alcohol, formalin, picric acid, etc. Most fixatives act by denaturation or precipitation of cell proteins or by making soluble components of cell insoluble. Fixing of smears makes it possible to store them for long periods of time without alteration of the morphology. Fixed unstained films can be kept for 5–10 days. Fixing also prevents the RBCs from hemolyzing when they come into contact with the water in which some of the stains are dissolved.

4. **What are the criteria for an ideal diluting fluid?**
   » It should neither cause hemolysis nor crenation of the red cells.
   » It must be isotonic.
   » It should contain a fixative to preserve the shape of the red cells and also to prevent autolysis of the cells so that count may be performed several hours after diluting.
   » It should prevent agglutination and it should not get spoiled on keeping.
   » It should contain a preservative to prevent growth of organisms.
   The fluids that satisfy most of these criteria are **Hayem's fluid, Dacie's fluid, 0.9% sodium chloride (isotonic saline) and Gower's solution**. Hayem's fluid is superior to the other two and hence commonly used to do RBC count.

5. **What are the functions of RBCs?**
   » Carries O_2 from lungs to tissues. Since they lack organelles like nucleus, mitochondria, ribosomes, etc., they use very little oxygen for their own metabolism.
   » Carries CO_2 from tissues to lungs for excretion.
   » Helps to maintain acid-base balance.
   » Contributes to the viscosity of blood.

6. **What is the normal life span of RBC?**
   In the circulating peripheral blood, the life span of RBC is about 120 days.

7. **How will you identify the RBC pipette? What is the unit on the markings in the pipette?**
   » It contains a red bead inside the bulb.
   » The bulb is larger than that of WBC pipette.
   » Markings are 0.5, 1 and 101.
   There is no unit for the markings.

8. **How will you differentiate an RBC pipette from a WBC pipette?**
   RBC pipette has markings 0.5 in the middle of the stem, 1 just below the bulb and 101 above the bulb; bulb is larger and contains a red bead; the end of the rubber tube contains mouthpiece that is red in color.
   WBC pipette has markings 0.5 and 1 in the stem and 11 above the bulb; bulb is smaller and contains a white bead; the mouthpiece is white in color **(Figs. 7.11 and 7.12)**.

9. **What is the reason for using two separate pipettes for doing RBC count and WBC count?**
   RBCs are more numerous than WBCs in blood. So different dilutions have to be made for RBC and WBC count. Hence two separate pipettes having different volumes should be used. For RBC count, blood has to be diluted 200 times since the RBC count is 5–6 millions/mm^3. For WBC count, blood need be diluted 20 times since the count is only 4,000–11,000 cells/mm^3 of blood.

10. **Name the diluting fluid for RBC count and give its composition. What are the functions of the ingredients?**
    Hayem's fluid (refer page 36).

11. **What is the significance of discarding few drops of fluid from the pipette before charging?**
    Discard at least three drops of fluid from the pipette before charging the counting chamber. This is because the stem is filled up with diluting fluid alone and contains no blood. It is necessary to remove this fluid before charging.

12. **Can you see leukocytes while doing RBC count?**
    Yes. Since leukocytes are not lysed, they can be seen along with red cells. But the WBC count is very less when compared to RBC count. The normal ratio of RBC: WBC is 700:1. Blood is diluted 200 times and so WBCs can rarely be seen while doing RBC count.

13. **How can we know that the distribution of cells is not even?**
    The number of cells in the five different squares should not differ widely from each other. The difference should not be more than 10–20 cells. If the difference is more, it means that the distribution of cells is not very even.

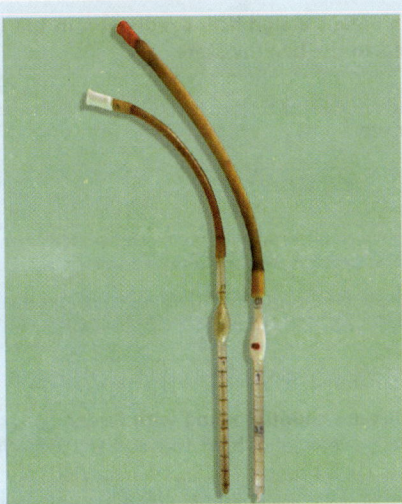

Fig. 7.11: WBC pipette on the left side and RBC pipette on the right side.

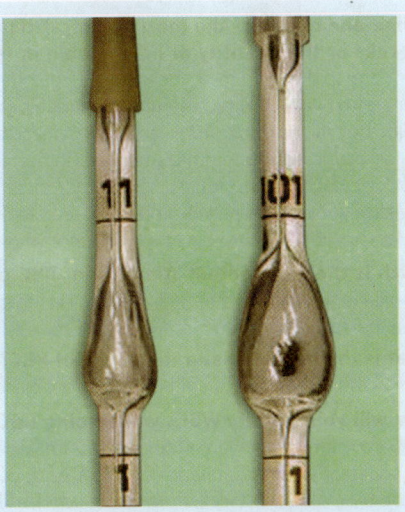

Fig. 7.12: Bulbs of WBC and RBC pipettes showing the markings above and below the bulbs. Note the difference in the size of the bulbs.

14. Dilution obtained in the RBC pipette is 1 in 200 and not 1 in 202. Why?
Mixing of blood with the diluting fluid occurs only in the bulb of the pipette and not in the stem. The stem contains only diluting fluid. Thus 100 volumes of diluted blood contains 0.5 volume of blood and 99.5 volumes of diluting fluid. That is, 0.5 in 100 or 1 in 200. Thus the dilution is 200 times.

15. What are the physiological and pathological variations in RBC count?
Refer page 39.

16. What is the difference between primary polycythemia (polycythemia vera) and secondary polycythemia?
Refer page 39.

17. What is relative polycythemia?
When there is dehydration, there will be increase in the RBC count. Actually the RBC count may be normal. Since the plasma volume is decreased, it gives a fall high RBC count.

18. What are the stages of erythropoiesis?

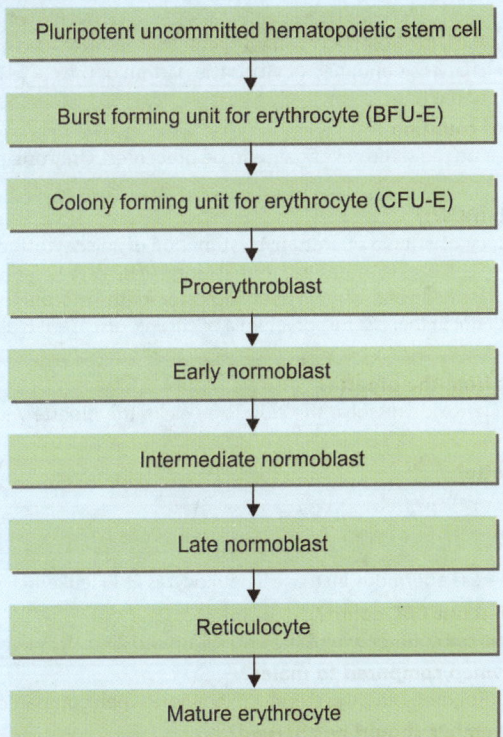

19. **Define anemia. Give the morphological classification of anemia.** Anemia means a significant reduction in the number of red cells or the quantity of hemoglobin in the blood or both as compared to the healthy state.
    According to the changes in mean corpuscular hemoglobin concentration (MCHC) and MCV 5 different types of anemia can be described. There is no hyperchromic anemia when MCHC is taken into consideration.
    - Normocytic normochromic anemia as in acute hemorrhage, aplastic anemia, etc.
    - Macrocytic normochromic anemia as in pernicious anemia.
    - Microcytic hypochromic anemia as in iron deficiency anemia, chronic hemorrhage, thalassemia, etc.
    - Microcytic normochromic anemia is seen in copper deficiency.
    - Macrocytic hypochromic anemia (dimorphic anemia) is seen in combined iron and folic acid/vitamin B_{12} deficiency.

20. **Which is the most potent stimulus for RBC production?**
    Hypoxia is the most potent stimulus for erythropoietin secretion from the kidney. Erythropoietin stimulates RBC production in the bone marrow.

21. **What is the normal maturation time of RBC?**
    Time taken for the conversion of proerythroblast to mature erythrocyte is called maturation time and it is normally 7 days.

22. **How will you identify WBCs while doing RBC count? What happens if WBCs are counted along with RBCs?**
    RBCs are round with even outline. WBCs are larger with uneven outline and have a halo around them. The ratio of RBC to WBC is 700:1 and so, there is hardly a chance of one WBC to come in the RBC counting area. But if it is counted as RBC, then the RBC count obtained will be more by 10,000 cells/mm^3 of blood. The RBC count is calculated by multiplying the total number of RBCs counted with 10,000.

23. **Give the sources and functions of erythropoietin.**
    The interstitial cells lining the peritubular capillaries of kidney produces 85% of erythropoietin and liver produces 15%. Hypoxia is the most potent stimulus for erythropoietin secretion. Functions of EPO:
    - EPO increases RBC production. Erythroid progenitor cells differentiate into pronormoblast under the influence of erythropoietin. Maximum EPO activity and sensitivity to EPO is seen during the conversion of CFU-E to pronormoblast.
    - It increases hemoglobin synthesis and potentiates the activity of δ-aminolevulinic acid synthetase.
    - EPO decreases maturation time of RBC.
    - It stimulates the release of mature erythrocytes from bone marrow into general circulation.

24. **What are the precautions to be taken while doing RBC count?**
    - While sucking blood and during dilution care must be taken to avoid air bubbles from getting into the pipette.
    - Blood should be taken exactly up to the 0.5 mark and diluting fluid up to the 101 mark
    - Discard 2–3 drops of fluid from the pipette before charging.
    - Fluid should not overflow into the moats while charging.
    - If the count is not performed immediately after the blood sample has been diluted and mixed, the contents of the pipette must be mixed again before the chamber is charged.
    - Do not keep the microscope tilted.

25. **What is Price-Jones curve?**
    Price-Jones measured the diameter of red blood cells by projecting a stained blood film on a paper and outlining their images with a pencil. Price-Jones curve is a graph in which the number of red cells is plotted along the X-axis and the diameter of the cells in the Y-axis. Its peak value is at about 7.2 μm. In microcytosis and macrocytosis the pattern of the curve may change or may even remain the same but the peak value shifts to the left or to the right respectively.

26. **What is the significance of 'rules of counting'?**
    If rules of counting are followed, counting the same cells again can be prevented. Only one pattern should be followed while counting (refer page 37 and 38).

27. **What is red cell distribution width (RDW)?**
    RDW gives a quantitative idea of anisocytosis. It is a quantitative estimation of anisocytosis and is computed as the standard deviation (in fl) or as coefficient of variation of red cell size distribution. Normal range of RDW is 42.5 ± 3.5 fl (standard deviation) or 12.8 ± 1.2% (as coefficient of variation). It is used for classifying anemia and as an indicator for the morphological analysis in the clinical laboratory. It is elevated in iron deficiency anemia, but not in thalassemia or anemia of chronic disease. It is also increased (above 17%) in megaloblastic anemia.

28. **How can you remove a blood clot from the pipette?**
    First using a strong acid or hydrogen peroxide dissolve the clot. Then clean the pipette with distilled water. For rapid drying pipette can be rinsed with alcohol or ether.

29. **What are the uses of the RBC pipette?**
    For doing
    - RBC count
    - Platelet count
    - WBC count in conditions where there is enormous increase in leukocytes as in leukemia

30. **What is the accurate method to find out RBC count?**
    Accurate method is by using electronic cell counter where the error is around 2%.

31. **Why RBC count is less in females when compared to males?**
    In males, testosterone stimulates erythropoiesis and the count will be more when compared to females.

32. **Why both sides of the counting chamber should be charged?**
    RBCs should be counted on both the sides and the average should be taken. This will reduce the error in counting the cells.

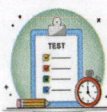

Objective Structured Practical Examination

I. Take blood in the RBC pipette and dilute it for doing RBC count
1. Take a clean and dry RBC pipette
2. Pour about 2 mL of Hayem's fluid in the watch glass.
3. Hold the mouthpiece of the RBC pipette between the lips and allow the pipette to hang down.
4. Sterilize the finger tip
5. The blood is obtained by a deep finger prick with a sterile lancet (stored venous sample can also be used).
6. Suck blood into the pipette accurately up to the 0.5 mark without any air bubbles.
7. Wipe off the blood sticking to the sides of the tip of the pipette.
8. Dip the tip of the pipette in the diluting fluid in the watch glass and suck the fluid accurately up to the 101 mark.
9. Hold the pipette horizontally and roll it between the palms to ensure thorough mixing.

II. Charge the Neubauer's counting chamber for doing RBC count using the diluted blood in the RBC pipette
1. Clean thoroughly the counting chamber and the cover slip
2. Place the coverslip on the platform of the counting chamber
3. Mix the fluid in the bulb of the RBC pipette by rolling it between the palms keeping it horizontally
4. Discard 2 or 3 drops of fluid from the pipette
5. Touch the tip of the pipette at the edge of the cover slip
6. The fluid starts moving by capillary action so that it spreads just beneath the coverslip.
7. Make sure that the fluid does not spill into the groove between the counting areas

Chapter 8

Red Blood Cell Indices—MCV, MCH and MCHC

LEARNING OBJECTIVES

- Calculate the different red blood cell indices
- Give the normal values of blood indices
- List the conditions where there is variation in the red cell indices

PY2.11: Estimate hemoglobin, red blood cell count, total leukocyte count, RBC indices, differential leukocyte count, blood groups, BT/CT.

INTRODUCTION

The features of red blood count (RBC) such as volume, number and color indicate the quality of blood and these features are referred to as blood indices. The blood indices are calculated from packed cell volume, hemoglobin concentration and the red cell count. The various blood indices are:

- Mean corpuscular volume (MCV)
- Mean corpuscular hemoglobin (MCH)
- Mean corpuscular hemoglobin concentration (MCHC)

MEAN CORPUSCULAR VOLUME OR MCV

Mean corpuscular volume (MCV) indicates the average volume of a single erythrocyte in cubic micrometer or femtolitres. It is calculated from the obtained PCV and RBC count. If the value for PCV of the blood sample obtained is 45%, then 1 mm³ of the blood contains 0.45 mm³ of RBC. If the number of red cells in the same sample of blood is 5 millions/mm³ of blood, then the packed cell volume occupied by the 5 millions of cells is 0.45 mm³. From this we calculate the volume occupied by one cell.

$$MCV = \frac{0.45 \text{ mm}^3}{5 \text{ millions}}$$

$[1 \text{ mm} = 1 \text{ mm} \times 1 \text{ mm} \times 1 \text{ mm}]$

$$OR \quad \frac{0.45 \times 1 \text{ mm} \times 1 \text{ mm} \times 1 \text{ mm}}{5,000,000}$$

$[1 \text{ mm} = 1,000 \text{ micrometer}]$

$$= \frac{0.45 \times 1,000 \text{ m} \times 1,000 \text{ m} \times 1,000 \text{ m}}{5,000,000}$$

$$= \frac{0.45 \times 1,000 \times 1,000 \times 1,000 \text{ μm}^3}{5,000,000}$$

$$MCV = \frac{0.45 \times 1,000}{5} = \frac{45 \times 10}{5} = 90 \text{ μm}^3 \text{ or in other words}$$

$$MCV = \frac{\text{Packed cell volume in 100 mL}}{\text{Number of red cells in millions per mm}^3 \text{ of blood}}$$

$\times 10 \text{ μm}^3$ or femtoliters

MCV can be measured directly with automated instruments.

MCV is an extremely useful value in the classification of anemia. It is expressed in **femtolitres (fl)** or μm³. One fl is 10^{-15} L. Normal value is 87–90 μm³ (fl) and the RBCs are referred to as normocytes. Cells with MCV more than 95 fl are called **macrocytes** and RBCs with MCV less than 80 fl are called **microcytes**.

MEAN CORPUSCULAR HEMOGLOBIN OR MCH

Mean corpuscular hemoglobin (MCH) is a measure of the average hemoglobin content per red cell. It indicates the amount or weight of hemoglobin expressed in picogram, present in a single red blood cell. The hemoglobin is estimated with a hemoglobinometer and the red cells are counted with a hemocytometer. Say the values obtained in a sample of blood are 15 grams of hemoglobin per 100 mL of blood and 5 millions cells per mm³ of blood. To calculate the MCH, we must divide the grams of hemoglobin in 100 mL of blood by the number of red cells in 100 mL of blood.

The number of cells in 1 mm³ = 5,000,000

1 cc or 1 mL = 10 mm × 10 mm × 10 mm = 1,000 mm³

Therefore, the number of cells in 1 mL = 5,000,000 × 1,000

The number of cells in 100 mL = 5,000,000 × 1,000 × 100

$$\text{So the MCH} = \frac{15\text{ g}}{5,000,000 \times 1,000 \times 100}$$

The following calculation converts gram into picogram or μμg

1 gram = 1,000 mg
= 1,000 × 1,000 micrograms
= 1,000 × 1,000 × 1,000 millimicrogram (nanograms)
= 1,000 × 1,000 × 1,000 × 1,000 micro microgram (picogram).

$$\text{So MCH} = \frac{15 \times 1000,000,000,000,000}{500,000,000,000} \text{ picogram or μμg}$$

$$\text{MCH} = \frac{15 \times 10}{5} = 30 \text{ picogram}$$

Or in other words,

$$\text{MCH} = \frac{\text{Hb in g/100 mL of blood}}{\text{Number of red cells in millions/mm}^3 \text{ of blood}} \times 10$$

Normal value of MCH is 30 picogram (pg or 10^{-12} g) and the RBCs are referred to as normochromic. It ranges from 27 to 33 pg. Cells with MCH less than 25 pg are referred to as hypochromic and when the value is increased it is referred to as hyperchromic. The hyperchromic state is always associated with macrocytosis. In health the red cells are fully saturated with hemoglobin and there is no room for any extra hemoglobin. The value for MCH can therefore increase only if the size of the cell is increased.

MEAN CORPUSCULAR HEMOGLOBIN CONCENTRATION OR MCHC

Mean corpuscular hemoglobin concentration (MCHC) is the amount of hemoglobin per 100 mL of packed red blood cells and it is expressed in percentage.

Normal value is 34 g/dL (32–38 g/dL) or 34%. For example, if hemoglobin content is 15 g% and PCV 45%,

$$\text{MCHC} = \frac{\text{Hemoglobin in g/100 mL} \times 100}{\text{PCV in 100 mL}}$$

$$= \frac{15 \times 100}{45} = 33.3\% \text{ (g of Hb/100 mL of RBC)}$$

MCHC is decreased in iron deficiency anemia but it is normal in megaloblastic anemia (vitamin B_{12} or folic acid deficiency).

If MCHC is within normal range, RBCs are said to be **normochromic**. Decrease in MCHC is referred to as **hypochromia**. Iron deficiency anemia is referred to as microcytic hypochromic anemia. Pernicious anemia is macrocytic normochromic anemia. In pernicious anemia, both MCV and MCH are increased so, MCHC is normal. Macrocytic hypochromic anemia is seen when, there is combined deficiency of iron and folic acid/vitamin B_{12}.

Anemia can never be hyperchromic because MCHC can never be more than 38%. This level is close to the solubility value for hemoglobin and further increase in hemoglobin may lead to its crystallization. Increased MCH does not necessarily mean that the cell is fully saturated with hemoglobin. Even if the MCH is more than normal, the large sized cell could have accommodated still more Hb, had it been healthy. To find out the degree of saturation, the cell size must also be considered. The index that indicates the degree of saturation of hemoglobin in the red cells is **mean corpuscular hemoglobin concentration** and this is expressed in terms of percentage. Thus an average cell of 90 μm³ volume contains 30 picogram of hemoglobin. Percentage saturation, i.e., the amount present in 100 volumes of cell mass will therefore be;

$$\frac{30 \times 100}{90} = 33 \text{ g of hemoglobin or the MCHC} = 33\%.$$

In other words, 45 (the PCV of 100 mL of blood) volumes of cells contain 15 g of hemoglobin.

100 volumes of cells therefore will contain,

$$\frac{15 \times 100}{45} = 33 \text{ g of hemoglobin or the MCHC} = 33\%.$$

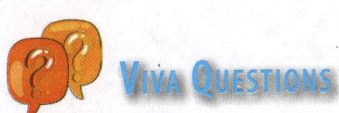

VIVA QUESTIONS

1. **Define MCV, MCH and MCHC giving the normal values.**
   Refer page 44 and 45.
2. **Mention the variations in the blood indices.**
   MCV is increased in megaloblastic anemia due to folic acid deficiency (nutritional anemia) and in pernicious anemia due to vitamin B_{12} deficiency. MCV is decreased in iron deficiency anemia, sideroblastic anemia, anemia due to chronic blood loss (bleeding piles, hook worm infestation, etc.) and in thalassemia. Deficient hemoglobin synthesis induces microcytosis.

MCH is increased in megaloblastic anemia and it is decreased in microcytic hypochromic anemia (iron deficiency anemia). In health the red cells are fully saturated with hemoglobin and there is no room for any extra hemoglobin. The value for MCH can therefore increase only if the size of the cell is increased.

MCHC is decreased in iron deficiency anemia. There is no condition where the actual MCHC is increased.

3. **Which is the best red blood cell index? Give your reason.**
   MCHC is the best blood index because, RBC count is not taken into consideration while calculating MCHC. It is calculated using hemoglobin content and PCV. PCV is more accurate than RBC count. RBC count using the microscope is subject to ±20% error. So it is not reliable.

4. **RBCs can never be hyperchromic. Give reason.**
   RBCs can never be hyperchromic because, MCHC can never be more than 38%. This level is close to the solubility value for hemoglobin and further increase in hemoglobin may lead to crystallization.

5. **Mention a condition where MCHC is likely to be increased.**
   The calculated value for MCHC is likely to be increased when the blood is hemolyzed and the hemoglobin estimation is higher while the number of cells and their volume (PCV) is decreased.

6. **Classify anemia based on blood indices**
   According to the changes in MCHC (mean corpuscular hemoglobin concentration) and MCV 5 different types of anemia can be described. There is no hyperchromic anemia when MCHC is taken into consideration.
   » Normocytic normochromic anemia
   » Macrocytic normochromic anemia
   » Microcytic hypochromic anemia
   » Microcytic normochromic anemia
   » Macrocytic hypochromic anemia (dimorphic anemia) is seen in combined iron and folic acid/vitamin B_{12} deficiency.

7. **Define macrocytosis and microcytosis.**
   Macrocytosis is the condition where MCV is increased (more than 96 fL). The red blood cells will be larger than normal. It is seen in folic acid deficiency and vitamin B_{12} deficiency.
   Microcytosis is a condition where the MCV is less than normal (less than 80 fL). It is commonly seen in iron deficiency anemia.

CALCULATION

I. **Calculate MCHC from the following data and comment on your report.**
   PCV: 45%; RBC count: 4.5 million/mm^3 of blood; hemoglobin content: 15 g/dL
   Ans: MCHC = 15/45 × 100 = 33.3%
   MCHC is found to be normal

II. **Calculate MCV and MCH from the following data and comment**
   PCV: 30%; RBC count: 4 million/mm^3 of blood; hemoglobin content: 9 g/dL
   Ans: MCV = 30/4 × 10 = 75 femtoliters
   MCH = 9/4 × 10 = 22.5
   MCV and MCH are less than normal. May be microcytic, hypochromic anemia (iron deficiency anemia)

Chapter 9: Determination of Specific Gravity of Blood

LEARNING OBJECTIVES

- Methods of determination of specific gravity of blood
- Define specific gravity and mention the factors that affect the specific gravity of blood
- List the conditions where there is alteration in the specific gravity of blood
- Describe the principle of determination of specific gravity of blood by Phillips and Vanslyke's copper sulphate method

PRINCIPLE

Specific gravity of blood is the ratio of the weight of blood to the weight of an equal volume of water at 4°C. It can be determined directly with a specific gravity bottle or a capillary pycnometer. Indirectly it is determined by the falling drop method. In this method the specific gravity of blood is determined by comparing the specific gravity of a drop of blood with that of solutions of known specific gravity.

Two miscible liquids of known but different specific gravities (water and copper sulfate solution; glycerin and water; chloroform and benzene) are mixed in varying proportions to give a series of solutions covering the expected range of specific gravities. A drop of blood is then allowed to fall in each of the solutions successively and its behavior in the solution is studied. Under ideal conditions the drop of blood remains steady and neither sinks nor floats over the solution if the specific gravities of both the solution and the blood drop are the same.

Phillips and Van Slyke's Copper Sulfate Method

In the copper sulfate method, a solution of copper sulfate of specific gravity 1,100 and water of specific gravity 1,000 are used. Stock solution of copper sulfate of specific gravity 1,100 is prepared by dissolving 170 g of blue vitriol ($CuSO_4 5H_2O$) in 1.0024 liters of distilled water. The temperature coefficient of expansion of the copper sulfate solution and blood are practically equal and hence no correction for temperature is required even if the experiment is conducted at room temperature. On adding the drop of blood to the solution, it gets covered by a layer of copper proteinate and remains discrete for sufficient length of time. Solutions having slight differences in their specific gravities can be prepared easily and accurate results obtained.

From the stock solution of copper sulfate with specific gravity 1,100, standard solutions of lower specific gravities ranging from 1,030 to 1,075 are prepared and taken in standard test tubes. A drop of blood is added from a height of about 1 cm above the fluid. The drop penetrates 2–3 cm deep into the solution in about 5 seconds irrespective of the specific gravity of the solution. The momentum is then lost and now the drop behaves according to its specific gravity relative to the solution. It remains steady if its specific gravity is the same as that of the solution; or rises up if its specific gravity is less and continues to sink down if its specific gravity is more than the solution. This behavior, i.e., steady, rising up or falling down continues for ten to fifteen seconds. It denotes the specific gravity of the blood drop in relation to the solution. After about 20 seconds from the moment of release of the drop into the solution, the drop becomes heavier than the standard solution (because of loss of water and formation of the copper proteinate on the surface) and sinks down to the bottom. Within one to two minutes, the solution becomes clear.

Advantages of Copper Sulfate

- The temperature coefficient of expansion of the copper sulfate solution and blood are practically equal and hence no correction for temperature is required.

- On keeping, the copper sulfate solution cleans itself as the blood settles down in a minute or two. The change in the specific gravity of the standard test solution caused by addition of the drop of blood is insignificant. So the same solution can be repeatedly used.
- Other solutions used are glycerin and water; chloroform and benzene. Copper sulfate is not hygroscopic as glycerin and neither volatile or inflammable as chloroform or benzene.
- Copper sulfate is cheap and easily available.

Requirements

Test tubes containing copper sulfate solutions of varying specific gravity, beaker containing oxalated blood, long glass dropper, and wooden rack to keep the test tubes.

Procedure

- Blood is obtained by a venipuncture and mixed with suitable anticoagulant. The anticoagulant added must be measured correctly. If very accurate results are required a correction may be applied for the same. With the 3:2 ammonium and potassium oxalate mixture the correction required is insignificant if only 1 mg is added per mL of blood.
- Prepare the standard solutions of different specific gravities ranging from 1,030 to 1,075, the increment in each tube being 0.005. If very accurate results are required many solutions differing by smaller values can be prepared.
- Mix the copper sulfate and water thoroughly while preparing each standard solution by repeated inversions closing the mouth with the clean palm of the hand.
- Label the test tube after preparing each of the standard solution.
- See that the solution is perfectly steady and not showing any movement.
- Mix the blood gently in order to mix the cells and plasma thoroughly well.
- Take blood in the glass dropper making sure that no air bubble enters the dropper. The same dropper should be used all along in one experiment so that the size of the blood drop will be the same.
- Confirm that the dropper delivers discrete drops.
- Start from the highest specific gravity standard solution.
- Hold the tip of the dropper about 1 cm above the copper sulfate level and put one discrete drop of blood into the center of the solution by pressing the rubber teat. Blood should not touch the sides of the tube.
- The drop must fall and break through the surface of the solution. If the solution is moving or contains dirt or if the drop contains air bubble or if the blood is coagulated, the blood tends to stick to the surface.
- The reading should be taken 15–20 sec after adding the drop of blood to copper sulfate solution. Observe the behavior of the drop after its initial descent. If the experiment is started from the solution of highest specific gravity the drop will stop for a moment and then start rising up. When it starts rising up it can be concluded that the specific gravity of the blood is less than that of the test solution. If the drop continues to fall down in this solution conclusion is that the specific gravity of blood is higher than this solution and solutions of higher specific gravity should be prepared.
- Continue the procedure till the test solution having the lowest specific gravity is reached.
- If in the solution with lowest specific gravity, the blood drop continues to fall down to the bottom the conclusion is that the specific gravity of the drop of blood is more than this test solution. If the drop rises up in this solution, another series of solutions of still lower specific gravities should be prepared.
- Note down the specific gravity of the test solution in which the drop remains suspended in the body of the solution for 10–15 seconds. It gives the specific gravity of the blood sample.

Normal Values of Specific Gravity

- **Venous blood:** 1,050–1,060
- **Red blood cells:** 1,085–1,090
- **Plasma:** 1,025–1,030

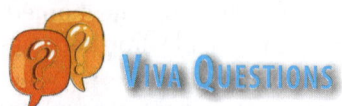

1. **Define specific gravity of blood. Give the normal value.**
   For definition, refer page 48.
   In health during resting conditions, the specific gravity of whole blood varies from 1,050 to 1,060. The specific gravity of the plasma varies from 1,025 to 1,030 and that of the red cells is about 1,090.
2. **What is the principle of Phillips and Vanslyke's copper sulphate method?**
   Refer page 47.

3. What are the factors that affect the specific gravity of blood?
- RBC count and hemoglobin concentration.
- Plasma protein concentration.
- Water and salt content of blood.

If packed cell volume or RBC count is more than normal the specific gravity will also be high. An increased concentration of proteins in blood can lead to a rise in the specific gravity. A decreased concentration of the proteins occurs in many conditions and leads to decrease in specific gravity. If plasma is examined separately, its specific gravity gives a direct indication about the concentration of the plasma proteins.

The specific gravity of the blood may change because of change in the concentration of water and salts. A reduced concentration of water and salts, due to dehydration in diseases like diarrhea, vomiting or in some physiological conditions like severe exercise, causes a rise in the specific gravity of the blood. This rise gives an indication of the severity of loss of water and salts.

Hemodilution due to increased amount of water and salts is usually transient or may occur during pregnancy and excessive secretion or administration of glucocorticoids. Hemodilution reduces the specific gravity.

4. Mention the variations in specific gravity of blood.

Physiological increase is seen in newborn, at high altitude, in males, after exercise and in hemoconcentration due to less water intake or excessive sweating.

Physiological decrease is seen in females due to low RBC count when compared to males; during pregnancy and in excess water intake due to hemodilution.

Pathological Increase
- Polycythemia
- Hemoconcentration as in dehydration (diarrhea, vomiting, burns)
- Hyperproteinemia

Pathological Decrease
- Anemia
- Hypoproteinemia
- Renal diseases with albuminuria, e.g., nephrotic syndrome
- Increase in glucocorticoid hormone level produces hemodilution.

5. What are the advantages of Phillips and Vanslyke's method?
- Copper sulfate is cheap, nontoxic and easily available.
- Apparatus is simple and easy to handle.
- If double oxalate is used as the anticoagulant reasonably accurate results are obtained.
- The same solution can be reused since the blood drop settles to the bottom and does not alter the specific gravity of the solution.
- Since the temperature coefficient of expansion of blood and copper sulfate is the same, no correction of temperature is needed.

10

Determination of Osmotic Fragility of Red Blood Cells

LEARNING OBJECTIVES

- Explain the principle of determining osmotic fragility of blood
- Mechanism of hemolysis of cells when exposed to hypotonic solution
- Define osmotic fragility and give the normal range
- List the common conditions where there is variation in osmotic fragility

PY2.12: Describe test for ESR, osmotic fragility, hematocrit; note the findings and interpret the test results.

PRINCIPLE

About 0.9% sodium chloride solution (normal saline) is isotonic with plasma. Red blood cells shrink in solutions with osmotic pressure greater than this and swell in solutions with osmotic pressure less than normal saline. When suspended in hypotonic solution, red cells swell and finally rupture (hemolyze) releasing hemoglobin, which colors the supernatant solution in the Kahn's tube red. The ease with which erythrocytes rupture or hemolyze when suspended in hypotonic solution is called **osmotic fragility**. Fragility is the susceptibility of the RBCs to rupture and release hemoglobin. Osmotic fragility of red cells can be assessed by measuring the amount of hemolysis that takes place when the red cells are placed in a series of increasingly hypotonic saline solutions.

APPARATUS

Small tubes called Kahn tubes, test tube stand, droppers, saline solution in serial dilution, oxalated or fresh blood.

PROCEDURE

- Place nine Kahn tubes on the rack in rows.
- Label them as N, 1, 2, 3, 4, 5, 6, 7 and W. Place 25 drops of 0.9% saline in N that serves as the control.
- Place 25 drops of 0.6% saline in tube 1 and then 23, 21, 19, 17, 15 and 13 drops of the same in consecutive tubes. Label the concentration of saline in each tube.
- Place 25 drops of distilled water in W.
- With a dropper add 2 drops of distilled water in the 2nd tube and then 4, 6, 8, 10 and 12 drops in each of the consecutive tubes to make the total volume in each of the tubes to 25 drops.
- Mix by inversion on dry fingers. The concentration of the saline in each of the middle seven tubes will be as follows: 1–0.6%, 2–0.55%, 3–0.5%, 4–0.45%, 5–0.4%, 6–0.35% and 7–0.3% respectively.
- Add one drop of the blood to all the nine tubes.
- Mix the blood with the saline by complete but gentle inversion (shaking may induce mechanical hemolysis and give false results).
- Keep the tubes on the stand undisturbed for one hour **(Fig. 10.1)**.
- Examine the color of the supernatant fluid in each of the tube. See whether the supernatant is clear, tinted red or uniformly red **(Fig. 10.2)**.
- Prepare a chart showing the tubes and the concentration.
- Observation is to be carried out without shaking the tubes while they are on the stand.

OBSERVATIONS

- Hold the rack with tubes and observe against diffuse light. Examine the tube marked N. All the cells are settled down at the bottom. The saline is colorless and

Chapter 10: Determination of Osmotic Fragility of Red Blood Cells

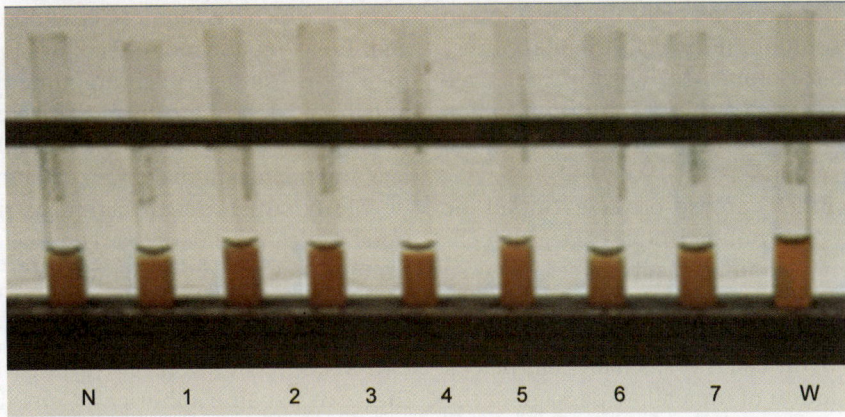

Fig. 10.1: Blood added to saline solutions of varying dilutions for determining the osmotic fragility of RBCs. [N: normal saline—(1) 0.6% NaCl; (2) 0.55% NaCl; (3) 0.5% NaCl; (4) 0.45% NaCl; (5) 0.4% NaCl; (6) 0.35% NaCl; (7) 0.3% NaCl; W: distilled water].

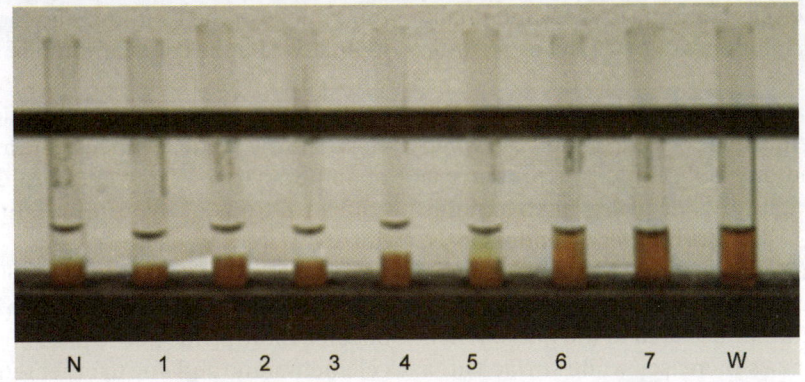

Fig. 10.2: Observation of osmotic fragility after one hour. Note that in the first 3 test tubes the supernatant solution is clear because hemolysis has not started. In the fourth test tube hemolysis has just started because the supernatant is tinted red. In the seventh test tube hemolysis is complete and the solution is uniformly red which denotes completion of hemolysis.

also clear. If this 0.9% saline shows a red color, i.e., if the cells are hemolyzed, the test should be repeated on a fresh sample of blood.

- Now examine the tube marked W. All the solution will be turned homogeneously red. The solution shows a little turbidity but no cells at the bottom. This indicates that the hemolysis is complete in distilled water.
- Now go on examining the tubes towards higher concentration one by one.
- Find out the tube of the highest concentration of the hypotonic saline that shows homogeneous red color and turbidity. It is the highest concentration of saline in which the cells are completely hemolyzed. No residue is left. Note down the number of the tube and find out its concentration.
- Continue to examine tubes of higher concentrations.
- Each of the tubes shows red color of the saline but the solution is not homogeneously turbid. The upper layer is clear while the lower layer is relatively turbid and shows the presence of intact cells. As the concentration increases the intensity of the red color of the upper layer gets reduced.
- Locate that tube of highest concentration which first shows a definite indication of the hemolysis, i.e., the supernatant will be tinted red.
- Osmotic fragility is expressed in terms of concentrations of saline solutions required (a) to initiate a noticeable hemolysis and (b) to complete hemolysis.

RESULT

The result is reported as follows:
Hemolysis started at the highest concentration of 0.40% and is complete at 0.35%.

DISCUSSION

The red cell membrane is semipermeable and through it many small substances like water and electrolytes can pass relatively freely.

Any iso-osmotic solution in which the cells are capable of surviving for some time without changing the cell size is called an 'isotonic solution'. If the cells are placed in a solution more concentrated than this, the excess of the salt draws out the water from the cells. Such a solution is called 'hypertonic solution'. If the cells are placed in a solution more dilute than isotonic, they absorb water, swell and ultimately rupture. Such a dilute solution is called 'hypotonic solution'. Isotonic solution for mammalian tissues is 0.9% sodium chloride.

All the isotonic solutions are iso-osmotic. But all the iso-osmotic solutions need not be isotonic, i.e., the cells will not survive in them. Solutions of substances like urea cannot maintain the integrity of the cells. Urea in solution can pass in and out of the cell membrane. Normally the concentration of urea in the cell is very small. Cells placed in the iso-osmotic solution of urea allow passage of the urea molecules into the cell. Water accompanies the urea molecules and the cells swell. This process continues till the intracellular and the extracellular concentrations of urea become equal. The cells continue to swell and finally rupture. Thus the urea solution can never act as isotonic solution.

Hemolysis is release of the hemoglobin from red blood cells into the plasma. Red cells are hemolyzed when they are placed in hypotonic solutions. This property is described as **osmotic fragility**. When placed in a hypotonic solution the red blood cells absorb water by endosmosis. As a result, the biconcave shape is lost and they become spherical. The biconcave shape of the red cell represents the maximum ratio of the surface area to the mass. When water is absorbed the mass increases while surface area remains the same. To accommodate all the mass in the same surface area the shape of the cell becomes spherical. The spherical shape represents the minimum ratio of surface area to mass. When the mass increases still further the cell membrane gets stretched like an elastic nylon net and the hemoglobin molecules escape through its widened pores. The cell, which has thus lost its hemoglobin, is called a ghost cell. Breaking down of the cell wall also leads to osmotic hemolysis. Younger RBCs are more resistant to hemolysis and the oldest cells are the most fragile ones. This is because the capacity of the older cells to pump out sodium ions is less and their sodium content will be high.

Many substances formed or introduced into the body can cause hemolysis. They are called the hemolytic agents. They act in various ways like reducing the surface tension or by dissolving the fat or by acting specifically as agglutinins, hemolysins, etc. The cells that are biconcave can accommodate larger quantities of water before they can become spherical. Cells that are more or less spherical can accommodate very small quantities of water. Biconcave cells therefore can withstand very low hypotonic solution. Spherical cells hemolyze even by slightly reducing the tonicity of the solution. The more fragile the cells, the higher will be the concentration of the hypotonic saline in which they show hemolysis.

Osmotic fragility is an indication of the shape of the cells. The more fragile the cells the more will be their degree of spherocytosis. They get hemolyzed in much higher concentrations of hypotonic saline when compared to normal biconcave flat red cells.

The ease with which RBCs rupture when subjected to mechanical stress is called **mechanical fragility**. The RBCs become more brittle due to pathological changes in the red cell membrane and due to other red cell disorders. The red cells are subjected to mechanical stress as they pass through capillaries and trabeculae of spleen and the abnormal cell becomes more fragile than the normal cell. For example, in sickle cell anemia, the cells become sickle shaped at low PO_2 and have a high mechanical fragility. However the osmotic fragility of the sickle cells is normal or even low.

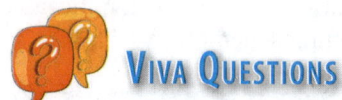

Viva Questions

1. **What is meant by osmotic fragility?**
   The ease with which RBCs rupture when suspended in hypotonic solution is called osmotic fragility. Breaking down of RBCs and release of hemoglobin is called hemolysis.
2. **What is the normal range of osmotic fragility?**
   Hemolysis starts in 0.45% and is completed in 0.35% sodium chloride solution.
3. **What is normal saline?**
   0.9% sodium chloride is isotonic with plasma and is called normal saline.
4. **Mention the variations in the fragility of RBC.**
   Increase in fragility is seen in spherocytosis, purpura, mismatched blood transfusion, glucose-6-phosphate-dehydrogenase (G-6-PD) deficiency, and in venous blood when compared to arterial blood (due to Hamburger phenomenon).
   Decrease in fragility is seen in iron deficiency anemia, thalassemia and pernicious anemia. The osmotic fragility of sickle cell is normal or even low but they have high mechanical fragility. Because of the abnormal shape, the sickle cells are subjected to deforming mechanical stresses as they pass through capillaries and may rupture. Increase in temperature within physiological limits decreases osmotic fragility.

5. **What are hemolysins?**
   Hemolysins are substances that produce hemolysis. Hemolysins or hemolytic agents may be chemical or biological agents.
   Chemicals: Ether, chloroform, bile salts, acids, alkali, and drugs like aspirin, etc.
   Biological hemolysins: Toxins of bacteria, snake venom, etc. Venom of cobra and certain insects contains lecithinase that dissolves lecithin present in the red cell membrane so that they are easily ruptured.

6. **Name some conditions that cause intravascular hemolysis.**
   Incompatible blood transfusion, spherocytic anemia, cobra bite, autoimmune hemolytic anemia, etc., cause intravascular hemolysis.

7. **What are the consequences of increased hemolysis in the body?**
   » When there is increased hemolysis, there is increased release of hemoglobin from the lysed RBCs into the blood. This hemoglobin is metabolized in the reticuloendothelial cells into bilirubin. This leads to hemolytic jaundice.
   » The released hemoglobin will be filtered by the kidney and it will form acid hematin. This will precipitate and block the renal tubules eventually leading to renal failure.
   » If renal failure is not treated it leads to uremia, coma and death.

8. **Which concentration of saline is isotonic with plasma?**
   0.9% sodium chloride solution is isotonic with plasma.

9. **Will all the red cells present in a sample of blood have the same osmotic fragility?**
   No. The older cells are more fragile than the younger ones because the amount of Na^+ inside the RBC will be more in older ones. This is because of less effectiveness of Na^+-K^+ pump to pump out Na^+. The younger ones are more resistant to rupture or they are less fragile.

Chapter 11

White Blood Cell Count or Total Leukocyte Count

LEARNING OBJECTIVES

- Perform total WBC count by hemocytometry
- Mention the composition of Turk's fluid and give the functions of each ingredient
- What is the normal range of total WBC count?
- List the precautions to be taken while doing TLC
- Adjustments of the microscope for doing WBC count
- The structure and functions of leukocytes

PY2.11: Estimate hemoglobin, red blood cell count, total leukocyte count, RBC indices, differential leukocyte count, blood groups, BT/CT.

PRINCIPLE

Estimation of the total number of the white cells has a definite clinical significance and hence is carried out frequently. The principle and the method of counting the white blood cells are similar to that of counting the red cells. The number of white cells in the blood is much less than RBCs (4,000–11,000 per mm^3 for WBC as compared to 5 millions per mm^3 of blood for RBC). There is usually only one WBC for every 500 RBC present. Therefore, the dilution required is much less. Since the WBC diluting fluid is not isotonic, the red blood cells will be lysed and so it is easier to see and count the WBCs. The leukocytes are made more distinct by the addition of stain in the diluting fluid.

APPARATUS

WBC pipette, Turk's fluid, Neubauer double counting chamber, special cover glass, microscope with low power objective, lancet or sterile needle, methylated spirit, cotton swab, etc.

WBC PIPETTE

The bulb of the WBC pipette is smaller than that of RBC pipette and has a capacity only 10 times that of its stem. It is marked with the number 11 at its top. In the middle of the stem there is a 0.5 mark and just below the bulb it is marked 1 (*see* **Figs. 7.2 and 7.10**). The bulb of the pipette contains a **white bead** to identify the pipette and also to mix the blood and diluting fluid thoroughly.

WBC DILUTING FLUID (TURK'S FLUID)

WBC diluting fluid is not isotonic as that of RBC diluting fluid. It contains **glacial acetic acid 0.2 mL, gentian violet 1% solution 0.1 mL** and distilled water is added to make the volume up to 100 mL. Glacial acetic acid is the purest form of acetic acid. This very dilute hypotonic acid solution quickly causes complete lysis of the red cells so that WBCs can be distinctly seen. Though the WBCs also rupture and lose their cytoplasm, they show their nuclei prominently fixed by the acid and stained by gentian violet. The number of white cells is counted in a relatively large amount of space and under the low power of the microscope. This makes the experiment more accurate and easy.

Stored blood is not recommended for doing total WBC count. Use of heparin is also contraindicated since it causes clumping of leukocytes.

Procedure

- WBC pipette is used for sucking blood. Suck blood with all precautions as for RBC count up to the 0.5 mark (in case of leukopenia, blood can be sucked up to the mark

1 instead of 0.5. The calculations should be modified accordingly).

- Dip the pipette in the diluting fluid and carefully suck diluting fluid exactly up to the 11 mark. When the diluting fluid is sucked into the pipette, the blood first enters the bulb followed by diluting fluid. When the fluid reaches the 11 mark, blood mixed with diluting fluid is present in the bulb and the stem contains only the diluting fluid. Therefore, fluid up to 1 mark does not take part in dilution. So 0.5 parts of blood are diluted 10 times, i.e., dilution is 1 in 20 or 20 times.
- Mix the fluid and the blood well by rolling the pipette between the palms.
- Wait for 3 minutes. During this time the red blood cells get hemolyzed by the acetic acid in the diluting fluid. When the red cells are not present in the field, it will be easy to identify the WBCs stained by gentian violet and count them.
- The blood for WBC count cannot be kept for long after dilution.
- Charge the counting chamber as for the red cell count.

Counting

- Mount the counting chamber on the stage of the microscope and fix it with the clips.
- Wait for 3 minutes in order to allow time for the cells to settle.
- The counting of the white blood cells is to be done under low power only. The condenser should be brought down and light should be reduced using the iris diaphragm attached to the condenser. If too much light is admitted; the WBCs will not be clearly visible.
- The nuclei of the cells appear prominent and stained. Under low power the entire field occupied by the 1 mm² area is clearly visible. The cells are sparsely distributed in this area. All of them can be easily and accurately counted (nucleated RBCs, dust particles, moulds and fragments of lysed RBCs may be mistaken for WBC). So make sure that the slide is very clean before charging. If there is doubt, nucleated RBCs can be identified by examining the peripheral smear of the subject.

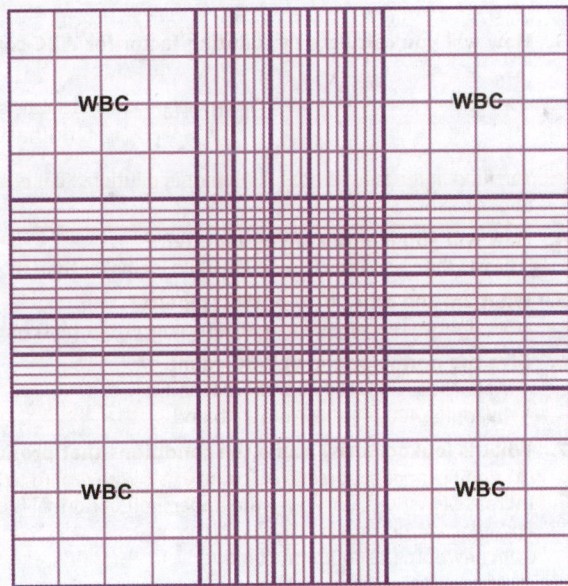

Fig. 11.1: WBC counting areas.

- In the Neubauer chamber there are four 1 mm² areas at the four corners of the ruled area (**Fig. 11.1**). Each is divided into 16 small squares. Bring each of these corner squares (1 square mm area) under the low power of the microscope and count the cells accurately in each of them and note the readings. Let the total number of cells counted in all the four corner squares be 'N'

Calculation

- Each of the 1 mm² area has a height of 1/10 mm and represents a volume of $1 \times 1 \times 1/10 = 1/10$ mm³.
- Since four such areas are counted, the total volume will be $1/10 \times 4 = 2/5$ mm³.
- If N is the sum representing the total number of cells counted then these cells are present in 2/5 cubic mm of the diluted blood.
- The number of cells in 1 cubic mm would be $N \times 5/2$.
- The blood was diluted 1 in 20. The number of cells in 1 cubic mm of the undiluted blood would therefore be equal to $N \times 5/2 \times 20$ or $N \times 50$.

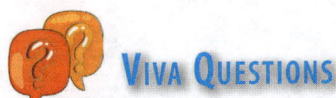 **VIVA QUESTIONS**

1. **How will you distinguish between dust particles and WBCs?**
   A halo will be seen around the stained nucleus of the WBC, which is not seen around dust particle. The halo or refractility around the WBCs is produced by glacial acetic acid (glacial means pure).
2. **What is the composition of Turk's fluid? Give the functions of the ingredients.**
   Dilute hypotonic glacial acetic acid lyses the RBCs so that the nucleus of WBC can be seen distinctly. Glacial acetic acid also fixes the nucleus of WBC. Gentian violet stains the nucleus of WBC.

3. **How will you calculate the diluting factor for WBC count?**

$$\text{Diluting factor} = \frac{\text{Final volume}}{\text{Original volume of blood taken}} = 10/0.5 = 20$$

The fluid in the stem is not taking part in dilution. So it is not taken for the final volume and hence 10 is taken even though the mark above the bulb is 11.

4. **How will you identify a WBC pipette?**
It has a white bead inside the bulb. Bulb is smaller than that of RBC pipette. Markings are 0.5, 1 and 11.

5. **What are the other uses of WBC pipette?**
WBC pipette is also used for doing absolute eosinophil count and sperm count. In severe cases of anemia it is used for doing RBC count.

6. **Give the normal range of WBC count.**
   » At birth: 18,000–20,000/mm³ of blood
   » In adults: 4000–11,000/mm³ of blood

7. **What is leukocytosis? Name the conditions that produce it.**
No significant variation in WBC count exists with regard to age and sex between 15 and 70 years.
Increase in WBC count above the upper limit of normal is called leukocytosis.
Physiological increase in WBC count is seen:
   » In newborn (18,000/mm³ of blood)
   » After strenuous exercise
   » In pregnancy and labor (12,000–15,000/mm³ of blood)
   » After a heavy protein meal
   » In stressful conditions like high fever, severe pain, etc.

Pathological increase in leukocyte count is seen in:
   » Acute and chronic bacterial infections
   » Infestations (presence of parasites in the body)
   » Leukemia
   » Hodgkin's disease
   » Severe hemorrhage and surgical trauma.

8. **What is leukemia? How will you distinguish between leukemia and leukocytosis?**
Leukemia is a malignant condition of bone marrow where there is abnormal, uncontrolled, purposeless proliferation of the precursor cells of leukocytes. Large number of blast cells or immature cells will be seen in circulation. WBC count will be in lakhs or millions. The abnormal cells are functionless.
In leukocytosis, there will be an increase in the number of WBCs but they will have normal morphology. The count will be only in thousands. No blast cells will be seen.

9. **What is leukemoid reaction?**
Leukemoid reaction is a condition where there is excessive leukocytosis resembling that of leukemia but not having clinical features of leukemia like hepatosplenomegaly, lymphadenopathy, etc. Blast cells are not seen in the peripheral smear and this helps to distinguish the blood changes from those in leukemia. Features of underlying disorders like severe infections, other malignant conditions, etc., will be present.

10. **What is leukopenia? Name the conditions producing leukopenia.**
Decrease in leukocyte count below the lower limit is called **leukopenia**. It is not seen normally and therefore leukopenia is always pathological and associated with disease. Causes are:
   » Drugs like sulfonamides, cytotoxic drugs like methotrexate, etc.
   » Hormones like ACTH.
   » Aplastic anemia due to suppression of bone marrow.
   » Bacterial infections like typhoid fever, paratyphoid fever and tuberculosis.
   » Viral infections like dengue, measles, influenza, etc.

11. **What are the properties of WBCs?**
   » Margination and diapedesis
   » Amoeboid movement
   » Chemotaxis
   » Opsonization
   » Phagocytosis

12. **What are the functions of leukocytes?**
   » Neutrophils form the first line of defense against invading organisms.
   » Monocytes form the second line of defense against invading organisms.
   » Eosinophils are involved in allergic conditions and they phagocytose and destroy antigen-antibody complexes, parasites, etc.
   » Lymphocytes are involved in immunity; B lymphocytes mediate humoral immunity and T lymphocytes mediate cellular immunity.

Chapter 11: White Blood Cell Count or Total Leukocyte Count

13. Why glacial acetic acid is used in Turkes fluid?
Water free or anhydrous acetic acid is called glacial acetic acid. Pure acetic acid should be used to view the WBCs with a clear refractility around it. This helps to identify leukocytes in a better way.

14. What are the types of leukemia?
Acute lymphoblastic leukemia (ALL) which is seen in children and young adults. There will be anemia, thrombocytopenia and marked increase in the number of leukocytes. 60–80% of cells are lymphoblasts.
Acute myeloblastic leukemia (AML) is seen in children and adults less than 40 years of age. More than 60% of leukocytes in the peripheral blood are myeloblasts.
Chronic myeloid leukemia (CML) is seen in adults usually in the fourth and fifth decades of life. There is marked increase in WBC count. Neutrophils and metamyelocytes predominate. Blast cells are seen rarely.
Chronic lymphocytic leukemia (CLL) is seen in adults over 50 years of age. Lymphocyte count is increased. More than 90% are lymphocytes.

# Objective Structured Practical Examination

I. Dilute the given blood sample for doing total leukocyte count
   » Carefully select the WBC pipette and make sure that it is clean and dry
   » Take Turke's fluid in the watch glass
   » After mixing the blood sample gently, suck blood in the WBC pipette exactly up to the 0.5 mark
   » Wipe the blood present outside the tip of the pipette with tissue paper
   » Suck diluting fluid exactly up to the 11 mark of the pipette
   » Mix the contents in the bulb by gently rolling the pipette between the palms

II. Charge the counting chamber with the diluted blood provided for doing total leukocyte count
   » Clean carefully the Neubauer counting chamber and the special coverslip
   » Place the coverslip on the platform of the counting chamber
   » Mix the contents in the bulb of the WBC pipette
   » Discard two drops of fluid from the pipette
   » Touch the tip of the pipette at the edge of the coverslip at an angle
   » Slowly release the fluid from the pipette till it spreads uniformly without air bubbles just beneath the coverslip
   » Fluid should not spill into the grooves

12

Differential Leukocyte Count

LEARNING OBJECTIVES

- List the precautions to be taken while preparing a blood smear
- Select a proper spreader slide to make a blood smear
- Make a blood smear using glass slide method or wedge method
- Enumerate the criteria for a good smear
- List the constituents of Leishman's stain and mention their functions
- State the principle of doing differential count
- Identify the different blood cells in the smear provided
- Describe the identifying features of each cell
- Explain the adjustments of the microscope for doing differential count
- List the other methods of making blood smear
- Mention the uses of a peripheral blood smear

PY2.11: Estimate hemoglobin, red blood cell count, total leukocyte count, RBC indices, differential leukocyte count, blood groups, BT/CT.

PRINCIPLE

Enumeration of each type of the white blood cells in a blood sample is called the differential count. It is done under an oil immersion objective on a stained film. The film prepared for this purpose should be made from a small but whole drop of freely flowing blood.

Blood cells contain structures that vary in their pH, some being acidic and others being basic or neutral. To stain these structures, two types of stains are used; one a basic stain and the other an acidic stain. Basic substances take up acid stain and are said to be acidophilic. Acid substances take up basic stain and are said to be basophilic. Nucleus contains nucleic acids and they take up basic stain and stains blue. The acidic granules of basophils contain heparin and other acid substances and they stain dark blue or almost black. Hemoglobin and the granules of eosinophils are basic in their reaction and stain with reddish acid stain and become pink or red. Neutrophils contain neutral substances that take up both the stains and stain lilac.

APPARATUS

- Microscope with an oil immersion objective and the mechanical stage.
- A counting machine (if available) or paper and pencil.
- 6 clean greaseless glass slides (the one that is used as spreader slide should have straight and smooth edge).
- Cedar wood oil, lancet, cotton swab, methylated spirit.
- Staining rack, Petri dish, Leishman's stain.

Preparation of Leishman's Stain

Stain that is used for doing differential count is Leishman's stain. It is prepared from a mixture of methylene blue and eosin. The resulting compound formed is called methylene azure or thiazine eosinate. It is a purplish red stain formed by combination of oxidation products of methylene blue and eosin.

The Leishman's stain is available ready for use as crystals. 0.15 g of the dry stain crystals is well ground. It is made up to 100 mL with acetone free methyl alcohol. Mix well till all the stain is completely dissolved. Do not filter. This solution taken in a glass-stoppered bottle is kept in sun to warm for two to three weeks. The stain improves on keeping and warming. All the apparatus to be used must be perfectly dry. The methyl alcohol should be acetone free; or else the stain deteriorates soon. In addition to this, acetone causes lysis of cells. In the stain, eosin and methylene blue exist as a complex called **thiazine eosinate** that is neutral. When water is added to the stain the complex breaks into eosin and methylene blue, which in turn stains the basophilic and acidophilic structures in the cells. The principle of staining depends upon the differential pH of the intracellular substances. Before staining the stain should be filtered.

METHODS OF MAKING A BLOOD SMEAR

- Glass slide or wedge method (since the smear appears like a wedge)
- Cover glass method
- Centrifugal blood smear method

Preparation of the Blood Smear by Glass Slide Method

- Puncture the fingertip with usual precautions.
- A small drop of blood should come out freely. Wipe off the first drop and allow another drop to be formed. The first drop may contain tissue cells from the puncture site.
- A slide is lifted by holding its edges along its length and touched to the drop at one end in the center at least 1 cm away from the narrow border.
- The slide is placed on the level surface of a table in such a way that the blood drop is on the right side.
- The spreader glass slide is held along its long edges to form an acute angle of 30–40° (on the right side) with the glass slide **(Fig. 12.1)**.
- The smooth edge of the spreader is made to touch the left end of the drop, which is then allowed to spread along the edge of the spreader **(Fig. 12.2)**.
- Now push the spreader ahead toward the left end with quick but uniform motion and a light but even pressure.

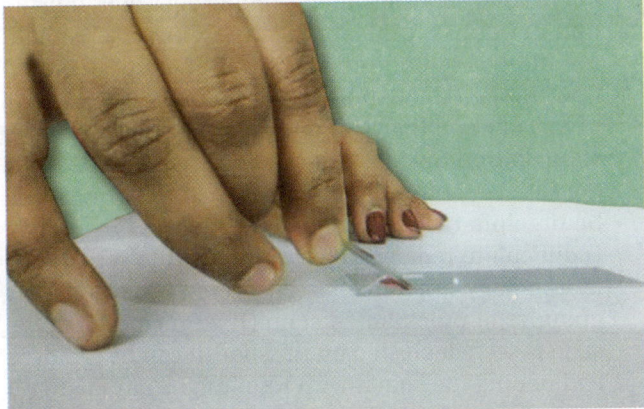

Fig. 12.1: Preparing a blood smear. Placing the spreader slide in front of the blood drop at an angle of 45°.

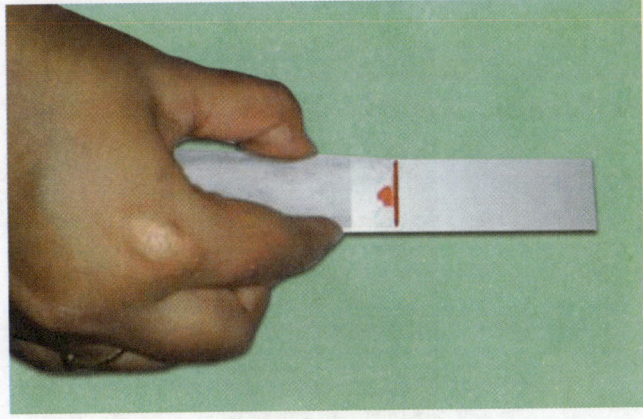

Fig. 12.2: Allow the blood drop to spread along the spreader slide.

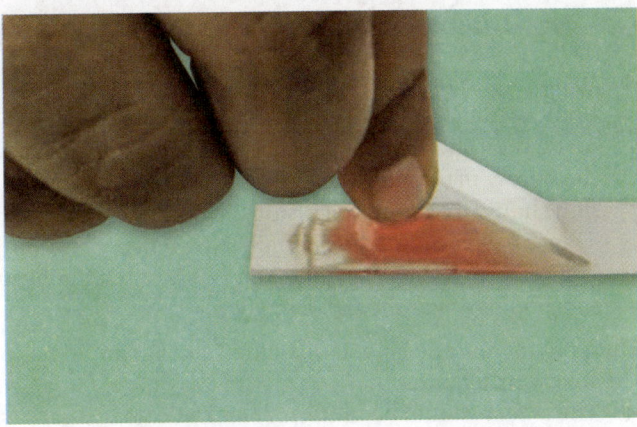

Fig. 12.3: Push the spreader slide toward the other end of the slide slowly and evenly to get a blood smear.

The blood follows the spreader to form a thin film **(Fig. 12.3)**. Holding the spreader more vertical and moving it rather slowly but evenly can obtain thinner films. If the movement is not uniform or if the angle is varied during movement good films are not obtained.

- Dry it quickly by waving in the air. The breeze from a fan will often help to hasten the drying. If the smear dries slowly, the resulting slow evaporation causes crenation and distortion of cells. Do not blow on the smear since water droplets may hemolyze the cells.
- Prepare at least three films in the same way from the same puncture site.
- First examine the smear against light and then under microscope.

When observed in good light an ideal smear should satisfy the following criteria:

- A good smear should be uniformly distributed over the slide in its middle third. When the film is well within the slide on all sides, all the cells present at the edges can be examined.
- It should not be too thick or too thin.

Fig. 12.4: A good unstained peripheral blood smear.

- It should be tongue shaped and should have a head, body and tail **(Fig. 12.4)**. Its head, i.e., the straight edge at the right should begin at least about 1 cm away from the border of the slide. The long horizontal edges of the film should be 5 mm well inside the border of the slide. This is called the body. The tail is the narrow end but it should not be too narrow. The WBCs show the best morphology near the tail of the film.

Under a microscope a good unstained smear should have the following features:
- The smear should be uniformly pink in color.
- The edges should be away from the border of the slide.
- The cells should be placed side by side and do not show rouleaux formation.
- The cells should show their morphology clearly. They should not be crenated, lysed or deformed.
- There should be no deposits, dust particles and fibrin threads in the smear.

Cover Glass Method of Preparing Blood Smear

Blood smears can also be made on glass cover slips (cover glasses). A drop of blood is spread between two cover glasses as they are pulled in opposite directions.

Advantage is that the WBCs will be evenly distributed.

Disadvantages:
- Cover slips are easily broken and it is difficult to label them
- It is a time consuming method
- The preparation should be done very carefully and need experience

Centrifugal Blood Smear Method

A slide spins in a centrifuge (specially made for spinning blood smeared slides) which facilitate rapid spreading of cells across a slide. A monolayer blood film of cells will be obtained. A drop of blood in a slide is centrifuged rapidly in a plane parallel to the plane of rotation of the centrifuge. Excess blood is spun off leaving a monolayer of well spread blood cells on the slide.

Fixing and Staining of Smear

- It is desirable to stain at least two good blood smears at a time.
- Place the slide in the petri-dish or on two parallel glass rods that are fixed across a sink.
- Put drop by drop the stain on the blood film until the film is completely covered. Count the drops added. Note the time. Take care that the stain does not dry on the slide if needed more stain can be added. This undiluted stain is allowed to act for one and a half minute. This is done to fix the film and methyl alcohol acts as the fixative. Methyl alcohol denatures the proteins and hardens the cell contents. The smear will stick firmly to the slide. Otherwise the film will be lost while washing. Fixing also prevents the RBCs from hemolyzing when they come in contact with water added during the staining procedure. Fixed unstained films can be kept for 5–10 days.
- After the one and half minute, add double the number of drops of distilled water using a dropper and dilute the stain. It is best to use buffer water with a pH 6.8 for diluting the stain. If the distilled water used is acidic or alkaline, the staining of different cells will not be proper. A scum or film with a metallic sheen will form on the surface of the diluted stain on the slide.
- Mix by rocking and by blowing through an ordinary pipette. Stain should not be allowed to dry. Wait for 7–8 minutes. To prevent drying, the slide should be rocked frequently.
- After seven minutes, wash the excess of the stain with distilled water (the stain must be flooded off the slide) followed by showing under running tap water until the film develops a pink appearance. The water should not directly fall on the stain from the tap. It should flow through the hand and then through the tail end of the smear. Otherwise the smear may peel off. The stain should never be poured off the slide because the surface scum will settle on the glass and there will be precipitated stain all over the blood film, which is difficult to remove. It is very difficult to see the cell morphology when the film is covered with numerous granules of precipitated stain (If a precipitate of the stain is seen deposited on the slide, it can be removed by flooding the smear with undiluted stain for 10–15 seconds and then washing it off by flooding the slide once more with distilled water).
- Drain the excess water from the slide.

Fig. 12.5: A stained peripheral smear.

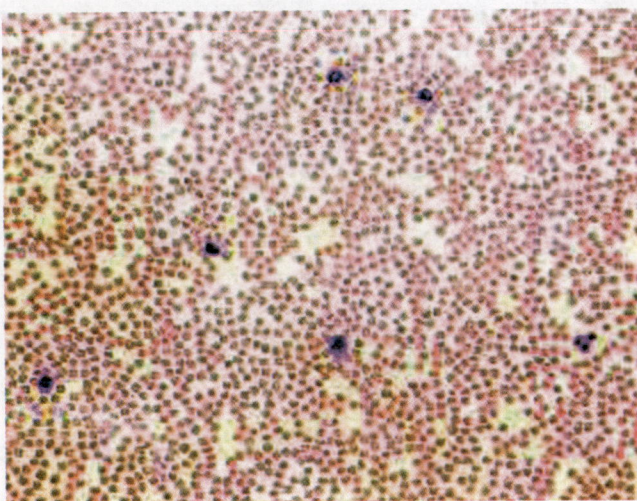

Fig. 12.6: Leishman's stained ideal blood smear under low power of the microscope.

- Wipe the backside of the slide with a clean and dry filter paper making sure that the blood film is not wiped off by mistake. Keep it in a vertical position to drain and dry **(Fig. 12.5)**.
- Examine the film under the low power of a microscope to decide whether it is good or not then observe under high power. Counting is done under oil immersion.
- If difficulty arises in identifying the surface of the slide on which smear is taken, hold it against light and view its reflexion. Tilt the slide and view the reflection in its various parts. The surface without the blood film shows a reflexion on all parts. The face on which the film is applied appears dull in that part and does not show the reflexion.

The blood film should be first observed under low power of the microscope **(Fig. 12.6)** to assess:
- The quality of the film, whether it is properly stained, degree of rouleaux formation, etc.
- The number and distribution of leukocytes.
- It also help to locate and select the proper fields to be used for counting under oil immersion.

A well-stained good film has the following characteristics under the oil immersion objective:
- No precipitate or granules on or between the cells.
- The red cells having an orange buff or pink color.
- The agranulocyte cytoplasm of a slate blue color.
- The neutrophil cytoplasm granules of a dull shade of lilac or light purple color.
- The nuclei and the basophilic granules should be of blue to purple color.
- The eosinophil granules of orange-red color.
  Certain parts of the cells have affinity for the basic portion of the stain, e.g., the nuclear chromatin being acid in character takes up basic portion, i.e., the methylene blue and stains deep blue. The basic protoplasmic material takes the acidic-eosin, i.e., pink dye; and the neutral material appears lilac or violet.

Distribution of Different WBCs in Different Parts of the Smear

There is uneven distribution of WBCs in the blood smear. The small lymphocytes are seen in relatively greater number in the central thicker portion of the smear and the larger WBCs like monocytes and granulocytes are seen in relatively greater number along the edges and the tail part of the smear because they are highly motile. The leukocytes in the tail portion of the smear are slightly flattened and show good morphologic detail.

Identification of Different Cells in the Peripheral Smear

Three types of cells are present in the blood: red blood cells or erythrocytes, white blood cells or leukocytes and platelets or the thrombocytes.

The White Blood Cells

Leukocytes are classified as follows:

Granulocytes: Neutrophils, eosinophils and basophils (mature granulocytes in the bone marrow are 20 times the number in the blood).

Agranulocytes: Lymphocytes and monocytes.
The differentiation between the granulocytes and the agranulocytes depends upon presence of granules in the cytoplasm after staining with Leishman or similar other stain. The agranulocytes, the lymphocytes and the

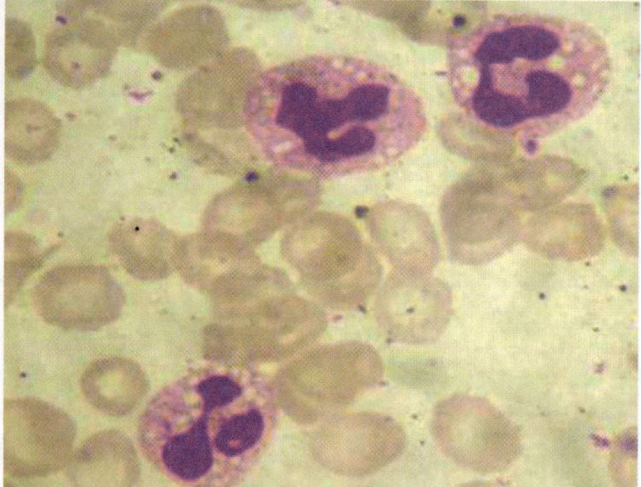

Fig. 12.7: Peripheral smear showing neutrophils.

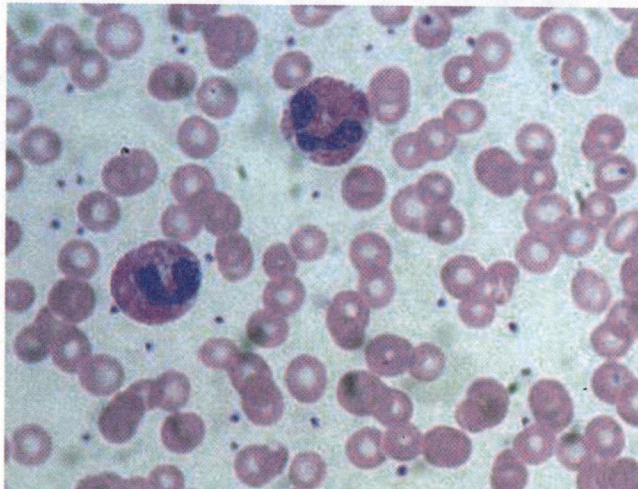

Fig. 12.8: Peripheral smear showing eosinophils (note the coarse orange red granules in the cytoplasm).

monocytes also contain fine granules in their cytoplasm, but these are not clearly seen after staining with the Leishman's stain.

Neutrophil

The neutrophil or the polymorphonuclear leukocyte is the predominant leukocyte of blood (50-70%). It is quite large (10-12 µm) when compared with the red cell (7-8 µm). The nucleus is stained blue and consists of three or four lobes joined by thin strands. The cytoplasm is only faintly lilac stained. It contains very fine granules **(Fig. 12.7)**. The granules are countless in number, uniform and scattered throughout the cytoplasm.

Eosinophil

The eosinophil has a size and shape similar to that of a polymorph; but its appearance is characteristic. The cytoplasm of this cell contains large round and reddish or orange granules, which are closely packed **(Fig. 12.8)**. The nucleus is bilobed and stained blue. These cells are few in number (1-4%).

Basophil

The basophil is the rare cell of blood (0-0.5%). It is a small cell (8-10 µm in diameter) containing a bilobed or 'S' shaped nucleus. The cytoplasm contains large basophilic granules, which may obscure the nucleus **(Fig. 12.9)**. The granules are water-soluble and may get washed off while staining. Unless established without any doubt, no cell in a blood smear should be identified as a basophil.

Lymphocyte

The next predominant leukocyte is the lymphocyte (20-40%). The lymphocytes are small cells with diameter

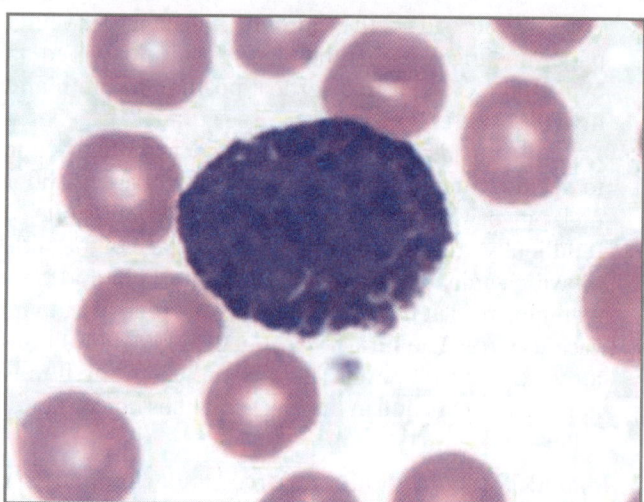

Fig. 12.9: Peripheral smear showing a basophil.

8-10 µm. But large lymphocytes are also present (4-8 %). The large lymphocytes have a diameter varying between 10 and 15 µm. The nucleus of both these types of lymphocytes is very big and occupies most of the cell. In case of the small lymphocyte it is so big that it occupies the whole of the cell and the cytoplasm is hardly visible. In case of the large lymphocyte a definite ring of cytoplasm is seen around the nucleus **(Fig. 12.10)**. The nucleus is usually round (but sometimes slightly indented) and occupies the central part of the cell. It is stained intensely blue. The cytoplasm when visible is stained pale or light blue.

Monocyte

The third predominant type of WBC is the monocyte (2-11%). The monocytes are the largest of the blood cells (18-20 µm in diameter). But when small they are confused with the large lymphocytes. The nucleus of a monocyte

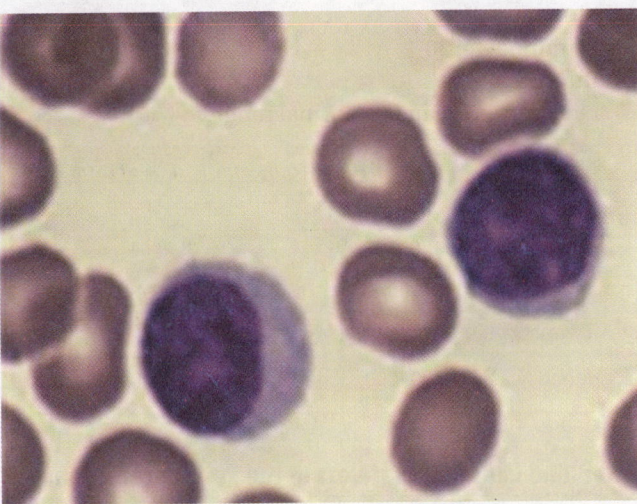

Fig. 12.10: Peripheral smear showing two lymphocytes.

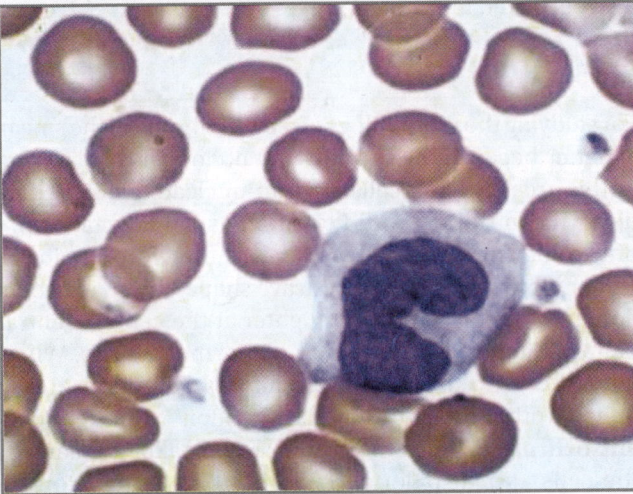

Fig. 12.11: Peripheral smear showing a monocyte.

is comparatively small, i.e., it fills only about half the available space. It is rarely rounded. It may be bean shaped, kidney shaped, horseshoe shaped or even may give an appearance of lobulation. It is stained blue **(Fig. 12.11)**. It is not homogeneously stained but presents a reticular appearance. *The cytoplasm* is abundant. An occasional red staining rod-like body, the Auer's body, if visible is a characteristic of the monocyte.

Differential Counting of Leukocytes

It is always desirable to do the differential count in a perfectly stained good smear. If the smear is bad, prepare another smear, stain it properly and examine it to obtain reliable results. Usually counting of WBCs is done by any of the following methods:

- ❖ Going lengthwise on the smear including both body and tail.
- ❖ Going back and forth sidewise on the smear including both the edges and the center.

Procedure

- ❖ Adjust the microscope for oil immersion.
- ❖ The surface on which the smear is taken should face the objective. The slide should not be kept with the film surface down. The cells in this case fail to come into view.
- ❖ Put a drop of cedar wood oil over the film and adjust the stage so that the oil immersion objective just touches the oil.
- ❖ Focus it properly by fine adjustment so that the cells can be seen clearly (*see* **Fig. 12.13**).
- ❖ Bring one corner; say the left upper corner of the film in view.
- ❖ Identify the cells seen.
- ❖ The counting machine (if available) shows different keys for different types of cells. Pressing the key records and also add the number of different leukocytes.
- ❖ If counting machine is not available, on a paper draw a table of 100 small squares and each cell counted can be entered in the small squares of the table, till 100 small squares are filled. After identifying every cell it is entered by writing a letter say 'N' for Neutrophil, 'E' for Eosinophil, 'B' for Basophil, 'L' for Lymphocyte, and 'M' for Monocyte and so on. By counting the number of neutrophils, eosinophils, basophils, lymphocytes and monocytes in all the 100 squares we will get the percentage of each cell. Record it in percentage.
- ❖ Identify all the white blood cells in view. Enter the observations. Do not ignore or omit any cell.
- ❖ With the help of the screw of the mechanical stage now shift the slide toward the left along the same horizontal axis to bring the adjacent field in view.
- ❖ Thus go on counting toward the right along the horizontal edge till you reach the right upper corner of the film. Do not leave any cell unidentified.
- ❖ Now shift the slide up and bring the lower adjacent field in view.
- ❖ Identify and enter the observations.
- ❖ Then go on counting toward the upper right till you reach the end.
- ❖ Then shift lower down and go on counting toward the left again and so on.

In a blood film, different leukocytes tend to lie in different parts of the film. The smallest cells, e.g., the lymphocytes tend to occupy the central part of the film while the larger ones, e.g., the neutrophils lie at the periphery. Neutrophils are also seen in more number toward the tail end of the smear because of its increased motility while preparing the film.

Precautions

- The stain should cover the whole of the smear and it should not get dried up.
- Observe the timings strictly.
- The amount of water added should be exactly double the amount of stain added.
- While washing do not pour off the stain from the slide, instead flood the slide with distilled water and allow it to flow out. Otherwise the stain will stick to the smear.
- When washing under tap water allow water to flow through your hand into the tail end of the smear till the smear becomes uniformly pink.
- While counting the cells, avoid recounting.
- The smear should be stained soon after making it provided, it is dry. If this is not possible, it should be fixed by dipping it in absolute methyl alcohol for 2–3 seconds and then air-dry it.

Calculations

- The counting machine directly gives the count of each type of cell.
- Otherwise the number of each type of the cell will have to be enumerated and summed up.
- Confirm that the total number of the cells counted and the sum total of all the types is the same.
- Express the results in terms of percentage of the white cells.
- If a total white cell count is simultaneously carried out calculate the number of each type of the cells also, i.e., the number of each cell per mm³ of blood. If the total leukocyte count is 6,000/mm³ of blood and the number of eosinophils counted is 3, then the absolute eosinophil count will be 3/100 × 6,000 = 180/mm³ of blood.

Table 12.1 shows box with 100 squares to enter differential count.

Result:
Neutrophil: 63%
Eosinophil: 3%
Basophil: nil
Monocyte: 4%
Lymphocyte: 30%

Inference:
Leukocytes are in the normal range.

Cell	Normal range (cells/mm³)	% of total WBC
Neutrophils	3,000–6,000	50–70
Eosinophils	150–300	1–4
Basophils	0–100	0.4
Lymphocytes	1,500–4,000	20–40
Monocytes	300–600	2–8

Red Blood Cells and Platelets in the Peripheral Smear

In a Leishman stained peripheral smear the morphology of red blood cells and the distribution of platelets should also be looked for.

Red Blood Cells

For studying the morphology of red cells the tail of the smear is better because the red cells are no longer overlapping in this area. The red cells are non-nucleated flat circular discs. When stained with Leishman's stain they take up a pink color. They are biconcave and are therefore thin in the center. Because of their biconcave shape, the stain seems darker at the periphery and lighter at the center (central pallor). Such RBCs are said to be normochromic. When the red cells in the blood film show variation in staining or color other than normal that variation is referred to as **anisochromia**. When the central area of pallor is enlarged, the cells appear paler and is said to be **hypochromic**. When the biconcave shape is lost the area of central pallor is diminished or even absent and the cells are said to be **hyperchromic**. Here there is no increase in the amount of hemoglobin in the RBC. But the cells will be larger.

When the size of the RBCs is within normal limits they are said to be **normocytic**. When the diameter is less than

Table 12.1: Box with 100 squares to enter differential count.									
N	L	N	N	N	M	L	N	N	L
N	N	L	N	N	L	L	N	E	N
N	N	N	E	L	L	N	N	L	N
N	L	L	N	N	N	L	N	N	N
L	N	M	L	N	N	L	N	L	N
N	L	N	L	L	N	N	N	N	L
M	N	N	L	N	N	N	L	N	N
N	N	L	N	N	N	L	N	N	E
N	N	N	L	N	L	N	N	N	N
N	L	L	N	M	N	N	L	N	L

Chapter 12: Differential Leukocyte Count

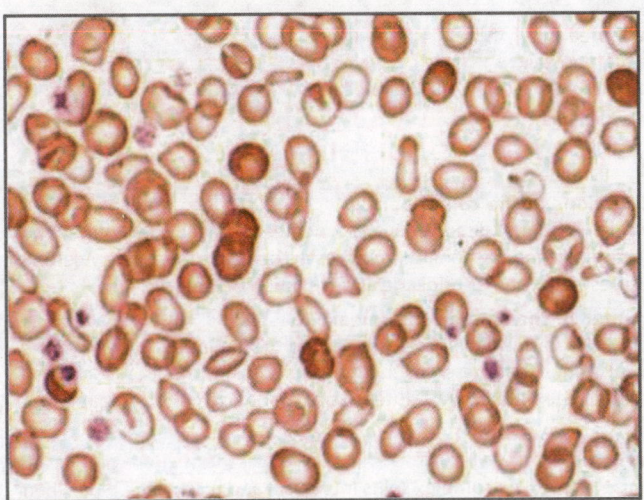

Fig. 12.12: A peripheral smear suggestive of microcytic, hypochromic anemia (iron deficiency anemia). Note the increase in the central pallor of RBCs and anisopoikilocytosis.

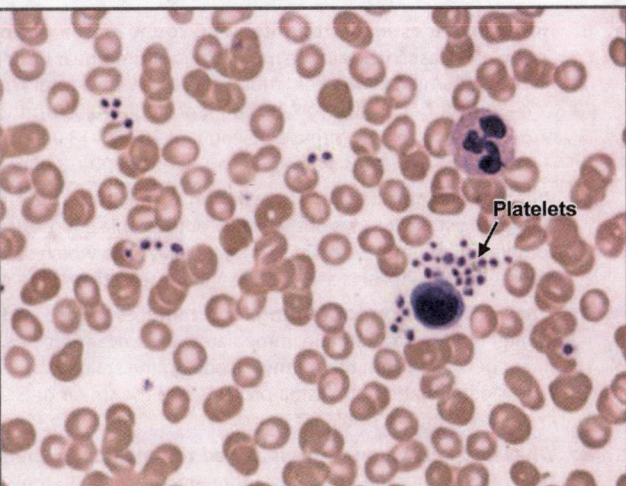

Fig. 12.13: Peripheral smear showing platelets (purple dots), erythrocytes, neutrophil and lymphocyte.

6 µm, they are called **microcytes** (e.g., iron deficiency anemia) and when the diameter is more than 8.5 µm, they are called **macrocytes** (e.g., pernicious anemia). Variation in the size of RBC is called anisocytosis. Microcytic hypochromic anemia is seen in iron deficiency and thalassemia.

Variation in the shape of RBCs is called **poikilocytosis** (**Fig. 12.12**). Normally RBCs are biconcave disks. Abnormal cells may assume various different shapes. Abnormally shaped RBCs include spherocytes, ovalocytes (elliptocytes), sickle cells, acanthocytes, etc.

The central pallor is not seen in vitamin B_{12} and folate deficiency but there will be anisocytosis and poikilocytosis along with macrocytosis. Nucleated red blood cells are found in the peripheral smear in severe anemia and also in leukemia.

Platelets or thrombocytes:
- Platelets are small, 2–4 µm in size.
- Usually they are seen in clumps in the smear which are purple colored (**Fig. 12.13**). If they are seen singly in the smear, it denotes reduction in platelet count.
- Each platelet in an average oil immersion field represents approximately 15,000 platelets/ mm^3 of blood. In normal blood, an average of 8–25 platelets should be seen in an oil immersion field after observing several fields.

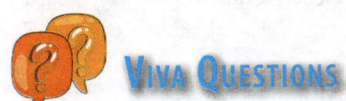

Viva Questions

1. **What are the different types of stains used for staining tissues?**
   Romanowsky stains are stains that are made up of combinations of acidic and basic dyes. Examples are Leishman's stain, Wright's stain, Giemsa's stain, Jenner's stain, etc. The basic stains used are methylene blue and toluidine blue. Acid stains are eosin, Azure I and Azure II.

2. **What are the uses of a peripheral blood smear?**
   » Differential leukocyte count helps in the detection of abnormal leukocytes as in leukemia (blast cells usually not seen in peripheral smear but seen in leukemia), other abnormalities of leukocytes, etc.
   » Toxic granules inside leukocytes suggest severe bacterial infection.
   » Helps to study the morphology of erythrocytes and can comment on the type of anemia.
   » Platelet count can be roughly estimated from a smear.
   » Thick smears can be used to detect malarial parasite (seen within the RBCs), microfilariae, etc.
   » Sex can be determined by the presence or absence of Barr body in the nucleus of neutrophils, but it needs special staining. It may also be visible in hematoxylin and eosin staining.

3. **How is Leishman's stain prepared?**
   Refer page 58.

4. **How will you select a spreader slide for making a blood smear?**
   Feel the edge along the breadth of the slide that is selected to be used as spreader slide. The edge should be very smooth. There are specially designed glass slides with a smooth edge and having breadth slightly less than that of usual glass slides.

5. **How can you estimate the total WBC count from a peripheral smear?**
   Observe at least 6 fields in the middle part of the smear under the high power.
   » 2–4 WBCs/high power field (hpf) correlates with a total WBC count of 4,000–7,000/ mm^3 of blood.
   » 4–6/hpf correlates with a WBC count of 7,000–10,000/mm^3.
   » 6–10/hpf correlates with a WBC count of 10,000–13,000/mm^3.
   » 10–20/hpf correlates with a WBC count of 13,000–18,000/mm^3.

6. **What is the composition of Leishman's stain? What are the functions of the components?**
   Leishman's stain consists of the stain complex thiazine-eosinate, which is neutral dissolved in acetone free methyl alcohol. When the complex splits, it forms eosin and methylene blue, which stains acidophilic and basophilic structures in the cell respectively. Acetone free methyl alcohol acts as a fixative and preservative. If acetone is present it causes shrinkage and crenation of the cells.

7. **What is the reason for waiting for 2 minutes before adding water to the stain in the smear?**
   If water is added to the stain immediately the smear gets peeled off while washing the slide later. During the 2 minutes of waiting, the smear gets fixed with the methyl alcohol in the stain. Fixative is a substance that preserves the morphology of the cells. Alcohol also causes denaturation of plasma proteins and the smear gets attached to the slide firmly. Diluted stain can be used if the smear is first fixed in absolute alcohol.

8. **What happens when water is added to the stain in the smear?**
   The complex thiazine-eosinate cannot enter the cells in their unionized state. The complex splits into eosin and methylene blue when water is added to the concentrated stain. Thiazine-eosinate is a neutral complex. When it splits, eosin stains eosinophilic structures in the cell and methylene blue stains basophilic structures like nucleus.

9. **What is the importance of the greenish scum on the top of the mixture of stain and water?**
   A metallic shiny greenish layer should form on the top of the mixture. Do not drain the mixture after 7 minutes by tilting the slide. If this is done, the greenish scum will stick to the surface of the smear and it will be difficult to count the cells. Instead add water to the mixture so that the scum flows off from the top without sticking to the smear.

10. **Why cedar wood oil is used for doing differential count?**
    Cedar wood oil has the same refractive index as that of glass. So minimal refraction occurs at the interface.

11. **What happens if the smear is not immediately prepared after placing the blood drop on the slide?**
    The blood will clot and the cells will not be uniformly distributed in the smear. A delay may lead to uneven distribution of leukocytes on the smear. Clumping of platelets also occurs.

12. **What are the adjustments of microscope for doing differential count?**
    Condenser completely raised, iris diaphragm fully open, plane mirror (if present) used and oil immersion objective (100x) brought in line.

13. **What are the criteria for a good blood smear?**
    Refer page 59.

14. **What is the significance of the angle between the spreader slide and the glass slide?**
    The angle between the spreader slide and the glass slide should be about 45° to get an ideal smear. Increasing the angle makes the smear thicker and decreasing the angle makes the smear thinner.

15. **Name the cells that can be seen in a field while doing DC?**
    Red blood cells, white blood cells and platelets are seen in a field. RBCs are red colored biconcave cells, which are the predominant cells in the peripheral smear. WBCs are nucleated cells larger than red blood cells. Platelets are seen as small purple dots singly and in groups.

16. **Which is the smallest of the formed elements of blood?**
    Platelets (2–4 µm in size).

17. **What are the functions of neutrophils, eosinophils, basophils, monocytes and lymphocytes?**
    Refer page 56 Q. No. 12.

18. **Mention the unique feature of a stained blood smear.**
    The stained smear can be preserved for rechecking for errors and also for evaluating the progress of the clinical status of the patient. The smear can also be used at a later date to assess the response of the patient to treatment. It can be preserved for years if stored carefully. Thus the peripheral smear becomes a permanent record. No other routine hematological test can be reassessed.

19. **How will you identify the different leukocytes?**
    » Neutrophils have multilobed nucleus and cytoplasm contains fine pink or lilac colored granules.
    » Eosinophils have bilobed or spectacle shaped nucleus and the cytoplasm contains coarse orange red granules.
    » Basophils are rarely seen in a normal smear. Care should be taken in identifying a basophil. When seen, the cell will be filled by large numerous slate gray or blue granules which may obscure the nucleus. Sometimes the granules get washed off while pouring water. Then the nucleus appears 'S' shaped or bilobed.
    » Lymphocytes may be large lymphocytes or small lymphocytes (most mature). Large lymphocytes are larger and have more cytoplasm with rounded or slightly indented nucleus. Small lymphocytes are smaller (of the size of RBC) with scanty cytoplasm and round nucleus that appears to fill the whole cell.
    » Monocytes are the largest of the leukocytes. It has a deeply indented or kidney-shaped nucleus and the cytoplasm will be slate gray in color.

20. **What are the variations seen in the differential count?**

Neutrophils
Neutrophilia is increase in neutrophil count greater than 10,000/mm^3 of blood. It is seen in the following conditions:
» Acute pyogenic bacterial infections like tonsillitis, appendicitis, septicemia, etc.
» Metabolic disturbances like diabetes mellitus, renal failure, etc.
» Necrotic lesions like myocardial infarction, burns, etc.
» Noninfective inflammatory conditions like gout, rheumatic fever, etc.
» Drugs like glucocorticoids, adrenaline, etc.
» Malignancies like chronic myeloid leukemia.

Neutropenia is decrease in neutrophil count below 2,500/mm^3 of blood:
» Bacterial infections like typhoid and paratyphoid fever; tuberculosis, brucellosis, etc. In typhoid and paratyphoid infections, there is depression of bone marrow and the neutrophil count falls first because its half-life in circulation is very less (only 7 hours). In tuberculosis, there is lymphocytosis and so a relative decrease in neutrophil count is observed.
» Viral infections like measles, influenza, hepatitis, infectious mononucleosis (IMN), AIDS, etc.
» Aplastic anemia due to bone marrow depression.
» Arsenic poisoning and therapy with drugs like chloromycetin, penicillin, cytotoxic drugs, anti-thyroid drugs, etc.
» Anaphylaxis and hypersensitivity.
» Hypersplenism where there is sequestration of neutrophils and also increased destruction.
» Autoimmune disorders like SLE where there is lymphocytosis.
» Vitamin B$_{12}$ and folate deficiency that interferes with DNA synthesis.
» Autoimmune neutropenia.
» Congenital neutropenia is found in early life and the more severely affected children die in the first 1–2 years of life from repeated infections.

Eosinophils
Eosinophilia (>500/mm^3)
» Allergic conditions like bronchial asthma, hay fever, food sensitivity, drug allergy, serum sickness, urticaria, etc.
» Worm infestations, e.g., roundworm, hookworm, tapeworm, filarial worm, etc.
» Drugs like penicillin.
» Skin diseases like eczema, dermatitis, scabies, etc.
» Tropical pulmonary eosinophilia and scarlet fever.
» Chronic myeloid leukemia.

Eosinopenia (eosinophil count less than 50/mm^3)
» Endocrine disorders like Cushing's syndrome where there is increase in glucocorticoid secretion; acromegaly, etc.
» ACTH and corticosteroid therapy, glucocorticoids cause margination and sequestration of circulating eosinophils, lowering the eosinophil count.
» Stress, as in acute infection, traumatic shock, severe exercise, burns, acute emotional stress, exposure to cold, etc.
» Aplastic anemia, SLE, eclampsia, etc.

Basophils
Basophilia (when the count is more than 100/mm^3).
» Viral infections like measles, chickenpox, influenza, etc.
» Chronic myeloid leukemia and myeloproliferative disorders.
» Polycythemia vera
» Myxedema
» Hypersensitivity states

Basopenia
» Cushing's disease and prolonged corticosteroid therapy.
» Acute pyogenic infections associated with neutrophilia.

Lymphocytes
Lymphocytosis is increase in lymphocyte count more than 4,000/mm^3 of blood:
» Chronic bacterial infections like tuberculosis, syphilis, etc., and acute bacterial infections like whooping cough and typhoid.
» Viral infections like chickenpox, mumps, measles, influenza and viral hepatitis.
» Infectious mononucleosis
» Chronic lymphatic leukemia
» Autoimmune conditions like myasthenia gravis and thyrotoxicosis.
» Relative lymphocytosis is due to a decrease in the number of other WBCs especially neutrophils.
» In children, lymphocyte count is high (40–60%).

Lymphopenia (count less than 1,500/mm^3)
» Corticosteroid and immunosuppressive therapy
» Aplastic anemia due to excessive radiation
» Acquired immunodeficiency syndrome (AIDS)
» Hypersplenism

Monocytes
Monocytosis is increase in monocyte count above 800/mm³ and is a rare condition. May be seen in:
» Protozoal like malaria, kala-azar, amoebiasis and rickettsial infections
» Bacterial infections like tuberculosis, typhoid, syphilis, brucellosis and subacute bacterial endocarditis.
» Monocytic leukemia and myeloproliferative disorders.
» Collagen vascular disorders like systemic lupus erythematosus (SLE).
» Infectious mononucleosis or glandular fever and Hodgkin's disease.

Monocytopenia is rare and is seen in aplastic anemia.

21. **What is shilling index?**
Schilling divided neutrophils into four groups—myelocytes, metamyelocytes, band forms and segmented cells. The bone marrow precursors of leukocytes in peripheral blood are also taken into account in finding out **Schilling index**. Schilling index is important to assess the severity of leukemia. In leukemia the bone marrow precursors will be present in plenty in the peripheral smear.
The percentages of bone marrow precursors normally present in peripheral blood are:
» Myelocyte—0%
» Metamyelocyte—0–1%
» Band form—2–6%
» Segmented forms—51–67%
The rest of the granulocytes will be mature in normal states.

22. **What is the significance of doing differential count?**
» DC helps to find out the type of leukocytes and to see whether there is increase or decrease in the number of any particular type.
» If the total count is known, then the absolute number of each WBC can be found out. For example, if the TC is 6,000/mm³ and percentage of neutrophils 60% then the absolute neutrophil count will be 60/100 × 6,000 = 3,600/mm³ of blood.
» DC helps in detecting viral, bacterial and parasitic infections. In each case there will be variation in the count of various cells.
» It also helps to study the effects of chemotherapy and radiation therapy.

23. **What is Arneth count?**
Arneth devised a technique by which neutrophils can be classified depending on the number of lobes in the nucleus. This is known as **Arneth count or Arneth index**. The neutrophils and their precursors are divided into five main classes, according to the number of lobes in their nuclei. If the number of lobes is less it comes under younger series of cells. If the number of lobes is more, the cells are older. **Shift to left**, i.e., more number of younger cells, is seen in pyogenic infections. If most of the neutrophils in peripheral blood show four or more lobes in the nucleus it is called **shift to right**. Shift to right is seen in pernicious anemia, neutropenia, etc. The younger forms will be absent in conditions of neutropenia caused by diminished formation of blood cells in bone marrow (pancytopenia) as in bone marrow depression.
100 neutrophils are counted and the number of cells in each group is expressed as percentage. The percentage of cells in group 1 and 2 and half of group 3 is normally about 60% (51–65%). This is referred to as **Arneth index**.
Younger Cells
» Single lobe—5%
» 2 lobes—30%
» 3 lobes—45%
Older Cells
» 4 lobes—18%
» 5 lobes—2%

24. **Define immunity. What are the types of immunity?**
Immunity is the ability of the body to resist foreign bodies like bacteria, viruses, parasites, toxic substances, cancer cells, etc. Immunity is of two types:
a. Innate immunity
b. Acquired immunity, which is of two types cellular immunity and humoral immunity. Cellular immunity is mediated by T-lymphocytes and humoral immunity by B-lymphocytes. B-lymphocytes divide to form plasma cells that secrete antibodies.

25. **What does double population of cells mean?**
In some blood films, the red blood cells seem to be of two distinct populations. For example, it may consist of very hypochromic cells as well as cells which are normally stained. This condition is referred to as **double population of cells**. This is seen in the smears of patients with anemia who have received a blood transfusion or in a patient with anemia who has been treated for the cause of anemia. The new cells produced will have normal morphology while the old cells will be abnormal.

26. **What is pancytopenia?**
Pancytopenia is a condition where all the formed elements of blood are reduced. It is seen in the following conditions:
» Aplastic anemia due drugs or excessive radiation
» Hypersplenism
» Disseminated tuberculosis
» In conditions of bone marrow infiltration like malignant lymphomas (Hodgkin's disease), multiple myeloma, secondary carcinoma, myelosclerosis, etc.

27. **What is agranulocytosis or granulocytopenia?**
Here, there is decrease in granulocyte count. So, there is relative increase in agranulocyte count and hence called **agranulocytosis**. Usually drugs that cause bone marrow depression cause this condition. Lymphocytes are released from the lymphatic tissue so their count will be normal.

28. **How will you identify the different leukocytes if there is difficulty in distinguishing them?**
    If there is difficulty in identifying the cells note the size of the cell.
    » The size of a red cell is always between 7 and 8 μm. Compare with the size of WBCs.
    » If a WBC seen is having a large round nucleus and is almost the size or slightly larger than the RBC the cell is possibly a small lymphocyte.
    » If the size is two times that of a red cell, the cell may be a granulocyte or a large lymphocyte or a small monocyte.
    » If the size of the WBC seen is very large when compared to RBC, the cell is possibly a monocyte.
    After determining the size, have a look at the nucleus.
    » Find out if the nucleus is single or lobed.
    » A small cell with a single round nucleus can be identified as a small lymphocyte. A similar larger one with large round nucleus is a large lymphocyte. The nucleus of a large lymphocyte never shows any lobes (rarely slight indentation may be seen).
    » If the cell is bigger (12–15 μm) and shows distinct lobes joined by strands it should be classified as a granulocyte.
    » Among the granulocytes, the eosinophils and the basophils usually show a bilobed nucleus, the lobes being joined by a thick connection and not by a strand.
    Then observe the granules in the cytoplasm.
    » The presence of eosinophilic and basophilic granules in the cytoplasm helps in the identification of granulocytes.
    » The color of the granules in the cytoplasm should be compared with the color of the nucleus. If the granules are distinctly pink or red as compared to the cytoplasm the cell is an eosinophil. If the color of the granules is more intensely blue than the nucleus, the cell is a basophil. Unless distinct, large, refractive, shining and orange colored granules are seen in the cytoplasm no cell should be identified as an eosinophil.
    » The polymorphonuclear leukocyte shows multiple lilac colored neutrophilic granules in the cytoplasm. Bilobed leukocytes with the cytoplasm containing fine lilac colored granules are likely to be a young bilobed polymorphonuclear neutrophil.
    If there is difficulty in distinguishing between a large lymphocyte and a small monocyte when the nucleus shows hardly any lobulation but only a slight indentation note the following points:
    » The nucleus of a monocyte is wrinkled; that of a lymphocyte is smooth and solid.
    » The lymphocyte nucleus shows deeply stained chromatin material; while the monocyte nucleus may show nucleoli.
    » The amount of cytoplasm is less in a lymphocyte, more in a monocyte.

29. **How can you roughly calculate the platelet count from the peripheral blood smear?**
    Each platelet in an average oil immersion field represents approximately 15,000 platelets/mm^3 of blood. In normal blood, an average of 8–25 platelets should be seen in an oil immersion field after observing several fields.

30. **How will you calculate the absolute leukocyte count?**
    Absolute leukocyte count is the number of each leukocyte per mm^3 of blood. For example, if the total leukocyte count is 6,000/mm^3 of blood and the number of eosinophils counted from the peripheral smear is 3, then the absolute eosinophil count will be $3/100 \times 6{,}000 = 180$/mm^3 of blood.

31. **What is the difference in the differential count in adults and children?**
    The percentage of lymphocytes will be more in children than in adults. In children, lymphocytes form 40 to 60% of the total leukocyte count.

32. **What is buffer water? Mention its use.**
    The water whose pH is 6.8 is buffer water for Leishman staining. To prepare buffer water, buffer tablet like phosphate buffer tablet is added to distilled water. The ratio depends on the pH of the buffer water to be prepared. Thiazine eosinate, the stain present in Leishman stain splits or ionizes to eosin and methylene blue completely at this pH. So buffer water is superior to distilled water in diluting Leishman stain.

33. **Why tap water is not used for dilution?**
    The impurities present in tap water give false appearance of granules in the leukocytes. So there will be difficulty in identifying different leukocytes. Tap water should never be used for dilution.

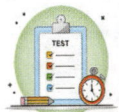

Objective Structured Practical Examination

I. **Prepare a blood smear with the given sample of blood.**
   » Take four clean glass slides
   » Select a spreader slide with smooth edge
   » Mix the blood sample gently
   » Place the glass slide on the table
   » Using a glass rod or a filler, place a drop of blood at one end of the slide
   » Fix the opposite end of the glass slide with the left hand
   » Place the smooth edge of the spreader slide in front of the blood drop at an angle of about 45°
   » Bring the spreader slide towards the blood drop till it touches the blood drop. Wait till the blood spread along the edge of the spreader
   » Push the spreader to the other end of the slide with a steady, smooth and quick movement
   » Wipe off the excess blood that is remaining at the other end
   » Dry the smear by waving it in air or by holding it under the fan

II. Stain the blood smear provided for doing differential leukocyte count.
- » See whether the smear provided is ideal for staining
- » Place the slide horizontally across the glass rods on the staining tray
- » Add 8–12 drops of Leishman stain on the smear and make sure that it completely covers the smear
- » Note the time
- » After 2 minutes, add distilled water using a filler, double the amount of stain added. Take care that it does not spill out
- » Mix the stain with the water by gently blowing air. Take care to avoid spilling of the mixture
- » After 7 minutes, add distilled water over the mixture so that the scum at the top flows off and it does not stick to the slide
- » Pour distilled water over the slide till the color of the smear becomes pink
- » Dry it in air

III. Examine the stained blood smear provided under oil immersion objective and focus an eosinophil.
- » Checks the smear provided under low power and high power objectives with proper adjustments of the microscope
- » Places a drop of cedar wood oil over the body of the smear and brings the oil immersion objective into position
- » Looks from the side and lowers the objective till it touches the oil
- » Adjusts the condenser and iris diaphragm for doing DC
- » Uses the fine adjustment screw and focuses an eosinophil

Chapter 13: Absolute Eosinophil Count by Hemocytometry

LEARNING OBJECTIVES

- Do the absolute eosinophil count using hemocytometry
- List the precautions to be taken during absolute eosinophil count
- Name the diluting fluid used, its composition and functions of each ingredient
- List the variations in eosinophil count
- Functions of eosinophils

INTRODUCTION

Absolute eosinophil count is done to diagnose diseases that specifically alter the eosinophil count only. It can be found out by direct and indirect methods. The direct method of absolute eosinophil count is done by hemocytometry. Indirect method is done by finding out the number of eosinophils as a percentage of the total leukocytes present in circulation. Two tests should be performed to calculate it by indirect method: (i) differential count and (ii) total count of leukocytes. It is time consuming and errors will be more. Direct absolute eosinophil count is more accurate.

PRINCIPLE

In the **direct method**, blood is diluted 10 times with diluting fluid in a WBC pipette. The diluting fluid selectively stains the eosinophils. RBCs are lysed by the dilute solution but eosinophils remain intact because of their high resistance to lysis. Eosinophil count is done under low power objective. The number of eosinophils in undiluted blood is then calculated, which gives the absolute eosinophil count.

APPARATUS

Hemocytometer with WBC pipette, diluting fluid (Dunger's fluid or Pilot's solution), microscope, lancet, spirit and cotton.

Composition of Dunger's Fluid

- Eosin (200 g/L)—10 mL
- 10% acetone—10 mL
- Distilled water—80 mL

Eosin stains the granules of eosinophils and acetone lyses RBCs.

Pilot's Solution

Each 100 mL of the solution contains
- Phloxine B (1% solution in water)—10 mL
- Propylene glycol—50 mL
- Sodium carbonate (1% solution in water)—1 mL
- Heparin—100 units
- Distilled water to make up the solution to 100 mL

Phloxin stains the eosinophil granules selectively, propylene glycol acts as solvent for the dye and it also lyses the RBCs, sodium carbonate enhances the staining of eosinophil granules, heparin act as anticoagulant and distilled water lyses all WBCs other than eosinophils (eosinophil membrane is more resistant to lysis).

Procedure

- Suck blood into the WBC pipette up to '1' mark.
- Suck Dunger's fluid up to '11' mark.
- Mix the contents well and wait for 10 minutes to allow time for staining of the eosinophils and lysis of the other cells.

Section 1: Hematology

- Charge the counting chamber after mixing the contents well.
- Count the eosinophils in all the 9 large squares under the low power of the microscope (only eosinophils are seen in the field because the stain stains only the eosinophils).

Calculation

- Volume of the 9 large squares—0.9 mm³
- Dilution—1/10
- Let the number of cells counted be N
- 0.9 mm³ of diluted blood contains N eosinophils
- So 1 mm³ of undiluted blood contains $\dfrac{N \times 10}{0.9}$

$$= N \times 11 \text{ eosinophils.}$$

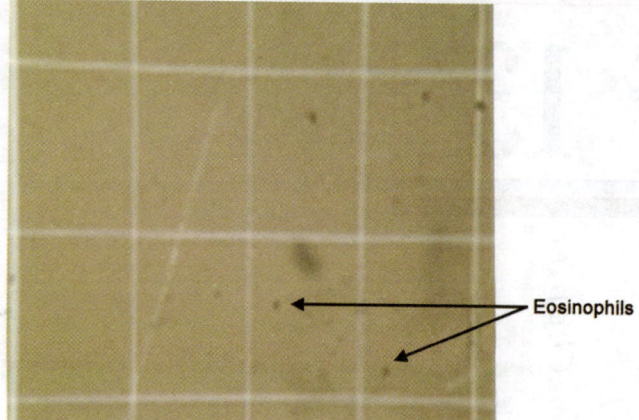

Fig. 13.1: Eosinophils are seen as prominent red dots.

Discussion

- Normal absolute eosinophil count is 150–400 cells/mm³ of blood.
- When the absolute eosinophil count is more than 600/mm³ it is referred to as **eosinophilia**.
- When the count is more than 4,000/mm³ of blood it is referred to as **marked eosinophilia**.
- Absolute eosinophil count can also be found out by multiplying the total WBC count by the percentage of eosinophils in the differential WBC count (indirect method). If the total count is 6,000 and the percentage of eosinophils 6%, then the absolute eosinophil count will be 6 × 6,000/100 = 360/mm³ of blood.
- The advantage of determining absolute eosinophil count is that it changes exclusively with variations in eosinophils only. When the eosinophils are expressed as percentage of total leukocyte count, the percentage remains unchanged even if there is increase or decrease in the number of all types of leukocytes. This is because 100 WBCs are counted not taking into consideration whether there is leukocytosis or leukopenia.
- Functions of eosinophils include phagocytosis especially of antigen-antibody complexes and help to limit allergic reactions. It also phagocytose and kills parasitic larvae like microfilaria. It is mainly involved in allergic reactions.

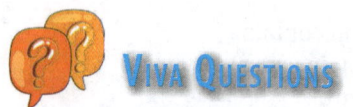

Viva Questions

1. **Name the two methods of doing absolute eosinophil count.**
   - Direct method using the principle of hemocytometry
   - Indirect method by calculating from differential leukocyte count and total leukocyte count
2. **What are the diluting fluids used for doing absolute eosinophil count?**
   - Dunger solution
   - Pilot solution
3. **Name the counting chambers that can be used to do absolute eosinophil count**
   - Neubauer counting chamber
   - Fuchs-Rosenthal counting chamber
   - Speir chamber
4. **What are the precautions for doing absolute eosinophil count?**
   - Counting should be done within 30 minutes of diluting the blood. This is because eosinophils will disintegrate in the diluting fluid after this time.
   - In order to mix the contents in the pipette, it should be rolled between the palm gently to prevent rupture of the eosinophil membrane.
   - Dust particles should not be mistaken for eosinophils. Eosinophils appear red in color.

5. **Name the contents in the eosinophil granules.**
   Two types of granules are seen in eosinophils:
   i. **Azurophilic granules** which are present in all granulocytes and contain acid hydrolases and other enzymes
   ii. **Specific granules** which contain the following:
      a. *Major basic protein (MBP)* kills larvae and adult parasites
      b. *Eosinophilic cationic proteins* (ECP) kills larvae and is also bactericidal
      c. *Eosinophil peroxidase (EPO)* participates in inflammatory reactions
      d. *Eosinophil derived neurotoxin (EDN)* interferes with the parasitic nervous system
      e. *Histaminases* break down histamine produced by mast cells
      f. *Aryl sulphatase B* is an enzyme that inactivates leukotrienes that are involved in hypersensitivity reactions
      g. *Lysophospholipase* is an enzyme that causes hydrolysis of intracellular lipoproteins

6. **What are the functions of eosinophils?**
   Refer page 72.

7. **What is Thorn test?**
   Absolute eosinophil count is taken as an index of ACTH activity in blood. In Cushing syndrome there is a reduction in eosinophil count. If ACTH is injected intramuscularly in a normal person, it results in reduction of the number of circulating eosinophils. This is called **Thorn test**. This test can be used to assess adrenocortical function. It is not a specific test and so not done nowadays.

8. **Mention the normal eosinophil count**
   » 3–5% of leukocytes
   » Normal absolute eosinophil count—150–400 cells/mm^3 of blood.

9. **Name the common conditions that produce eosinophilia and eosinopenia.**
   Refer page 67.

10. **What is the merit of direct absolute eosinophil count over indirect count?**
    While doing eosinophil count using differential count, the percentage of eosinophils remains unchanged even if there is leukocytosis or leukopenia. We are counting 100 WBCs and finding out the number of eosinophils in them. Then we find out the total leukocyte count. The percentage remains unchanged in the indirect count. But absolute eosinophil count changes only with variation in eosinophils only.

Chapter 14

Reticulocyte Count

LEARNING OBJECTIVES

- State the principle of doing reticulocyte count
- Perform reticulocyte count of your own blood
- The precautions for reticulocyte count
- State the normal reticulocyte count in different age groups
- List the causes of variation in reticulocyte count
- Name the stain used for reticulocyte count and mention the principle of staining

PY2.13: Describe steps for reticulocyte and platelet count.

PRINCIPLE

Reticulocytes are immature red cells, which contain remnants of ribosomes and RNA. The ribonucleoproteins have the property of reacting with certain basic dyes to form a blue precipitate of granules or filaments. Largest amount of dark blue reticulum is found in the most immature reticulocytes. Staining of ribonucleic acid requires special staining technique. A supravital stain such as brilliant cresyl blue or new methylene blue is used.

Brilliant cresyl blue stain contains:
- Brilliant cresyl blue—1 g
- Sodium chloride—0.7 g
- Sodium citrate—0.6 g
- Distilled water up to 100 mL

Brilliant cresyl blue stains the RNA of reticulocytes, citrate prevents clotting of blood and normal saline provides isotonicity to the solution.

New methylene blue stain:
This stain is prepared as a 1% solution in isotonic saline and then diluted to 100 mL with 3.8% sodium citrate. New methylene blue stains the reticulum present in the cytoplasm more deeply than brilliant cresyl blue.
- New methylene blue stains the RNA of reticulocytes
- Sodium citrate prevents coagulation of blood
- Sodium chloride makes the solution isotonic

PROCEDURE

Wet Method or Cover Slip Preparation

Mix one drop of blood and one drop of stain on a grease-free glass slide. Put a cover glass and wait for 10–20 minutes. Cover it with a petri-dish containing moist filter paper so that the solution does not get evaporated. If the slides are incubated at 37°C for 15 minutes to simulate the living conditions, the stain may better penetrate the reticulocytes and stains the RNA more deeply. Observe under the high power of the microscope. Count 1,000 red blood cells and note the number of reticulocytes counted. RBCs with blue granular or reticular precipitate in the cytoplasm are reticulocytes. They will be slightly larger than the mature RBCs. The reticulocyte count is expressed as the percentage of the total RBCs that are counted.

Smear Preparation (Dry Preparation)

Take 2–3 drops of the supravital stain in a test tube and to it add equal amount of blood and incubate it at 37°C for 15 minutes. After gently mixing the contents make a thick smear on a clean grease-free glass slide. After drying observe under the oil immersion objective using cedar wood oil. Identify the reticulocytes by their large size and presence of filamentous strands and dots stained deep blue in the cytoplasm. Count 1,000 RBCs in different fields and record the number of reticulocytes seen among these RBCs. This method is most widely practiced.

Because of the large number of cells in each field, inserting a circular piece of paper with a central perforation in front of the eyepiece can reduce the size of the field. This will allow easy counting of cells and avoids recounting.

Let the number of reticulocytes per 1,000 RBCs be 'n'

$$\text{The percentage of reticulocytes} = \frac{n \times 100}{1000}$$

Automated Electronic Method

The reticulocytes are stained with a fluorochrome dye that specifically stains RNA. When exposed to ultraviolet light the cells show fluorescence and the cells are counted in machines.

Advantages

- Takes very little time since the machine counts thousands of reticulocytes in just a few seconds.
- It is an accurate method
- Easy procedure for the technician

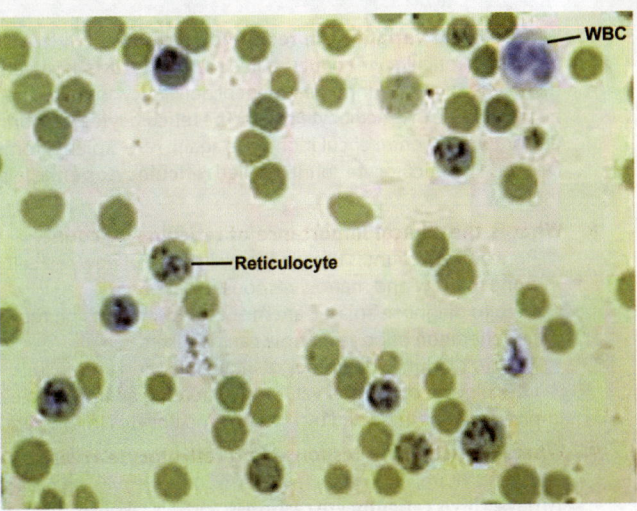

Fig. 14.1: Supravital staining showing reticulocytes (note the network of blue strands inside the reticulocytes).

DISCUSSION

Reticulocytes are immature red cells that contain remains of ribonucleic acid. It is about 8 μm in diameter, irregular and polylobulated due to extrusion of nucleus. Cytoplasm contains small amount of basophilic material consisting of remnants of organelles like ribosomes, mitochondria and Golgi complex. Reticulocyte cannot be seen in a Leishman-stained blood smear because methyl alcohol destroys the ribonuclear protein. **Supravital staining** with brilliant cresyl blue causes ribosomal RNA to precipitate into a network of blue strands, hence the name reticulocyte **(Fig. 14.1)**. Reticulocyte becomes mature RBC within 32–48 hours. Reticulocytes remain in the bone marrow till mature because of their adhesive property. They have a coating of globulin especially transferrin.

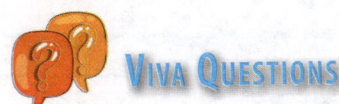

VIVA QUESTIONS

1. **What does supravital staining mean? What is its difference from intravital staining?**
   Vital staining is staining of the cells or tissues in a living state. It includes intravital staining and supravital staining. Staining of living cells outside the body (in vitro) is supravital staining. Incubating the blood with certain stains while the cells are still alive is called **supravital staining**. Other living cells in vitro can also be stained by supravital staining. Supravital staining can be done only on unfixed and living cells. Brilliant cresyl blue and new methylene blue are examples of supravital stains. **Intravital stains** are used for staining living cells in vivo by injecting colloidal solution of dyes. Trypan blue, Lugol's iodine, toluidine blue are examples of intravital stains. This is not done nowadays.

2. **Why reticulocytes are not seen in Leishman-stained smears?**
   The reticulocytes can be demonstrated only by supravital staining. In the Leishman-stained smear, the cells are fixed by methyl alcohol.

3. **What are the indications for doing reticulocyte count?**
   Reticulocyte count is indicated for assessing the erythroid activity of bone marrow and for checking the therapeutic response in anemia.

4. **Name two supravital stains and their composition and functions of the contents.**
   Refer page 74.

5. **What is the difference between methylene blue and new methylene blue stains?**
   New methylene blue ($C_{36}H_{44}Cl_4N_6S_2Nn$) is chemically different from methylene blue ($C_{16}H_{18}ClN_3S$) stain. Methylene blue is a poor reticulocyte stain. New methylene blue is a supravital stain. Mixed with whole blood, RNA and DNA stain deep blue with new methylene blue. Azure B is a substitute for new methylene blue.

6. **What is the normal reticulocyte count? How will you find out the absolute reticulocyte count?**
   Adult—0.5–1%
   Fetus—30–50%
   At birth—2–6% and one week after birth count comes to adult level
   Absolute reticulocyte count = reticulocyte percent × red cell count/100
   $= 1 \times 5,000,000/mm^3/100 = 50,000/mm^3$ of blood
   Normal range of absolute reticulocyte count is 25,000–100,000/mm^3 of blood.

7. **What are the variations in reticulocyte count?**
   Increase in reticulocyte count is called **reticulocytosis**. It is seen in conditions of increased erythropoietic activity. For example, in hypoxia, hemolytic anemia, during treatment of deficiency anemia, after splenectomy, after acute hemorrhage and after severe exercise there will be an increase in reticulocyte count. The reticulocytes are normally trapped in the trabeculae of spleen where they mature into RBC in a day or two and enter circulation once again. After splenectomy this does not occur and hence an increase in reticulocyte count is seen. Decrease in reticulocyte count is called **reticulocytopenia**. It is seen in aplastic anemia, myxedema, hypopituitarism and cytotoxic drug therapy.

8. **What is the clinical importance of reticulocyte count?**
   » Reticulocyte count is used in the evaluation of new red cell production and is helpful in determining the hemopoietic activity of the bone marrow and marrow response to anemia.
   » Help to diagnose aplastic anemia. Very low counts on repeated tests after treatment indicate bone marrow suppression.
   » Regeneration of bone marrow can be tested.
   » Help to diagnose deficiency of vitamin B_{12} and folic acid.
   » Reticulocyte count is of value while treating anemia especially megaloblastic anemia.
   Improvement is indicated by a rise in reticulocytes in the peripheral blood.

9. **What is reticulocyte response and reticulocyte crisis?**
   Following vitamin B_{12} injection in pernicious anemia, reticulocytes start to appear in circulation by 4–5 days and maximum is reached by 10 days. This is **reticulocyte response** and it is taken as the earliest sign of clinical improvement. There will be increase in the number of circulating reticulocytes up to 30–40%. After 10 days, reticulocyte count gradually declines while RBC count rises steadily. Reticulocyte response is also seen while treating other forms of anemia like iron deficiency anemia. A reticulocyte response to a particular therapy confirms the diagnosis of the deficiency of the substance. It also helps to assess the response of the patient to the treatment for anemia. In conditions of acute hemolysis or in periods of recovery from severe anemia, the RBC production is sharply increased and the reticulocyte count may go up to 25–30%. This is known as **reticulocyte crisis**. During the course of pernicious anemia there will be periods of remission and relapse. The increase in reticulocyte count seen during periods of remission is also called reticulocyte crisis.

10. **What is the life span of reticulocyte in circulation?**
    24 hours.

11. **What is the absolute reticulocyte count?**
    Normal range of absolute reticulocyte count is 25,000–100,000/mm^3 of blood.

12. **How can you reduce the size of the microscopic field? What is its importance?**
    Place a small circular piece of paper preferably black paper in the eye piece in which a hole of 5 mm diameter has been made at the center. When the size of the field is reduced, it will be more easy to count the cells and it also helps to avoid recounting of cells.

13. **What is the principle and advantages of automated method of reticulocyte count?**
    Refer page 75.

Chapter 15

Platelet Count

LEARNING OBJECTIVES

- Perform platelet count using Rees-Ecker method
- The composition and functions of Rees-Ecker fluid
- Mention the precautions to be taken while performing the above method
- State the importance of doing platelet count
- List the common conditions that alter platelet count
- Mention other methods of performing platelet count

PY2.13: Describe steps for reticulocyte and platelet count.

APPARATUS

Improved Neubauer double counting chamber, RBC pipette, thick cover slip, spirit, lancet and Rees-Ecker fluid (platelet diluting fluid).

Composition of Rees-Ecker Diluting Fluid

- Sodium citrate—3.8 g
- Formalin (1% solution)—0.2 mL
- Brilliant cresyl blue—50 mg
- Distilled water up to 100 mL

Freshly prepared solution should be used. The solution can be stored at 2–4°C for a maximum of one week but it should be filtered before use. Sodium citrate acts as anticoagulant. Formalin helps in fixation of cells and it also prevents bacterial and fungal growth. It also lyses RBCs. Brilliant cresyl blue forms a background in which the platelets can be identified easily. It does not stain the platelets and is used only for the identification of the diluent. *Freshly prepared solution should be used; otherwise formaldehyde gets converted to formic acid that destroys the platelets.*

Brecher-Cronkite method can also be used for platelet count. Here **1% ammonium oxalate** in distilled water is used as the platelet diluting fluid. Ammonium oxalate acts as anticoagulant by preventing platelet adhesion and it also preserves the platelets. The hypotonic solution destroys the RBCs. The principle is based on phase contrast microscopy. The advantages of this method are (i) identification of platelet is easier and (ii) error encountered is low.

Procedure

- A drop of 14% magnesium sulfate is placed on the sterilized finger tip.
- Prick the fingertip through the magnesium sulfate solution to minimize platelet loss due to adhesion and aggregation at the site of injury (venous blood anticoagulated with EDTA is best for doing platelet count).
- If venous blood is used the errors in the platelet count will be less. This is because the platelets may clump at the puncture site in finger prick method. So the platelet count obtained will be less than that of venous blood. The venous blood can be anticoagulated using EDTA because EDTA reduces platelet clumping tendency. The test should be performed within 2 hours of collecting blood.
- Suck blood up to the 0.5 mark of RBC pipette.
- Wipe off excess blood from the sides of the tip of the pipette.
- Immediately suck the platelet diluting fluid up to the 101 mark (the fluid should be filtered before use).
- By gently rotating the pipette by placing it between the palms horizontally, mix the blood with the diluting fluid thoroughly. The bead in the bulb facilitates this.

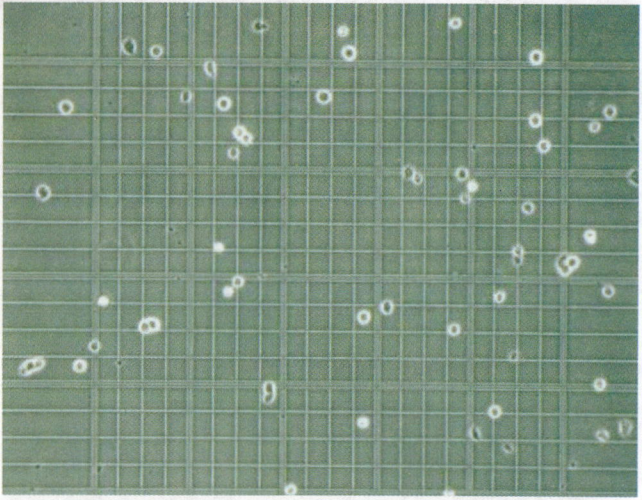

Fig. 15.1: Platelets seen as refractile bodies under the microscope (using 1% ammonium oxalate as the diluting fluid).

- Wait for 10–15 minutes and discard first few drops of fluid from the pipette.
- Place the cover slip over the ruled area of the chamber and charge both the counting areas of the counting chamber.
- Cover the chamber with a petri-dish containing wet filter paper to prevent drying up of the fluid in the counting chamber. Wait for 15–20 minutes for the platelets to settle down to the surface of the chamber so that all of them will be on the same plane of focus.
- Under high power objective of the microscope count the number of platelets in all the 25 squares of area 1 mm × 1 mm in the center of the ruled area of the chamber (RBC counting areas).
- The platelets appear as tiny highly refractile rounded structures about 2–4 μm in diameter. They can be seen clearly by reducing the amount of light by adjusting the iris diaphragm **(Fig. 15.1)**.
- Count the number of platelets in both the ruled areas on either side of the chamber. Find out the average. The difference in count in both areas should be minimum.
- Take care that the chamber or the diluting fluid does not contain dust particles since they may be mistaken for platelets.
- The number of platelets in 1 mm³ of undiluted blood is calculated.

Calculation

- Let 'N' be the number of platelets counted in the 25 squares of the RBC counting area.
- Total area of 25 squares is 1 mm².
- Depth between the counting area and cover slip is 1/10 mm.
- Volume of fluid present in the 25 small squares is 1 mm² × 1/10 mm = 1/10 mm³.
- 1/10 mm³ of diluted blood contains 'N' platelets.
- So 1 mm³ of diluted blood contains 10N platelets.
- Dilution is 200 times.
- Therefore 1 mm³ of undiluted blood contains 10N × 200 = 2,000N platelets.

Precautions

- Observe all precautions taken for RBC count.
- The diluting fluid should be filtered just before the experiment. The hemocytometer and the cover glass should be very clean. If dust particles or bacteria are present, they may be mistaken for platelets.

AUTOMATED ANALYZER

Automated electronic particle counters can also do platelet count. This method is more accurate than the manual method. Electronic cell counter is usually used. The diluted blood is allowed to pass through an aperture. The particles between 2 and 10 μm³ (fL) are counted as platelets.

DISCUSSION

Platelets are cytoplasmic fragments derived from bone marrow megakaryocytes. Platelets play an important role in blood coagulation and hemostasis. Normal platelet count is 2–4 lakhs/ mm³ of blood. It has a half-life of 4–8 days.

Platelets cannot be counted from a Leishman-stained smear because they are seen clumped together. Platelet count can be accurately done if phase contrast microscope is used.

Variation in Platelet Count

Thrombocytosis is a condition where there is increase in platelet count (>4,50,000/mm³ of blood). A large increase in platelet count can lead to the risk of thrombosis in blood vessels. Thrombocytosis is seen in the following conditions:
- After splenectomy
- After exercise due to splenic contraction
- During infections
- Immediately after hemorrhage as in childbirth, surgery, injury, etc.
- During stress due to release of epinephrine which causes splenic contraction
- Polycythemia vera
- Iron deficiency anemia
- Chronic myeloid leukemia

Thrombocytopenia is decrease in platelet count (less than 1,50,000/mm³ of blood). It is one of the most common causes of uncontrolled bleeding. It is associated with small hemorrhages (petechial rashes) in the skin and mucous membrane and bleeding from gum and nose. It is seen in the following conditions:
- Viral infections like dengue fever, measles
- Drug hypersensitivity
- Acute leukemia

- Aplastic anemia due to bone marrow depression
- Megaloblastic anemia
- Idiopathic thrombocytopenic purpura (ITP) which is an autoimmune disease where antibodies are produced against platelets which destroys the platelets.
- Hypersplenism (enlarged spleen).

Thrombasthenia is a condition where the platelet count is normal but the platelet function is abnormal. Here also the bleeding time will be prolonged. Drugs such as aspirin also decrease platelet function and this is the reason why aspirin is prescribed to patients with arterial thrombosis in order to prevent heart attacks.

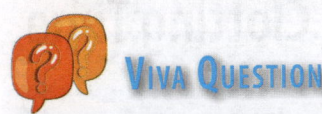

Viva Questions

1. **What is the normal platelet count?**
   1.5–4.5 lakhs/mm^3 of blood.

2. **Name the contents of the alpha granules of platelets.**
   Platelet derived growth factor (PDGF), platelet factor 3 (PF$_3$), fibronectin, plasminogen, fibrinogen, clotting factor V, thrombospondin, α$_2$ plasmin inhibitor and hydrolases.

3. **What are the contents of dense granules?**
   Serotonin, ADP and calcium ions.

4. **Enumerate the functions of platelets.**
   » Temporary arrest of bleeding by the formation of platelet plug by virtue of its properties like adhesion, aggregation and platelet activation.
   » Clotting of blood and clot retraction.
   » Phagocytosis of small particles like carbon particles, immune complexes and viruses.
   » Storage and transport of substances like serotonin, heparin, etc.

5. **What is thrombocytosis? Name the conditions producing it.**
   Refer page 78.

6. **What is thrombocytopenia? Name the conditions producing it.**
   Refer page 78.

7. **Name the constituents of Rees-Ecker diluting fluid.**
   Refer page 77.

8. **What are the steps in the formation of platelets?**
   Platelets are formed in the red bone marrow. The myeloid stem cell develops into CFU-GM, which in turn develops into megakaryoblast and then into megakaryocyte. Megakaryocytes are the largest cells in the bone marrow, the diameter being 100 mm. The megakaryocyte breaks up into 2,000–3,000 small cytoplasmic fragments. Each fragment enclosed in the cell membrane form a platelet. About 30–40% of platelets formed in the bone marrow are stored in the spleen. The rest are released into the circulation.

9. **Why platelet count is decreased in hypersplenism?**
   Half-life of platelets is 4–8 days. They are destroyed in the spleen. So in hypersplenism, their count is decreased.

10. **What is purpura?**
    Purpura is a clinical condition characterized by spontaneous hemorrhage beneath the skin and mucous membrane. It may be due to decrease in platelet count (thrombocytopenic purpura), abnormality in platelet function (thrombasthenic purpura) or it can be due to vascular defect. Thrombocytopenic purpura can be graded into three:
    » Mild purpura—platelet count will be 30,000–50,000/mm^3 and the bleeding will be mild.
    » Moderate purpura—platelet count will be less than 10,000/mm^3 and the bleeding will be severe.
    » Fulminating purpura—platelet count less than 1,000/mm^3 of blood and there will be uncontrolled internal bleeding.

11. **Why is venous blood preferred to capillary blood for doing platelet count?**
    Refer page 77.

12. **How can you differentiate between dirt particles and platelets?**
    The platelets appear as tiny highly refractile rounded structures about 2–4 μm in diameter. They can be seen clearly by reducing the amount of light by adjusting the iris diaphragm.

13. **Name the other counting chamber used to do platelet count?**
    Spencer-Brightline counting chamber which has a metallic surface is used. The metallic surface makes it easier to identify the platelets. The distribution of platelets is also uniform since the surface of the chamber is smoother.

14. **What is the life span of platelet in circulation?**
    8–12 days in circulation. Half life of platelets is 4 days.

15. **What is the standard dilution of platelet count?**
    1:100 times.

16. **How will you find out the platelet count from a peripheral blood smear?**
    Platelets in 10 oil immersion fields are counted and the average is found out.
    Estimated platelet count per μL = Average count in 10 fields × 15,000

Chapter 16

Determination of Bleeding Time and Clotting Time

LEARNING OBJECTIVES

- Determine your own bleeding time using Duke method
- Determine clotting time of your blood by capillary tube method
- Give the normal values of bleeding time and clotting time and enumerate their variations
- What are the precautions to be taken while determining bleeding time and clotting time
- Name the tests done to assess the efficiency of intrinsic and extrinsic pathway of blood coagulation
- Enumerate the specific blood tests done to diagnose hemophilia
- List the steps of blood coagulation

PY2.11: Estimate hemoglobin, red blood cell count, total leukocyte count, RBC indices, differential leukocyte count, blood groups, BT/CT.
PY2.8: Describe the physiological basis of hemostasis and anticoagulants. Describe bleeding and clotting disorders (hemophilia, purpura).

BLEEDING TIME

Principle

A deep prick is made on the skin and the time for which it bleeds is noted. Bleeding stops when a platelet plug is formed at the site of injury in the vessel wall.

Methods

- Finger prick method
- Duke's method
- Ivy's method

Finger Prick Method

- Give a deep prick on the tip of left ring finger with a lancet after cleaning the area with spirit.
- Immediately start a stop watch.
- Gently touch the pricked area with filter paper and see whether blood spots are formed in the filter paper at 10 seconds interval. Fresh areas of filter paper should be used.
- Stop the stop-watch when no more blood spots are formed in the filter paper and note the time which gives the bleeding time (**Fig. 16.1**).
- *Normal bleeding time by this method is low and is about 1–3 minutes.*

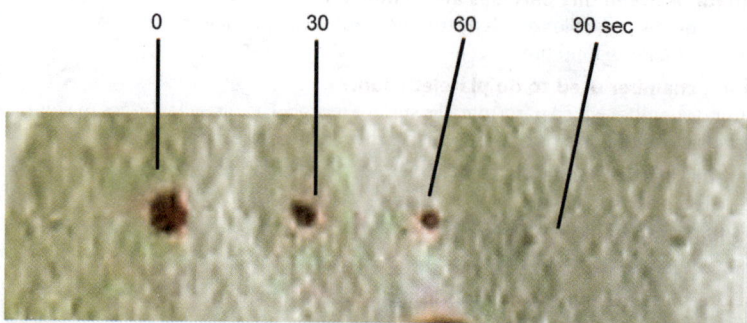

Fig. 16.1: Bleeding time by finger prick method. Here the bleeding time is one and a half minute.

Duke's Method
- Clean the tip of ear lobe with spirit and allow it to dry.
- Using a lancet give a deep prick on the lower edge of the ear lobe to a depth of approximately 3 mm.
- Immediately start a stopwatch.
- Touch the bleeding site with filter paper, repeat touching the area on new areas of the filter paper every 10–20 seconds.
- Stop the stopwatch when no stain is formed on the filter paper and note the time.

Normal bleeding time by Duke's method is 3–5 minutes.

Ivy's Method
- Clean an area in the flexor aspect of the forearm which is devoid of superficial veins with spirit and allow it to dry.
- Tie the cuff of sphygmomanometer around the upper arm of the subject and inflate it up to 40 mm Hg and maintain this pressure throughout the test.
- Give a deep prick on the clean skin about 3 mm deep and start the stopwatch.
- Gently touch the bleeding area with filter paper every 30 seconds as in the previous method
- Do not rub the skin or remove any clot that has formed.
- Stop the stopwatch when no blood stain is seen on the filter paper after a gentle touch and note the time.

Normal bleeding time by Ivy's method is 3–8 minutes and is the method of choice. Bleeding time is more accurate by this method.

Discussion
Time in minutes, which it takes for a standardized skin wound to stop bleeding, is the bleeding time. Continuous bleeding from cuts, wounds, following tooth extraction, etc., suggests defect in bleeding time and clotting time.

Normal bleeding time is 2–6 minutes and it is prolonged in:
- Thrombocytopenia
- Defective platelet function as in thrombasthenia.
- Aplastic anemia
- Liver diseases which produces deficiency of clotting factors.
- Abnormality of blood vessel wall as in dengue fever, vasculitis, etc.
- Following therapy with anticoagulant drugs like aspirin, warfarin, etc.
- Disseminated intravascular coagulation where the clotting factors get used up.

CLOTTING TIME

Principle
The time taken by whole blood to clot when it is taken out of the body is the clotting time. Determination of clotting time is a screening test for coagulation disorders and is a measure of the plasma clotting factors.

Methods
- Capillary tube method (Wright's method)
- Lee and White's method

Capillary Tube Method
- Prick the fingertip with a lancet after cleaning the area with spirit.
- Start the stopwatch immediately.
- Wipe off the first drop of blood.
- Fill two long capillary tubes with the free flowing blood from the site of puncture.
- After two minutes carefully break the capillary tube at one cm distance every 15 seconds till a thin fibrin strand is formed between the two broken ends (**Fig. 16.2**).
- Stop the stopwatch and find out the time, which gives the clotting time. Normal clotting time—1–5 minutes.

Lee and White Method
- Take 3 mL of venous blood into a plastic syringe from a forearm vein after cleaning the area.
- Start the stopwatch immediately.
- Transfer 1 mL of blood each into 3 glass tubes which are kept at 37°C in a water bath.
- After 3 minutes tilt the tubes one by one every 30 seconds.
- Find out the time when the tube can be tilted without spilling the contents which gives the clotting time.
- Normal clotting time by this method is 5–10 minutes.

Other Tests Used to Measure the Efficiency of Coagulation
- **One stage (Quick's) prothrombin time:** Oxalated venous blood is mixed with an excess of thromboplastin

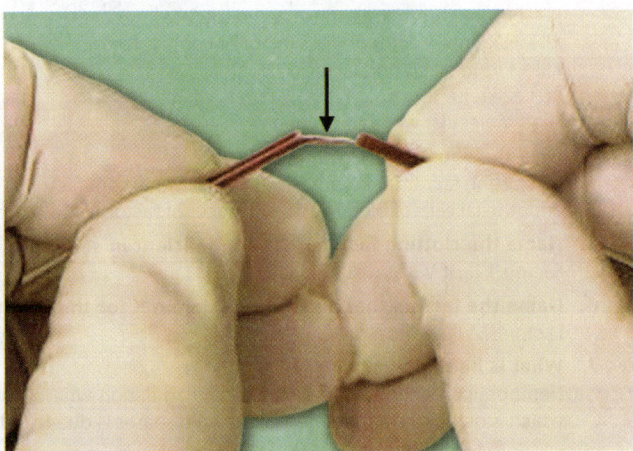

Fig. 16.2: The broken capillary ends connected by fibrin threads.

obtained from tissues. The mixture is then recalcified and the time taken for the formation of clot is measured. Instead of whole blood, plasma of the subject can be used. Prothrombin time is done frequently while treating cases of thrombosis with dicoumarol and fibrinolytic drugs. Normal value is 16 seconds.
- **Thromboplastin generation test:** It is done to test the integrity of the extrinsic pathway of coagulation.
- **Clot retraction time:** It is measured by observing the clot and liberation of serum at 37°C. Normal value 30–60 minutes.
- **Platelet count:** 2–4 lakhs.

DISCUSSION

The time it takes for whole blood immediately taken in a capillary tube or a container to clot is the clotting time. Clotting time is prolonged in the following conditions:
- Deficiency of coagulation factors as in hemophilia, vitamin K deficiency, afibrinogenemia, etc.
- Administration of anticoagulants like heparin, aspirin, etc.
- Disseminated intravascular coagulation.

VIVA QUESTIONS

1. **What are the common tests to assess blood coagulation? Give the normal values. Bleeding time:** 1–4 minutes bleeding time is said to be prolonged when it is >8 minutes as in purpura, von Willebrand disease, etc.
   Clotting time: 4–11 minutes
   Prothrombin time (PT): 16 seconds. It measures the efficiency of extrinsic pathway and the common pathway of coagulation. Clotting time of plasma is found out after adding tissue extract containing tissue thromboplastin (factor III). It measures the efficacy of clotting factors I, V, VII, X and XIII.
   Activated partial thromboplastin time (APTT): 40 seconds. It measures the efficiency of intrinsic and common pathway.
   Platelet count: 2–4 lakhs/mm^3 of blood
   Clot retraction time: 30–60 minutes.

2. **What is the clinical significance of doing bleeding time and clotting time?**
   » These tests are routinely done before any surgery, biopsy, etc.
   » It is done before anticoagulant therapy in patients who are at the risk of developing thromboembolism as in atrial fibrillation.
   » These tests are periodically assessed while the patient is on anticoagulant therapy.
   » Diseases like hemophilia can be detected early before complications occur.

3. **Enumerate the clotting factors.**
   I—Fibrinogen
   II—Prothrombin
   III—Thromboplastin or tissue factor
   IV—Ca^{2+}
   V—Labile factor or proaccelerin
   VI—Now this factor is discarded
   VII—Stable factor or proconvertin
   VIII—Antihemophilic factor-A
   IX—Christmas factor or antihemophilic factor-B
   X—Stuart Prower factor
   XI—Plasma thromboplastin antecedent (PTA)
   XII—Hageman factor or glass factor or contact factor
   XIII—Fibrin stabilizing factor
   Prekallikrein
   High molecular weight kininogen

4. **Give the sources of clotting factors.**
   All clotting factors are synthesized in the liver except factor III, IV and VIII. Factors III and VIII are synthesized by platelets and damaged endothelial cells of blood vessels. Sources of factor IV (Ca^{2+}) are diet and bone.

5. **Name the clotting factors that are deficient in serum.**
   Factors I, III, V, VIII and XIII

6. **Name the factors that depend on vitamin K for their synthesis in the liver.**
   Factors II, VII, IX and X

7. **What is hemophilia?**
   Hemophilia is an inherited disorder of coagulation where some clotting factors are deficient. Hemophilia A or classical hemophilia which is one of the commonest bleeding diseases is due to deficiency of factor VIII. Hemophilia B or Christmas disease that is clinically

indistinguishable from hemophilia A is due to deficiency of factor IX. Both these conditions are inherited as sex linked (X-linked) recessive trait and are seen only in males (in very rare situations females may be affected). Hemophilia C is due to deficiency of factor XI and it occurs with equal frequency in males and females. The gene controlling the synthesis of this factor is located in one of the autosomal chromosomes. Hemophilia C is not that severe.

8. **What is the difference between hemophilia and purpura?**
   In hemophilia, bleeding time is normal but clotting time is prolonged. Hemophilia may be due to deficiency of clotting factors VIII, IX or XI. In purpura, bleeding time is prolonged but clotting time is normal. It may be due to thrombocytopenia, defective platelet function or due to vascular defects. Purple spots are seen in the skin in purpura due to subcutaneous hemorrhage.

9. **What are the blood tests to confirm hemophilia?**
   Clotting time, activated partial thromboplastin time (APTT), prothrombin time and bleeding time are determined to confirm hemophilia. Clotting time and APTT are pro- longed in hemophilia due to deficiency of clotting factor VIII (classical hemophilia or hemophilia-A). Prothrombin time and bleeding time are normal in hemophilia. Factor VIII assay can also be done to assess the severity of the disease.

10. **How will you treat hemophilia?**
    » Fresh blood or fresh plasma transfusion is done because factor VIII, which is a labile factor, is destroyed rapidly on storage.
    » Cryoprecipitate (fresh frozen plasma) of factor VIII is available and is given intravenously.
    » For Christmas disease, stored blood also can be given because factor IX is a stable factor and is not lost during storage.

11. **What is hemostasis? Enumerate the steps in hemostasis.**
    Hemostasis means arrest of bleeding by physiological process. It includes temporary hemostasis and permanent hemostasis. Temporary hemostasis includes vascular spasm by serotonin released from platelets at the site of injury and platelet plug formation. Permanent hemostasis includes coagulation of blood and clot retraction.
    Coagulation is the conversion of temporary platelet plug into a definitive clot. It includes complex cascades of reactions in which, clotting factors activate one another, i.e., a series of autocatalytic reactions occur. Once the process is initiated, the reactions act in a positive feedback manner to form a large quantity of product. The fundamental reaction in clotting is conversion of soluble plasma protein fibrinogen into insoluble fibrin.
    Coagulation occurs by two pathways: (1) intrinsic pathway and (2) extrinsic pathway. The final step is conversion of prothrombin to thrombin. Thrombin converts soluble fibrinogen into insoluble fibrin threads, which form the clot.

12. **Name the clotting pathway involved in capillary tube method.**
    Intrinsic pathway of coagulation is involved since blood comes in contact with water wettable surface like glass.

13. **What is the effect of body temperature on bleeding time?**
    Bleeding time will be prolonged when body temperature is more than normal. This is because the vessels are in a dilated state at high temperature to increase heat loss and it will take longer time for the vessels to constrict and stop bleeding.

14. **What is zero time?**
    The time of puncture of the skin to estimate bleeding time is called zero time. Bleeding time is calculated from zero time to the time when there is no stain in the filter paper.

15. **How will you find out the bleeding time if stopwatch is not available?**
    Note the time of prick and mark it as zero time. After every 30 seconds gently touch the bleeding site with filter paper and continue this till there is no blood stain in the filter paper. Each blood stain in the filter paper represents 30 seconds of blood flow from the site of prick. Count the total number of blood stains on the filter paper and multiply it with ½. This gives the bleeding time in minutes.

16. **Which are the steps in coagulation that do not require calcium ions?**
    Conversion of factors XII and XI to their active forms and conversion of fibrinogen to fibrin monomer do not require calcium ions.

17. **Even if Ca^{2+} is necessary for coagulation, calcium deficiency does not produce coagulation defects. Why?**
    Only traces of Ca^{2+} are necessary for coagulation. When there is severe hypocalcemia it produces other symptoms like tetany, convulsions etc., before it affects coagulation.

18. **Name few conditions where bleeding time is prolonged but clotting time normal.**
    Thrombocytopenia, thrombasthenia, von Willebrand disease, vitamin C deficiency, following treatment with large doses of aspirin, corticosteroids; purpura due to vessel wall defects, increased body temperature, etc.

19. **What is purpura?**
    Purpura is a condition characterized by petechial hemorrhage into the skin, mucous membrane and internal organs due to capillary abnormality or abnormality of platelets.

20. **Name the conditions where bleeding time is normal but clotting time prolonged.**
    Hemophilia, liver diseases like cirrhosis, obstructive jaundice, vitamin K deficiency, anticoagulant overdose, and following blood transfusion with citrated blood.

21. **Name the blood tests done to assess platelet function.**
    » Platelet count
    » Bleeding time
    » Clotting time
    » Clot retraction time
    » Platelet aggregation and adhesiveness tests

22. **What is the difference between hemostasis and homeostasis?**
    Hemostasis is arrest of bleeding when there is injury to blood vessel. Homeostasis is maintaining a constant internal environment (milieu interior). Hemostasis is an essential component of homeostasis.

23. **Explain the test done in purpura to assess the integrity of blood vessels.**
    Capillary fragility test of Hess or tourniquet test:
    This test is done to assess the integrity of the blood vessels, i.e., the ability of the capillaries to withstand increased stress. The blood pressure cuff is tied in the arm and is kept inflated to a pressure of 100 mm Hg for about 5 minutes. If more than 10 petechial hemorrhages appear in the forearm there is defect in the integrity of blood vessels as in vasculitis.

24. **What is thrombocytopenia? Name a few conditions.**
    Decrease in the number of platelets from normal is called thrombocytopenia. In thrombocytopenia, bleeding time is prolonged when platelet count is less than 1 lakh/mm^3 of blood, easy bruising occurs when the platelet count is less than 50,000/mm^3 and spontaneous bleeding occur when the count is less than 20,000/mm^3 of blood. It is seen in infections like dengue fever, autoimmunity, hypersplenism, etc.

25. **Explain purpura.**
    Purpura is defined as small purple bleeding spots under the skin or mucous membrane due to hemorrhage from small blood vessels. It can be due to platelet defects or vascular defects (**Fig. 16.3**).

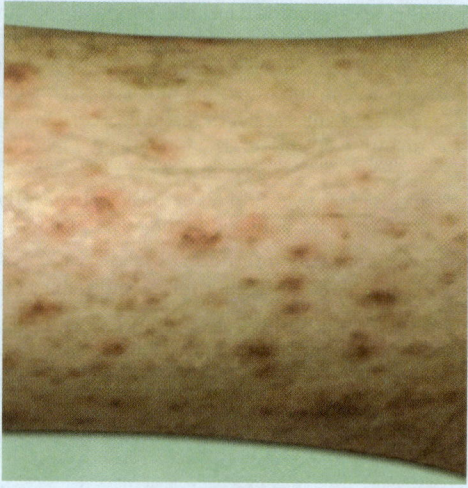

Fig. 16.3: Purpura.

» *Primary thrombocytopenic purpura or idiopathic thrombocytopenic purpura* (ITP) may be due to autoimmunity (antibodies are produced against platelets) or it may be hereditary or congenital, which usually occurs in children. Splenectomy (removal of spleen) is done in severe cases of primary thrombocytopenic purpura.
» *Secondary thrombocytopenic purpura* may be due to drugs, infections, bone marrow depression, leukemia and hypersplenism. In hypersplenism, there will be increased destruction of platelets in the spleen.

Thrombasthenic purpura: It is due to abnormal platelets in circulation. Here, the platelet count is normal, but there is defect in platelet adhesion and aggregation. This condition can also be due to abnormal functioning of platelets as in leukemia, von Willebrand disease, etc.
Vascular defects like vasculitis, drugs like steroids, severe sun exposure, cytomegalovirus infection etc. can lead to purpura. This is called **non-thrombocytopenic purpura**.

26. **What is the difference between thrombus and embolus?**
    Damage to the endothelium of blood vessels will expose the underlying collagen. Platelets stick to this collagen through vWF and platelet become activated and finally a platelet plug will be formed. Clotting occurs simultaneously and this clot is called **thrombus**. Formation of thrombus is called thrombosis.
    Sometimes the thrombus gets detached from the vessel wall and gets carried through the blood stream and this clot is called **embolus**. Air bubbles, fat from broken bones, tissue debris, etc., transported through blood are also called emboli. Emboli originating in arteries may get lodged in small arteries of vital organs like coronary vessels and leads to conditions like myocardial infarction. If the embolus originates from a vein, it reaches the lungs and cause pulmonary embolism.

Chapter 17: Determination of Blood Group

LEARNING OBJECTIVES

- Determine the blood group using anti-A, anti-B and anti-D sera
- Describe the significance of determination of blood group
- List the different blood group systems
- State Landsteiner's laws
- The indications of blood transfusion
- Explain the hazards of blood transfusion
- Explain the concept of universal donor and universal recipient
- Describe the principle of cross matching
- Importance of other blood group systems
- Describe the inheritance of ABO and Rh blood group systems
- Describe major and minor cross matching
- Explain the pathophysiology of erythroblastosis fetalis
- What are the changes that occur in the blood during storage?
- What is autologous transfusion?

PY2.11: Estimate hemoglobin, red blood cell count, total leukocyte count, RBC indices, differential leukocyte count, blood groups, BT/CT.
PY2.9: Describe different blood groups and discuss the clinical importance of blood grouping, blood banking and transfusion.

PRINCIPLE

There are more than 300 blood group systems but ABO and Rh systems are of importance since these are inherited characters that give rise to antigen-antibody reaction. The red cells contain different types of antigens (agglutinogens) and plasma contains antibodies (agglutinins). To determine the blood group of a subject, the red cells of the subject are allowed to react with sera containing known antibody.

APPARATUS

Glass slides, 0.9% saline, antiserum A, B and D, glass-marking pencil. In order to identify the sera, anti-'A' serum is given a **blue color** by adding patent blue and anti-'B' serum is **yellow** in color by adding tartrazine. The coloring agents have no other function. Anti-'D' serum is colorless **(Fig. 17.1)**.

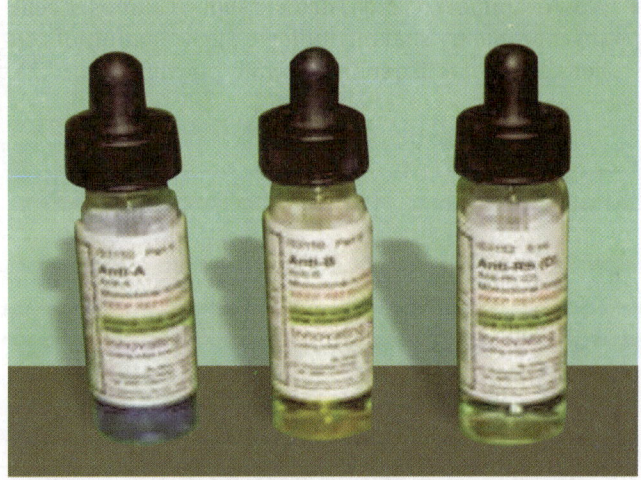

Fig. 17.1: Anti-A (blue), anti-B (yellow) and anti-D (colorless) sera.

PROCEDURE

- Take four glass slides and label them with glass marking pencil as A, B, D and C.
- A red cell suspension is prepared. In a China dish take 3 mL of 0.9 % saline and a drop of fresh capillary blood

from the person whose blood group is to be determined. A red cell suspension (i.e., 1–2 volumes of cells per 100 volumes of saline) of cells is thus made. Mix the blood and the saline gently and thoroughly.
- Place anti-'A' serum on the slide labeled A. Anti-'A' serum is obtained from the blood of a person belonging to the blood group B; and anti-'B' serum from an A group person.
- With a separate clean and dry pipette place anti-B serum on the slide labeled B.
- Place anti-D serum on the slide labeled D.
- With another clean and dry pipette place a drop of 0.9% saline on the slide labeled C that acts as the control.
- Now add one drop of the red cell suspension of the unknown blood to each of the antiserum on the three slides and to the saline on the slide C.
- The dropper should not touch the serum.
- Mix the cells and the serum by rocking and tilting or by mixing with three separate glass rods.
- Wait for 6–10 minutes.
- Examine each slide after 6 minutes. Compare with the slide labelled C. The antigen-antibody reaction may not be complete before 6 minutes.

OBSERVATIONS

- Examination is carried out both by the naked eye and under simple microscope. A hand lens can also be used.
- First examine slide C. It should not show any clumping. Rarely rouleaux formation may be present. It can be differentiated from clumping by shaking the slide. The cells will separate if it is rouleaux.
- Now examine A, B and D marked slides. Clumps of cells inseparable by shaking indicate agglutination of red cells. It appears like sprinkled chilly powder (**Fig. 17.2**).
- Confirm the results using a hand lens or observe under a simple microscope.
- Clumping in the three slides indicates presence of both agglutinogens (antigens) in the red cells, i.e., the cells belong to blood group AB and is Rh positive.
- Clumping in the slide labeled 'A' indicates the presence of 'A' agglutinogen in the red cell membrane and the blood group is A.
- Clumping in the slide labeled B indicates the presence of 'B' agglutinogen in the cells and the blood group is B.
- Absence of clumping in all the three slides indicates absence of 'A', 'B' and 'D' agglutinogens and the blood group is O negative. If agglutination is present in the slide marked D, but absent in the other slides the blood group is O positive.
- Clumping in the slide labeled D indicates presence of 'D' antigen in the red blood cell and the person is Rh positive.
- If there is no clumping in slide D, the person is Rh negative (**Fig. 17.3**).

DISCUSSION

Landsteiner in 1900 first classified people into four groups; A, B, AB and O. The antigens present in the red cell membrane are called **agglutinogens** and the antibodies against them present in the plasma are called **agglutinins**. The agglutinogen is present not only in the red blood cells but also in the tissue cells and their secretions. Such persons whose secretions contain blood group antigens are called secretors. They inherit the secretory gene. Those who do not inherit the secretor gene are non-secretors and their secretions do not contain the blood group antigens.

The ABO System

The A, B and the O antigens are mucopolysaccharides. A group people have 'A' agglutinogen in their red blood cells and the 'beta' agglutinin in their plasma. B group people have 'B' agglutinogen in their cells and the 'alpha' agglutinin in their plasma. AB group people have both 'A' and 'B' agglutinogens on their red cells and no alpha and beta agglutinins in their plasma. O group people have no A and B agglutinogens, but only 'H' agglutinogen in their cells. Their plasma contains both the alpha and beta agglutinins.

The Rh System

Three pairs of alleles 'Cc', 'Dd' and 'Ee' exist and their combinations make several blood groups in the Rh system. The terms Rh positive and Rh negative are based upon the presence or absence of the 'D' agglutinogen. This agglutinogen is highly antigenic, i.e., it can evoke a high

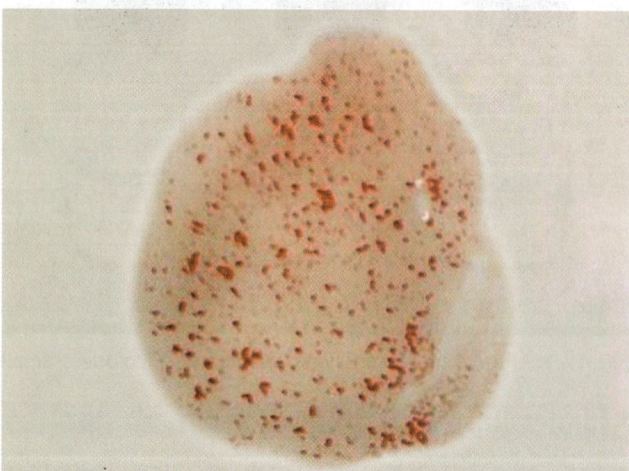

Fig. 17.2: Slide showing agglutination of RBCs (note the sprinkled red chilly powder appearance).

Chapter 17: Determination of Blood Group

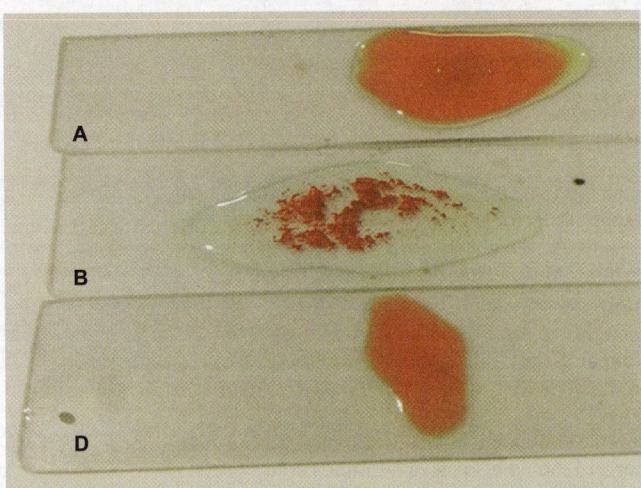

Fig. 17.3: Since there is agglutination only in slide B the blood group of this individual is B negative. Slide B contains anti-B serum (α-antibodies); it leads to agglutination of red cells which contains B antigens on their membrane. Slide A contains anti-A serum and slide D contains anti-D antibodies. Since there is no agglutination in these two slides the person is not A group and is not Rh positive.

antibody titer, when injected into a person not having the 'D' agglutinogen (Rh-negative person).

When an Rh-negative mother conceives an Rh-positive child; the Rh antigen may enter the mother's body through the placenta and immunize her. The Rh-antibodies are developed in her plasma. These Rh antibodies cross the placenta and combine with the Rh antigen in the baby's red cells and cause hemolysis. Various hemolytic diseases of the newborns, abortions and sterility in females have been attributed to this cause. Antigenic reactions are usually associated with the antigen D.

Rh-positive blood transfusion should never be given to an Rh-negative woman who is in the childbearing age. This will make her sensitive to Rh antigen and if she become pregnant with Rh positive babies she will lose all her babies. Rh-positive transfusion is likely to produce severe hemolytic reactions if given for a second time to an Rh-negative person.

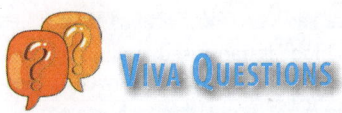

Viva Questions

1. **What is the importance of blood group determination?**
   Besides blood transfusion and Rh incompatibility, knowledge of blood groups is very important for the following purposes:
   » Study of human genetics
   » In cases of disputed paternity
   » Anthropology, i.e., to study of origin and development of man
   » Association and proneness to diseases; e.g., in 'A' group people, the incidence of pernicious anemia and diabetes mellitus is more than in others. Group A people also tend to suffer from gastric carcinoma more than group O people; while group O people show a greater tendency to suffer from duodenal ulcer.

2. **What is blood transfusion? What are its indications?**
   Collecting blood from a healthy person and injecting it into the vein of another person who needs blood is called blood transfusion. The person who donates blood is called a donor and the person who receives it is called the recipient. In conditions like hemorrhage, shock and anemia blood transfusion is a lifesaving procedure.

3. **What are the various components of blood?**
   » Packed red cells
   » Platelet concentrate
   » Buffy coat
   » Plasma
   » Cryoprecipitate (contains mainly factor VIII and fibrinogen)
   » Plasma protein solution (PPS).

4. **How is blood stored in blood bank?**
   Optimum storage temperature for whole blood is 4 ± 2°C. Anticoagulants usually used are acid-citrate-dextrose (ACD)—15 mL/100 mL of blood or citrate phosphate dextrose (CPD) solution. It can be stored for 3 weeks. Plasma stored at 4°C can be preserved for 1–2 years. Powdered plasma can be stored for 10 years. Blood banks are now referred to as centers of transfusion medicine.
   Stored blood is not suitable in cases of WBC and platelet deficiency because blood stored for more than 24 hours contains no viable leukocytes and platelets.

5. **What is the composition of ACD?**
   » Acid citrate—0.48 g
   » Trisodium citrate—1.32 g
   » Dextrose—1.47 g
   » Distilled water to make up the volume to 100 mL

6. **What is preservation injury?**
   During preservation of blood, certain defects occur in blood collectively called preservation injuries. It includes:
   » Loss of ATP.
   » Decrease in 2,3-DPG in RBC, i.e., shift to left of oxygen dissociation curve.
   » Hyperkalemia due to leaking out of K^+ from RBC into plasma. Plasma potassium concentration increases to 20–30 mEq/L by 2 weeks of storage.
   » Increase in intracellular Na^+ concentration to 30–40 mEq/L, which leads to increased cell size and increased fragility.
   » Concentration of the coagulation factors decrease on storage, especially factor VIII.
   » Decrease in pH due to formation of lactic acid.
   » Citrate toxicity leads to hypocalcemia. Ca^{2+} is precipitated as calcium citrate and ionic calcium level falls.

7. **What are the precautions to be taken during blood transfusion?**
   » Blood transfusion is indicated only in cases of loss of blood and anemia.
   » The donor should be healthy and diseases like syphilis, malaria, hepatitis, AIDS, etc., should be excluded before collecting blood.
   » 350–500 mL of blood can be donated at a time depending upon the body weight. People weighing less than 45 kg are exempted.
   » PCV and Hb should be within the normal range.
   » The blood should be collected, preserved and transfused using sterile equipment and with complete aseptic precautions.
   » After bleeding, the donor should be asked to take rest for an hour and should be given a nutritious drink.
   » 480 mL of blood is mixed with 120 mL of an anticoagulant mixture called acid-citrate-dextrose (ACD).
   » The blood is stored in this form at 4°C. It can be used for about 21 days if kept under aseptic conditions.
   » Before blood transfusion is done, a cross matching should be undertaken even if the donor and the recipient belong to the same blood group.

8. **What are the complications of blood transfusion?**
   Complications are divided into *hemolytic reactions* and *nonhemolytic reactions*. Hemolytic reactions are due to incompatible blood transfusion and it leads to agglutination and destruction of red blood cells with release of hemoglobin.
   Nonhemolytic reactions include fever, shivering, etc., if the transfusion set is not sterile. Excess transfusion of whole blood may lead to volume over load and cardiac failure. Hyperkalemia is seen when stored blood is transfused. If not properly tested, transfusion leads to spread of infectious diseases like AIDS, hepatitis, syphilis, malaria, etc.

9. **What is autologous transfusion or predonation?**
   In elective surgeries, blood is collected from the same patient a few weeks before surgery and this blood is transfused during surgery. This is called autologous transfusion or predonation. This helps to avoid transmission of diseases from another person as well as the risk of transfusion reaction.

10. **What is erythroblastosis fetalis?**
    If an Rh-negative mother carries an Rh-positive fetus, during delivery and in rare cases during pregnancy, some amount of fetal blood leaks into the maternal circulation. The Rh-positive RBCs will stimulate the production of anti-Rh antibodies in the mother. The antibodies belong to IgG type, which can cross the placenta and enter the fetal circulation. These antibodies cause agglutination of fetal RBCs leading to hemolysis and the condition is called hemolytic disease of newborn (HDN). Since there is increased destruction of red cells, there is increased erythropoiesis and large number of blast cells will be present in fetal blood and it is hence called erythroblastosis fetalis. Other manifestations include hydrops fetalis, kernicterus, etc.

11. **How can you prevent HDN?**
    Immediately after delivery of an Rh-positive baby by an Rh-negative mother, she should be given an injection of anti-D antibodies. These antibodies will destroy the Rh-positive fetal red cells that have entered the mother's circulation before these cells can sensitize the mother to produce antibodies against the Rh antigen.

12. **ABO incompatibility is rare during pregnancy. Why?**
    The α and β antibodies of the ABO system belong to IgM type and they cannot cross the placenta because of their large size. So they are less likely to produce hemolytic reactions in the fetus even if there is ABO incompatibility between mother and fetus.

13. **If an Rh-positive mother carries an Rh-negative baby usually no complications occur. Why?**
    Even if some amount of mother's Rh-positive blood leaks into the fetal circulation during pregnancy as in conditions like placental insufficiency, the Rh antigen cannot stimulate the production of antibodies in the fetus because the fetus does not have the capacity to produce antibodies. The ability to produce antibodies develops only few weeks after birth. Moreover, normally, maternal RBCs do not cross the placenta.

14. **Why is cell suspension used instead of whole blood in determining blood group?**
    Cell suspension is used because:
    » Dilution of cells allows easy detection of clumping when present.
    » Plasma factors, likely to interfere with agglutination are diluted.

15. **What is cross matching? What are the types?**
    » Mixing the donor's cells with the recipient's plasma and look for agglutination (major cross matching).
    » Mixing the recipient's cells with the donor's plasma (minor cross matching).

16. **What is the advantage of carrying out the test for determining blood group by test tube method?**
    The test can also be carried out in small test tubes. The advantage of using test tubes is that, in cases of doubt, the test tubes are centrifuged for one minute. The cells will sediment. The tubes are then shaken. If agglutination has not occurred, the cells disperse and form an even suspension. If agglutination has occurred red particles of clumps are clearly observed.

17. **Even though there are several blood group systems, only ABO system and Rh system are taken into consideration before every blood transfusion. Why?**
    This is because the agglutinogens of these systems are highly antigenic. The MN system and P system of agglutinogens are peculiar because of their inability to evoke agglutinins in human beings. These blood groups are therefore usually ignored for blood transfusion purposes.

18. **Blood group 'O' is regarded as the universal donor even though it contains anti-A and anti-B antibodies. Why?**
    During transfusion a comparatively small quantity of blood (about 450 mL) from the donor is mixed with a large quantity (about 4,000 to 5,000 mL) of the recipient's blood. The donor's plasma that contains the antibodies is thus diluted in the recipient's blood and the agglutinins present in the transfused blood therefore fail to act on the red cells of the recipient.

19. **What is dangerous 'O' group?**
    In some O group individuals, the antibody titer (α and β antibodies) will be very high and this may lead to agglutination of the recipient's red blood cells if he is not belonging to O group. This can be prevented by cross matching before blood transfusion.

20. **State Landsteiner's laws.**
    » Landsteiner's **first law** states that *if an antigen is present on the RBC membrane, the corresponding antibody will be absent in the plasma*.
    » Landsteiner's **second law** states that *if an antigen is absent on the RBC membrane, the corresponding antibody will be present in the plasma*. Thus, type A blood contains anti-B antibody, type B contains anti-A antibody, AB group contains no antibodies and type O contains both anti-A and anti-B antibodies in plasma. Second law is not applicable to the Rh system.

21. **What is Bombay group?**
    If the genotype is hh, the precursor substance remains as such and H antigen is not formed. Even if the person has genes coding for A or B antigen, these antigens are not formed because H antigen (H-Ag) is the substrate for A and B antigens. They may be genetically A or B or AB group. These people without H-Ag who are grouped under O group due to the absence of A or B antigens are called Bombay group or Bombay phenotype. As A, B or H antigens are absent on the RBC membrane of the Bombay group people, their plasma contains anti-A (α), anti-B (β) and anti-H antibodies according to Landsteiner's first law.
    Due to the presence of all the antibodies, especially anti-H antibodies, these people cannot be transfused with any other blood other than Bombay group. Frequency of Bombay phenotype in India is 1:13,000.

22. **Describe the inheritance of blood group systems?**
    The position of a gene on a chromosome is called its locus. Every individual has a locus on each of the paired chromosomes for a gene of the ABO system. A person belonging to blood group 'A' (phenotype-A) may have the corresponding 'A' genes on both the loci, i.e., genotype-AA, a homozygous individual; or he may have 'A' gene on one chromosome and 'O' gene on the other one of the homologous pair, i.e., genotype-AO, a heterozygous individual. The 'A' gene is described as dominant and the 'O' gene as recessive and so the phenotype will be A. B group individuals have genotype BB or BO and phenotype B. The genes received by him from his father and mother determine the genotype of an individual. The phenotype is determined by the dominant of the two genes. The genotype 'AA' individual can have children all of whom possess 'A' gene ('A' is dominant); while the genotype 'AO' individual may have children, 50% of whom possess 'A' gene and 50% 'O' gene. A person having blood group AB, has 'A' gene on one locus and 'B' gene on the locus of the other chromosome of the pair and the phenotype will be AB since both genes are dominant. O group individuals do not possess either A gene or B gene on the paired chromosomes. They have only O gene.
    Three pairs of alleles 'Cc', 'Dd' and 'Ee' exist and their combinations make several blood groups in the Rh system. The terms Rh-positive and Rh-negative are based upon the presence or absence of the 'D' agglutinogen because it is highly antigenic.

23. **What is the difference between rouleaux and agglutination?**
    Rouleaux formation is a reversible phenomenon. It is due to temporary attachment of RBCs at their broad surface when there is stagnation of blood flow. Agglutination is due to antigen antibody reaction and is irreversible and leads to hemolysis.

24. **Mention the source of antibodies for blood group determination.**
    Normal blood donors are used as the source of supply of naturally occurring antibodies, such as those of ABO systems. Antibodies for the Coombs serum are obtained from rabbits. Monoclonal antibodies to blood groups produced by hybridomas are in use. Mouse hybridomas produce anti-A and anti-B monoclonal antibodies.

25. **What are cold and warm antibodies?**
    Since antibodies of the ABO system work best at temperatures below the body temperature, they are known as cold agglutinins. Antibodies of Rh system react with antigens best at body temperature. Hence they are called warm antibodies.

26. **Now we do not use the terms universal donor and universal recipient. Why?**
    These terms are not valid because it is applicable only to ABO blood group system. But there are other blood group systems like Rh system which can produce incompatibility and reactions. So cross matching is a must before any blood transfusion.

Section 2: Clinical Examination

18. General Examination
19. Physical Examination
20. Determination of Arterial Blood Pressure
21. Examination of the Respiratory System
22. Examination of Cardiovascular System
23. Recording of Arterial Pulse
24. Examination of Abdomen
25. Examination of Nervous System
26. Examination of the Sensory System
27. Examination of Motor System
28. Examination of the Cranial Nerves
29. Examination of Reflexes

Chapter 18

General Examination

LEARNING OBJECTIVES

- The student should communicate with the subject or patient properly
- Take a relevant history
- Do a proper general examination in a volunteer

PY11.13: Obtain history and perform general examination in the volunteer/simulated environment.

INTRODUCTION

General examination of the subject is the examination of the general state of the subject. It is done before examining a particular system because general examination if done along with a properly elicited history, gives an idea about the system which is most affected. It also gives an idea about the physical condition of the subject. The personal details of the subject should be recorded first like name, age, sex, occupation and address. Some conditions like lead poisoning, asbestosis, silicosis, etc., may be related to the patient's occupation. Inhalation of asbestos for a long time leads to malignant mesothelioma, a tumor of the pleura. Address is also important since certain diseases like tuberculosis, filariasis, etc., may be endemic in that area.

General examination should be done in the presence of good daylight rather than artificial light with the subject relaxed. Change in skin color as in mild jaundice is difficult to recognize in artificial light. While examining, the right handed examiner should stand on the right side of the subject since it is easier to examine the jugular veins, apex beat, etc., in this position.

General examination includes the following:
- Overall appearance
- Posture and gait
- Build and nourishment
- Height and weight
- Look for anemia (pallor), jaundice (icterus), cyanosis, clubbing, lymphadenopathy and edema
- Examination of skin and hair
- Pulse
- Blood pressure
- Jugular venous pressure
- Respiratory rate
- Body temperature

Overall Appearance, Posture and Gait

See whether the subject look well, mildly ill or severely ill. Posture and gait can be assessed as the subject walks into the room.

Build and Nourishment

Observe whether the subject is well built and well nourished. Assess the skeletal framework of the subject and compare it with the normal for his age. See whether he is well built, moderately built or ill built and report. Noting whether he is lean or stout can assess nourishment. Calculate the body mass index (BMI) using the formula:

$$BMI = Weight\ in\ kg/Height\ in\ m^2$$

Those who are suffering from malnutrition, loss of appetite (anorexia), diseases that lead to weight loss like malignancies, tuberculosis, etc., will be ill built. Features of poor nutrition include cracked skin, loss of hair, poor wound healing and edema. Glossitis (inflammation of tongue with loss of papillae) and angular stomatitis (cracking of angles of mouth) suggest vitamin B and iron deficiency.

Height and Weight

Height is measured in centimeters and weight in kilogram. The average height of an adult male is about 170 cm and that of female is 160 cm. Weight of an adult male ranges between 55–75 kg and female between 45–65 kg. By calculating the body mass index (BMI), obesity can be ruled out. If obese note it down.

Anemia (Pallor)

Anemia is pallor of skin and mucous membrane due to reduction in the hemoglobin content of blood. Observe the color of the lower palpebral conjunctiva **(Fig. 18.1)**. Normally it will be red. If it is pale it suggests anemia. The color of gums can also be noted in fair skinned individuals. Other areas to look for anemia include nail bed, palm and sole. If the palmar crease color is lighter than the surrounding skin when the hand is hyperextended, it indicates a hemoglobin level less than 7 g/100 mL of blood.

Anemia can be due to decreased production of red blood cells as in deficiency anemia, bone marrow suppression; or it can be due to increased RBC destruction as in hemolytic anemia; or it can be due to acute blood loss as in accidents, chronic blood loss due to hookworm infestation and bleeding piles.

Jaundice (Icterus)

Yellowish discoloration of skin, mucous membrane and sclera due to increase in the amount of bilirubin in blood (more than 2 mg/100 mL of blood) is called icterus **(Fig. 18.2)**. The upper sclera, under aspect of tongue, skin, and nails are observed for yellowish discoloration in good sunlight. Icterus can be missed if the patient is examined in artificial light.

Bilirubin specifically stains elastic fibers and sclera contains plenty of elastic fibers. Elevate the upper eyelids

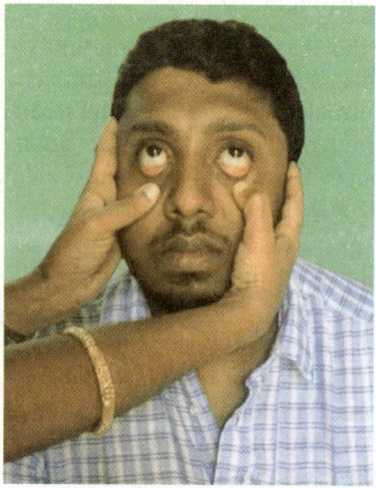

Fig. 18.1: Looking for anemia in the conjunctiva.

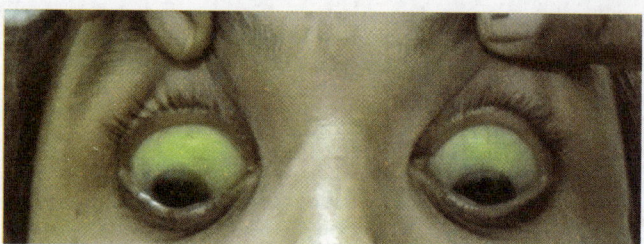

Fig. 18.2: Jaundice (note the yellowish discoloration of sclera).

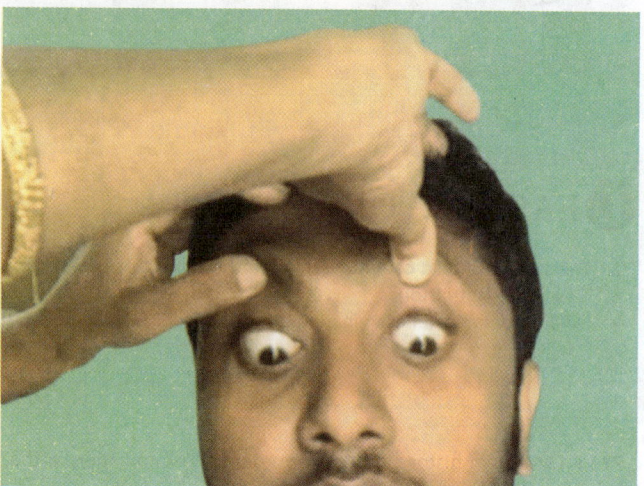

Fig. 18.3: Looking for icterus (jaundice) of eyes.

and ask the subject to look down to see the upper sclera clearly **(Fig. 18.3)**. Scleral icterus indicates a serum bilirubin more than 2.5 mg/dL.

Jaundice can be due to increased hemolysis (hemolytic or prehepatic jaundice) when the color will be lemon yellow; or it can be due to liver diseases like hepatitis, cirrhosis, etc. (hepatocellular jaundice) where the color will be orange yellow; or it can be due to obstruction of the biliary system (posthepatic or obstructive jaundice), the color will be greenish yellow. Normal bilirubin content of blood is 0.2–1.2 mg/dL. Yellowish discoloration of skin is also seen in carotinemia as in hypothyroidism, but here the sclera will not be stained yellow.

Cyanosis

Bluish discoloration of skin and mucous membrane due to increase in the concentration of reduced hemoglobin above 5 g/100 mL of capillary blood is cyanosis. Cyanosis can be central cyanosis or peripheral cyanosis. Central cyanosis is due to defective oxygenation of blood in the lungs or due to right to left shunt in the heart. Peripheral cyanosis is due to stagnation of blood in the periphery especially when exposed to cold. The cyanosed extremity will be cold and tongue is unaffected in peripheral cyanosis.

Observe the tongue and lips for central cyanosis; and the fingertip, tip of nose, ear lobes, nail bed and toes for peripheral cyanosis **(Fig. 18.4)**. The extremities will be

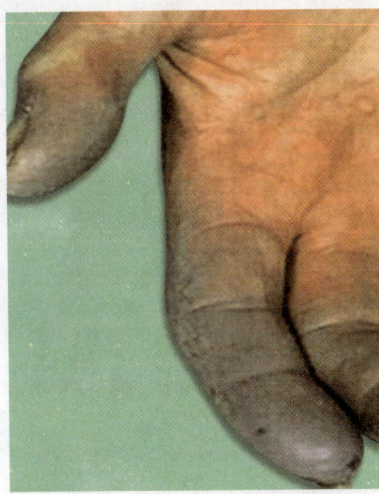

Fig. 18.4: Peripheral cyanosis.

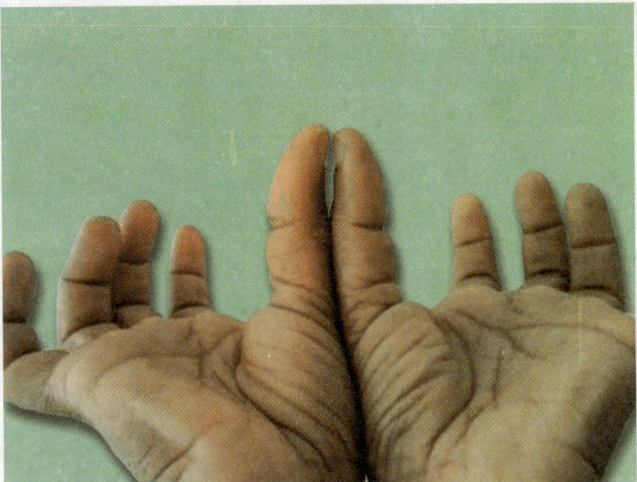

Fig. 18.5: Looking for clubbing of fingers (Shamroth's sign).

warm in central cyanosis but it will be cold in peripheral cyanosis. Cyanosis is not present in severe anemia because at least 5 g/dL of reduced hemoglobin is necessary to produce central cyanosis and the hemoglobin content in the anemic patient will be very less.

Methemoglobinemia, sulfhemoglobinemia, or carboxyhemoglobinemia may be mistaken for cyanosis. But in these conditions, patient will not be dyspneic.

Clubbing

Inspect the nail bed angle of the index finger by keeping the finger horizontally at the eye level of the examiner. Normally, the level of the proximal margins of the nail is slightly lower than that of the nail fold when examined from the side. There will be a rhomboid space between the two thumb nail beds when both the thumbs are kept against each other known as Shamroth's sign **(Fig. 18.5)**.

In certain conditions, the tissues in the nail bed and finger pulp hypertrophy giving rise to convexity of the nail and nail bed. This leads to obliteration of the angle between the nail and the skin at the root of the nail in the fingers and toes and is called clubbing **(Fig. 18.6)**. Hyperplasia of the soft tissues beneath the nail is usually due to chronic hypoxia. The tip of fingers and toes appear to be club shaped or drum stick shaped in advanced cases. When clubbing occurs, the Shamroth's sign disappears.

Clubbing is seen in chronic lung diseases like chronic obstructive pulmonary disease (COPD), lung cancer, pulmonary interstitial fibrosis, bronchiectasis, lung abscess; cardiac conditions like congenital cyanotic heart disease, subacute bacterial endocarditis (SABE), etc.

Lymphadenopathy

Lymph nodes should be gently palpated by a circular motion of the fingertips and slowly increase the pressure. Examine

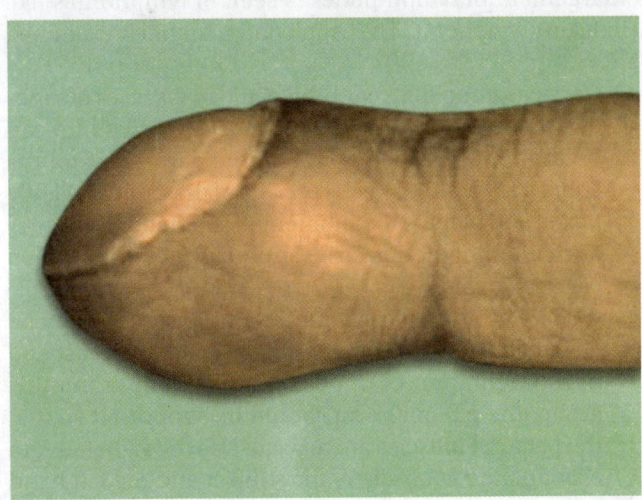

Fig. 18.6: Clubbing of finger (note the obliteration of the nail bed angle).

the cervical and axillary nodes with the subject in the sitting posture and the abdominal and inguinal nodes in the supine position. Palpate one group of nodes on one side and then palpate the corresponding group on the opposite side. See whether there is enlargement and tenderness of the various lymph nodes. In the majority of the healthy individuals the glands are not palpable. In some, the glands may be palpable with difficulty and in few others, their presence could be very easily felt. If a particular group of node is palpable, it is always associated with some evident sign of disease in the part examined. The lymph nodes that drain a particular organ or tissue will be affected if there is some pathology in that part.

Determine the size, position, consistency, mobility, and tenderness of the different groups of lymph nodes. The enlarged lymph nodes will be tender if there is infection of the part being drained, whereas malignant lymphadenopathy is usually non-tender. Generalized

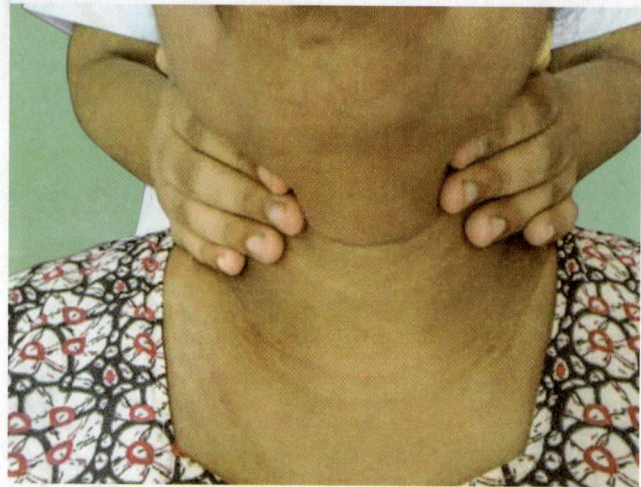

Fig. 18.7: Examination of cervical lymph nodes.

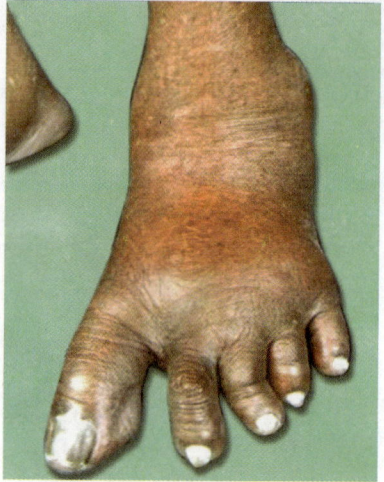

Fig. 18.8: Edema of dorsum of foot.

enlargement of lymph nodes is seen in lymphomas like Hodgkin's lymphoma. The lymph nodes routinely examined are:

- Cervical group that may be affected in diseases of lungs like tuberculosis, lung cancer, etc. Cervical group can be examined properly by standing at the back of the subject **(Fig. 18.7)**. Keep the neck of the subject slightly flexed and palpate the submental, submandibular, pre-auricular, jugulodigastric, supraclavicular and deep cervical nodes.
- Axillary group (apical, anterior and posterior) may be affected in diseases of breast like cancer of breast and in inflammation of upper limb. For examining this group, the patient's arm should be supported so that the pectoral muscles are relaxed. Use the right hand to examine the left axilla of the subject and the left hand to examine the right axilla. Palpate for the nodes in the apex of the axilla and slide the fingers downwards against the chest wall to feel for lymphadenopathy. Then examine the inside of the anterior and posterior axillary folds to feel the pectoral and subscapular lymph nodes.
- Epitrochlear glands is usually affected in leprosy.
- Inguinal group, which may be affected in conditions affecting the lower limbs, anal canal, external genitalia, buttocks and lower vagina.
- Popliteal nodes are examined by palpating deep in the popliteal fossa with the knee flexed using both hands of the examiner.

Edema

Edema is collection of excess fluid in the extracellular space. The skin will be swollen and shiny and the normal wrinkles will be obliterated **(Fig. 18.8)**. If the person is bed ridden edema is seen in the back especially over the presacral region. If he is ambulant, edema occurs in the lower extremities especially in the dorsum of feet and around the ankle joint.

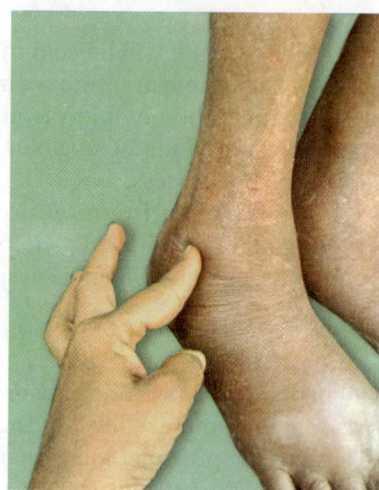

Fig. 18.9: Looking for pitting edema over the lateral malleolus.

Apply moderate pressure with the flat of the thumb for 30 seconds on the skin especially over a bony area (shin of tibia, medial or lateral malleolus, dorsum of foot, sacrum) and see whether there is pitting **(Fig. 18.9)**. If a pit appears in the area, it is pitting edema. Pit is formed due to displacement of fluid from the area of pressure. If a depression is not formed over the edematous area on applying pressure, it is non-pitting edema. **Pitting edema (Fig. 18.10)** is seen in hypoproteinemia as in malnutrition and nephrotic syndrome, in inflammatory conditions, congestive cardiac failure (CCF) etc. **Non-pitting edema** is seen in late filariasis and in myxedema. **Anasarca** refers to gross generalized edema.

Skin, Hair and Nails

Examine the exposed skin and look for temperature, hydration, color, discoloration like hypopigmentation, hyperpigmentation, cyanosis; cutaneous eruptions, etc. The skin will be dry, rough, thick and yellowish in hypothyroidism.

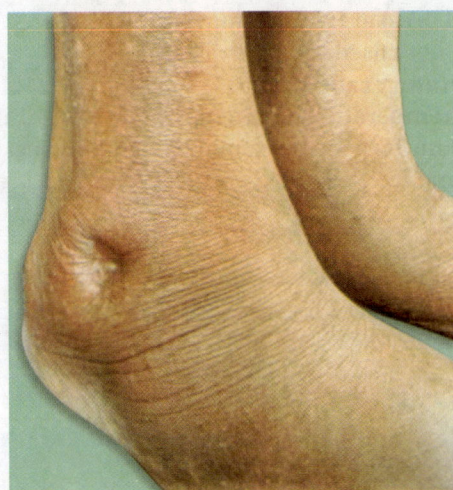

Fig. 18.10: Pitting edema in a patient with cardiac failure. Note the depression formed over the edema after firm fingertip pressure is applied.

It will be moist and warm in hyperthyroidism. Localized warmth of skin is seen if there is regional inflammation. Hypopigmented patches should be examined thoroughly to rule out leprosy. Purpura if present should be noted. Color, texture and distribution of hair should also be noted. Hirsutism (increased facial hair) is observed in females with glucocorticoid excess. Examine the nails and see if it is normal. Report if they are discolored, brittle or if there is clubbing or koilonychia.

Pulse

Pulse is defined as the expansile wave transmitted from the aorta to the peripheral arteries due to intermittent ejection of blood from the left ventricle into the already full aorta. Palpate all the peripheral pulses like radial pulse, carotid pulse, femoral pulse, popliteal pulse, dorsalis pedis pulse and posterior tibial pulse. To find out the pulse rate the radial pulse is examined. The right radial pulse of the subject is palpated with the tip of index, middle and ring fingers of the left hand of the examiner. Rate, rhythm, character, volume and condition of the vessel wall are looked for. If the rhythm is regular, count the number of beats for 15 seconds and multiply it with 4 to get the pulse rate. Irregular and very slow pulses require palpation for a full minute. If cardiovascular disease is suspected, look for radio-femoral delay. See whether there is time lapse between the appearance of radial and femoral pulsations (for details refer examination of cardiovascular system).

Blood Pressure

Record the blood pressure in the sitting or lying down posture from the subject's arm or thigh using a sphygmomanometer. Standing BP should also be recorded to rule out orthostatic hypotension. First do the palpatory method and then the auscultatory method to avoid auscultatory gap. The manometer should be at the same level of the cuff on the subject's arm and the observer's eyes. Express the blood pressure as systolic pressure/diastolic pressure in mm of Hg (details of measurement of blood pressure is given in Chapter 20).

Jugular Venous Pressure (JVP)

The right internal jugular vein is observed with the subject inclined in bed at 45°. Note the upper level of jugular venous pulse. Normally the JVP is not visible above the clavicle. If visible in this position, JVP is raised. The vertical height from the sternal angle to the upper level of the venous pulse is measured in centimeters and is expressed as jugular venous pressure (refer page 119 and **Fig. 22.5**).

Respiratory Rate

Place the right palm of the examiner on the abdomen of the subject when he is relaxed and count the number of respiratory movements for one minute.

Temperature

Body temperature may be recorded in the mouth, axilla or rectum using a clinical thermometer with centigrade or Fahrenheit scale. Normal oral temperature varies between $37.2 \pm 0.5°C$. The rectal temperature (core temperature) will be 0.5°C higher and axillary temperature 0.5°C lower than oral temperature. In women ovulation is associated with 0.5°C rise in temperature due to the thermogenic action of progesterone.

Clean the thermometer with antiseptic solution. Shake it well so that the mercury column falls below the lower mark. To measure the oral temperature, the subject is asked to hold the thermometer under the tongue supported by the lips for 1–2 minutes. Lips should be closely shut and the subject should breathe through the nose. The subject should avoid hot or cold drinks immediately before taking the oral temperature. In the axilla, the skin should not be moist with perspiration.

Temperature is expressed in °C or °F indicating the site and time. For example, 37°C in the axilla at 11 am.

Normal Report Pattern of General Examination

Name:
Age: (Express in days, months or years)
Sex:
Occupation:
Address:

General Examination

- Moderately built and well nourished
- **Height:** 160 cm

- **Weight:** 60 kg
- No pallor, no icterus, no cyanosis, no clubbing of fingers or toes, and no edema
- No lymphadenopathy
- Skin, hair and nails are normal in appearance
- **Pulse:** 70/min, regular, normal in volume and character, no vessel wall thickening, no radiofemoral delay, all peripheral pulsations felt normally on both sides
- **Blood pressure:** 110/70 mm Hg
- JVP is not raised
- **Respiratory rate:** 15/min
- **Body temperature:** Oral temperature is 98.4°F at 10 am.

Impression: On general examination, the subject appears to be normal.

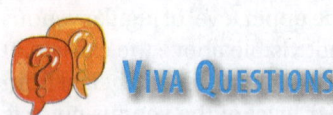

Viva Questions

1. **Why do you prefer natural light instead of artificial light?**
   General examination should be done in the presence of good daylight rather than artificial light with the subject relaxed. Change in skin color as in mild jaundice is difficult to recognize in artificial light.

2. **What is the significance of general examination?**
   Before any systemic examination a general physical examination should be carried out on the subject. This will give a clue regarding the systems that may be involved in the disease. Detailed general examination should be confined to the signs and symptoms the patient is having. For example, if he comes with complains of breathing difficulty a detailed general examination related to respiratory system should be done like respiratory rate, type of breathing, cyanosis, clubbing, cervical lympadenopathy, temperature, etc.

3. **Define anemia, cyanosis, edema and jaundice.**
   Refer page 94 and 96.

4. **Why is it advisable for the examiner to stand on the right side of the subject?**
   While examining, the right handed examiner should stand on the right side of the subject since it is easier to examine the jugular veins, apex beat, etc., in this position.

5. **The hands of the examiner should be warm while palpating. Give the reason.**
   The patient feels comfortable only while examining with a warm hand. The muscles beneath a cold hand will contract and the area becomes rigid making it difficult to get information regarding the underlying structures.

6. **Enumerate the conditions that should be followed before a clinical examination?**
   » Examine the subject in naturally well-lit room
   » Ask the subject to sit or lie in a comfortable relaxed position
   » Explain the procedure you are going to perform clearly to the subject in advance
   » If the subject is a female, and the examiner a male, always ask one relative or a female attender to be with the subject during the examination.
   » Always stand on the right side of the subject while examining if the examiner is right handed.
   » If complete exposure of the private parts of the body becomes necessary, cover the subject with a gown or blanket after examination.

Chapter 19

Physical Examination

LEARNING OBJECTIVES

- Evaluate the systemic examination of the subject by inspection, palpation, percussion and auscultation
- Discuss the rules of percussion

INTRODUCTION

The complaints of the patient about his illness like headache, nausea, etc., are called **symptoms**. On examining the subject, the doctor observes certain findings like pallor, jaundice, cyanosis, etc., those are called **signs**. A group of signs and symptoms appearing together is described as a **syndrome**. Examination of a sick patient is called **clinical examination or physical examination**. It includes the following aspects; inspection, palpation, percussion and auscultation, which are to be done in the correct sequential order.

INSPECTION

Inspection, i.e., observation should start as soon as the subject enters the room. Information like gait, physical attitude, etc., can be assessed by inspection only. Good daylight is ideal for inspection. For proper inspection, the body surface should be bare. The right and left sides of the body should always be compared with each other. During inspection if a particular finding is observed, the following points should be noted; the situation, size, shape, surface, i.e., the appearance of the skin overlying the area, movements as in respiratory movements, etc.

Active and reflex movements of the limbs, head, neck and face are studied systematically. A healthy person performs the necessary movements to assume a comfortable posture. Involuntary and purposeless movements are absent in health. Voluntary movements occurring at each joint have definite ranges in various directions. Limitation of movement and associated pain, or exaggeration of the ranges might occur in disease.

PALPATION

Palpation is examination by touching the subject gently. It is carried out by touching or feeling with the flat surface of fingers or palm of hands. The hands must be clean and the nails trimmed so that the patient is not harmed.

Place the right hand of the examiner flat on the body surface to be palpated **(Fig. 19.1)**. For the examination of the superficial structures, light pressure is sufficient which is called superficial palpation; for the examination of the deeper structures, sufficient pressure might be required which is called deep palpation. Ask the subject to relax before palpation so that the muscles will be lax.

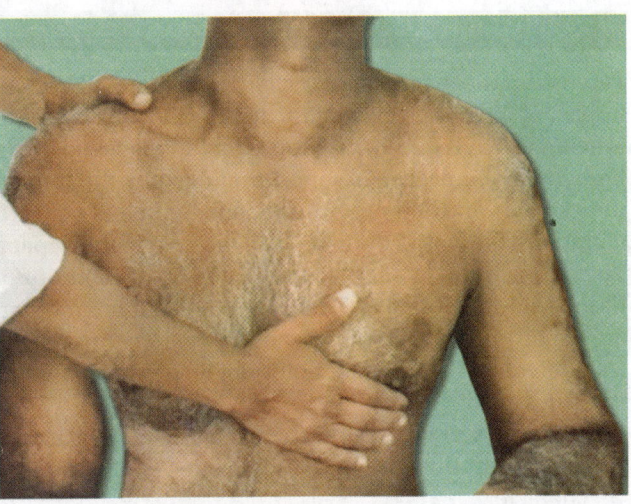

Fig. 19.1: Palpation of the chest.

During palpation the following are looked for:
- Temperature of the area to be examined is assessed by applying the back of the fingers to the surface of the subject's body.
- The findings obtained by inspection are verified during palpation. The flat of the palm is moved lightly on the surface to be examined. Presence of nodules is more accurately judged by palpation. For example, enlarged lymph nodes are better appreciated by palpation.
- **Movements:** Their extent, rate, rhythm, duration, force and direction are assessed. Movements are studied in detail by palpation. Movements of voluntary muscles include passive movements and active movements. Passive movements are carried out at the various joints and their ranges in various directions are carefully noted. Active movements are carried out against resistance and power of the muscles is determined. Examination of the respiratory movements is very important when testing the integrity of the respiratory system.
- **Vibrations:** Vocal fremitus, thrill, etc., are looked for. Vocal fremitus is explained under respiratory system and thrill in cardiovascular system.
- **Edema:** When there is accumulation of excessive tissue fluid a moderate degree of pressure leaves a relatively permanent depression, which is called pitting on pressure. The clinical condition is called edema. Edema may be pitting or non-pitting.
- **Tenderness:** Tenderness is defined as pain on the area of touch or pressure. In healthy persons no part is tender to touch. Only the testes and the eyeballs are tender on moderate pressure and the abdominal viscera on very heavy pressure. If tenderness is located, the area over which it exists should be identified.
- If prominent dilated blood vessels are observed, find out the direction of flow of blood. Emptying the vessel and blocking the flow at either end one at a time helps to find out the direction of flow in superficial vessels.

PERCUSSION

Percussion means tapping or giving an impact. When an impact or a tap is given with the finger to a body, a sound is heard which is due to the audible vibrations set up in the body by the impact. The sound produced by the impact depends upon the amount of tissue, which is set into vibrations, the type of the tissue and the force of the impact. The stronger the impact the larger will be the amount of tissue set into vibration. The tissues present in an organ are usually not homogeneous and the percussion note is also different. The different notes obtained on percussion in tissues are of three types:
1. Hollow viscera like stomach containing gas give a note that is described as tympanitic which is of a musical character.
2. An organ like lung in which air is trapped in tiny compartments gives a note, which is described as resonant.
3. Solid viscera like liver containing no air and made up of soft fleshy material, or if fluid is present as in pleural effusion give a note, which is described as dull.

Rules of Percussion

- Usually the middle finger of the right and the left hand are used for percussion. Place the middle finger of the left hand on the part to be percussed and press firmly against it, with slight hyperextension of the distal interphalangeal joint. This finger is called the **pleximeter**. There should be no airspace between the body surface and the finger. Other fingers of the left hand should be separated apart and should not touch the surface. The pleximeter finger should be placed parallel to the border of the organ to be percussed.
- The percussion stroke is given on the finger placed on the surface by the tip of the middle finger of the right hand. This finger is called **plexor**. The impact is given to the middle phalanx of the pleximeter **(Fig. 19.2)**. The movement should be at the wrist rather than at the elbow.
- Percussion is always carried out from a resonant area towards a dull area. While percussing on bones, the whole bone is acting as a pleximeter, e.g., percussing over the clavicle.
- The tip of the middle finger should strike the surface to be percussed in a perpendicular direction. The percussion movement is carried out by the flexion and extension of the wrist joint. The movement should not be from the elbow or shoulder joint. As soon as the percussion stroke is given the finger should be lifted up, else it will damp the vibrations set up.

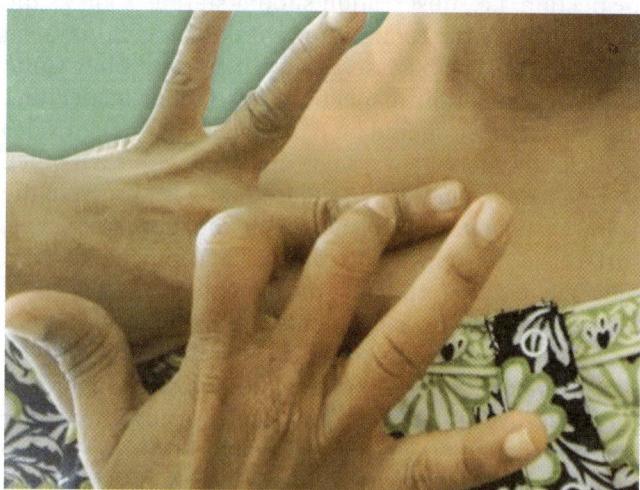

Fig. 19.2: Correct technique of percussion.

❖ The stroke can be given directly on the body surface to be examined. This is direct percussion, which is carried out over hard structures like bones.

AUSCULTATION

Auscultation means listening to the sounds produced in the body with the help of a stethoscope **(Fig. 19.3)**. The sounds might be those, which are produced naturally like the heart sounds or produced by external forces like the Korotkoff's sounds heard while recording blood pressure or produced vocally and conducted through the body tissues like vocal resonance.

Auscultation is carried out with the help of a stethoscope where the two ears are used. While using fetoscope in hearing fetal heart sounds, only one ear is used.

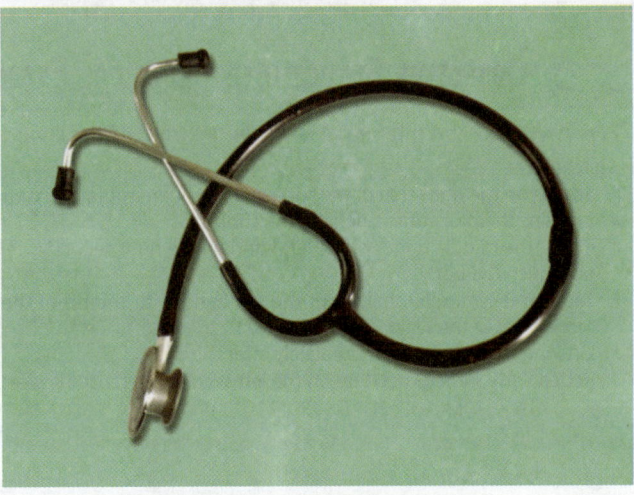

Fig. 19.3: Stethoscope.

Parts of the Stethoscope

❖ Ear piece
❖ Conducting tubes
❖ Chest piece

The ear frame is a metallic structure consisting of two tubes joined by a flat curved strip, which acts as a spring to pull together the upper ends of the two tubes. Each tube has an upper horizontal limb, which bears a curvature similar to that of the external auditory meatus. It runs medially, downward and forwards **(Fig. 19.3)**. The tip of each tube entering the meatus is covered with a smooth soft plastic cap to protect the wall of the meatus.

The conducting tube is a flexible and soft pressure tubing made of rubber or some synthetic material. The total length of the stethoscope should be about 50 cm from the ear tips to the chest piece. The inner diameter of the tube should be 3 mm and should not change at the joints.

Chest piece: On one side of the combined chest piece is a bell shaped chest piece and on the other side is a diaphragm type of chest piece. Any one of the two could be placed in position with the help of a lock arrangement. The mouth of the bell shaped chest piece is conical and is covered by a ring of rubber or any other material, which is a bad conductor of heat. The bell shaped chest piece has a comparatively smaller diameter. It does not cause any amplification of the sound. All the sounds conducted to the ear are of the same intensity. Low-pitched sounds are heard best with this chest piece.

The diaphragm type chest piece is flat and is fitted with a diaphragm of a celluloid material. It has a large mouth. The diaphragm causes amplification of the sounds and they are heard much louder than the original one. The diaphragm cannot amplify all the frequencies equally and the high-pitched sounds are heard well.

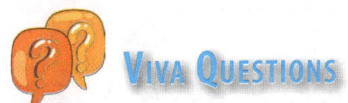

Viva Questions

1. **What is percussion? What are the rules of percussion?**
   Refer page 100.
2. **Why percussion is done from a resonant area towards a dull area?**
   Resonant sounds are clear, low pitched, hollow sounds and almost loud to hear from a distance. Dull sound is not very clear and need to be heard very close to the area. A dull sound indicates the presence of a solid mass under the percussing surface. The change from resonance to dullness is easy to differentiate. For example, to percuss out the upper border of liver, first percuss from the lower lung field on the right side down towards the diaphragm.
3. **Who invented stethoscope? What are its components?**
   Stethoscope was invented by Rene Laennec, a French physician in 1816.

OBJECTIVE STRUCTURED PRACTICAL EXAMINATION

Percuss the second intercostal space in the front of the subject.

Checklist:
» Stands on the right side of the subject and ask the subject to remove the clothes on the upper part of chest
» Explains the procedure briefly to the subject
» Places the middle finger of the left hand on the right second intercostal space firmly after identifying the space. The other fingers should not touch the body
» Taps on the middle phalanx of the left hand with the tip of the middle finger of the right hand perpendicularly with the percussion movement at the wrist joint
» Lifts the striking finger immedialely after the tap.
» Repeats the same procedure on the left second intercostal space

20
Chapter

Determination of Arterial Blood Pressure

LEARNING OBJECTIVES

- Determine blood pressure by palpatory and auscultatory methods
- Discuss the advantages of palpatory method
- Enumerate the precautions to be taken while recording blood pressure
- Define blood pressure and give its normal value in adults
- Describe the physiological basis of Korotkoff sounds
- What is auscultatory gap? Mention its significance
- Enumerate the determinants of arterial BP
- Explain sinoaortic mechanism or baroreceptor reflex
- Discuss the variations in BP with exercise and change in posture

PY5.12: Record blood pressure and pulse at rest and in different grades of exercise and postures in a volunteer.

AIM

To measure the blood pressure of the given subject.

PRINCIPLE OF MANUAL BLOOD PRESSURE MEASUREMENT

When a large artery like the brachial artery is partially compressed by applying air pressure using the cuff of the manometer, blood flow through the narrowed vessel become turbulent. Turbulent flow creates noises that can be auscultated with a stethoscope and the sounds are referred to as Korotkoff sounds. The values in the long limb of the manometer at which these noises change in intensity correlate with systemic arterial pressures.

Sphygmomanometer

The arterial blood pressure is determined indirectly using a sphygmomanometer devised by Riva-Rocci. Automated blood pressure monitors are also available. Sphygmomanometer consists of three parts:
1. A mercury manometer
2. A rubber bag covered with a linen cuff
3. A rubber pump with a one way-valve

Mercury Manometer

One limb of the manometer is long and graduated while the other limb is very short and broad and it acts as the mercury reservoir. The graduations on the long limb start from 0 at the base and end at 250 at the top and this limb is open at the upper end. This open end is fitted with a valve that prevents spilling of mercury when the apparatus is inverted. The short limb of the manometer contains mercury that can be pushed into the long limb by inflating the rubber bag. Mercury level can be raised in the long limb up to the 250 mark. The readings are marked in even numbers. Smallest division corresponds to a reading of 2 mm Hg. The mercury reservoir can be connected to the rubber bag by rubber tubing.

Rubber Bag with a Linen Cuff

The inflatable rubber bag is soft and is covered by a linen cuff that is longer and broader than the rubber bag called Riva-Rocci cuff (**Fig. 20.1**). The cavity of the rubber bag is connected to two rubber tubes. One tube is fitted with a metal adapter, which forms an airtight joint with the reservoir of the manometer. The other tube is connected

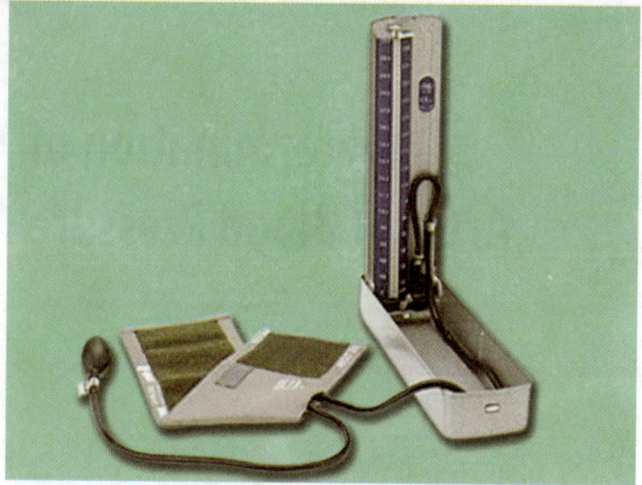

Fig. 20.1: Sphygmomanometer.

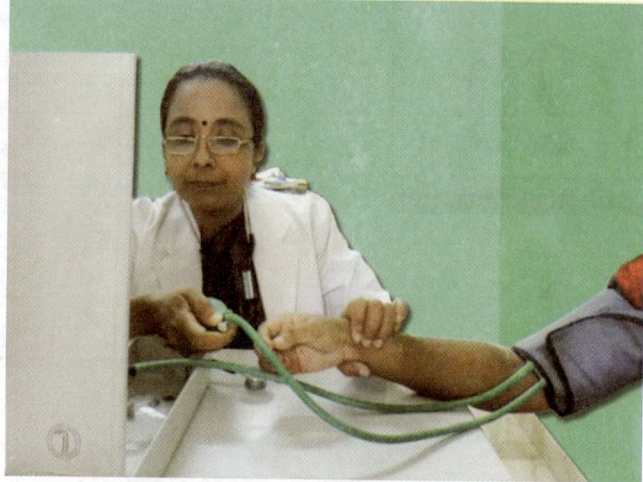

Fig. 20.2: Determination of arterial blood pressure by palpatory method.

to the rubber pump. The size of the rubber bag varies. The rubber bag should have sufficient length to cover 80% of the arm circumference. It should have a breadth half of its length. For most adult subjects, a standard rubber bag (12.5 cm wide and 23 cm long) is sufficient, but obese subjects require a wider thigh cuff (15 cm width) or the blood pressure will be overestimated. For children, different sized cuffs are available. The one, which covers most of the upper arm leaving a gap of 1 cm below the axilla and above the anterior cubital fossa, can be selected.

Rubber Pump

It is a thick and flexible rubber balloon, oval in shape and of a size that fits in the fist. It has two openings that are provided with valves. These valves direct the flow of air in one direction. The end of the pump through which the air goes out is connected to an adapter that communicates with the rubber tubing of the rubber bag. It is provided with a screw which when loosened allows escape of air to the outside.

METHODS OF SPHYGMOMANOMETRY

Palpatory Method

The palpatory method of BP recording should always precede the auscultatory method. The blood pressure measurement is done in either of the arms or thighs with the subject in the sitting or lying down posture. Avoid caffeine, eating and smoking half an hour before recording blood pressure since these factors may affect the reading.

The cuff is tied firmly around the bare upper arm in such a way that the rubber bag is placed over the brachial artery and fixed in position. The cuff should not be tied too tightly or too loosely. Make sure that the cuff is 2.5–3 cm above the cubital fossa. Connect the tube of the cuff to the manometer. Press the pump to inflate the bag. The mercury will rise in the vertical limb. Inflate the bag to raise the mercury column to about 200 mm level. Now release the screw and deflate the bag slowly.

As the rubber bag is filled with air, the pressure is transmitted to the limb and indirectly to the underlying artery. It is necessary to compress a sufficient length of artery to measure the blood pressure accurately. When the pressure applied over the artery is equal to or a little more than the blood pressure, the blood flow stops. On releasing the pressure, the flow is reestablished.

In the palpatory method, the radial pulse is felt to detect the presence of flow. After tying the cuff feel for the pulse. The cuff is then inflated fairly rapidly to increase the air pressure in the cuff 20–30 mm Hg above the point at which the radial pulse disappears. With the help of the screw valve in the rubber pump, air is slowly let out of the cuff to reduce the pressure while watching the mercury level in the long limb of the manometer (**Fig. 20.2**). The mercury level at which the pulse is felt first is taken as the systolic blood pressure reading. By the palpatory method only the rough systolic blood pressure can be measured. The diastolic blood pressure cannot be measured by this method.

The reading obtained by the palpatory method is about 5 mm Hg lower than the actual systolic BP. After doing the palpatory method, the cuff should be completely deflated and rest should be given to the subject's arm.

Oscillatory Method

Air is pumped into the rubber bag to a level above that of the systolic pressure obtained by the palpatory method. The mercury level is then watched while the pressure is being slowly reduced. When the pressure becomes equal to the systolic pressure the slowly falling mercury level starts oscillating. The level at which the first oscillation appears is taken as the systolic blood pressure. As the pressure is reduced further, the oscillations increase in amplitude.

They reach a maximum and then the amplitude decrease and finally disappear. The pressure at which the mercury level shows maximum amplitude of the oscillations is taken as the diastolic blood pressure reading. This method is not accurate and is unreliable.

Auscultatory Method

The Russian physician, **Korotkoff**, introduced the auscultatory method in 1905. After tying the cuff in position, feel the pulse of the brachial artery in the anterior cubital fossa. Usually it is felt medial to the tendon of the biceps muscle. The chest piece of a stethoscope is placed lightly over the palpable part of the brachial artery in the cubital fossa. Under normal conditions, no sounds can be heard through the stethoscope when it is placed over an unobstructed artery. This is because streamline or laminar flow of blood does not produce sound. The pressure in the cuff is raised to a level about 10 mm Hg above the systolic pressure obtained by the palpatory method. Now deflate the cuff and the pressure is reduced slowly at 2–3 mm Hg/sec until the Korotkoff sounds produced in the vessel are heard through the stethoscope **(Fig. 20.3)**.

While the pressure in the cuff is more than the blood pressure there is no flow of blood through the vessel and no sound is produced. As the cuff pressure decreases and becomes equal to or just less than the systolic blood pressure, blood flows through the obliterated vessel in spurts during each systole and a sound is produced with each heartbeat. These sounds were first described by a Russian scientist named Korotkoff and are named after him. As the pressure in the cuff is progressively reduced the character of the sounds change. Five phases are there.

The **first phase** starts from the beginning of production of the sound. This occurs when a jet of blood is able to pass through the obliterated part of the vessel first time as the cuff pressure is reduced. The sound appears suddenly and is usually clearly heard as a tapping sound. The mercury level in the manometer at which this first abrupt sound is heard is taken as the systolic blood pressure. The sound becomes louder and louder as the level in the manometer falls progressively till the pressure is reduced by about 10 mm of mercury. At this stage the sound acquires a murmurish quality. This is the end of the first phase.

When the systolic blood pressure is very high, the sound first produced will be a faint tap and then it disappears. So this sound may be missed. As the pressure in the bag is reduced further the sound reappears and becomes louder and audible at a much lower level. This reading is then mistakenly taken as the systolic blood pressure reading. The difference between this reading and the true systolic reading is referred to as the **auscultatory gap**.

The **second phase** starts when the sound acquires the murmurish quality. It continues during the fall of next 15 mm of mercury.

At the end of the second phase the sound becomes clearer and louder. This is the beginning of the **third phase**. It continues during the fall of next 15 mm of mercury pressure.

At the beginning of the fourth phase, the sound suddenly becomes muffled. This phase continues for a fall of about 5 mm of mercury. The level of the mercury in the manometer at the time the sound gets suddenly muffled is taken as the diastolic blood pressure level.

At the end of the **fourth phase** the sound may slowly or suddenly disappear and this is taken as the **fifth phase**. Some consider this value as the diastolic pressure. In conditions like aortic regurgitation the sounds continue to be heard even at very low levels. In such cases the level of muffling is taken as the diastolic pressure. Usually phase 4 is taken as the diastolic blood pressure if phase 5 is very low and the difference between phase 4 and phase 5 is more than 10 mm Hg.

Normally, the first occurrence of the sound is taken as the systolic blood pressure and the sudden muffling of the sound or its disappearance is taken as the diastolic blood pressure. Before confirming the blood pressure take two more readings. Make sure that the cuff is deflated and sufficient rest is given to the arm after taking each reading.

A difference in the systolic blood pressure of more than 10 mm Hg or diastolic pressure of more than 6 mm Hg between the right and left upper limbs is clinically significant.

RECORDING OF BLOOD PRESSURE IN DIFFERENT POSTURES AND AFTER EXERCISE

Record the blood pressure in the sitting posture, lying down posture and in the standing posture and note the difference in blood pressure in different postures. While recording BP, the cuff and the manometer should be at the level of the heart **(Fig. 20.4)**. Blood pressure should be recorded

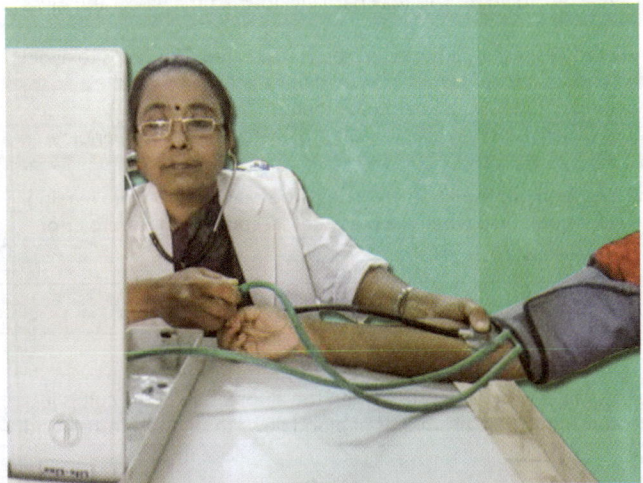

Fig. 20.3: Recording of blood pressure by auscultatory method.

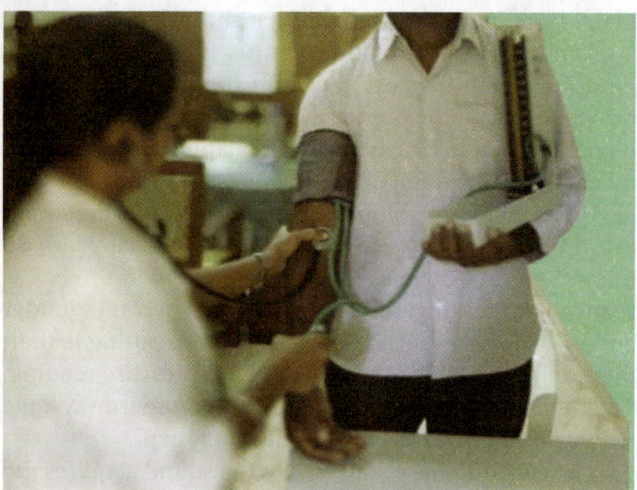

Fig. 20.4: Recording of blood pressure in the standing posture (note that the manometer is at the heart level).

within a few seconds after change in posture. Otherwise due to the operation of compensatory mechanisms, BP will come back to the original value within 2–3 minutes. Every time the position of the subject is changed, disconnect the tubing from the manometer and leave the cuff attached to the arm. Join the two before recording the pressure. Then after mild to moderate exercise for about 5 minutes again record the blood pressure and note the changes in systolic and diastolic pressure.

Measure the blood pressure in the leg while the subject is lying down. This is done by tying the cuff round the mid-thigh level and the subject should lie in the prone position. Hold the knee slightly flexed so that the muscles around the popliteal fossa are relaxed. Palpate the popliteal artery and place the stethoscope over it and hear the sounds in the popliteal artery when the cuff is deflated. Ideally a large sized cuff is necessary to measure the blood pressure in the thigh.

If there is a difference of more than 20 mm Hg in the blood pressure recorded in the upper and lower limbs, it is clinically significant.

SAMPLE REPORT PATTERN

- Blood pressure in the sitting posture
  - Palpatory method—110 mm Hg
  - Auscultatory method—116/78 mm Hg
- Blood pressure in the supine position—120/76 mm Hg
- Blood pressure in the standing posture—114/80 mm Hg
- Blood pressure after exercise—140/84 mm Hg

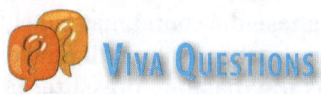

Viva Questions

1. **What are the precautions to be taken while recording blood pressure?**
   - Sufficient rest should be given to the subject before recording BP. Anxiety increases systolic BP.
   - The cuff and the manometer should be at the level of heart
   - The cuff should not be tied too tightly or too loosely
   - The two tubes connected to the cuff should be directed downwards and should come on the medial side of the arm. This makes sure that the rubber bag is over the brachial artery.
   - Look for zero error in the manometer
   - The manometer should face the examiner and not the subject
   - Inflation should be done quickly and deflation slowly
   - The cuff should be deflated completely after taking each reading
   - Do not press the diaphragm of the stethoscope over the artery while recording BP. This may partially obstruct the vessel and gives a false reading
   - Systolic pressure should be first estimated before auscultatory method especially if hypertension is suspected. This helps to avoid auscultatory gap.
   - If the Korotkoff sounds are less audible, repeated closing and opening of the fist can accentuate them.
   - The mercury reservoir should be locked before closing the apparatus. Otherwise it may lead to spilling of mercury from the manometer.

2. **What is 'zero error' mercury manometer?**
   When the BP cuff is completely deflated, the mercury column in the long limb of the manometer should be exactly at the zero reading. If it is above or below the zero reading, false higher or lower values will be obtained when the pressure is recorded. This is zero error.

3. **What are the advantages of palpatory method?**
   - The systolic pressure can be estimated roughly
   - Auscultatory gap can be avoided in hypertensive individuals

4. **What are the disadvantages of palpatory method?**
   - Diastolic pressure cannot be estimated
   - Systolic BP obtained will be 5–10 mm Hg lower than the actual systolic BP. This is because when the air pressure in the cuff is just below the brachial artery pressure (this is the actual systolic pressure), only a small amount of blood flows through the artery and this is not sufficient enough to produce a pulse wave to be felt.

5. While recording BP, the cuff and the manometer should be at the level of the heart. Give reason.
The blood pressure in any vessel above the level of heart will be less and that in vessels below the level of the heart will be more than in vessels at the level of heart. This is due to the effect of gravity. The change in mean blood pressure will be 0.77 mm Hg for each cm vertical distance above or below the heart.

6. The cuff should not be left inflated for long periods. Why?
- It produces pain and discomfort to the arm since the arm suffers from ischemia.
- If the person is suffering from purpura, it produces subcutaneous bleeding.
- In conditions producing hypocalcemia like hypoparathyroidism, tetany may be precipitated.
- If the artery is kept occluded for long periods it produces reflex spasm of the blood vessel and a high reading will be obtained.

7. Define blood pressure. Give the normal value in an adult at rest.
Blood pressure is defined as the lateral pressure exerted on the walls of the vessel by the contained blood. Normal value in a young adult is 120/70 mm Hg.

8. What is pulse pressure? Give one condition where it is widened.
Difference between systolic pressure and diastolic pressure is pulse pressure. It is increased in hyperthyroidism. Excess thyroxine increases heart rate and force of contraction thereby increasing cardiac output and systolic BP. It produces peripheral vasodilatation due to increased metabolism (BMR) leading to decrease in peripheral resistance and decrease in diastolic BP. This leads to widening of pulse pressure.

9. What is mean arterial pressure? Give its significance.
Mean arterial pressure is the average pressure during a cardiac cycle. It is diastolic pressure + 1/3 pulse pressure. Normal value in an adult is 90–100 mm Hg.
- Mean pressure determines tissue perfusion
- The cardiovascular reflexes like baroreceptor reflex are sensitive to changes in mean arterial pressure.

10. What is auscultatory gap or silent gap?
In some hypertensive individuals, the systolic pressure will be very high. While doing auscultatory method, when the cuff pressure is reduced from very high values, the Korotkoff sound will appear for a brief period and then it disappears. Again it reappears after the cuff pressure is further reduced and disappears when the pressure reaches the diastolic value. The silent period during which sound is not heard between the first appearance and its first disappearance is called auscultatory gap or silent gap. The exact cause is not known and it is seen only when the systolic BP is very high. If the systolic pressure is not assessed initially by the palpatory method, the cuff pressure may not be raised to the original systolic value and the systolic pressure will be taken as the value at which the sound appear after the silent gap. This gives a false low reading.

11. What are Korotkoff sounds? Mention its physiological basis.
Blood flow through a normal straight vessel is silent and the flow is referred to as laminar or streamline. When the blood vessel is compressed by inflating the cuff of the sphygmomanometer, blood flow completely stops in the vessel and no sound is heard. When the cuff pressure is slowly reduced, sounds can be heard through the stethoscope placed over the brachial artery distal to the obstruction. These sounds are called Korotkoff sounds. As the cuff pressure is decreased, first a fine tapping sound appears which changes in quality to loud tapping and then to a murmurish quality. The sounds are heard because the flow becomes turbulent when it occurs through a narrowed vessel. Turbulent flow produces sounds. The sounds disappear when the flow is reestablished completely, i.e., when the cuff pressure is equal to the diastolic blood pressure.

12. What is hypertension? Mention the types.
Hypertension is increase in blood pressure above the normal range for the particular age and sex of the individual. It can be primary (essential or idiopathic hypertension) and secondary hypertension. The cause of primary hypertension is not clear and 80% of hypertensive belongs to this group and women predominate. Secondary hypertension is secondary to diseases like atherosclerosis, renal artery stenosis, glomerulonephritis, pheochromocytoma, Cushing syndrome, etc.

13. What is orthostatic hypotension? What is the test for orthostatic hypotension?
When some individuals stand up from the lying down posture there will be sudden fall in blood pressure due to pooling of blood in the lower extremities and they may feel giddy or may even faint. This is due to improper baroreceptor reflex, which is one of the most important immediate compensatory mechanisms that operate when there is a fall in blood pressure.
First check BP in the supine position. Three minutes after standing up, BP is again checked. In orthostatic hypotension, there will be a sustained drop in systolic pressure by more than 20 mm Hg and diastolic pressure of more than 10 mm Hg from the lying down posture after 3 minutes of standing up. Heart rate should not increase by more than 30 beats/min above base line on standing up.

14. What is "white coat" hypertension?
Doctors and healthcare workers usually wear white overcoats. In some people who have normal blood pressure, will have a higher reading when they approach the examiner. This is called white coat hypertension. This is because, people become anxious or stressed when they approach the doctor. This can be managed by proper lifestyle changes. In the long run, these people are prone to develop hypertension.

15. What is the reason for slight fall in the diastolic BP after severe isotonic exercise? During exercise there is decrease in peripheral resistance (PR) and slight decrease in diastolic BP due to the following reasons:
- There will be accumulation of vasodilator metabolites like lactic acid, adenosine, etc., in the skeletal muscles which produces vasodilation of muscle blood vessels and decrease PR
- The body temperature increases and to remove excess heat there will be cutaneous vasodilatation, which leads to decrease in peripheral resistance
- There is stimulation of sympathetic cholinergic fibers supplying the skeletal muscles that produces vasodilatation.

16. **What are the changes observed in the BP readings when there is a change in posture from the sitting posture?**
   In the standing posture, systolic blood pressure will be less than that of sitting posture and diastolic BP will be maximum. This is because on standing up there is pooling of blood in the lower extremities, which decreases venous return and cardiac output. So the systolic pressure falls. When the mean arterial pressure decreases, baroreceptor reflex come into play leading to increased sympathetic discharge and vasoconstriction. This increases peripheral resistance and diastolic pressure.
   In the lying down posture, systolic pressure will be maximum and diastolic pressure minimum.

OBJECTIVE STRUCTURED PRACTICAL EXAMINATION

I. **Record the blood pressure of the subject by palpatory method in the sitting posture.**
   » Explain the procedure to the subject
   » Expose the right hand up to the shoulder
   » Wrap the BP cuff firmly around the right upper arm 2 cm above the cubital fossa with the rubber tube coming medially
   » Place the BP apparatus on the table and open the stop cock and check the zero level
   » Palpate the radial artery and feel the radial pulse using the left hand
   » Close the screw of the rubber bulb and inflate the cuff slowly until the radial pulse disappears
   » Using the screw, release the pressure in the cuff slowly till the radial pulse reappears. Note down the reading

II. **Record the blood pressure of the subject in the lying down posture.**
   » Explain the procedure to the subject
   » Expose the right hand up to the shoulder
   » Wrap the BP cuff firmly around the right upper arm 2 cm above the cubital fossa with the rubber tube coming medially
   » Place the BP apparatus on the cot and open the stop cock and check the zero level
   » Record BP by palpatory method
   » Deflate the cuff
   » Place the chest piece of the stethoscope over the brachial artery
   » Inflates the BP cuff to a value 10 mm Hg above that obtained by palpatory method
   » Release the pressure in the cuff slowly till the systolic and diastolic pressures are recorded. Remove the cuff and close the stop cock.

Chapter 21: Examination of the Respiratory System

LEARNING OBJECTIVES

- Examine the respiratory system of the subject
- Test the vocal fremitus and vocal resonance of the subject
- Perform percussion and auscultation of the lung areas of the subject
- Perform the systemic examination of the respiratory system by palpatory method
- Describe the different types of breath sounds

PY6.9: Demonstrate the correct clinical examination of the respiratory system in a normal volunteer or simulated environment.

INTRODUCTION

First do a general examination with special emphasis to dyspnea, cough, change in voice, cyanosis, clubbing of fingers, edema and cervical, supraclavicular and axillary lymphadenopathy. Most patients with respiratory disease will present with chest pain, difficulty in breathing, cough, wheeze or excess sputum. Family history of similar illness and occupational history should also be taken. Inhalation of asbestos in industries leads to severe lung illness later. The clinical examination of the respiratory system consists of examination of the lungs and the trachea.

INSPECTION

Upper Respiratory Tract

Using a torch examine the nose and throat. Look for any block, discharge, congestion or other abnormalities.

Trachea

Note the position of trachea. Normally it is central. Note whether there is shift to the right or left, which can be due to diseases of the lungs.

Examination of Chest

For describing the findings specifically, the chest wall is divided into different areas bilaterally and each area is examined separately.

Front

- Supraclavicular area
- Clavicular area
- Infraclavicular area
- Mammary area
- Inframammary area

Side

- Axillary area
- Infra-axillary area

Back

- Suprascapular
- Interscapular
- Upper interscapular
- Middle
- Lower
- Infrascapular

Shape of the Chest

Ask the subject to remove the clothes that cover the chest. A female subject should be examined behind a screen in the presence of a bystander. The subject should sit straight on a stool. Inspect the chest from the front, side and the back under good light. The subject can also be in the supine position, inclined at an angle of 45° supported by headrest or pillows or he can be in the standing posture. Compare the right and the left sides of the chest for symmetry. Normally the two sides are symmetrical. The cross section of the chest is elliptical normally, i.e., the breadth of the chest is wider than the anteroposterior diameter, ratio being 7:5.

The angle of Louis (Ludwig's angle) can be seen at the junction of manubrium with the body of the sternum. This corresponds to the second rib. Observe the supraclavicular and the infraclavicular fossae, which are seen as smooth shallow hollows. Observe the intercostal space and see whether there is drawing in of intercostal space during inspiration. On the back note the scapular prominences, the suprascapular, interscapular and the infrascapular regions. Look for any abnormality.

The chest may be distorted by disease of the ribs or spinal vertebrae or by the underlying lung tissue. Abnormal shapes of the chest include pectus excavatum, pigeon chest, barrel-shaped chest where the cross section of chest become circular due to overinflated lungs as in chronic obstructive lung disease (COPD), kyphosis (forward bending of vertebral column), scoliosis (lateral bending), kyphoscoliosis, etc.

Respiratory Rate

Count the respiratory rate by altering the attention of the subject. The rate in a relaxed adult varies from 14 to 16 breaths per minute. Exertion, nervousness and fear can change the rate even in healthy subjects.

Rhythm of Respiration

Normally respiration is even and regular. Inspiration is followed by expiration without any pause. There is a pause at the end of expiration. The duration of inspiration is longer than the duration of expiration. Abnormalities in rhythm include Cheyne-Stokes breathing (seen in severe cardiac failure, narcotic drug poisoning, and neurological disorders), central sleep apnea, obstructive sleep apnea, etc.

Type of Breathing

Both the abdomen and the thorax move during respiration. In the males, the respiratory movements are abdominothoracic, i.e., the abdominal movements are more prominent when compared to the thoracic movements. In the females, the respiratory movements are thoracoabdominal, i.e., the thorax moves more than that of the abdomen during respiration especially during pregnancy.

Chest Movements

Look for chest movements during respiration from all sides, i.e., side-to-side movements, vertical and anteroposterior and see if the chest movements are symmetrical. Ask the subject to raise his arms and rest them on his head. Compare the movements on the right and the left sides. The movements are normally symmetrical. If there is an abnormality on one side of the chest, the movement seems to be diminished on that side. See whether the accessory muscles of respiration are working. If there is a drawing-in of the intercostal spaces with inspiration (intercostal retraction), it may indicate severe upper airway obstruction.

Pulsations

If visible, note the position of apex beat over the precordium. See whether there are visible pulsations over the chest other than apex beat. Dilated veins on the chest should also be noted. The venous pulses in the neck should be inspected. Chronic obstructive pulmonary disease (COPD) may lead to chronic pulmonary hypertension and right heart failure. A raised jugular venous pressure (JVP) is seen in this condition.

PALPATION

Confirm the findings of inspection during palpation.

Position of Trachea

Verify whether trachea is central. Subject should be in the sitting position, neck slightly flexed with the chin remaining in the midline of the body. Place the index finger and the ring finger of the right hand of the examiner over the sternoclavicular joints of the subject. Palpate the trachea with the middle finger from thyroid cartilage to the suprasternal notch and note whether there is any deviation **(Fig. 21.1)**. Normally in some healthy individuals trachea may be slightly deviated to the right.

Deviation of trachea can be due to push or pull of the mediastinum from the right or left sides. Trachea can be shifted to the right if there is collapse or fibrosis of right lung (pull) or pleural effusion or pneumothorax of the left lung (push).

Apex Beat

Palpate for the apex beat in the lower part of the precordium with the subject in the supine position and record its exact position. Displacement of the apex beat without displacement of the trachea may be due to scoliosis or due to enlargement of the left ventricle. A significant displacement of the apex beat and the trachea suggest that

Chapter 21: Examination of the Respiratory System

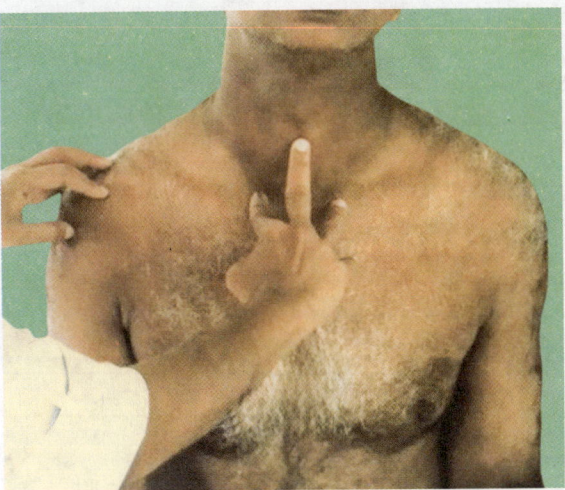

Fig. 21.1: Examining the position of trachea.

the position of the mediastinum has been altered by disease of the lungs or pleura.

Chest Measurements and Chest Expansion

Measure the various parameters of the chest like chest circumference, transverse diameter and anteroposterior diameter in centimeters. Take the measurements at the end of forced expiration and at the end of deep inspiration. The anteroposterior and transverse dimensions are taken at the level of fourth intercostal space with the help of books applied to the chest wall. The help of an assistant is needed.

Chest expansion can be measured using a tape placed at the level of the nipples in males and below the level of nipples in females. At the end of forced expiration take the circumference in cm. Ask the subject to take a deep inspiration and find out the difference. Normally chest expansion is 5–8 cm in a healthy young man. A value of less than 3 cm in male and less than 2.5 cm in female are abnormal. It is decreased in pulmonary fibrosis, asthma, deformities of thoracic cage, etc.

Respiratory Rate

Place the palm of the right hand over the abdomen of the subject while he is in the supine position and count the number of movements for one minute. The subject should not be aware that the examiner is counting his respiratory rate.

Chest Movements during Respiration

The extent of movements must be examined in different areas of the chest and a comparison should be carried out with the opposite side simultaneously.

- Place the partially spread out fingers of both the hands on symmetrical areas on either side of the rib cage and bring the tips of the two extended thumbs in the midline **(Figs. 21.2A and B)**.
- Now fix the fingers rigidly on the chest wall without exerting pressure on the chest wall. The fingers of the two hands should touch the chest but the thumbs should not touch the chest wall.
- Ask the subject to take a deep inspiration. When the subject breathes in, because of the lateral expansion of the chest, the two thumbs recede away equally from the midline.
- If one thumb remains closer to the midline, it suggests diminished chest expansion on that side. This can be due to underlying lung disease or disease of the rib cage.
- The extent of movements is more in the lower part of the chest than in the upper part. Maximum expansion occurs in the lateral bases of the lungs. The movements are equal in similar areas on either side of the body, anteriorly as well as posteriorly.

Vocal Fremitus

Vocal fremitus usually referred to, as tactile vocal fremitus is a vibratory sensation felt by the hand placed on the chest wall while the subject is talking. The vibrations caused by

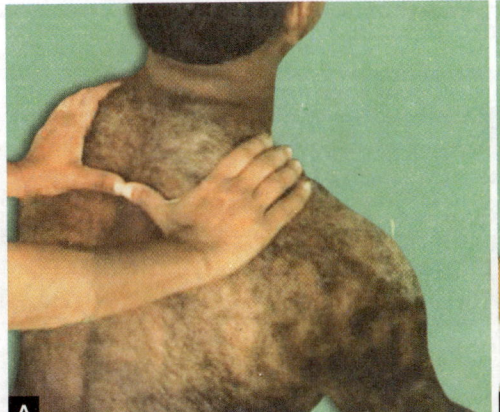 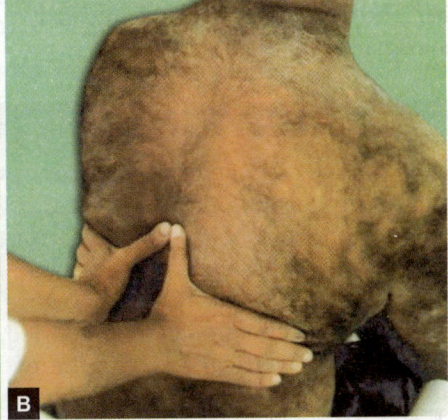

Figs. 21.2A and B: Examination of chest movements in the suprascapular (A) and infrascapular (B) areas.

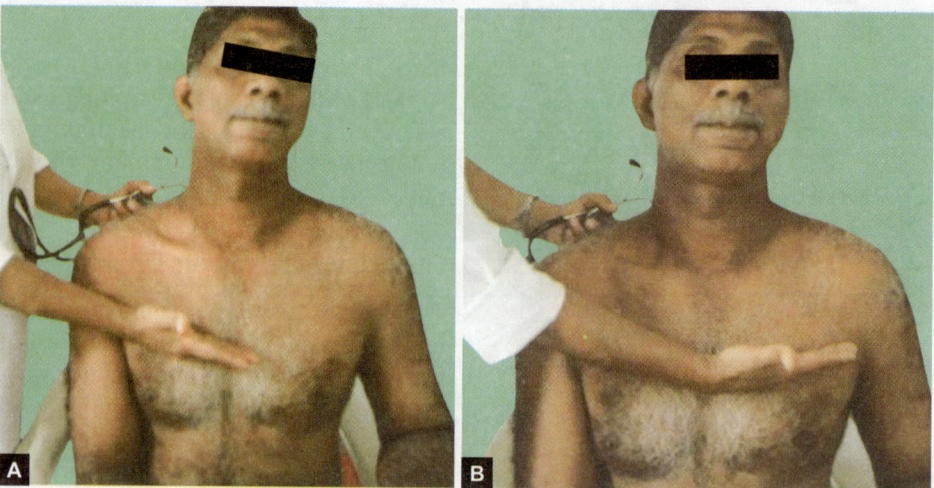

Figs. 21.3A and B: Testing for vocal fremitus.

the vocal cords are conducted through the lung tissue to the chest wall and are perceived by the hand. The intensity of sensation depends upon the structure and conductivity of the underlying tissues. Thus, a consolidated lung tissue conducts the sound better and the sensation of vibrations felt is more when compared to other normal areas. Presence of fluid in the pleural cavity, which separates the lung tissue from the chest wall, dampens the vibrations and does not allow the sensation to be felt. Then the vocal fremitus is decreased or not felt.

Place the ulnar border of the hand horizontally in the intercostal space on the area over the chest to be examined and ask the subject to say repeatedly ninety-nine or any number (Figs. 21.3A and B). Feel for the vibratory sense. Place the palm on the symmetrical intercostal space on the opposite side. Feel the sensation. Repeat two or three times and compare the sensations on both sides. The fremitus should be felt equally on any two symmetrical areas on the two sides. Similarly compare the fremitus in different symmetrical areas of the chest. The fremitus is felt well on the front than on the back. This is because the muscles on the back are thicker. The fremitus is felt best in the axillary regions. It is felt maximally over the trachea.

PERCUSSION

Auenbrugger devised this method. Percussion can assess the consistency of the underlying tissue by listening to the type of percussion note heard. The different percussion notes heard in different situations are resonant, hyper-resonant, dull, stony dull and tympanitic note. By percussion, the borders of the lung can be defined, the percussion notes on symmetrical areas on the two sides can be compared and one can confirm that a resonant note is heard all over the normal lung tissue. If performed repeatedly and inexpertly, percussion can be uncomfortable for the patient.

To obtain the resonant note in individuals with different builds, the strength of the percussion stroke should be increased with increase in the muscle mass and fatty tissue. Even then the resonance obtained is not the same in different individuals. Different areas of chest give different degrees of resonances.

- Ask the subject to sit relaxed with head and shoulders erect. Chest should be bare.
- Percuss directly on the clavicle on the medial side of the midclavicular line (Fig. 21.4).
- Following the rules of percussion (refer Chapter 20), percuss the supraclavicular fossae, first intercostal space and then each intercostal space lower down. The pleximeter finger should be placed firmly parallel to the intercostal space (Fig. 21.5). While percussing one side, compare with the opposite side at the same time.
- Percuss the lateral wall of chest while the subject places his arms over his head.
- Percuss the posterior chest wall while the subject inclines his head forwards and arms across the chest

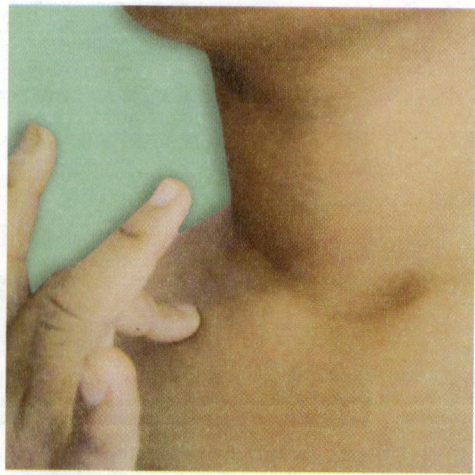

Fig. 21.4: Direct percussion over the clavicle.

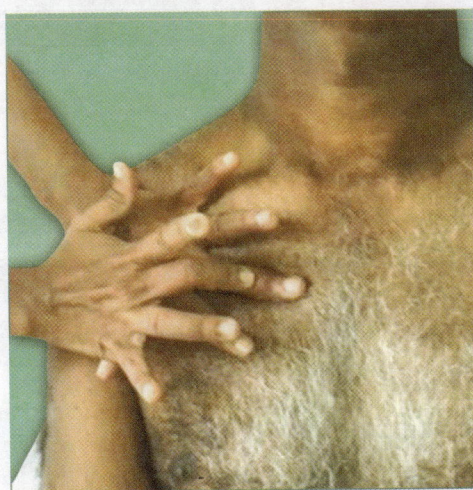

Fig. 21.5: Percussion over the chest wall in the right second intercostal space.

with the hands touching the opposite shoulder tips. This shifts the scapula laterally. Percuss from apices downwards.

- On percussion, it is seen that the apex of each lung extends 3 cm above the clavicle and gives a resonant note. The lower border of each lung lies in the 4th intercostal space in the midline in front, in the 6th space in the midclavicular line, in the 8th space in the midaxillary line, in the 10th space in the midscapular line on the back and in the 11th space in the paravertebral line at the end of normal inspiration.
- An impaired resonance is obtained over two spaces below these levels, after which this note becomes dull on the right side. This is because of the presence of liver. On deep inspiration this impaired resonance is improved to clearer and louder resonance because of inflation of the lung tissue and the liver will be pushed down.
- On the left side, the heart dullness disturbs the border in the midline. The lower border of the left lung extends a little lower as compared to the right; on the right side the liver raises it by about 2 cm as compared to the left.
- A tympanitic note in the 5th space replaces the resonant note of the lower border of the left lung. The stomach causes the tympanitic note (drum like note).

Impaired resonance is obtained in fibrosis and a dull note is obtained in consolidation. In pleural effusion and empyema, stony dullness (as if percussing over the thighs) is obtained on percussion. Hyper-resonant note is obtained in pneumothorax.

AUSCULTATION

With a stethoscope certain audible sounds are produced during breathing. During auscultation the following points should be noted:
- Breath sounds
- Abnormal breath sounds
- Added sounds
- Vocal resonance

Breath Sounds

Note the intensity and type of breath sounds. See whether the intensity is normal and equal bilaterally. Record if it is diminished or absent.

Two types of breath sounds are heard using a stethoscope, vesicular and bronchial breath sounds. The sound heard over the normal lung tissue is described as 'vesicular breath sounds'. Vesicular breath sounds are low pitched and rustling in character. Duration of inspiration is more than that of expiration and there is no pause in between. The sound heard over the trachea or over the large bronchi is described as 'bronchial breath sounds', which is harsh and high pitched. Expiration is either equal to the duration of inspiration or prolonged with a definite pause in between. Variations in the intensity and the mixtures of the two types of sounds in various proportions occur in different regions. These breath sounds are produced due to the turbulence in the air column during the entry and exit of air in the lungs.

Ask the subject to breathe in and out slowly and deeply through the mouth to eliminate the sounds produced in the nose and throat. Auscultate all the chest areas mentioned above comparing with the opposite side. Compare the intensity and quality of the sound in all areas. If possible compare the duration of inspiration and expiration during each breath. Pure vesicular breath sounds are heard in the axillary and infra-axillary areas. Bronchial breathing is heard when the stethoscope is placed over the trachea.

Abnormal Breath Sounds

Abnormal breath sounds are heard in diseased conditions of lungs. When the stethoscope is placed over an area of consolidation, high-pitched bronchial breath sounds are heard and it is referred to as **tubular breath sound**. When placed over cavities in lung, low-pitched bronchial breathing is heard, which is referred to as **cavernous breath sounds**. Breath sounds may be diminished or absent in conditions like pleural thickening, pleural effusion and pneumothorax.

Added Sounds or Adventitious Sounds

Added sounds include **rhonchi (wheezes), crepitation (crackle or rale) and pleural rub**. Wheezes are heard when there is narrowing of respiratory passage as in the case of bronchial asthma. Crackles are heard when there is secretion in the respiratory passage as in the case of bronchitis. Crepitation is also heard when there is sudden opening of collapsed alveoli. Fine crepitation is heard over the lung bases in pulmonary edema.

In pleural inflammation as in pleurisy, the inflamed pleural surfaces rub against each other producing a rubbing sound referred to as pleural friction rub. It may be heard during both inspiration and expiration.

Vocal Resonance

Vocal resonance is the sound of the subject's voice heard through a stethoscope placed on his chest wall. The sound created in the larynx by the vocal cords is conducted through the trachea and the bronchial tubes to the lung tissue and then to the chest wall where it is heard. The intensity of the resonance heard will depend upon the loudness and the depth of the subject's voice and the conductivity of the lung tissue for the sound. The subject's voice being constant a change in the resonance (as compared to a paired area on the opposite side) signifies an increased or decreased conduction through the lung tissue. Depending upon the conductivity of the tissues, different areas give different degree of vocal resonance in a healthy person.

Place the stethoscope over the area to be examined. Ask the subject to say repeatedly one, one, one. While listening through the stethoscope, ascertain the place from where the sound is coming.

- If it seems to come from the mouth of the subject and not from the chest wall it means that the vocal resonance is absent. This is seen when auscultated over the liver area.
- If the sound seems to be heard as if coming deep from the chest but not from the chest piece of the stethoscope it means that the vocal resonance is faintly heard. This is seen when auscultated over the pectoral muscles.
- If the sound appears to be heard from the chest piece of the stethoscope as a weak, muffled and distant rumble with the individual syllables slurred and indistinguishable, it means that the vocal resonance is normal. This is heard over areas all over the lung tissue where vesicular breathing is heard.
- If the sound is heard nearer the ear than the chest piece, it means that the vocal resonance is increased. This is heard over areas where bronchial breathing is heard.
- If the sound is heard in the earpiece but the individual words or syllables are indistinguishable, it means that the vocal resonance is extremely increased. Normally it is heard over the trachea. This phenomenon is described as **bronchophony** if it is heard over the lung tissue.
- When auscultated over the trachea, even a whisper is clearly audible. This phenomenon is described as **whispering pectoriloquy**, if this is present when auscultated over the lung parenchyma. Here the whispered sounds are transmitted to the chest wall with sufficient clarity to maintain the syllabic character and the individual syllables or words are clearly distinguishable as if uttered directly into the examiner's ears. Whispered sounds are normally inaudible over the lung parenchyma.

REPORT PATTERN

- Name:
- Age:
- Sex:
- Occupation:
- Address:

GENERAL EXAMINATION

Normally built and nourished, no pallor, icterus, cyanosis, clubbing, edema or lymphadenopathy.

Pulse: 72/min, regular, normal in volume and character, no vessel wall thickening, no radio-femoral delay.

Blood pressure: 110/70 mm Hg

Oral temperature: 37°C at 10 am

RESPIRATORY SYSTEM EXAMINATION

Upper respiratory tract—normal.

Inspection (Both Sides of the Chest to be Compared)

- Shape of chest—bilaterally symmetrical and elliptical in cross section
- Position of trachea—central
- Apex beat—not visible
- Type of breathing—abdominothoracic
- Respiratory rate—18/min, regular
- Chest movements—equal on both sides
- No visible pulsations over the chest

Palpation

- Trachea—central
- Apex beat—felt in the left fifth intercostal space half an inch medial to the midclavicular line
- Chest movements—equal on both sides in all areas
- Chest expansion—5 cm
- Vocal fremitus—normal and equal on all corresponding areas of chest

Percussion

Normal percussion note heard in all lung areas bilaterally.

Auscultation

- Breath sounds—vesicular breath sounds heard over all lung fields
- Vocal resonance—normal on both sides
- No adventitious sounds heard

Impression: The respiratory system of the subject appears to be normal.

Viva Questions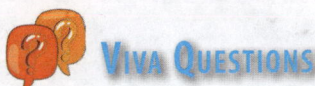

1. **What are the differences between vesicular breathing and bronchial breathing?**
   » *Intensity*: Vesicular breathing is low in intensity; bronchial breathing is much louder when compared to the vesicular breathing.
   » *Relation with the phase of respiration*: In case of vesicular breathing, respiratory sounds are heard well during inspiration, while in case of bronchial breathing they are heard better during expiration.
   » *Pause between inspiration and expiration*: In case of the vesicular breathing, there is no pause between inspiration and expiration. In case of the bronchial breathing, there is a definite pause between inspiration and expiration.
   » *Duration of the phases*: In the vesicular breathing, the inspiratory sound is twice as long as the expiratory sound. In case of the bronchial breathing the durations of the inspiratory and the expiratory sounds are equal.
   » *Character of the sound*: In the vesicular breathing the inspiratory sound is more intense than the expiratory sound. In case of the bronchial breathing the expiratory sound and the inspiratory sound are of the same intensity. Vesicular breathing has a rustling character whereas bronchial breathing is harsh in character.

2. **Mention the rules of percussion.**
   Refer page 100.

3. **What are the differences between bronchial breath sounds and vesicular breath sounds?**
   Refer page 113.

4. **What is the difference between vocal fremitus and vocal resonance? Mention the conditions where they are altered.**
   Refer page 111 and 114.

5. **What are added sounds?**
   Refer page 113.

6. **What is the difference between bronchophony and whispering pectoriloquy?**
   Refer page 114.

Objective Structured Practical Examination

I. **Test the vocal fremitus in the subject provided**
   » Explain the procedure to the subject
   » Place the ulnar aspect of the right hand above the clavicle and ask the subject to say 99 several times and feel the vibration
   » Repeats the procedure on the opposite side and compares
   » Then ulnar border of hand is placed in all the intercostal areas and ask to say 99, 99, 99 comparing with the opposite side
   » On the back the interscapular and infrascapular areas should also be examined on both sides

II. **Assess the chest movements during respiration**
   » Explain the procedure to the subject and ask him to remove the cloths from the chest area
   » Place the partially spread out fingers of both the hands on symmetrical areas on either side of the rib cage and bring the tips of the two extended thumbs in the midline
   » Ask the subject to take a deep inspiration.
   » See whether both the thumbs move equally to either side from the midline.
   » See whether the movements are equal in similar areas on either side of the body, anteriorly as well as posteriorly.

Chapter 22

Examination of Cardiovascular System

LEARNING OBJECTIVES

- Examine the radial pulse of the subject in a sequential order and comment
- Define precordium and apex beat
- Locate the apex beat of the subject
- Percuss out the borders of the heart
- Demonstrate elicitation of parasternal heave
- Identify the different auscultatory areas over the precordium
- Auscultate the heart sounds and identify the quality
- Examine the right jugular vein and if JVP is elevated measure it

PY5.15: Demonstrate the correct clinical examination of the cardiovascular system in a normal volunteer or simulated environment.

INTRODUCTION

First do a general examination with special emphasis to dyspnea, cyanosis, clubbing of fingers, edema and jugular venous pressure. Most patients with cardiovascular disease will present with difficulty in breathing, palpitation, and chest pain especially on exertion, raised JVP, cyanosis or edema. Clubbing is present in congenital cyanotic heart disease and infective endocarditis. Pitting edema in the dependent parts is a cardinal feature of congestive heart failure.

Examination of cardiovascular system is done under the following headings:
- Arterial pulse
- Recording of blood pressure
- Venous pulse
- Examination of precordium

EXAMINATION OF ARTERIAL PULSE

Arterial pulse is an expansile wave transmitted along the arteries due to ejection of blood from the left ventricle into the already full aorta, and which is transmitted along the vessel wall and is felt in the peripheral arteries. Usually the radial artery is examined.

The patient should be at complete physical and mental rest for at least 3 minutes before examining the pulse. The radial pulse on the right side should be examined. The pulse on the left side must also be examined in cardiac patients.

The right forearm of the subject is held in the semiprone position with the wrist and elbow slightly flexed. The radial pulse should be felt against the head of radius with the tips of the middle three fingers of the examiner's left hand **(Fig. 22.1)**. The following points should be noted.
- Rate
- Rhythm

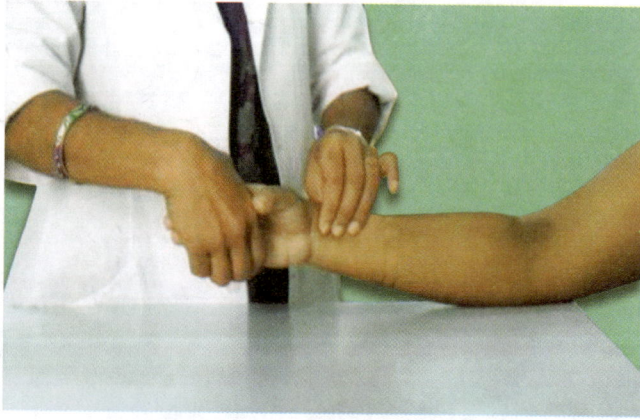

Fig. 22.1: Palpation of radial pulse.

- ❖ Volume
- ❖ Character
- ❖ Symmetry (equality on both sides)
- ❖ Condition of the vessel wall
- ❖ Radiofemoral delay
- ❖ Palpation of other peripheral pulses

Rate

The pulse is counted for complete one minute and is expressed in beats per minute. If it is counted for 15 sec and multiplied by 4 it may not be accurate because of sinus arrhythmia (heart rate is increased during inspiration and decreased during expiration). The normal pulse rate ranges between 60–100 beats/min (average 80/min). Increase in pulse rate above 100/min is **tachycardia** (seen in exercise, anxiety, excitement, fever, thyrotoxicosis, tachyarrhythmia and circulatory shock) and decrease in heart rate below 60/min is **bradycardia** (seen in athletes, myxedema and in heart blocks).

Rhythm

See whether the pulse beats at regular intervals. Comment as regular or irregular. If irregular, see whether it is **regularly irregular or irregularly irregular**. An irregular rhythm may be due to atrial fibrillation, frequent ectopic beats, or due to paroxysmal arrhythmias. Sinus arrhythmia is increase in the pulse rate during inspiration and decrease during expiration. It is a physiological phenomenon caused by a change in vagal tone affecting the sinoatrial node, during each respiratory cycle. The variation is markedly observed in children and during sleep. If the pulse is irregular, look for **pulse deficit**. The examiner auscultates the heart rate while an assistant counts the pulse rate for the same minute. The difference between heart rate and pulse rate is called pulse deficit. Pulse deficit is seen in atrial and ventricular fibrillation.

Volume

Volume of the pulse is defined as the amplitude of expansion of the vessel wall produced by the pulse wave. Feeling the volume of the pulse can assess the pulse pressure. The pulse may have a normal, high or low volume. It is constant from beat to beat. The volume of the pulse is a measure of the amount of blood flowing through the artery during each beat. It is directly related to the stroke volume. Low volume pulse is felt in circulatory shock and heart failure. In circulatory shock pulse is referred to as **weak and thready** (low-volume). High volume pulse is felt during exercise, in old age and in aortic regurgitation. In aortic regurgitation the pulse is described as collapsing pulse. Pulses alternans and pulses paradoxes are volume abnormalities.

Character of the Pulse

Character describes the volume, tension and waveform of the pulse. Tension is the pressure required to obliterate the pulse and it can be normal, increased or decreased. Character of the pulse is usually evaluated at the right carotid artery in the neck or the radial artery. It can be better studied by sphygmography. An upstroke and a down stroke can be recorded for each pulse wave **(Fig. 22.2)**. The normal pulse waveform is catacrotic. Abnormalities in pulse character include anacrotic pulse, dicrotic pulse, bisferiens pulse and collapsing pulse.

Abnormal Pulses (Fig. 22.3)

- ❖ **Collapsing or water hammer or Corrigan's pulse** characterized by rapid upstroke and rapid down stroke

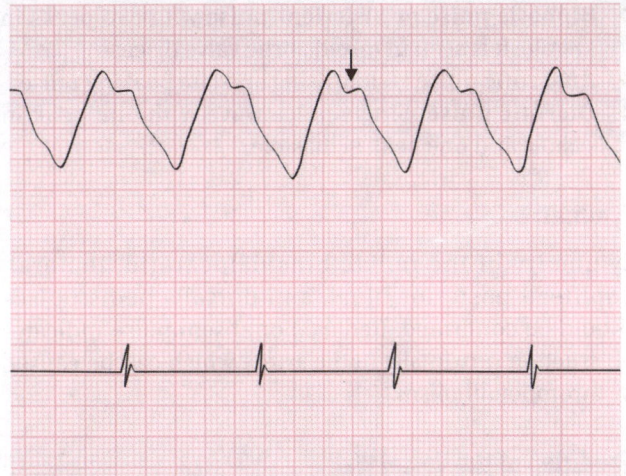

Fig. 22.2: Arterial pulse recorded in a physiograph from the finger (upstroke of each wave is the anacrotic limb, down stroke is the catacrotic limb. In the down stroke, note the dicrotic notch represented by the arrow).

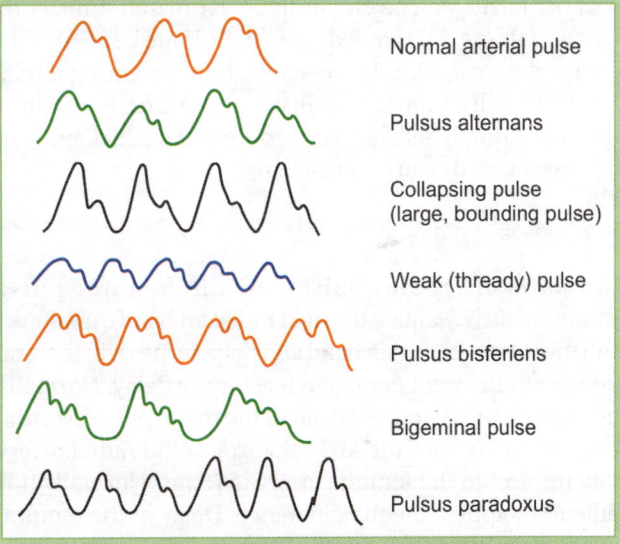

Fig. 22.3: Abnormal arterial pulses.

of the pulse wave. It is a large volume pulse and is seen in aortic regurgitation and patent ductus arteriosus. For the examination of collapsing pulse, feel for the radial artery with the distal aspect of the examiner's right palm. The collapsing pulse can be exaggerated at the radial artery by lifting the arm. Elevate the limb vertically up to 90° swiftly, to feel for a thud or collapse.

- **Pulses paradoxus** are seen in large pericardial effusion and in constrictive pericarditis (at the end of deep inspiration, pulse becomes weaker or even disappears). It is called paradox because heart sounds may be heard on auscultation of the precordium at a time when no pulse is palpable at the site of radial artery.
- **Pulses alternans** where a high volume pulse is followed by a low volume pulse due to left ventricular failure (e.g., myocardial infarction of left ventricle).
- **Biphasic pulse or bisferiens pulse** with two peaks in systole. It is seen in mixed aortic valve disease.
- **Anacrotic pulse** is slow rising and late peaking pulse.
- **Dicrotic pulse**: Single pulse wave with one peak in systole and one peak in diastole.

Symmetry

Symmetry of the radial, brachial, carotid, femoral, popliteal, posterior tibial, and dorsalis pedis pulses should be confirmed. Reduced or absent pulse indicates obstruction proximally in the artery which can be caused by thromboembolism.

Condition of the Vessel Wall

The radial artery is palpated with the index, middle and ring finger of the right hand of the examiner. Compress the artery with the index finger or the proximal finger and empty the vessel by squeezing distally with the ring finger or the distal finger. The middle finger is pressed sufficiently hard and the vessel is rolled against the bone beneath it, to feel for the texture of the vessel wall. In the young adults the vessel wall cannot be felt distinctly. In elderly people it may be distinctly felt as a cord as a result of thickening of the vessel wall due to atherosclerosis.

Radiofemoral Delay

Compare the radial pulse and the femoral pulse simultaneously. Palpate the right radial artery of the subject with the fingers of the left hand and palpate the right femoral artery with the right hand and feel for the delay. Normally the femoral pulse comes ahead of the radial pulse. Normal delay of pulse from the arch of aorta to the radial artery is 80 ms and to the femoral artery is 75 ms. Normally it is difficult to appreciate the difference. Delay of the femoral pulse when compared with the radial pulse is seen in coarctation of aorta.

Palpation of Other Peripheral Vessels

- **Carotid artery:** With the subject in the supine position, gently palpate the carotid artery with the thumb at the level of the thyroid cartilage against the transverse process of sixth cervical vertebra. To examine the left carotid use the right thumb and vice versa. Both the carotids should not be palpated simultaneously.
- **Femoral artery:** Palpate the artery with three fingers or the thumb at the midpoint between anterior superior iliac spine and the pubic symphysis.
- **Popliteal artery:** Flex the supine subject's knee at 120° and place the fingertips of both the hands of the examiner on the popliteal fossa with the thumbs resting on the subject's patella. Feel for the popliteal artery.
- **Posterior tibial artery:** Palpate the artery at a distance of 1 cm behind the medial malleolus with the foot relaxed between plantar and dorsiflexion.
- **Dorsalis pedis artery:** Palpate the artery against the tarsal bones in the first intermetatarsal space proximally.
- **Brachial artery:** Palpate the anterior cubital fossa by partially flexing the elbow joint and by placing the fingers medial to the insertion of biceps tendon.
- **Superficial temporal artery:** Place the fingers above the zygomatic arch in front of the tragus of the ear and palpate the artery on both sides.

MEASUREMENT OF ARTERIAL BLOOD PRESSURE

Blood pressure is the lateral force exerted by the blood column per unit area of vascular wall and is expressed in mm of mercury. It is recorded using a sphygmomanometer with the subject in the sitting or lying down posture. Both palpatory and auscultatory methods should be done (details given in Chapter 20).

JUGULAR VENOUS PRESSURE (JVP)

Jugular venous pressure is defined as the height of the vertical column of blood in the internal jugular vein, above the sternal angle measured in centimeters. The right internal jugular vein is examined under good light with the subject reclined at an angle of about 45° with the horizontal. The head should rest on a pillow and chin should be in the midline. Elevate the chin slightly to stretch the skin over the lower neck and supraclavicular area. The internal jugular vein lies adjacent to the medial border of the sternocleidomastoid muscle.

The right internal jugular vein reflects the right atrial pressure (central venous pressure) as it is directly in line with the right atrium. In normal individuals jugular venous pulse (JVP) is not visible in the neck in the above-mentioned position of the subject, because it is just below the clavicle. If visible, it indicates elevation of right atrial pressure. If visible, mainly two waves can be distinguished in the venous

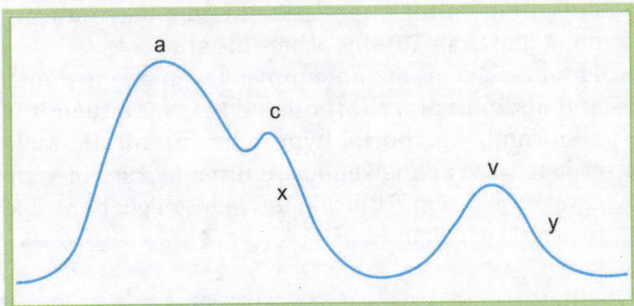

Fig. 22.4: Waves of jugular venous pulse.

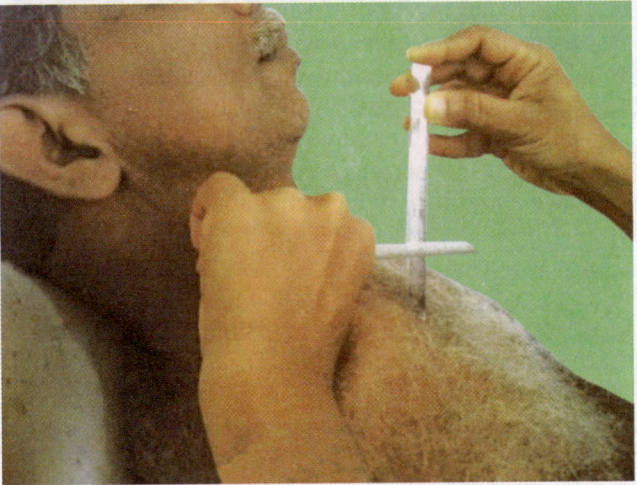

Fig. 22.5: Measurement of JVP.

pulse 'a' and 'v' waves. The 'c' wave of jugular venous pulse tracing is a very small wave and it is not visible over the neck. JVP may be visible normally when the subject is in the supine position.

Since the jugular vein reflects right atrial pressure the **jugular pulse tracing** also has the same waves as that of atrial pressure changes, i.e., a, c, v which are positive waves and x and y descend **(Fig. 22.4)**. The perpendicular level at which pulsation is obtained over the jugular vein depends on the hydrostatic pressure in the right atrium. Normally it corresponds to manubrium sterni in the erect posture. So it is not visible in the erect posture. When the person is reclined at an angle of 45°, the pulsation cannot be seen above the clavicle. If the pulsation is seen above the clavicle at this angle, then there is increase in the right atrial pressure and it indicates some pathology. Normal jugular venous pressure (central venous pressure) is 6 mm Hg.

View the jugular pulse waves and time the waves with the carotid pulse by simultaneously palpating the left carotid artery with the left hand, which is passed behind the subject's neck. The 'a' wave comes just before the carotid pulse while the 'v' wave comes with the carotid pulse or follows the carotid pulsation. The 'a' wave is produced by atrial systole. In atrial fibrillation, there is no 'a' wave and the JVP loses its double waveform.

Measurement of JVP

The jugular venous pressure is measured in centimeters vertically from the sternal angle to the upper level of the venous waveform. To measure the JVP, a scale is placed vertically from the sternal angle and a second scale is placed horizontally at the upper level of the vertical oscillating column of blood. The distance from the sternal angle to the horizontal scale is measured in cm **(Fig. 22.5)**.

The normal upper limit is 4 cm. This is about 9 cm above the right atrium and corresponds to a pressure of 6 mm Hg. Elevation of JVP indicates a raised right atrial pressure or superior vena caval obstruction.

Hepatojugular Reflux

With the subject inclined at an angle of 45°, the examiner who is standing on the right side of the subject should apply firm pressure over the mid-abdomen for at least 30 seconds. In normal individuals the rise in jugular venous pressure will be less than 3 cm and it is not sustained, returning to normal in less than 3 cardiac cycles. In right heart failure, a sustained rise in JVP more than 3 cm is obtained.

EXAMINATION OF PRECORDIUM

Inspection

Chest should be bare when the precordium is examined. Precordium is the part of the chest overlying the heart. The subject should lie relaxed on an examination couch in the supine position or at 45° to the horizontal. Look for the following:
- Shape of precordium
- Position of the apical impulse
- Other visible pulsations over the chest

During inspection observe the shape of the precordium and see whether there is any bulging or depression of precordium or other deformities. See whether the apex beat is visible. Mention the position in relation to nipple in the male. In addition, look for pulsations outside the precordium like the carotid pulsations in the neck and the veins and venous pulsations in the neck. Look for pulsations in the supraclavicular, suprasternal, second intercostal spaces and the epigastrium. See whether there are dilated veins over the thorax and the abdomen.
- Cardiac impulse refers to the diffuse movements occurring in the precordium due to the impact of heart against the chest wall during ventricular systole. Apex beat is seen as forceful, repetitive, rhythmic bulging movement in the left and lower part of the area of cardiac impulse. The rate will be same as that of the pulse rate. It may not be visible because of obesity, thick muscular chest wall, if the apex beat lies behind a rib, in scoliosis and after deep inspiration when the lungs cover the

heart. It may not be visible on the left side if the heart is on the right side (dextrocardia).
- When the cardiac impulse is not visible, the subject should be examined in the sitting position while bending forward or while lying down on his left side. The impulse is normally seen in the fifth left intercostal space about half an inch medial to the midclavicular line. In children, it is usually in the 4th intercostal space; and in persons with long, narrow chest it may be in the 6th space. It will be very prominent in thin individuals.
- The carotid pulsations are visible on either side in the anterior triangle of the neck by the side of the sternomastoid muscles especially in thin individuals. They synchronize with the cardiac impulse in rate and rhythm.
- The external jugular veins are seen on the surface in the posterior triangle of the neck. They are seen when they are full with blood. The height of the column of blood in these veins can be regarded as a measure of the venous blood pressure.
- The venous pulsations are seen over the jugular veins better on the right side. The pulsations are prominent at the lowest level in the supraclavicular fossa where the veins enter the deeper tissues to join the superior vena cava. The pulsations are more marked if the veins are full. In the erect posture the column sinks to the level of the manubrium sterni and venous pulsations are hardly seen. Only the carotid pulsations are visible in this position. In the supine recumbent position with the neck slightly flexed and turned a little to the left, the venous pulsations are seen prominently.
- The carotid pulsations are normally seen in thin individuals and in anxiety. Pathologically carotid pulsations will be prominent in conditions like thyrotoxicosis, aortic regurgitation and in aneurysms of aorta.
- Pulsations in the suprasternal notch may indicate unfolding or aneurysms of arch of aorta.
- Prominent veins are not normally seen on the thorax and abdominal wall. If dilated veins are seen it is abnormal, e.g., portal hypertension, intrathoracic growth obstructing venous return and inferior vena caval obstruction. Thin and tiny veins might be visible in people with fair skin.

Palpation

- Confirm the findings obtained by inspection.
- If apex beat is palpable, locate its exact position using the pulp of the fingers with the subject preferably in the supine position. Palpation should be started from the axillary region, using whole of the palm **(Fig. 22.6A)**. Once a definite impulse is felt, the apex beat should be located carefully using the index or middle finger **(Fig. 22.6B)**. If the apex beat is not felt try it at the end of expiration or in the left lateral position. If it is not felt on the left side look on the right side. The cardiac impulse may be felt forcefully, moderately or feebly. It is felt as a tap coming from inside the chest towards the anterior wall. The junction of the manubrium with the body of the sternum is called sternal angle or angle of Louis. The second costal cartilage articulates with the sternum at the sternal angle. The intercostal space immediately below this rib is the second intercostal space. Vertical line drawn from the center of the clavicle downwards is the midclavicular line.
- Place the ulnar border of the right hand parallel to the left sternal border and see whether there is a left parasternal heave **(Fig. 22.7)**. Right ventricular enlargement produces a systolic thrust (heave) in the left parasternal area. There will be systolic elevation of left costochondral junction. Subject should be in supine position.

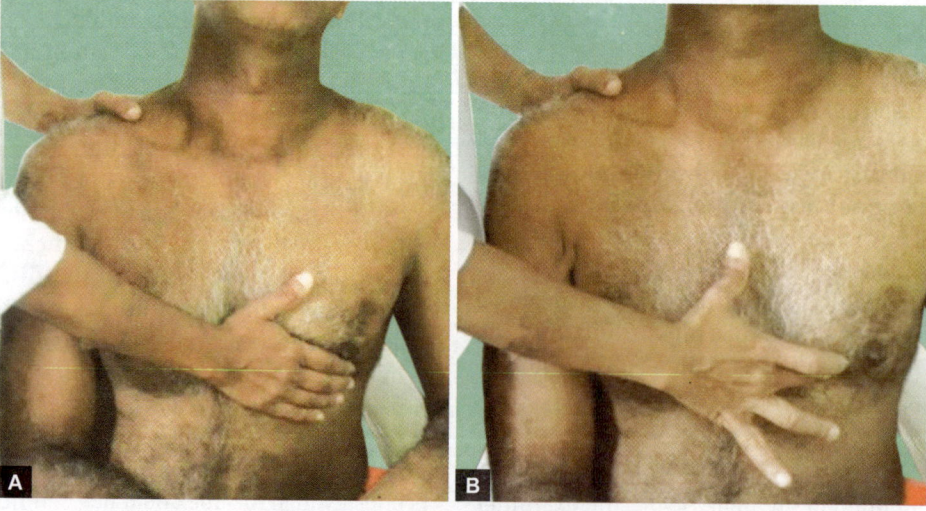

Figs. 22.6A and B: Locating the apex beat.

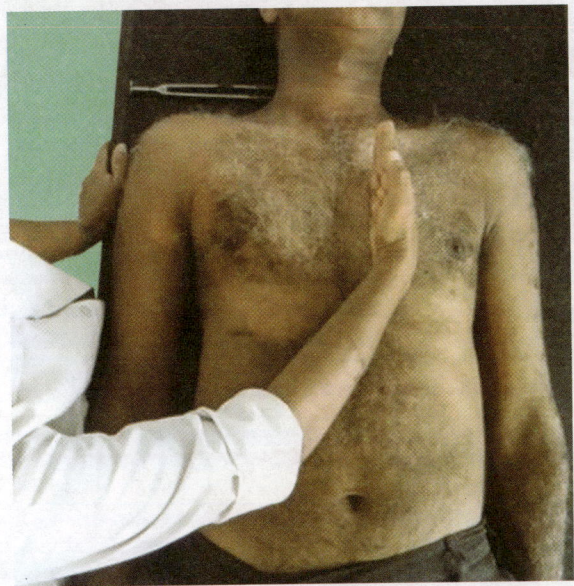

Fig. 22.7: Looking for left parasternal heave with subject in the supine position.

- Place the palm flat over the precordium and feel for any vibrations and thrills. The turbulent flow responsible for murmurs may produce palpable vibrations on the chest wall called thrills. Thrills are palpable murmurs. These should not be present in health. It is felt prominently in aortic stenosis, ventricular septal defect and patent ductus arteriosus.
- Feel for the carotid pulsations, which are felt as expansile waves. Venous pulsations in the neck are clearly seen than felt. By emptying the vein and compressing it at either end it may be confirmed that it fills from the head end towards the chest.
- Look for other palpable pulsations in the precordium, intercostal spaces and epigastrium. Epigastric pulsations are felt in aneurysms of abdominal aorta and in heart failure due to pulsatile liver. It may be felt normally in very thin individuals.
- If there are dilated veins over the chest and abdomen find out the direction of flow of blood.

Percussion

Percussion can define the borders of the heart mainly the right and left borders. Gross enlargement or shift in the position of the heart can be made out. Percussion is also useful to identify pericardial effusion and right atrial enlargement. While percussing the heart, a moderate force should be used.
- The subject should be in the supine position.
- The left border of the heart is percussed first.
- Start percussing in the 5th left intercostal space from the midaxillary line (vertical line descending from the center of axilla).
- Place the pleximeter finger in the space parallel to the ribs and percuss. A resonant note is heard normally.
- Continue percussing shifting the pleximeter finger towards the right by 1 cm.
- When the area of cardiac impulse is reached a dull note will be heard. The heart tissue gives a dull note. Mark the point with ink.
- Now repeat the same procedure on the 4th intercostal space. Mark the point where the dull note is heard.
- Repeat the procedure in the 3rd space and then on the 2nd space, till the clavicle is reached. Join the points to draw a line. It defines the left border of the heart. It begins in the third intercostal space 2–3 cm to the left of the midsternal line and extends 7–8 cm to the left of the midsternal line and ends just medial to the midclavicular line in the fifth intercostal space.
- To mark out the right border of the heart place the pleximeter finger on the right side of the chest in the 2nd intercostal space 4–5 cm away from the sternum. Percuss. A resonant note is obtained.
- Percuss in the same vertical line in each lower intercostal space. Listen to the note.
- In the 5th space a dull note is heard. This is due to liver.
- Find out the lowest space where a resonant note is heard. From this space, start percussing towards the left, while listening to the percussion note produced. A resonant note is heard till the sternum is reached.
- Repeat the percussion over each space above till the sternum is reached. The resonant note is heard all over till the sternum is reached.
- The right border of the heart corresponds to the right sternal border.

Percussion cannot define the upper border and the inferior border of the heart accurately. The upper border cannot be percussed out accurately as the dullness of the heart tissue continues with the dullness of the great vessels. Joining the lower point of the left and right borders and the upper points in the same gives the upper and lower borders of the heart. Percussion of the great arteries should be carried out medially from the midclavicular line on either side along the second intercostal space. Both the second intercostal spaces are always resonant. Dullness here is a sign of disease.

Auscultation

By auscultation we listen to the heart sounds, i.e., the sounds produced in the heart and the great vessels. The sounds are produced mainly due to the closure of the heart valves and are heard all over the precordium. Ideally auscultation should be done in a sound proof room with a good stethoscope.

Clinically the chest is auscultated to hear the sounds clearly over four main areas. These areas are called the valvular areas of auscultation. These areas do not

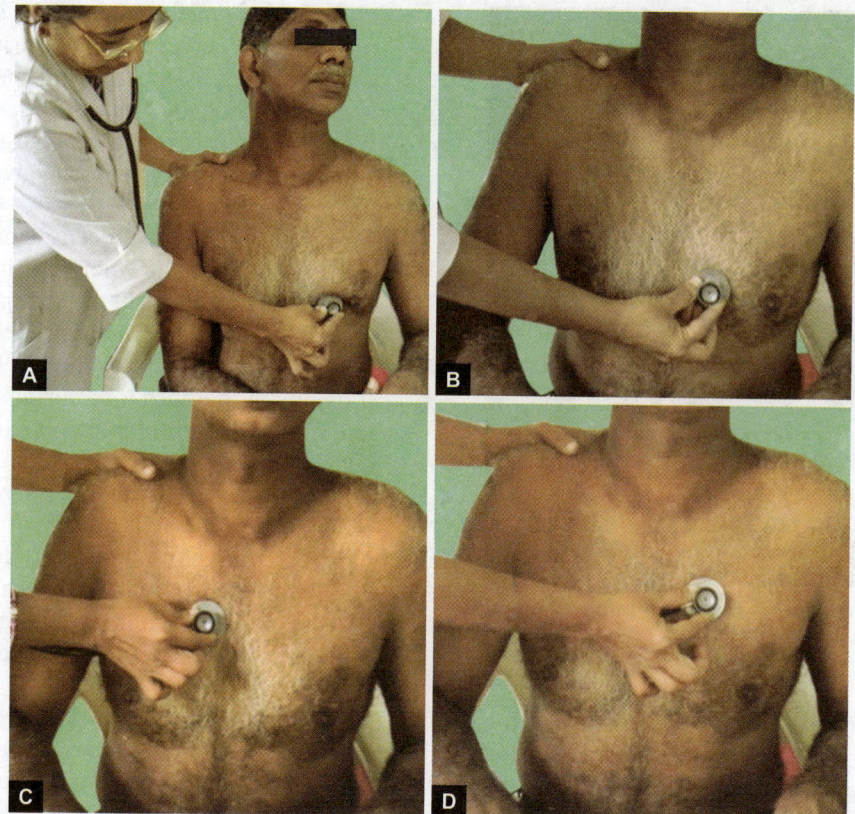

Figs. 22.8A to D: Areas for auscultation: (A) Mitral area over the apex beat; (B) Tricuspid area at the lower end of sternum on the left side; (C) Aortic area in the second right intercostal space near the sternal border; (D) Pulmonary area in the second left intercostal space near the sternal border.

correspond to the anatomical location of the respective valves. The sound produced by each valve of the heart is heard best in each of these areas.

The areas are (**Figs. 22.8A to D**):
- The mitral area overlying the apex-beat.
- The tricuspid area lies just to the left of the lower end of the sternum in the fifth intercostal space.
- The aortic area at the right 2nd intercostal space close to the sternal border.
- The pulmonary area in the left 2nd intercostal space near the sternal border.
  - On auscultation, two sounds are heard all over the chest. There occurs a pause after the occurrence of the two sounds and again they are repeated.
  - The sound that occurs first is the first heart sound, which can be mimicked as 'lubb' and the one that follows it in rapid succession, is the second heart sound, which is mimicked as 'dup'. It occurs as 'lubb dup', 'lubb dup' in succession.
  - In children, a short and faint 3rd heart sound may sometimes be audible in mitral area, which immediately follows the second sound.
  - Abnormal sounds heard over the precordium include murmur and friction rub or pericardial rub. A friction rub occurs in pericarditis. Murmurs are caused by turbulent flow within the heart and great vessels. Murmurs may also indicate valve disease or abnormal communications between the right and left sides of the heart (e.g., septal defects).
  - Heart murmurs are defined by four characteristics: Loudness, quality, location and timing. Loudness reflects the degree of turbulence. This relates to its frequency and is described as low, medium or high-pitched. The location of the murmur on the chest wall depends on its site of origin. Murmurs are timed according to the phase of systole or diastole during which they are audible. Systolic murmurs are ejection systolic, midsystolic, pansystolic or late systolic; diastolic murmurs are either early diastolic, mid-diastolic or late diastolic (presystolic) in timing. Continuous murmurs are heard both during systole and diastole of the cardiac cycle as in the case of patent ductus arteriosus.
  - Finally auscultate for carotid and femoral arterial bruits. Bruits are vibrating sounds that can be heard while auscultating over arteries in which there is turbulent blood flow. It may be due to arterial narrowing.

REPORT PATTERN

Name:
Age:
Sex:
Occupation and address:

General Examination

Consciousness: Conscious
Orientation: Well oriented
Built and nourishment: Normally built and nourished; no pallor, icterus, cyanosis, edema, dyspnea, clubbing or lymphadenopathy.
Body temperature: 37°C
Respiratory rate: 16/min, regular, abdominothoracic
Pulse: 70/min, regular, normal in volume and character, no thickening of vessel wall, no radiofemoral/brachiofemoral delay. All other peripheral pulsations are felt equally on both sides.

Blood pressure in the right upper limb in supine position:
Palpatory method—116 mm Hg
Auscultatory method—120/80 mm Hg

Cardiovascular System Examination

Inspection

Shape of chest: Normal
Trachea: Appears to be central
Apex beat: Not visible (if visible indicate the site)
JVP: Not raised
Visible pulsations: No visible pulsations over the chest
 Engorged veins in neck, chest and abdomen: No dilated veins over the neck, chest and abdomen.

Palpation

Trachea: Centrally placed
Apex beat: Apex beat felt in the fifth left intercostal space half an inch medial to the midclavicular line
Thrills: No thrills
Parasternal heave: No parasternal heave

Percussion

Heart borders are within normal limits.

Auscultation

Mitral area, tricuspid area, pulmonary area and aortic area: First and second heart sounds heard normally in the mitral, tricuspid, aortic and pulmonary areas. No murmur or other abnormal sounds. No carotid or femoral arterial bruits.

Impression

The cardiovascular system of the subject appears to be normal.

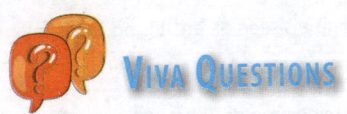

VIVA QUESTIONS

1. **What are the causes of first heart sound?**
   » Closure of the mitral and the tricuspid valves.
   » Contraction of the ventricular musculature.
   » Vibrations set up in the mediastinum.

2. **What are the causes of second heart sound?**
   » Closure of the aortic and the pulmonary valves.
   » Vibrations of blood vessels.
   » Turbulence produced in the blood column.

3. **What are the causes for third and fourth heart sounds? Give the conditions in which it is audible.**
   » The third heart sound is due to gushing of blood into the ventricles during the diastole at the end of the isovolumetric relaxation phase. It is heard in children and young adults. It also occurs in high output states caused by exercise, anemia, fever, pregnancy and thyrotoxicosis.
   » The fourth heart sound is due to the atrial systole. It is not an audible heart sound. It can only be recorded by phonocardiography. In the elderly, S4 is sometimes physiological. Pathological S4 occurs in hypertension, aortic stenosis, and hypertrophic cardiomyopathy.

4. **How will you distinguish between first and second heart sounds?**
   » The first heart sound is almost synchronous with the carotid pulsation or the apex beat while the second sound follows it. Thus the sounds can be recognized as the first and the second sound.
   » The first sound is referred to as systolic sound because it is associated with the ventricular systole. The first heart sound is longer in duration when compared to the second and louder. But it is low pitched. The first sound is heard well in the mitral and tricuspid areas.
   » The second is called diastolic sound because it indicates the beginning of the diastole. The second sound is high pitched, of short duration and less in loudness. The second sound is heard well in the pulmonary and aortic areas.

5. **What are the variations in pulse rate with age and sex?**
   When the pulse rate is decreased the condition is called bradycardia. A rapid pulse rate is called tachycardia.
   Age: The pulse rate varies with age. In the fetus, the heart rate is about 140 per minute. In a newly born infant it is about 130, at the age of five it is about 90, at the age of 10 years 80, at the age of 15 years 75, and at the age of 20 it comes to about 70–72 per minute. It remains constant throughout the life after this age.
   Sex: The pulse rate is about five beats more in the adult woman than in the adult man.
   Athletes show a rate of 50–60/min due to well-developed vagal tone.

6. **Name the conditions where JVP is elevated.**
   » Tricuspid valve stenosis
   » Congestive cardiac failure
   » Constrictive pericarditis
   » Cardiac tamponade
   » Superior vena cava obstruction
   » Right ventricular infarction
   » Pulmonary embolism
   In constrictive pericarditis and in cardiac tamponade, inspiration produces a paradoxical rise in the JVP referred to as Kussmaul's sign. This is because the increased venous return that occurs during inspiration cannot be accommodated within the constrained right side of the heart.

7. **What are the abnormalities seen in the waveform of JVP?**
   » Giant 'a' wave occurs in forceful atrial contraction against a stenosed tricuspid valve or a non-compliant hypertrophied right ventricle.
   » Cannon 'a' wave is caused by atrial systole against a closed tricuspid valve. It occurs in complete heart block and in ventricular tachycardia.
   » Giant 'v' wave is seen in tricuspid regurgitation.
   » Prominent 'x' and 'y' descents occur in constrictive pericarditis.

8. **How will you distinguish between arterial and venous pulse?**
   » Venous pulse is better seen than felt whereas arterial pulse is better felt than seen.
   » Venous pulse has a definite upper level, which falls during inspiration.
   » Venous pulse varies with posture.
   » Hepatojugular reflux is seen in venous pulse. When moderate pressure is applied over the right hypochondrium, there will be a slight increase in the JVP due to increased venous return.
   » The double wave form of JVP is not seen in arterial pulse.

9. **Why is external jugular vein not selected to assess venous pressure?**
   » Valves are present in the course of external jugular vein and so it may not reflect the exact right atrial pressure.
   » External jugular vein passes through more fascial planes and so, it is subjected to external compression as it passes under the clavicle.

10. **Define apex beat. Give its normal location.**
    Apex beat is the lowermost and outermost point over the precordium where a definite cardiac impulse is seen or felt. It is normally felt in the fifth left intercostal space ½ an inch medial to the midclavicular line.

11. **Mention the conditions where the apex beat is displaced from the normal site.**
    Apex beat may be on the right side in dextrocardia. Shift to left of apex beat is seen in left ventricular hypertrophy. Chest wall deformities such as pectus excavatum may compress the heart and displace the apex to the left and this can be mistaken for cardiac enlargement. Shift of apex beat can also be due to push or pull due to diseases of the surrounding viscera. Pushing can be due to pleural effusion or pneumothorax. Pulling of the apex beat can be due to pulmonary fibrosis or collapse of the lung.

12. **What is the difference between thrill, murmur and bruit? What are the types of murmur?**
    Palpable murmur over the precordium is called thrill. Murmur is an abnormal sound auscultated over the precordium. The types of murmurs are systolic murmurs, diastolic and pan systolic murmur. Bruit is a vibrating sound heard over arteries on auscultation.

13. **What does physiological splitting mean? What is the reason for the physiological split of second heart sound? What is the reason for its widening in deep inspiration?**
    Aortic valve close first because the pressure difference is more on the aortic side. Pulmonary vascular resistance is 1/10th that of systemic resistance. So, the right ventricular ejection starts earlier and is completed slightly later than left ventricular ejection. So, the pulmonary valve closes after the closure of aortic valve. The splitting of the second sound (aortic and pulmonary components) is normal and is called **physiological splitting** and it is present during inspiration.
    If the person takes a deep inspiration, the splitting widens, i.e., A_2 appears earlier and P_2 occurs a little late than normal. This is because of increase in the negativity of intrathoracic pressure and the resulting increase in the venous return to the right atrium. End-diastolic volume in the right ventricle is increased leading to an increase in the ejection period. Thus, P_2 will be a little delayed from normal, i.e., it is postponed. On the left side, increased negativity of intrathoracic pressure causes increase in the volume of left atrium leading to a decrease in the pressure in the left atrium. The pressure gradient becomes less between atrium and ventricle on the left. This leads to decrease in ventricular filling and there will be a reduction in the ventricular ejection time and so, A_2 is preponed than that of normal. During forced expiration, opposite of the above changes occur and the splitting becomes narrow. Exaggerated splitting is seen in right bundle branch block. Reversed splitting (splitting is seen during expiration and not during inspiration) occurs in left bundle branch block.

14. **Define arterial pulse. Mention three abnormal pulses.**
    Definition (refer page 117).
    » Collapsing pulse in aortic regurgitation.
    » Pulsus alternans or alternating pulse is seen in severe left ventricular failure.
    » Biphasic pulse with two systolic peaks is seen in mixed aortic valve disease.
15. **What is the reason for high volume pulse in old age?**
    In old age, due to atherosclerosis the systolic pressure increases. There is not much increase in the diastolic pressure normally. So, the pulse pressure increases. This results in high volume pulse.
16. **What are the precautions to be taken while examining pulse?**
    » The subject should rest and relax for about 5 minutes before examining the pulse.
    » Pulse should be counted for one whole minute.
    » If pulse is irregular look for pulse deficit by counting the heart rate simultaneously.
    » Pulses on both sides should be compared.
    » Radiofemoral delay should not be missed.
17. **What is Hepatojugular reflux?**
    Refer page 119 and 120.

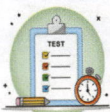

OBJECTIVE STRUCTURED PRACTICAL EXAMINATION

I. Examine the radial pulse of the subject and comment
1. Stand on the right side of the subject
2. Hold the right hand of the subject in a semipronated and semiflexed position and support the hand
3. Place the examiners middle three fingers on the radial artery of the subject just above the wrist
4. Count the pulse for one minute and note the volume and character of the pulse also
5. Palpate for the artery using the middle three fingers and see whether it is thickened
6. Compare with the pulse of the opposite side
7. Check for radiofemoral delay
8. Write down the findings

II. Locate the apex beat of the subject and comment
1. Expose the chest
2. Inspect the precordium for visible pulsation in the 5th left intercostal space
3. Place the palm on the precordium over the mitral area and feel for pulsation
4. If felt, use the ulnar border of the hand to confirm the pulsation
5. Using the tip of the middle finger carefully locate the exact position where a definite pulsation is felt and mark that area
6. Count the intercostal space and locate the exact position of the apex beat from the midclavicular line

III. Auscultate the aortic area for heart sounds
1. Explain the procedure to the subject and ask him to expose the chest
2. The right second intercostal space is identified
3. Checks whether the diaphragm of the stethoscope is functioning properly by gently tapping over it after keeping the ear piece in the ear
4. Place the diaphragm over the second right intercostal space close to the sternal border
5. Listens to the heart sounds carefully

Chapter 23

Recording of Arterial Pulse

LEARNING OBJECTIVES

- Examine the radial pulse in the proper sequence
- Define arterial pulse
- Mention the clinical importance of examination of radial pulse
- List the abnormalities of pulse giving examples
- Mention the names of the arterial pulses that are examined clinically

PY5.16: Record the arterial pulse in a normal volunteer using physiograph.

AIM

To record the arterial pulse from the fingertip using physiograph.

APPARATUS: PHYSIOGRAPH

Physiograph is an instrument which can be used for recording several physiological parameters like arterial pulse, venous pulse, blood pressure, respiratory volumes and capacities, respiratory movements, skeletal muscle and cardiac muscle contractions, etc., a transducer converts different forms of energies into electrical impulses.

The physiograph consists of a main console which has coupler housing for lodging various couplers for different experiments.

Console Side

On one side of the console, there are three sockets. The top one is for the stimulator which provides electrical pulses and time base. The lower two sockets are IN and OUT sockets for connecting more than one physiograph to the same equipment. This side of the console also has three screw driver controls marked as 'Gain', 'Damping' and 'Offset'.

On the other side of the console, a fuse and a Mains lead can be seen. In front of them there is a slot for paper stack.

Console Front

Here we can see MAINS ON/OFF switch, speed range selector knob, speed selector push buttons and window for paper feeding and pen lift knob.

Console Top

On the top of the console, are seen pens and ink wells, slot for receiving paper, guides, thumb screw and bearing, coupler housing and the main amplifier.

The main amplifier consists of;
- 50 Hz filter on/off
- Sensitivity selector
- Pen position control

PROCEDURE

- After switching off the mains, plug in the coupler for recording pulse in the coupler housing.
- Fill the ink wells, lift the pens and check the ink flow.
- Put the stack of chart in the paper receptacle through the slot. The chart side should face down and the paper end facing the window. Fold the paper end into 'V' and with fingers of one hand slide the paper upwards, and pull it out from the slot in the console with the other hand. Slide the paper under the two guides and under the ball bearing lifting the ball bearing manipulating the thumb screw. Depress the ball bearing on the paper by the thumb screw for paper movement.

- Connect the pulse transducer to the subject by wrapping it around the finger tip. Connect the other end of the transducer to the coupler.
- Connect the physiograph stimulator to the physiograph and adjust it to record the time base.
- Put console mains 'ON' select desired chart speed and sensitivity.
- Put pens, on chart paper manipulating the pen lift knob.
- Run paper a few centimetres, using thumb screw. Adjust pen position to centre with pen position control. Set base line while the paper is moving, stop paper, using thumb screw.
- Put coupler 'ON' and run paper. Record the normal arterial pulse and calculate the rate and note the rhythm and character of the pulse.

DISCUSSION

Peripheral Pulse Tracing

Peripheral pulse tracing consists of an up-stroke, peak and a down-stroke. Up-stroke is called **anacrotic limb**, down-stroke **catacrotic limb** and the notch seen in the down-stroke is called **dicrotic notch (Fig. 23.1)**. Anacrotic limb is due to ejection of blood from the ventricle during systole. The factors affecting the height of anacrotic limb are:
- Stroke volume
- Duration of cardiac cycle
- Diastolic pressure
- Distensibility of the vessel wall

Catacrotic limb is due to diastole and elastic recoil of vessel wall.

Dicrotic notch is due to backflow of blood in the aorta at the beginning of diastole and it corresponds to the incisura of aortic pressure curve. It marks the end of ventricular systole.

ABNORMALITIES OF ARTERIAL PULSE

- **Rate:** Increase in the pulse rate denotes tachycardia and decrease in the pulse rate denotes bradycardia.
- **Volume** and force of pulse
  - Rapid and thready pulse (small, weak pulse) occurs in hypotension or circulatory shock. This is seen in severe heart failure, hypovolemia and severe aortic stenosis.
  - Increase in the volume of pulse is seen in exercise and ventricular hypertrophy.
- **Rhythm of pulse:** Irregular pulse is seen in ectopic beats, atrial fibrillation and other arrhythmias.
- Other abnormal pulses **(Fig. 23.2)**
  - *Pulsus alternans:* There is a beat to beat alternation in pulse size and intensity. Here alternating strong and weak beats are felt but the rhythm is basically regular. It is indicative of left ventricular systolic impairment (left sided heart failure).
  - **Water hammer pulse** or Corrigan's pulse or collapsing pulse or large bounding pulse where the pulse is bounding and forceful, rapidly increasing and subsequently collapsing seen in aortic insufficiency, anemia, hyperthyroidism, etc. The pulse pressure is increased. Causes are increased stroke volume, decreased peripheral resistance, or both.
  - **Bisferiens pulse** is an arterial pulse with a double systolic peak. It is seen in aortic regurgitation.
  - **Pulsus bigeminus** is characterized by groups of two heart beats close together followed by a longer pause. This is a disorder of rhythm and is caused by a normal beat alternating with a premature contraction. The stroke volume of the premature

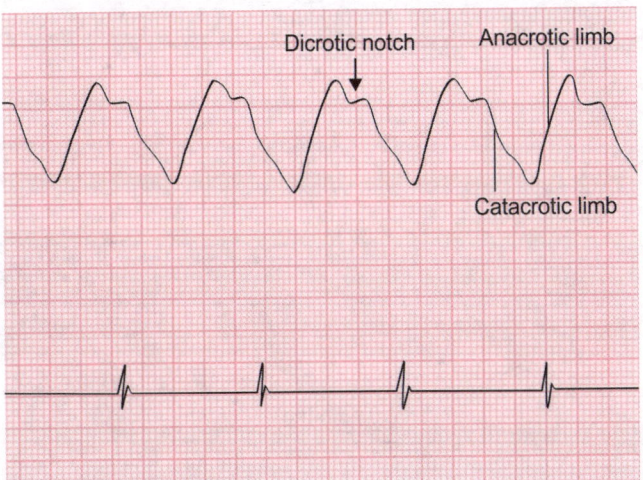

Fig. 23.1: Arterial pulse tracing using physiograph.

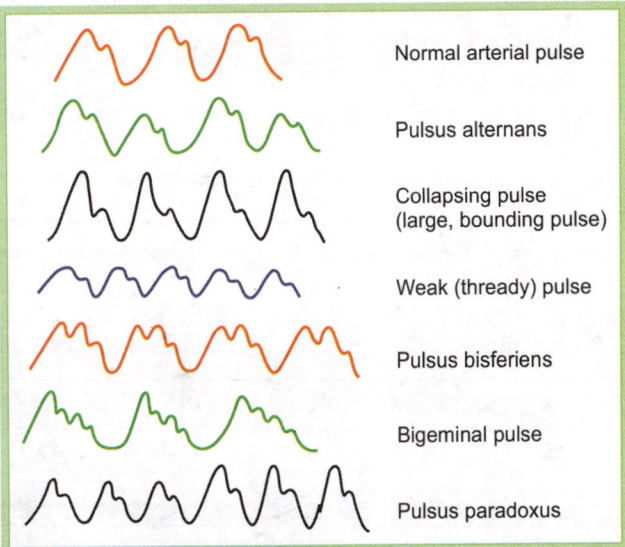

Fig. 23.2: Abnormal arterial pulses compared with normal pulse recording.

beat is less and so the second pulse is weaker than the first and sometimes may not be palpable. It is seen in regularly occurring ventricular premature beats as in digitalis toxicity, myocardial infarction, electrolyte imbalance, hypothyroidism, etc.

- **Pulsus paradoxus** where the pulse disappears in deep inspiration and appears in expiration. It is seen in pericardial effusion, cardiac tamponade and in exacerbations of chronic obstructive pulmonary disease. There is a palpable decrease in the amplitude of the pulse in quiet inspiration. The systolic pressure decreases by more than 10 mm Hg during inspiration.
- **Weak thready pulse** is seen in hypotension or circulatory shock. The features are weak pulse, tachycardia, shallow breathing and unconsciousness. Weak thready pulse is difficult to be felt, it is felt as a small thread under the palpating finger. It will be usually rapid.

Chapter 24

Examination of Abdomen

LEARNING OBJECTIVES

- Explain the clinical importance of examination of abdomen
- Show the different quadrants of the abdomen and name them
- Demonstrate the steps to palpate the liver and spleen
- Demonstrate the technique to look for shifting dullness
- Auscultate the abdomen to check bowel sounds and explain its clinical significance

PY4.10: Demonstrate the correct clinical examination of the abdomen in a normal volunteer or simulated environment.

AIM

To examine and report the findings in the abdomen of the subject.

REQUIREMENTS

Stethoscope, sphygmomanometer, measuring tape, torch and knee hammer.

PROCEDURE

Any systemic examination should be preceded by the general examination. The points relevant to the gastrointestinal system should be examined in a detailed manner like pallor, icterus, clubbing, edema, lymphadenopathy, pulse rate and blood pressure.

Oral cavity should always be checked to assess the health of teeth, gums, tongue, tonsils and oropharynx.

ABDOMINAL EXAMINATION

The abdomen is divided into 9 areas by two horizontal and two lateral vertical lines as shown in the figure. The areas are **right hypochondriac, right lumbar, right inguinal, epigastric, umbilical, suprapubic, left hypochondriac, left lumbar and left inguinal.**

The two lateral lines pass from the mid-inguinal point below to cross the costal margin close to the tip of the ninth costal cartilage.

The two horizontal lines, the subcostal and the interiliac, pass across the abdomen to connect the lowest points on the costal margin and the tubercles of the iliac crest respectively.

The subject is asked to lie down and expose the abdomen. The examiner's hand should be kept warm while examining the abdomen.

The abdominal examination of the subject is carried out in the following order:
- Inspection
- Palpation
- Percussion
- Auscultation

INSPECTION

Shape of the Abdomen

Look for normal abdominal contour whether it is flat or scaphoid. Look for fullness or distension.

Sunken or scaphoid abdomen is seen in:
- Severe malnutrition
- Starvation
- Malignancy

Generalized fullness or distension may be due to:
- Fat
- Fluid

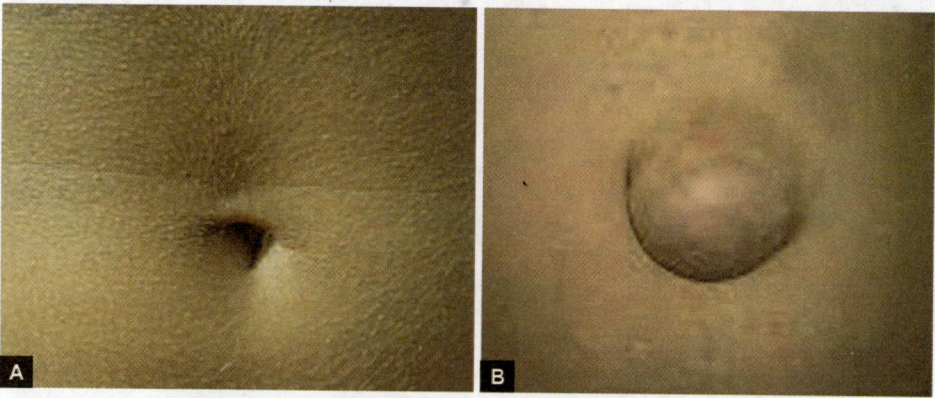

Figs. 24.1A and B: (A) Normal umbilicus; (B) Umbilical hernia.

- Flatus
- Feces
- Fetus

Localized distension may be symmetrical or asymmetrical
- Symmetrical distension may be due to small bowel obstruction.
- Asymmetrical distension may be due to gross enlargement of spleen, liver or ovary.

Umbilicus (Figs. 24.1A and B)

- Normal appearance of umbilicus is slightly retracted and inverted.
- Everted umbilicus may be due to umbilical hernia.

Movements of Abdominal Wall

- Normally, the abdominal wall rises during inspiration and falls during expiration. The movements should be equal on both sides.
- The abdominal movement are absent or markedly diminished in generalized peritonitis

Visible Pulsations on the Abdomen

It is a normal finding in very thin subjects.

Visible Peristalsis

- Visible peristalsis is seen normally in very thin elderly people with lax abdominal muscles.
- Obstruction of the pylorus due to fibrosis, chronic duodenal ulceration, carcinoma of stomach in the pyloric antrum leads to visible peristalsis.
- In obstruction of the distal small intestine, peristalsis will be seen locally with distended coils of the small intestine.

Skin and Surface of the Abdomen (Figs. 24.2A to D)

- In marked abdominal distension, the skin is smooth and shiny.
- Striae atrophica or gravidarum—they are white or pink wrinkled linear marks on the abdominal skin produced due to gross stretching of the skin with the rupture of the elastic fibers. Pregnancy, ascites, wasting diseases and severe dieting are some of the causes.
- Wide purple striae are seen in Cushing syndrome and in excessive steroid treatment.
- See whether scars are present or not. Old scars appear whitish, recent scars appear red or pink in color.
- Look for superficial prominent veins
    - Thin veins seen over costal margin has no significance.
    - Veins are prominent over the abdomen in inferior vena caval obstruction.
    - They are also prominent in portal hypertension due to venous anastomosis.
- Look for pigmentation of the abdominal wall. Linea nigra in the midline below the umbilicus is a sign of pregnancy.

PALPATION

Palpation of the abdomen is carried out to evaluate internal organs and to identify the sources of pain, if pain is present. If there is pain, start palpation from the non-painful area and observe the patient's face during palpation, as it may give clue regarding the intensity and location of pain. If the subject does not complain of pain, start palpation from the left iliac region lightly (superficial palpation) and work anticlockwise to end in the suprapubic region. Deep palpation in all areas may be done to assess intra-abdominal organs and to elicit the following signs.

Abdominal Guarding

Abdominal guarding may be **voluntary or involuntary**. If the subject voluntarily contracts the abdominal muscles, ask him to lie relaxed. Voluntary guarding may also be due to pain and the patient contracts the abdominal muscles in order to avoid pain during the examination.

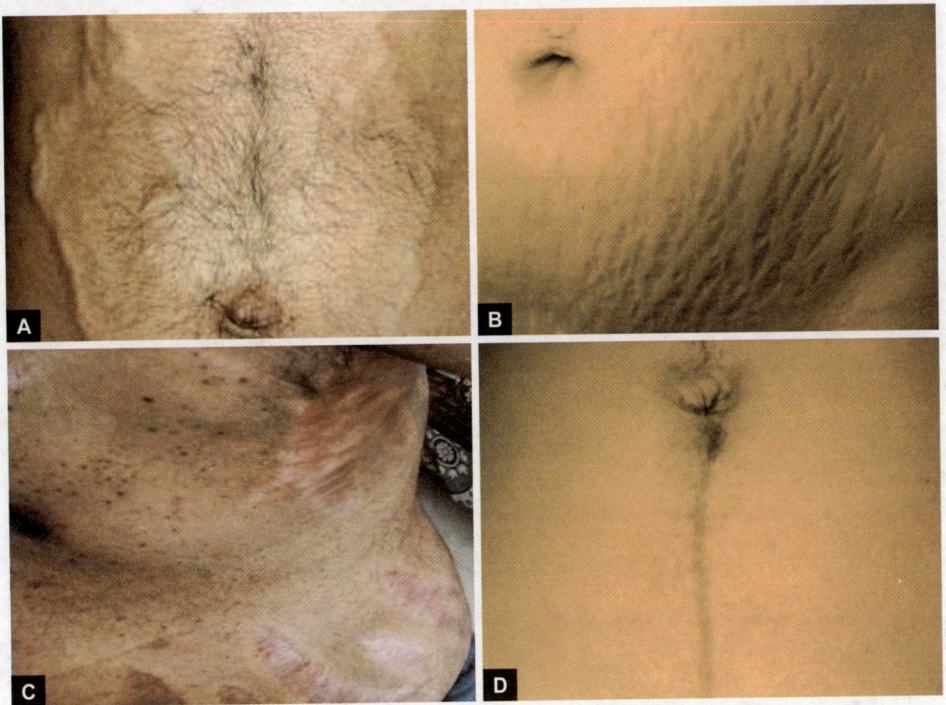

Figs. 24.2A to D: (A) Prominent veins on the abdominal wall; (B) Striae gravidarum; (C) Wide purple striae in Cushing syndrome; (D) Linea nigra.

Voluntary guarding is usually generalized over the entire abdomen. Involuntary muscle guarding (rigidity) may be due to peritoneal inflammation and is often localized to a particular quadrant of the abdomen.

Rebound Tenderness

Abrupt pain is felt in this condition when the compression of the abdomen is released suddenly. This is because of the irritation of the receptors in the parietal peritoneum.

Palpation of Left Kidney

To palpate the left kidney, right hand is placed anteriorly in the left lumbar region while the left hand is placed posteriorly in the left loin. Ask the subject to take a deep inhalation and press the left hand forward and the right hand backward, upward and inward.

The left kidney is not palpable unless either low in position or enlarged. Its lower pole when palpable is felt as a rounded, firm swelling between both right and left hands. That is, it is bimanually palpable. It can be pushed from one hand to the other in an action which is called balloting.

Spleen (Figs. 24.3A and B)

Place the flat of the left hand over the lowermost rib cage posterolaterally. The right hand is placed beneath the costal margin well out to the left **(Figs. 24.3A and B)**. Press in deeply with the fingers of the right hand beneath the costal margin at the same time exerting considerable pressure medially and downwards with the left hand. Then ask the subject to breathe in deeply. Repeat the procedure with the right hand being more and more medially beneath the costal margin in each occasion.

Right Kidney

- Feel for the right kidney in much the same way as that of the left.
- Place the right hand horizontally in the right lumbar region anteriorly with the left hand placed posteriorly in the right loin **(Fig. 24.4)**.
- Push forwards with the left hand and press the right hand inward and upward.
- Ask the subject to take a deep inspiration.
- Lower pole of right kidney, unlike the left, is commonly palpable in thin individuals.

Liver

- Sit beside the right hand side of the subject, place both hands side by side flat on the abdomen in the right subcostal region lateral to the rectus with the fingers pointing towards the ribs. If resistance is felt, move the hands further down until resistance disappears.
- Ask the subject to breathe in deeply and at the height of inspiration, press the fingers firmly inwards and upwards. During deep inspiration, the diaphragm moves the liver down towards the examiner's hand **(Fig. 24.5)**.

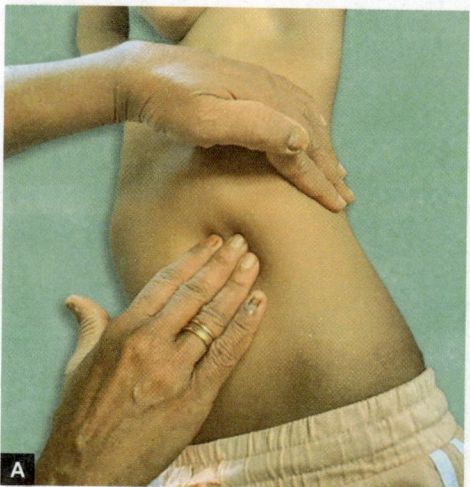 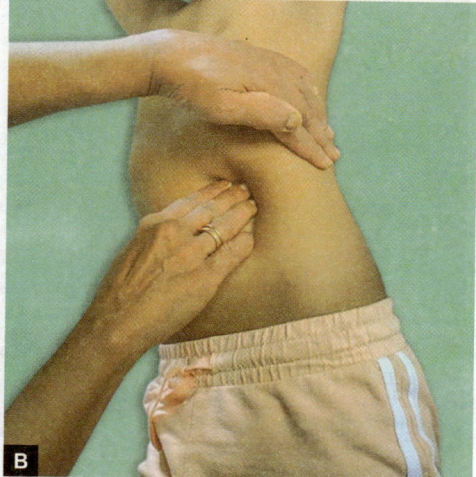

Figs. 24.3A and B: (A) Palpation of spleen; (B) Deeper palpation of spleen.

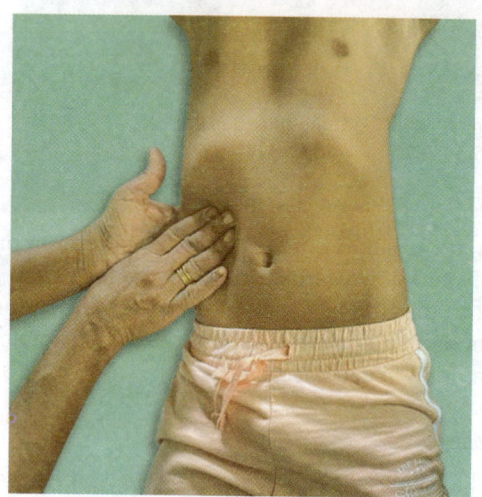

Fig. 24.4: Palpation of right kidney.

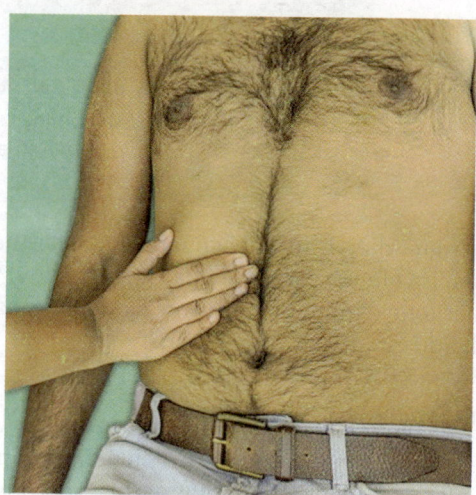

Fig. 24.6: Palpation of liver.

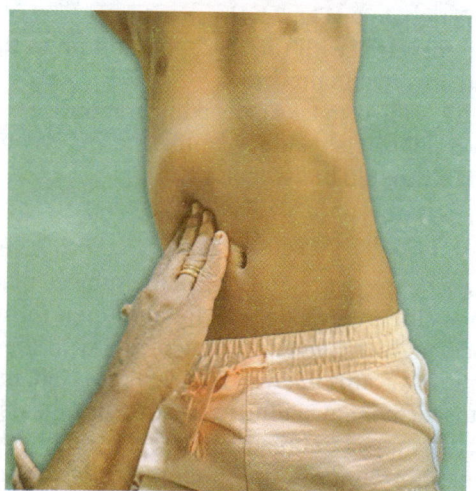

Fig. 24.5: Palpation of liver.

- Alternate method: Place the right hand below and parallel to the right subcostal margin. Liver-edge will be felt against the radial border of the index finger during inspiration **(Fig. 24.6)**.
- Normally the liver is not palpable in healthy individuals. If palpable it will be felt as a sharp regular border which slides beneath the fingers.

Gallbladder

- Gallbladder is palpated in the same way as the liver
- Normal gallbladder cannot be felt
- Distended gallbladder may be palpated as a firm, smooth or globular swelling with distinct borders just lateral to the edge of rectus abdominis near the tip of the ninth costal cartilage. It moves with respiration.

Urinary Bladder

- Normally urinary bladder is not palpable.
- When distended, it is felt as a smooth, firm, regular, oval swelling in the suprapubic region.

Palpation of Inguinal Lymph Nodes

Inguinal lymph nodes are enlarged in conditions affecting the anal canal, external genitalia, buttocks and lower vagina.

PERCUSSION

Normal percussion note over most parts of the abdomen is resonant or tympanic except over the liver, where the note is dull.

Boundaries of Abdominal Organs

Liver (Fig. 24.7)

- The upper and the lower borders of right lobe of liver can be mapped out accurately by percussion.
- Start anteriorly at the fourth right intercostal space where the note will be resonant over the lungs and work vertically downwards.
- The note becomes dull at the upper border of fifth intercostal space on the right side.
- The dullness extends down to the lower border at or just below the right subcostal margin, giving a normal liver vertical height of 10–14 cm. In normal subjects, the liver is fully covered by ribs.
- Enlargement of the liver is called hepatomegaly. The length of the liver will be more than 16 cm in the midclavicular line.

Reduced dullness is seen in:
- Severe emphysema
- Large right pneumothorax

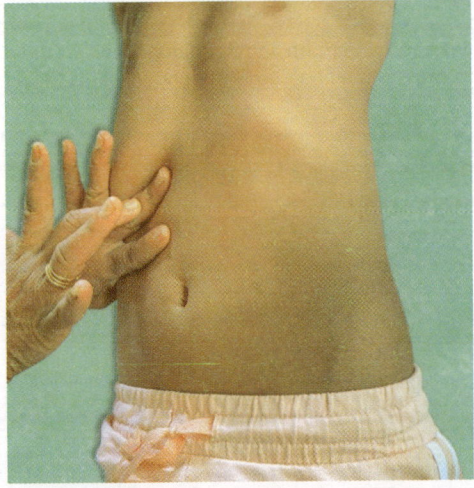

Fig. 24.7: Percussion of lower border of liver.

- After laparotomy
- After laparoscopy

Spleen

Dullness in an enlarged spleen extends from the left lower ribs into the left hypochondrium and the left lumbar region.

Urinary Bladder

Dullness on percussion over the suprapubic region is seen in urinary retention.

Testing for shifting dullness

The patient should be in the supine position
- Place the fingers of the examiner in the longitudinal axis on the midline near the umbilicus and begin percussion moving the fingers laterally towards the right flank.
- When dullness is first detected, keep the fingers in that position and ask the patient to roll on their left side.
- Wait for a few seconds for any peritoneal fluid to redistribute.
- If ascitis is present, the percussion note should have become resonant.
- This shift in the area of dullness can be confirmed by finding the left border of dullness with the patient still on his left side and seeing whether it shifts when the patient returns to the supine position.

Testing for Fluid Thrill

- The patient should be in the supine position.
- Place one hand flat over the lumbar region of one side and ask an assistant to put the side of their hand longitudinally and firmly in the midline of the abdomen.
- Then flick or tap the opposite lumbar region.
- A fluid thrill or wave is felt as a definite and unmistakable impulse by the detecting hand held flat in the lumbar region.
- Fluid thrill is felt in case of ascitis.

AUSCULTATION

Usually auscultation of the abdomen should be done prior to palpation and percussion. This is because manipulation of the abdomen may induce changes in the bowel sounds.

Bowel Sounds

- Place the stethoscope over the abdominal wall just to the right of the umbilicus.
- Normal bowel sounds are heard as intermittent, low or medium pitched gurgles interspersed with an occasional high pitched noise or tinkle every 5–10 seconds.
- Bowel sounds are exaggerated in small bowel obstruction.
- In generalized peritonitis, the abdomen will be silent.

Vascular Bruit

- Vascular bruit is heard over the following areas
- Above and to the left of umbilicus sound arising from aorta
- In the iliac fossa from iliac arteries
- In the epigastrium from celiac or superior mesenteric arteries
- Lateral to the mid abdomen from the renal arteries
- Hepatic bruit is heard over the liver
- Bruit is heard in stenosis and aneurysms

REPORT PATTERN

Write down the details of the subject:
- General examination
- Examination of abdomen
    1. Inspection
    2. Palpation
    3. Percussion
    4. Auscultation

IMPRESSION

The abdomen of the subject appears to be normal.

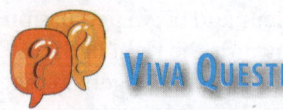

VIVA QUESTIONS

1. **List the common causes of prominent veins over the abdomen.**
    » In portal hypertension as in cirrhosis liver, distended veins around the umbilicus will be seen. This is called caput medusae which is due to development of anastomoses between portal vein and systemic veins.
    » Obstruction of inferior vena cava produces distended veins on the abdominal wall and chest wall **(Fig. 24.2A)**.
    » In thin, fair individuals, small veins may be visible over the abdominal wall.
2. **Is the liver and spleen palpable normally?**
    No. It has to be enlarged 2 or 3 times its normal size for the spleen to become palpable. Enlargement of liver is called hepatomegaly.
3. **How do you know that there is fluid accumulation in the abdominal cavity?**
    Accumulation of fluid in the abdominal cavity is called ascites. If there is fluid accumulation in the peritoneal cavity, two signs can be elicited: (a) shifting dullness; (b) fluid thrill. Refer page 132.
4. **Name a few conditions where the liver dullness is not appreciated at the right fifth intercostal space?**
    Emphysema, severe pneumothorax, presence of air in the peritoneal cavity as in perforated gastric ulcer.

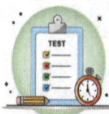

OBJECTIVE STRUCTURED PRACTICAL EXAMINATION

I. **Palpate the liver of the subject provided**
   » Explain the procedure to the subject briefly and ask him to expose his abdomen.
   » Stand on the right side of the subject and makes sure that the palms are warm
   » Ask the subject to lie in the supine position and breathe quietly
   » Places the right hand on the subcostal area of the subject on the right side of abdomen with fingers pointing towards the ribs
   » Asks the subject to take a deep breath and at the end of deep inspiration presses the fingers inwards and upwards to feel for the lower border of liver
II. **Palpate the spleen of the subject**
III. **Percuss out the lower border of liver in the subject provided**

25

Examination of Nervous System

LEARNING OBJECTIVES

- Examine the higher functions of the subject
- Enumerate the abnormalities of gait

INTRODUCTION

The functions of the nervous system include sensory functions, higher functions and motor functions. Before examining the subject, note if there is any abnormality in gait, difficulties with speech, hypokinetic or hyperkinetic movements. By a routine neurological examination it is difficult to identify and characterize disorders of the autonomic nervous system. So during history taking, enquire about autonomic functions like bladder and bowel control and sexual function. Examination of nervous system is carried out under the following headings:

- General examination
- Higher functions
- Sensory system
- Motor system
- Reflexes
- Cranial nerves

EXAMINATION OF HIGHER FUNCTIONS

Note down the subject's educational status, occupation, handedness, and knowledge of languages.

Higher functions include mental state, memory, speech, and posture and gait. The mental state of the individual can be assessed during history taking and general examination.

MENTAL STATE

General Appearance and Behavior

See whether the subject appears well, moderately ill or severely ill. Watch his dress, personal hygiene and his interest in the surroundings. See whether he is cooperative or indifferent. Look for behavioral abnormalities like aggressiveness.

Emotional Behavior (Mood)

Watch the subject's mood and see whether he is normal. Look for restlessness, anxiety, depression, euphoria, and inability to concentrate.

Sleep

Inquire about sleep, its duration, early awakening, narcolepsy, etc. Insomnia is a feature of depression. Ask about dreams and its nature. Dreams are frequent in anxious subjects.

Orientation in Place, Person and Time

See whether the subject can appreciate his surroundings. Ask him to say where he is, who he is, the approximate time without looking at the watch, the day of the week or month. Disorientation is an important sign of organic brain disease, but it is also seen in psychiatric disorders.

Attention and Level of Consciousness

Observe whether the subject is attentive to questions put to him, to environmental cues and to the bystanders.

Observe his response to tactile, painful, thermal and visual stimuli presented to him and assess his level of consciousness. See whether he is alert, confused, delirious, drowsy, or in stupor or coma.

- **Dementia:** The person is awake and alert but is confused in time, place and person. He has loss of memory.

- **Somnolence:** Person can be aroused by painful stimuli and may respond to commands verbally. He is somewhat confused but mentally clear.
- **Lethargy or drowsiness:** The patient is unable to maintain wakeful state in the absence of external stimulus.
- **Stupor:** Person can be aroused by painful stimuli but may not respond to commands. Restlessness and spontaneous movements may be seen.
- **Semi-coma:** Painful stimuli may cause withdrawal movements. No other responses.
- **Coma:** Deeply unconscious. No response to the most painful stimulus.

Intelligence

Taking the educational and occupational history can assess intelligence. He can be asked to solve simple mathematical problems.

Delusions and Hallucinations

Delusions are false beliefs that continue to be held despite evidence to the contrary such as misinterpretations, suspicions, etc. For example, he may feel that others are making fun of him.

Hallucinations are perceptions that are not based on any real external stimulus. They are false impressions referred to the organs of special senses like hearing, vision and smell in the absence of any stimulus. The person may see large insects crawling over the wall or ghost figures, which they believe to be true. He may perceive abnormal smells or hear voices to which he may respond but no one else hears it. Auditory hallucinations occur in disorders like schizophrenia, organic brain disease and manic-depressive illness.

Illusion is misperception of a stimulus.

MEMORY

Ask the subject about an event that occurred while coming to the hospital. Give him some common objects and ask him to name them and to say their use. Recent memory is lost in some neurological disorders and in Alzheimer's disease. Amnesia is loss of memory.

Memory is the ability to recall events that has been learnt. It can be recent memory or short-term memory and remote or long-term memory. Recent memory is recalling events that occurred seconds to hours before. Remote memory involves recollection of events that occurred in the remote past. Ask him about his place of birth, his school days, some past events, childhood hobbies, etc. It is lost in severe brain damage and in psychiatric disorders.

SPEECH

Ask the subject some questions and observe how he speaks. While taking the history and during general examination speech defects, if any can be detected. Note for any abnormalities. Speech means expression of feelings, ideas and thoughts by using words. For normal speech, the cerebral cortex as well as the motor mechanisms that control articulation (uttering of words) must be perfect. Sensory speech is understanding of spoken or written speech.

Motor speech includes production of sound and writing of words.

Types of Speech Disorders

Dysphonia is an abnormality in the production of sounds by the vocal cords. Dysphonia is seen in vocal cord paresis (partial paralysis) and in Parkinson's disease.

Anarthria means inability to speak, **dysarthria** means difficulty in articulation. Both indicate damage or lesions of phonation apparatus and its nerve supply. Dysarthria is seen in upper motor neuron disorder that affects the muscles of tongue, pharynx and face. It is also seen in cerebellar lesions due to ataxia, in Parkinsonism due to hypokinetic movements, in bulbar palsy where the muscles supplied by the seventh to twelfth cranial nerves are affected and in myasthenia gravis.

Aphasia or dysphasia indicates an acquired disorder of speech caused by lesion in the cerebrum while the speech apparatus and its nerve supply are intact. Aphasia can be considered as a defect in symbol formation and expression. In aphasia speech may be absent or it will not be sensible. The most common cause of dysphasia is dominant hemisphere stroke. It is also an important feature of neurodegenerative dementias.

POSTURE AND GAIT

First observe the subject standing. Look for abnormalities of posture. Stance is the manner in which a person stands. Gait refers to the manner, style or pattern of walking. For the maintenance of normal stance and gait, the musculoskeletal apparatus, motor pathways, proprioceptive sensations, cerebellar functions, intact vestibular system, muscle tone and basal ganglia are essential.

If the subject has difficulty in walking, first rule out any local causes that affect locomotion like osteoarthritis of hip. The subject with the legs exposed and with bare feet is asked to walk for some distance in a straight line, turn round and walk back again. Note how he walks, whether he is deviating to one side or other. If he deviates to one side note the side of deviation. Maintenance of normal posture and equilibrium is an integration of proprioceptive, vestibular, cerebellar, basal ganglia and cerebral cortical function.

Abnormalities in Posture and Gait

- **Spastic gait or hemiplegic gait** is seen in patients with hemiplegia. The posture is typical with the spastic arm held adducted at the shoulder with the elbow flexed and the forearm in front of the chest with flexion at the wrist and fingers. The spastic leg is stiff with impaired knee flexion and ankle dorsiflexion. He walks with abduction of the leg to bring the plantar-flexed foot round and forward when taking a step (circumduction). Otherwise his foot drags on the ground since the knee cannot be flexed.
- **Stamping gait** is seen in tabes dorsalis (neurosyphilis). The patient raises each foot and briskly brings it down on the ground with a thump. It occurs due to sensory ataxia. He may be steady as long as he can see the ground and his feet. The moment he closes his eyes, he will lose balance.
- **Drunken or reeling gait or ataxic gait** (wide-based unsteady gait with irregular sized paces and potential to topple in any direction) is due to ataxia in cerebellar lesion. He walks in a clumsy manner zigzagging like a drunkard. The ataxia is present even if the eyes are open.
- **Kyphotic posture and festinant gait** is seen in Parkinson's disease. Walks with short steps initially, which may get bigger. There will be acceleration of rate of steps once walking is initiated (festinant gait). When gently pushed forward, he may not be able to stop immediately. Swinging of arms will be reduced or absent while walking.
- **Waddling gait** is seen in myopathies and muscular dystrophies due to weak gluteus medius muscle.
- **High stepping gait (foot drop)** is seen in common peroneal nerve palsy and in weakness of the extensor muscles of the feet. The leg has to be lifted abnormally high to make a step.

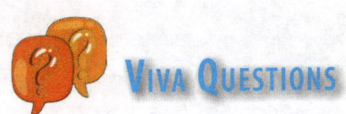

Viva Questions

1. **What is aphasia? Classify dysphasia or aphasia.**
   Aphasia or dysphasia is defect in speech, writing or reading due to lesions in the speech centers of cerebral cortex. There is loss of production or comprehension of spoken and/or written language. *It is not due to defects of vision or hearing or due to motor paralysis.*
   Aphasia is classified into:
   » *Sensory aphasia or receptive aphasia* can be due to a lesion in the Wernicke's area or auditory association area (area 22) or visual association area (area 18, 19) or the arcuate fasciculus in the dominant hemisphere. Here, the ability to understand what is heard or read is absent depending on the area involved. Inability to understand spoken speech is **word deafness**. Inability to understand written speech is **word blindness or alexia**. In sensory aphasia, the person is not able to communicate with others but he can say something without any meaning, i.e., the speech is fluent and the patient may speak a lot. So it is called fluent aphasia.
   » *Motor aphasia or non-fluent aphasia*: In **motor aphasia**, the person is not able to speak or write or both but there is fairly good comprehension of speech. Inability to write is **agraphia**. Damage to the Broca's speech area in the categorical hemisphere (dominant hemisphere) results in non-fluent aphasia or motor aphasia. The patient is not able to properly articulate and form words. Speech is limited and effortful. They know what they wish to say but cannot speak.
   » *Global aphasia*: Global aphasia where both motor and sensory speech centers are affected combines the features of sensory and motor aphasias. Comprehension and speech are completely lost.

   Head's classification of aphasia
   a. *Verbal aphasia*: The ability of expressing an idea in words is lost.
   b. *Syntactical aphasia*: The ability of fluent speech is lost. There are mistakes in arrangement of words and there will be no grammar.
   c. *Nominal aphasia*: The ability of naming correctly even the well-known objects is lost.
   d. *Semantic aphasia*: The ability of understanding the meaning of written or heard speech is lost.

2. **What are the abnormal gaits observed?**
   Refer page 137.

3. **What is the difference between dysphasia and dysarthria?**
   Refer page 136.

4. **What is the difference between delusion and hallucination?**
   Refer page 136.

Chapter 26

Examination of the Sensory System

LEARNING OBJECTIVES

- Classify sensory receptors
- Test the sensation of light touch, tactile localization and two-point discrimination in the upper limbs of the given subject
- Trace the pathway for touch and fast pain
- Test the sensation of pain in the upper limbs of the subject
- Test the vibration sense and stereognosis in the upper limbs of the subject provided
- Define anesthesia

PY10.11: Demonstrate the correct clinical examination of the nervous system: sensory system in a normal volunteer.

REQUIREMENTS

Cotton wool or hair esthesiometer, sterile sharp pins, hot and cold water, tuning fork.

METHOD

Examination of sensory system cannot be carried out if the patient is in coma and stupor. Different body parts are examined in the following sequence, upper limbs, neck, chest, abdomen, lower limbs and the back. Similar areas on the right and the left sides of the limbs and the body are examined alternately to compare them with each other.

Modalities Tested

- Superficial sensations
  - Light touch or fine touch
  - Pressure
  - Temperature
  - Pain
- Deep sensations
  - Sense of position
  - Joint sense (sense of passive movement)
  - Vibration sense
  - Deep pain or pressure pain
- Cortical sensations
  - Tactile localization
  - Two-point discrimination
  - Stereognosis
  - Graphesthesia
  - Double simultaneous stimulation

TOUCH SENSATION

Fine Touch and Tactile Localization (Fig. 26.1)

- Twist the cotton wool to form a wisp.
- Expose similar areas on the two sides of the body.
- First show the wisp to the subject, touch the skin with it and ask him to point out exactly where he feels the touch.
- Then ask him to close his eyes and ask him to say yes and to point out the exact location as soon as he feels it.
- Touch the various symmetrical areas of the skin on either side alternately. Abnormal findings are recorded.

Two-Point Discrimination

Compass esthesiometer is used to test two-point discrimination (Blunt dividers can also be used). Each limb of the compass is bifurcated to possess two points, one blunt end to test for the touch sensation and the other sharp point for testing pain sensation. The angle between the two limbs and hence the distance between them can be measured

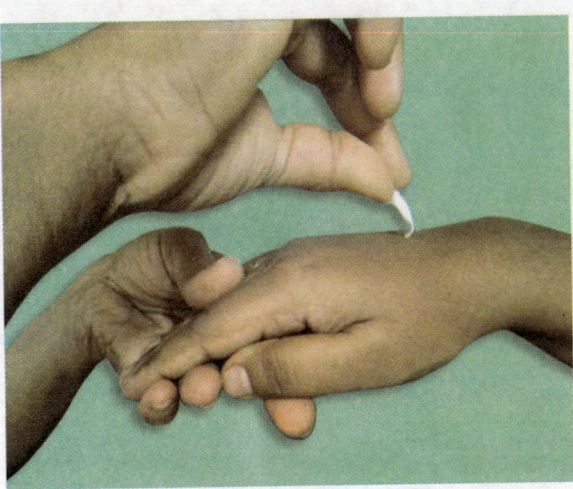

Fig. 26.1: Testing for fine touch sensation on the hand.

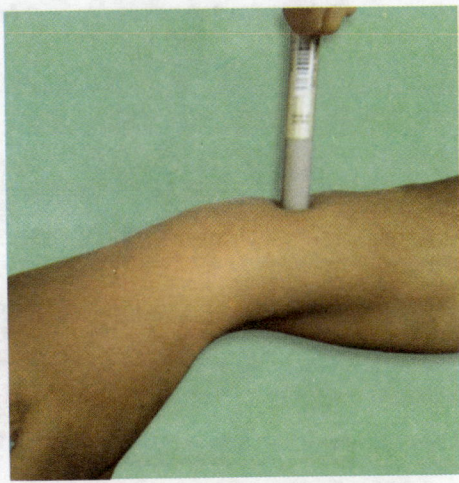

Fig. 26.2: Testing for pressure sensation.

along a graduated arc. The instrument is used to determine the minimum distance between two points, which could be recognized as distinct touches or pains when stimulated simultaneously. To start with, the two limbs are separated apart and are simultaneously touched while the subject has closed his eyes. He is asked to recognize whether he feels two points or only one. The distance between the two limbs of the compass is then reduced and the test is repeated.

The ability to distinguish between two touch points differs in different parts of the body. Normal discrimination possible is 3–8 mm on the finger tips, 3 cm on the dorsum of the hand, 5 cm on the back of the body. This test helps to detect lesions of sensory cortex and dorsal column.

Pressure

Strong touch stimuli applied from outside are recognized as pressure by the deeper tissues. Press upon the deeper tissues and the muscles with a blunt object **(Fig. 26.2)**. Ask the subject whether he feels the pressure or not. There is not much difference between touch and pressure sense. Touch is felt from the skin and pressure is felt from the deeper structures. Therefore, pure pressure without touch cannot be created in health.

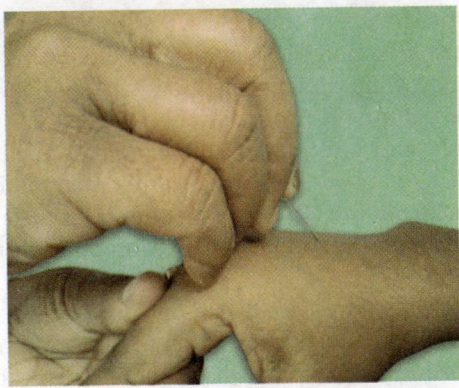

Fig. 26.3: Testing for superficial pain on the hand.

PAIN SENSATION

Superficial Pain

It is examined by pinprick on a pattern same as that for touch **(Fig. 26.3)**. Care should be taken not to inflict unnecessary pain.

Deep Pain or Pressure Pain

Examine for deep pain by applying intense pressure upon the muscles, tendons and the joints. The pressure must be sufficiently hard to induce pain, e.g., squeeze the muscle or tendon to inflict deep pain **(Fig. 26.4)**.

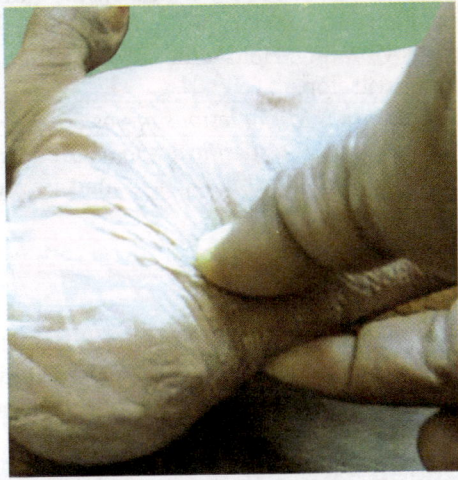

Fig. 26.4: Testing for pressure pain by squeezing the Achilles tendon.

VIBRATION SENSE

- ❖ Sensation of vibrations results from stimulation of the touch and the pressure receptors in a peculiar pattern.
- ❖ A vibrating tuning fork of low frequency is placed on the surface of the body preferably over the bone.

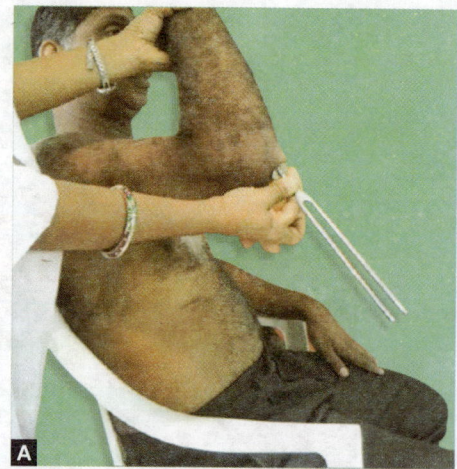
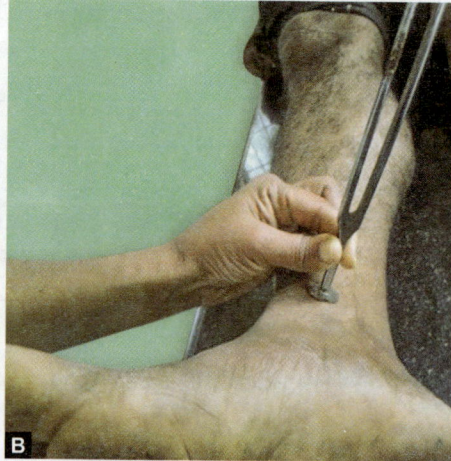

Figs. 26.5A and B: Testing for vibration sense over the olecranon process (A) and medial malleolus (B).

- Ask the subject to close his eyes. Initially train him to identify vibration sense by placing the tuning fork on his body while vibrating and not.
- Strike a tuning fork of frequency 100 Hz on the palm of the hand and place the base of the tuning fork touching flat over bony parts of the area to be tested **(Figs. 26.5A and B)**. The bone intensifies the stimulus by mechanically conducting the vibrations over a large area.
- In the upper limb start distally and proceed proximally. Start on the distal phalanx, then wrist and then elbow. In the lower limb, test the distal phalanx of big toe, then the medial malleolus and upper part of tibia.
- Ask the subject to say whether he feels the vibrations.
- Do not touch the twangs of the tuning fork with the hand while it is vibrating. Hold it on its foot. Otherwise the vibrations will stop.
- *Vibration sense is lost in lesions of posterior column of spinal cord and it is a specific test to assess the integrity of dorsal column pathway*. It is also impaired in polyneuropathy.

TEMPERATURE

Clinically the temperature sensation is tested with the help of test tubes containing hot (about 40°C) and cold (about 10°C) water. Test different parts of the body on either side.

STEREOGNOSIS

Ask the subject to close his eyes and give in his palm (right and left tested separately) various familiar objects like pen, chalk, coins, keys, etc., and ask him to identify each object **(Fig. 26.6)**. Stereognosis is recognition of size, shape, and form of objects by feeling them with fingers. It is a higher function requiring an intact sensory association area in the cerebral cortex. Loss of stereognosis is called **astereognosis** and it occurs in parietal lobe lesions.

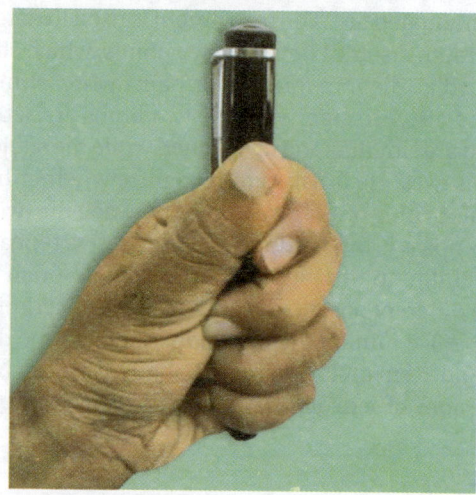

Fig. 26.6: Testing for stereognosis using a pen.

APPRECIATION OF PASSIVE MOVEMENT AND SENSE OF POSITION (PROPRIOCEPTION)

The sense of position and appreciation of passive movement also depends upon intact touch and pressure senses.

Sense of Passive Movement

- For testing the appreciation of passive movement, move a digit or limb of the subject passively with the subject's eyes closed. The joint to be tested is fixed proximally by holding it with the thumb and index finger of the examiner, so that the movement imparted to the joint is not felt proximally. Ask him to respond by saying 'up' or 'down' each time a movement is made **(Fig. 26.7)**. Do it on both sides. A normal person should be able to detect even 1° of movement at the terminal interphalangeal joint of the thumb and great toe and 100° at other joints.
- An inclined plane can also be used. With eyes closed the subject's forearm is placed on the board. Slowly pull

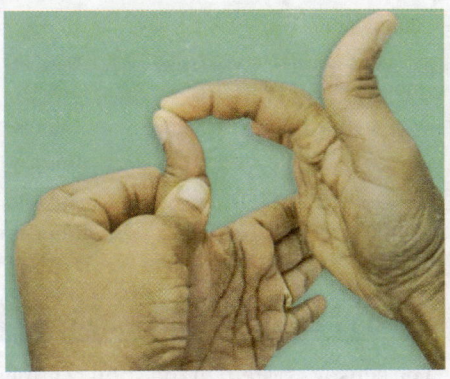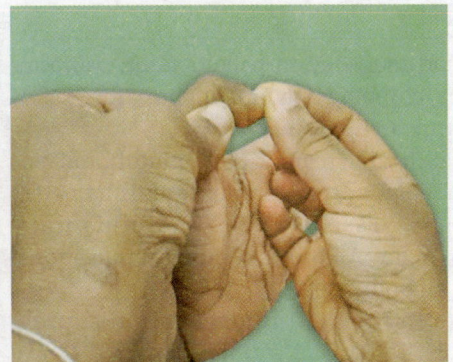

Fig. 26.7: Testing sense of passive movement by asking the subject to tell the position of his finger with eyes closed.

the string connected to the board. The board moves upwards and the degree of movement can be noted on the scale attached. Normally movement through 10° is appreciated.

Sense of Position

- To test the sense of position, keep the index finger or thumb of the right hand of the person in one position and ask him to bring the other finger in the same position with his eyes closed **(Fig. 26.8)**. Similarly do it with the big toe.
- Proprioceptive loss is the basis of **sensory ataxia**. The term ataxia refers to imperfect control over voluntary actions. Sensory ataxia may be mistaken for cerebellar ataxia. To distinguish between the two, *Romberg's test* can be done. Ask the subject to stand with his feet side by side with his eyes open. If he does not lose his balance, ask him to close his eyes taking care that he does not fall (*refer* **Fig. 27.6**). If he loses balance with his eyes closed, Romberg's sign is positive, i.e., he has sensory ataxia. When the eyes are open, visual sensation helps him to maintain posture. When visual cues are removed, the person becomes unsteady and tends to fall. Sensory ataxia is seen in diseases affecting the posterior column such as tabes dorsalis, subacute combined degeneration of spinal cord, etc. In cerebellar ataxia he will lose balance even when his eyes are kept open and the incoordination seen here is referred to as **motor ataxia**.
- Impaired proprioception occurs in large fiber sensory neuropathies, lesions of posterior column of spinal cord and in lesions of sensory cortex.

GRAPHESTHESIA

It is the ability to recognize letters or numbers written on the skin with a blunt point like pencil, key, etc. Letters and numbers are traced out on the palm, anterior aspect of forearm, thigh, or lower leg. Figures like triangles, rectangles and letters can be used. The letters or numbers should be written in the subject's reading direction. Compare both sides.

DOUBLE SIMULTANEOUS STIMULATION

It is the ability to perceive two identical stimuli applied on both sides of the body in mirror image points. Use tips of index fingers or blunt pins. Explain that a stimulus will be applied either on one side or both sides simultaneously. The subject is instructed to respond by saying one or two. In sensory inattention, there will be inability to perceive the stimuli as two on the opposite side of lesion even though each can be separately identified.

TEST THE SENSORY CRANIAL NERVES (I, II, VIII) AND THE SENSORY PARTS OF MIXED NERVES

Discussed in examination of cranial nerves.

REPORT PATTERN OF A NORMAL SUBJECT

Name:
Age:
Sex:
Occupation and address:

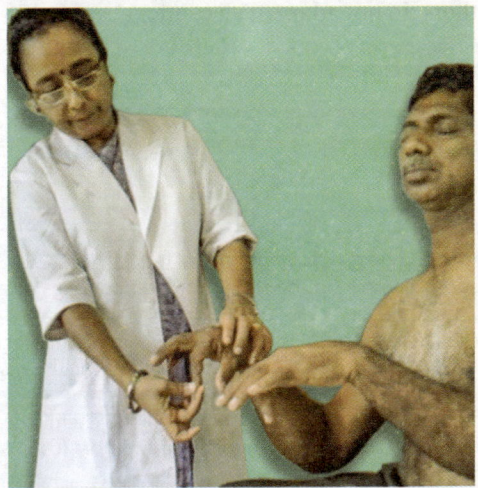

Fig. 26.8: Testing for sense of position.

General Examination

- Normally built and nourished; no pallor, icterus, cyanosis, edema, dyspnea, clubbing or lymphadenopathy.
- Body temperature: 37°C
- Respiratory rate: 16/min, regular, abdominothoracic
- Pulse: 70/min, regular, normal in volume and character, no thickening of vessel wall, no radiofemoral/brachiofemoral delay. All other peripheral pulsations are felt equally on both sides.
- Blood pressure in the right upper limb in supine position:
  - Palpatory method—116 mm Hg
  - Auscultatory method—120/80 mm Hg

Higher Functions

- General appearance and behavior: Normal
- Level of consciousness: Conscious
- Mental and emotional state: Normal
- Orientation in time and place: Well oriented
- Memory and intelligence: Normal
- Sleep: Normal
- Gait: Normal
- Speech: Normal
- Delusions and hallucinations: Absent
- Right handed

Sensory System Examination

Sensibility	Right side of the body	Left side of the body
Touch		
◆ Light touch	Normal	Normal
◆ Pressure	Normal	Normal
◆ Tactile localization	Normal	Normal
◆ Two-point discrimination	Normal	Normal
Pain		
◆ Superficial pain	Normal	Normal
◆ Deep or pressure pain	Normal	Normal
Temperature	Normal	Normal
Sense of position and passive movement	Normal	Normal
Vibration sense	Normal	Normal
Stereognosis	Normal	Normal
Abnormal sensations	Absent	Absent
Sensory cranial nerves	Normal	Normal

IMPRESSION

The sensory system of the subject appears to be normal.

DISCUSSION

Knowledge about the external as well as the internal environment is obtained through the sensory system. It consists of the receptors, the sensory or afferent nerves, the posterior root ganglia and their homologous ganglia in the cranial nerves, the relay centers in the posterior horn of the spinal cord or in the medulla, pons and midbrain, the tracts in the spinal cord, medulla, pons and midbrain; the thalamus, the sensory radiations and the sensory cortex in the postcentral gyrus.

Receptors respond to the various changes in our environment. When stimulated by adequate stimulus, it initiates a nerve impulse along its afferent nerve. The smallest strength of the stimulus, which is capable of stimulating the sensory unit, is called the **adequate stimulus** or the intensity threshold for the sensory unit. The receptor possesses a transducer mechanism. It converts the energy of stimulus into an electrical potential. The *potential* generated causes depolarization of the afferent nerve fiber and the nerve impulse initiated continues along the nerve fiber.

The area of the skin supplied by the afferent fibers from a single segment of the spinal cord is called a **dermatome**.

Some receptors adapt very quickly (phasic receptors) while others do not adapt at all (tonic receptors).

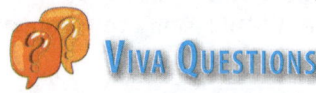

Viva Questions

1. **How will you classify receptors?**
   Receptors are classified in different ways
   » *Classification based upon the source of stimulus and the site of the receptor.*
   - Telereceptors or distance receptors: Source of stimulation away from the body, e.g., rods and cones of retina.
   - Exteroceptors: Source of stimulation outside the body and the sensory receptors on the surface of the body, e.g., cutaneous receptors for touch, pain, etc.
   - Interoceptor: Source of stimulation inside the body and the sensory receptors situated in the viscera, e.g., carotid sinus receptors.
   - Proprioceptors: Source of stimulus inside the body and the receptors inside the muscles, tendons, and joints and in the vestibular apparatus, e.g., muscle spindle, hair cells of crista ampullaris.
   » *Classification based upon the nature of stimulus:* Photoreceptors (light), chemoreceptors (smell, changes in blood chemistry), touch receptors, baroreceptors (intravascular pressure), mechanoreceptors (stretch), nociceptors (injury), osmoreceptors (osmolarity of body fluids).

2. **What is the difference between sense and sensation?**
   The various ways by which information is gained about the environment are called senses. Senses are classified as general and special senses. The general senses include touch, pain and temperature. The special senses are olfaction, taste, hearing and vision. Sensation means the feeling or understanding of different types of sensations. A definite type of a sensation is called a **modality**. Specific stimulus acting upon a specific type of sensory unit possessing a special pathway reaching a specific area in the cerebral cortex evokes a modality. Each type of sense like smell, taste, hearing, vision, touch, pain and temperature constitute at least one separate modality of sensation.

3. **Give the difference between tactile localization and two-point discrimination.**
   The ability to locate accurately the source of stimulus at a particular point on the body surface is called localization; and the ability of distinguishing it from a similar other point source situated nearby constitutes two-point discrimination. These depend upon the number of sensory units in a given area and the extensiveness of their topographical representation in the cerebral cortex. Thus the fingertips and the lips have the maximum sensitivity, while the visceral sensations are usually vague. Defective localization of touch sensation is called allochiria.

4. **What are the abnormalities in touch and pain sensation?**
   Absence of sense of touch, pain and temperature is called **anesthesia**. Hair esthesiometer is used to demarcate exactly any anesthetic area if detected, as in leprosy. Reduced sensitivity for these sensations is called **hypoesthesia** while increased sensitivity is **hyperesthesia**. Loss of one type of sensation independent of the others due to lesion of some areas in the spinal cord (e.g., syringomyelia) is called **dissociated anesthesia**. **Paresthesia** is wrong interpretation of sensations or abnormal sensations like numbness, pins and needles sensation, sensation of insects crawling over the body, etc.
   Analgesia is absence of pain sensitivity. **Hyperalgesia** is increased sensitivity or reduced threshold for pain.

5. **What is paradoxical cold fiber discharge?**
   The cold receptors are stimulated maximally at body temperatures between 25°C and 30°C. But these fibers also get stimulated at temperatures above 45°C producing a sensation of pain. This is referred to as the paradoxical response of cold fibers.

6. **What is the accuracy of localization of different sensations?**
   » Superficial pain can be localized but less accurately than the touch.
   » Pressure is touch from deeper tissues. But it is localized still less accurately than the pain. The subject should be able to distinguish between pressure and superficial touch because pressure cannot be caused without touch.
   » Localization of the deep pain is still more difficult. Very often it gets referred to some superficial parts of the body belonging to the same dermatome.
   » Sensations are lost in lesions of sensory pathways and in lesions of sensory cortex. Cerebral hemisphere lesions give rise to sensory loss, which is referred to as cortical sensory loss. Cortical sensations like tactile localization, discrimination and stereognosis are lost in lesions of parietal cortex but crude sensations like crude touch, and pain and temperature can be appreciated to some extent at the thalamic level.

7. **What is meant by adaptation of receptors?**
   On continued stimulation for a variable time, sensory units may reduce their frequency of discharge or ultimately may even cease to initiate the impulse. This is due to accommodation and fatigue. For accommodation to occur there must be a slow rate of change of stimulus and for fatigue to occur there must be a prolonged continuous activity.

8. **Name the sensations lost when there is lesion to the dorsal column.**
   Fine touch, tactile localization, tactile discrimination, light pressure, vibration sense and conscious proprioception.

9. **Which are the sensations lost when there is lesion of the spinothalamic pathway? Which side of the body will be affected? Why?**
   Lesion of lateral spinothalamic pathway leads to loss of pain, temperature, itching, tickling and visceral sensations from the opposite side of the body. Involvement of anterior spinothalamic pathway leads to loss of crude touch sensation from the opposite side. The opposite side is affected because both are crossed pathways.

10. **What are the features of superficial pain?**
    » It arises from the skin
    » It is sharp and pricking in character
    » Can be well localized, i.e., limited to a well-defined area
    » There will be reflex withdrawal of the part

11. **Enumerate the features of deep somatic pain.**
    » It arises from the muscles, bones and tendons and is extremely painful
    » It is dull and aching and difficult to localize

12. **Discuss the features of visceral pain.**
    » Occurs when the pain receptors in the viscera are stimulated due to damage or distension of internal organs
    » It is vague, not localized, or clearly defined as in menstrual pain
    » The pain may radiate to a distant site
    » Sometimes it will be referred to another site other than the organ involved
    » Visceral pain may produce nausea, vomiting, sweating, fall in blood pressure and fainting

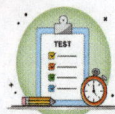

Objective Structured Practical Examination

I. Test the fine touch sensation in the left upper limb of the subject
» Explain the instructions briefly to the subject and ask him to sit
» Expose the left upper limb of the subject
» Ask the subject to close his eyes
» Take a cotton wisp and touches the different parts of the left upper limb from finger tips onwards and asks the subject to say 'yes' when he feels the touch
» Occasionally without touching asks the subject whether he is being touched

II. Test the vibration sense in the left upper limb of the subject
» Tells the procedure briefly to the subject
» Ask him to sit on a stool
» Select a tuning fork of frequency 128 Hz and strike one of its prongs on the edge of the table to set it into vibration
» Place the base of the tuning fork on any bony prominence of the subject in some other part of the body to make him familiar of the vibration sense
» Place the base of the vibrating tuning fork on the knuckles, head of radius, olecranon process of the elbow and each time asks the subject to respond.

Chapter 27

Examination of Motor System

LEARNING OBJECTIVES

- Test the integrity of the motor system in the given subject
- Name the descending pathways
- Explain the origin, course and termination of the pyramidal tract
- Differentiate between upper motor neuron and lower motor neuron lesions

PY10.11: Demonstrate the correct clinical examination of the motor system in a normal volunteer or a simulated environment.

INTRODUCTION

Clinical examination of the motor system consists of the following aspects:
- Inspection
- Bulk of the muscle
- Muscle tone
- Coordination of movement
- Power of muscles
- Gait
- Abnormal movements if any

INSPECTION

Complete exposure of the limbs, shoulders and trunk are required for proper examination of the motor system. Observe the muscles of the limbs and trunk. Compare the two sides by placing the limbs in symmetrical position. Wasting of muscle is a common sign of disease. Muscle atrophy may be due to disuse, thyrotoxicosis (thyrotoxic myopathy), other myopathies, peripheral motor nerve disease, muscle denervation, motor neuron disease, poliomyelitis, syringomyelia, etc. Also look for hypertrophy. See whether it is true hypertrophy or pseudohypertrophy.

Look for twitches within a muscle at rest. Fasciculation is spontaneous contractions of the muscle fibers of individual motor units within a muscle at rest. It is seen in peripheral neuro pathies, amyotrophic lateral sclerosis, etc. Look for tremor when the subject is at rest. Resting tremor is seen in Parkinson's disease.

BULK OF MUSCLE

- Bulk of the muscle can be roughly estimated clinically by inspection. Minor abnormalities can be detected only by measurement.
- Feel the muscles with the hand. Wasted muscles have a soft and flabby feel except when fibrosed.
- Measure the circumference of the limbs with a tape at certain definite points and compare with the opposite side. Unilateral wasting can be detected. A difference of up to 1 cm between the dominant and the nondominant limbs is not significant.
- In the upper limbs, the circumference is measured 5 inches above the olecranon and 4 inches below it.
- In the lower limbs, the circumference is measured 9 inches above the knee joint and 6 inches below it.
- Muscle atrophy is seen due to disuse, in lower motor neuron lesion, etc. Hypertrophy of muscles occurs with isometric exercise, and in disease conditions like muscle dystrophy and pseudohypertrophy. In muscle dystrophy, the muscles are weak even though the muscle bulk is increased. In 'pseudohypertrophy', there is degeneration of muscle with replacement of muscle tissue by fat. The muscles have a rubbery consistency.
- Differentiate wasting from thinning. Wasted muscles have a soft and flabby feel. It is associated with weakness. Thinning is not associated with weakness, flaccidity or loss of reflexes.

MUSCLE TONE

Tone is the resistance of a muscle to passive stretch. A certain degree of reflex contraction of skeletal muscles induced by gravity and the slight stretch of the muscle always exists at rest normally. This small and continued contraction of the muscles at rest is described as muscle tone. Some of the motor units from the different muscles function alternately to maintain a particular posture. So, muscle tone does not produce fatigue. Tone in the muscle is a reflex phenomenon. The reflex involved is **stretch reflex** or myotatic reflex. Damage to any part of the reflex arc abolishes muscle tone.

The tone in a group of muscles depends upon their location in the body and the position assumed by the subject. The tone will be more in the muscles involved in the maintenance of a particular posture. Normal tone can be fully appreciated only by examining patients with hypertonia and hypotonia. The two forms of pathological hypertonia are spasticity (seen in upper motor neuron disease) and rigidity (seen in extrapyramidal diseases like parkinsonism).

Subject should be in the supine position, lying relaxed. Talking to the subject about things of mutual interest may distract attention.

The muscle tone is examined by:
- Noting the posture and position of different joints of the body
- Feeling the muscles
- Testing the resistance to passive movements
- Looking for pendular movement

Position of Joints

Examine the position of the various joints of the subject at rest and in different postures. Normally under resting conditions, the various joints of the body are kept in a partially flexed position. If a joint remains in an overflexed or overextended position at rest it denotes alteration in the tone. Overflexion may be caused by an exaggerated tone in the flexors or reduced tone in the extensors. The reverse of it causes overextension.

Ask the subject to assume different postures. Normally, he can maintain it for some time. Inability to assume quickly a new posture or inability to maintain it for some time may be due to change of the tone in the muscles involved in the act.

If the tone is increased, see whether it is spasticity or rigidity. In spasticity the affected upper limb will have a characteristic posture. It will be flexed at the elbow, wrist and fingers.

Feel of the Muscles

Ask the subject to relax completely. Feel the muscles by grasping them between the fingers. See whether they feel soft, flabby, elastic, firm or hard. Try to move them from side to side. In health muscles have an elastic feel. The feel becomes tough when the muscle contracts actively. The belly of a relaxed muscle can be moved slightly from side to side. When the tone is increased, the muscles are felt hard and rigid. When the tone is decreased, they are felt soft and flabby.

Resistance to Passive Movements

Ask the subject to relax the muscles of his limbs and the examiner should try to passively move his joints of the upper and lower extremities through the full range of its movements. Hold the limb and carry out all the movements occurring at the various joints (**Fig. 27.1**). Assess the resistance offered by the muscles to move the joints. In health a small but definite force is required to carry out the passive movements. The same degree of force is required over the complete range of movement.

Tone is expressed as normal tone, hypotonia (if reduced) or hypertonia (if tone is increased). When the tone is increased more resistance is felt. When the tone is decreased the resistance is reduced and even hyperextension may be possible. Hypertonia may be spasticity or rigidity.

In the upper limbs, do flexion and extension of fingers, wrist, elbow; supination and pronation of forearm; and adduction and abduction of shoulder. In the lower limbs, do flexion and extension of hip, knee and ankle and adduction and abduction of hip. While doing this, palpate the muscle, hypotonic muscles are flabby and hypertonic muscles are stiff to feel. Hypotonia is seen in lower motor neuron lesion, neuronal shock and in cerebellar lesion.

In **spasticity**, there will be more resistance to passive extension of the joints of the upper limb than to passive flexion. Hold the patient's elbow and hand and extend the elbow briskly from a fully flexed to a full-extended position. The initial resistance will suddenly reduce and the spastic arm will give way, as does a clasp knife. This is referred to

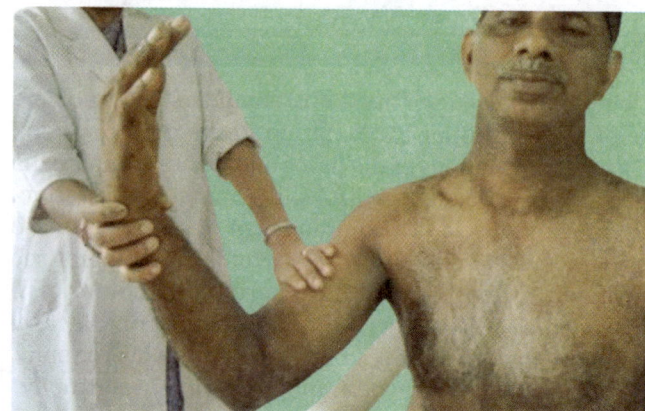

Fig. 27.1: Testing for resistance to passive movement. While passively flexing the elbow, note the tone of flexors and by passively extending the elbow, note the tone of the extensors.

as **clasp knife phenomenon**. In the leg, spasticity typically affects the adductors and extensors. Clonus can be elicited in spasticity. Brisk passive dorsiflexion of the ankle elicits a succession of involuntary brief repetitive contractions of the calf muscle until pressure on the sole of the foot is removed.

In case of pyramidal tract lesion, pronator spasticity (resistance offered on attempted supination of forearm at the radioulnar joint while doing alternating supination and pronation) and adductor spasticity (resistance on abducting the thigh while doing alternating abduction and adduction), are the most prominent and early appearing signs.

Rigidity is a feature of extrapyramidal lesions. Rigidity may be lead pipe rigidity or cogwheel rigidity. In **lead pipe rigidity**, the resistance is felt throughout the passive movement. Resistance to passive movement is equally increased in both agonistic and antagonistic muscles so that resistance is felt uniformly throughout the movement. It is better elicited in the lower limbs. In **cogwheel rigidity**, the rigidity is modified by tremor and the resistance will be intermittent. The muscle contracts in jerks due to combination of tremor and rigidity like the movement of a cogwheel. It is best elicited in the forearm by doing alternate supination pronation and wrist flexion-extension.

Pendular Movement of Extremities

The subject is seated on a tall stool and his lower limb below the knee should hang freely. Now swing it to and fro with sufficient force and quickness. In health, the extremity swings freely and two or three pendular movements occur and the swinging stops. If the tone is increased, more force is required to swing the extremity and the number of the pendular movements is decreased. Less force is required to swing the limb when the tone is decreased and the pendular movements are increased in number. Pendular movements become more evident if the knee jerk is elicited.

COORDINATION OF MOVEMENT

Coordination of movement depends upon the precision of rate, range, direction and force of each component of a voluntary act. It depends on information reaching the cerebellum from muscle and joint receptors, an intact dorsal column pathway, cerebellum and its tracts and a normal muscle tone. An idea about the coordination of movement can be obtained by observing the patient while he is undressing, picking up objects, etc. To test coordination of upper limbs, finger-nose test, finger-to-finger test and diadochokinesis test are done. Look for rebound phenomenon, past pointing and dysdiadochokinesis. For lower limbs, heel-knee test, Romberg's test and straight line tests (tandem walking; **Fig. 27.7**) are done. Normal findings in the supine position do not exclude a cerebellar lesion.

In the Upper Limbs

Finger-Nose Test

- Ask the subject to place the tip of his index finger on the tip of his nose. Ask him to touch the examiner's fingertip held in front of him at about half a meter distance. Now ask him to touch the tip of his nose again.
- If he can do it, change the position and distance of the examiner's finger and repeat and instruct him to carry out the test at faster and faster speeds.
- Repeat the test with the other arm.
- Repeat the test while his eyes are closed.
- Ask the subject to keep his arm outstretched. Then ask him to touch the tip of his nose with the index finger of the outstretched arm first with eyes open (**Figs. 27.2A and B**) and then with eyes closed (**Figs. 27.3A and B**).
- In cerebellar ataxia, as the finger approaches the nose it shows action tremor which is referred to as **intention tremor**. The tremor is of low frequency and large amplitude and it becomes more marked in amplitude as the patient's finger approaches the nose or the examiner's finger.
- In sensory ataxia as in tabes dorsalis, the movement tends to be smooth with the eyes open. But when the eyes are closed, the finger hesitates before touching the nose.

Finger-to-Finger Test

Ask the subject to touch the fingertips of his own two hands while they are extended and spread out. It can also be done to assess the coordination of movement of hands.

Pronation and Supination (Diadochokinesis)

Rapid alternating movements are tested (**Figs. 27.4A and B**). Ask the subject to pat his knee alternately with the palm and dorsum of his hand on either side simultaneously and rapidly. Ask him to rapidly pronate and supinate his forearm. Both sides are tested separately. If he is unable to do the rapid alternating movement, the condition is called **adiadochokinesis or dysdiadochokinesis**. This is because they cannot start or stop movements quickly and the movements are slow and irregular. This is an important sign of cerebellar ataxia.

Rebound Phenomenon

The subject's arm should be kept adducted at the shoulder, forearm supinated and semiflexed at the elbow and hand made into a fist. He is asked to flex his elbow against resistance. The examiner should release the resistance suddenly. If the patient is unable to check the flexion of the elbow it is abnormal, and is described as a **positive rebound phenomenon**.

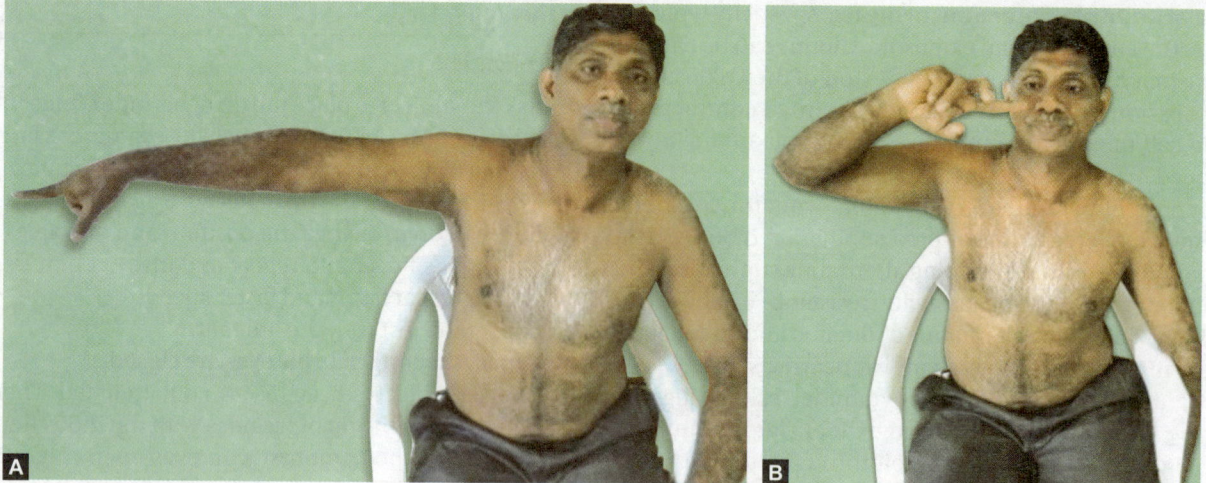

Figs. 27.2A and B: Finger-nose test of right hand with eyes open.

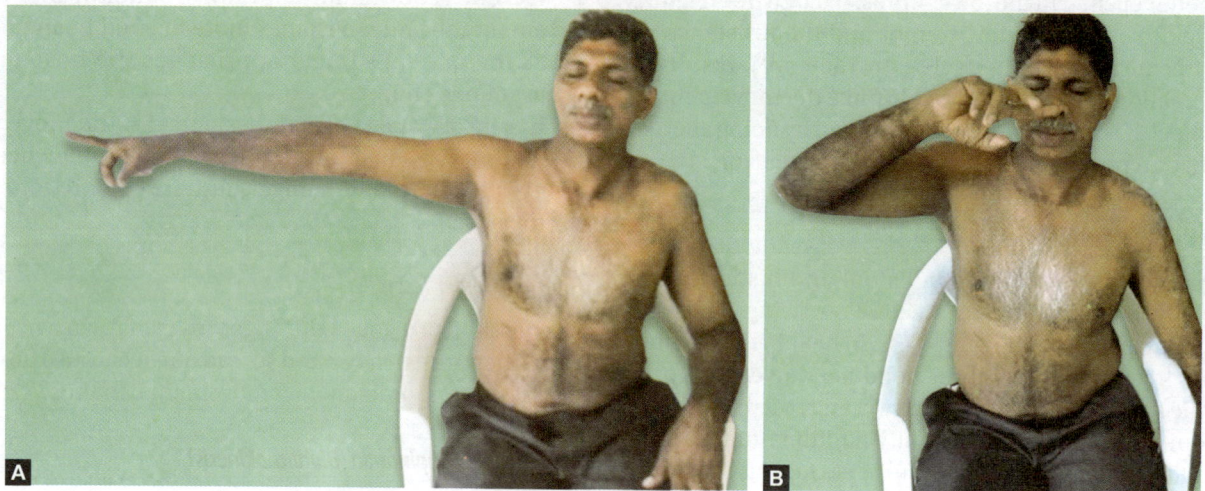

Figs. 27.3A and B: Finger-nose test with eyes closed.

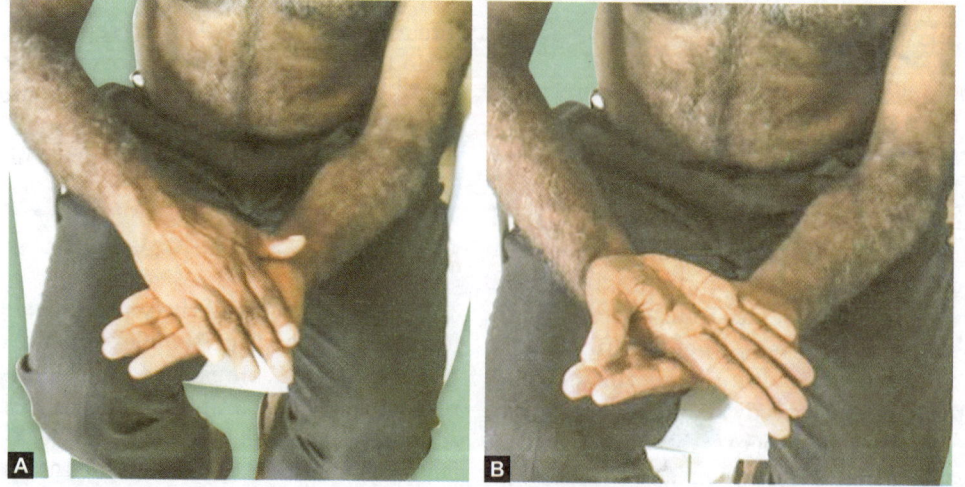

Figs. 27.4A and B: Looking for diadochokinesis by rapidly pronating (A) and supinating (B) the forearm.

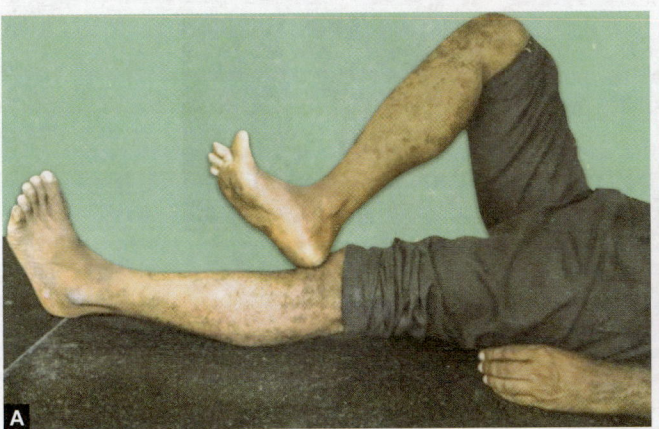 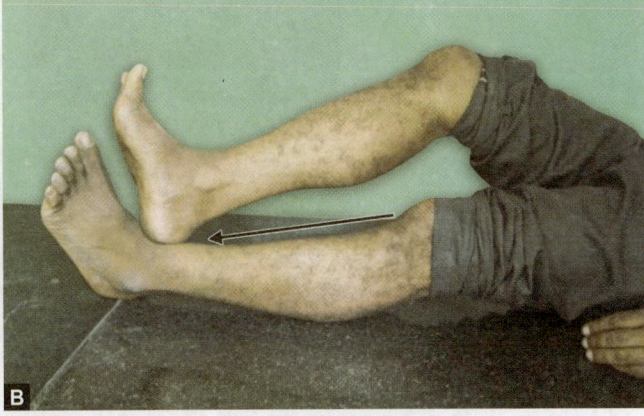

Figs. 27.5A and B: Heel-knee test.

Past Pointing

Ask the subject to sit opposite the examiner and hold his hand horizontally, so that his index finger touches the tip of the examiners finger. Then ask him to raise his hand vertically upwards, and bring it down to touch the tip of the examiner's finger first with eyes open and then with eyes closed. In unilateral cerebellar lesions, the ipsilateral hand deviates laterally due to incoordination.

In the Lower Limb

Heel-Knee Test or Heel-Shin Test

Ask the supine subject to lift one leg and place the heel of that leg on the knee or shin of the other leg and slide it down over the shin and over the dorsum of the foot toward the big toe **(Figs. 27.5A and B)**. The test is done with eyes open and closed. It should be repeated on the opposite side. In cerebellar disease, the heel is carried up to overshoot the knee. As the heel is dragged down, it begins to execute an action tremor. Proprioception should also be tested because proprioceptive loss (sensory ataxia) can give rise to signs, which look just like cerebellar incoordination. In sensory ataxia, the patient may raise his head to look at the legs during testing.

Romberg's Test

Ask the subject to stand erect with the feet touching each other first with eyes open and then with eyes closed. A healthy subject can stand without swaying **(Fig. 27.6)**. A subject who cannot do so and falls when eyes are closed is described as having the **Romberg's sign positive**. This is a test to assess the position sense in the legs. The increase in swaying caused by the closure of eyes is very marked in proprioceptive sensory loss (tabes dorsalis). In cerebellar ataxia, the person sways even with the eyes open. This test is not specific to assess cerebellar function.

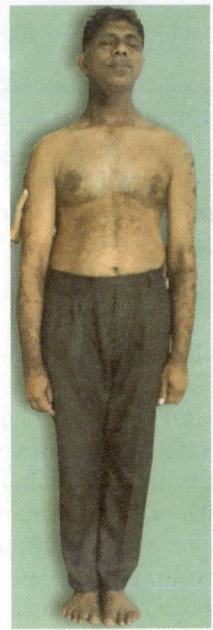

Fig. 27.6: Romberg's test.

Straight-Line Test (Tandem Walking)

Ask the subject to walk along a straight line first with eyes open and then with eyes closed. All healthy subjects walk accurately along a straight line with eyes open. When the eyes are closed a little difficulty may be observed, but the subject does not make any mistake and is able to complete his walk correctly. Tandem walking can also be tested. He is asked to walk along a line, placing the heel of one foot directly in front of the toes of the foot behind first with eyes open and then with eyes closed **(Figs. 27.7A and B)**. If incoordination is present, the subject deviates to one or the other side and walk in a zigzag manner. In sensory ataxia, patient does better with eyes open. In unilateral cerebellar lesion, patient falls to the same side of lesion.

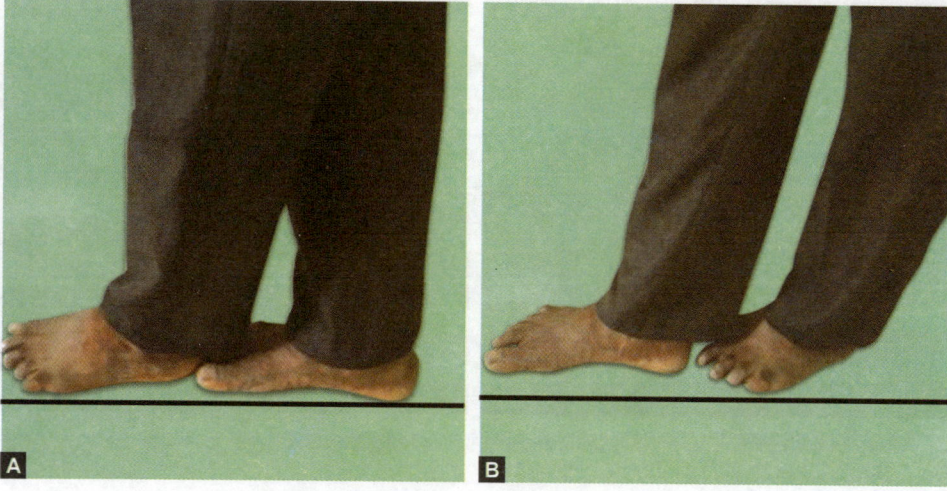

Figs. 27.7A and B: Tandem walking.

Speech

Ask the subject to utter some words and see whether he can pronounce it clearly. See whether there is pause in between the syllables of a word. In cerebellar lesion, speech is referred to as **scanning speech** due to incoordination of the action of muscles involved in speech.

Incoordination

- Lack of coordination occurs because of errors in the rate, range, direction and force of movement. In a complex movement, different components of the movement occur at wrong times and an attempt to compensate results in irregular and jerky movements. Most commonly lack of coordination is associated with cerebellar disease. **Ataxia** is inability to effect a movement smoothly and accurately. Ataxia is of two types—cerebellar ataxia and sensory ataxia.
- **Past pointing** indicates difficulty in measurement and appreciation of distance and it is referred to as **dysmetria**.
- **Asynergia** means lack of simultaneous action in the various muscles carrying out the same movement.
- Inability to perform alternate movements rapidly, e.g., pronation and supination or flexion and extension is called **adiadochokinesia**.
- Inability to utter words smoothly results in pauses between syllables during pronunciation of one word. It is described as **scanning speech**.
- **Decomposition of movements** is lack of smoothness in the movements with divisions and pauses in between.
- Defects in coordination also occur due to damage to the sensory system. It is usually associated with diseases or lesions of the dorsal column of spinal cord like tabes dorsalis.

The condition is called **sensory ataxia**. The sensory ataxia may be compensated by the sense of vision. Therefore, incoordination may become apparent only when the eyes are closed or when the person is in the dark.

MUSCLE POWER OR STRENGTH OF THE MUSCLES

Normal muscle power is defined as the strength of the muscles observed in a healthy person during a maximum contraction. During examination the active movements both unopposed and against resistance are examined. When a muscle of one side is tested, compare the strength of the similar muscle on the opposite side. To test the power of the muscles of the upper limbs, the subject can be in the sitting or supine position and for lower limbs, supine position is needed.

In suspected UMN lesions, the main movements about a joint are tested like flexion and extension of the elbow joints. In lesions of the pyramidal tract, weakness predominantly affects hip flexors, dorsiflexors of foot, shoulder abductors and wrist and elbow extensors. In suspected LMN lesions, individual muscles should be tested separately to localize the lesion in the peripheral nervous system.

Muscle Groups to be Tested

- Flexors and extensors of neck
- Adductors, abductors, flexors, extensors and rotators of the shoulder joint
- Flexors and extensors of elbow, wrist and fingers
- Handgrip
- Abdominal muscles
- Extensors of spine
- Adductors, abductors, flexors and extensors of hip
- Flexors and extensors of knee

- Muscles involved in dorsiflexion, plantar flexion, eversion and inversion of ankle
- Flexors and extensors of toes

MUSCLES OF UPPER LIMB

Muscles of Fingers and Wrist Movements Abductor Pollicis Brevis (Median Nerve C8, T1)

The subject is asked to place his hand on the table. Ask him to abduct his thumb in a plane perpendicular to that of the palm passively and then against resistance offered by the examiner **(Fig. 27.8)**. The muscle will become prominent and the tension can be felt.

Adductors of Thumb

The subject is asked to grasp a paper or card between the thumb and the radial border of index finger. Pulling on the paper can assess the strength of adductors. Normally the paper will not come off **(Fig. 27.9)**.

Opponens Pollicis (Median Nerve)

Ask him to touch the tip of the little finger with the tip of his thumb against resistance and feel for the power **(Fig. 27.10)**.

Dorsal Interossei (Ulnar Nerve; T1)

Asking the subject to abduct his fingers against resistance can test the dorsal interossei.

Palmar Interossei (Ulnar Nerve; T1)

Place the subject's hand flat on the table and ask him to adduct the fingers against resistance.

Lumbricals [Median Nerve (Lateral 2) and Ulnar Nerve (Medial 2)]

Ask the subject to hold the fingers straight with flexion at metacarpophalangeal joints and extension at the interphalangeal joints **(Fig. 27.11)**. Feel for the strength

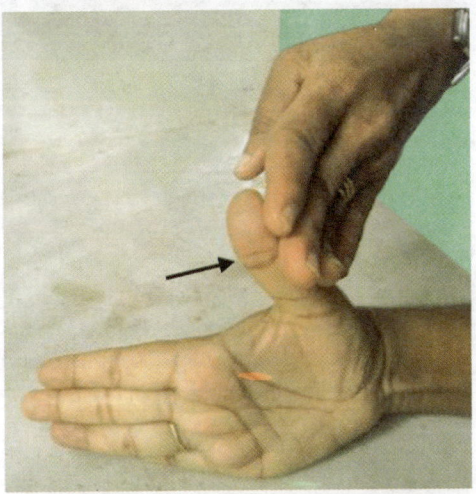

Fig. 27.8: Testing abductor pollicis brevis.

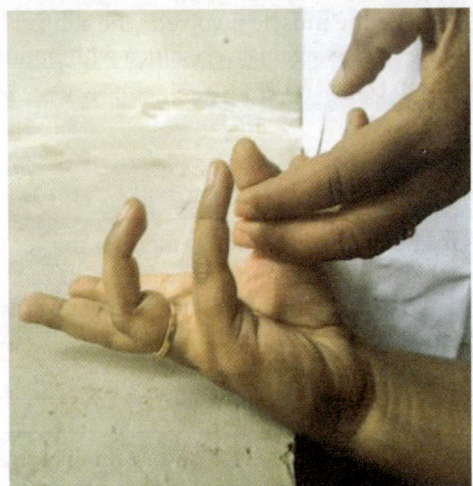

Fig. 27.10: Testing opponens pollicis.

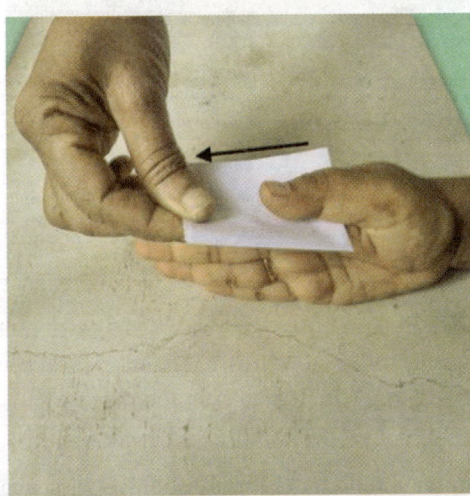

Fig. 27.9: Adductors of thumb.

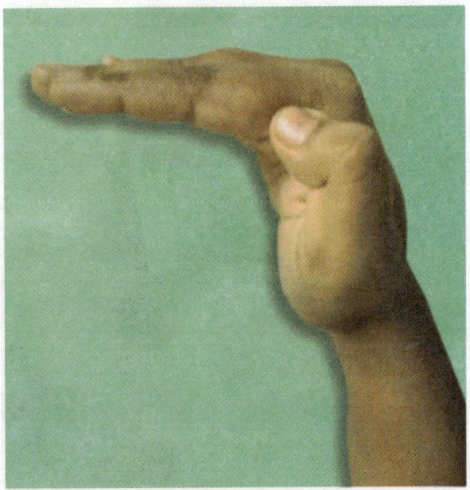

Fig. 27.11: Testing of interossei and lumbricals.

when the subject flexes his metacarpophalangeal joints and extend the interphalangeal joints against resistance.

Abductor Digiti Minimi (Ulnar Nerve; C8, T1)

Action is abduction of fifth finger. Ask the subject to spread out his fingers. The examiner should try to adduct the subject's little finger against resistance offered by the subject.

Flexors of the Fingers
(Median Nerve and Ulnar Nerve; C7, 8 and T1)

This is tested by handgrip. Flexor digitorum profundus is the muscle involved (first and second fingers supplied by median nerve and ring finger and little finger by ulnar nerve). Ask the subject to squeeze the examiner's middle and index fingers with his fingers (**Fig. 27.12**).

Extensors of Fingers

Extensor digitorum communis (posterior interosseous nerve; C7, C8) is the muscle involved. The subject is asked to extend the fingers against resistance with hands in the prone position (**Fig. 27.13**).

Flexors of the Wrist
(Median Nerve and Ulnar Nerve; C7, 8)

Flexors are flexor carpi radialis (median nerve; C6, C7) and flexor carpi ulnaris (ulnar nerve; C7, C8, T1). Ask the subject to make a fist and to flex his wrist against resistance (**Fig. 27.14**).

Extensors of the Wrist (Radial Nerve; C6, 7)

Extensors of wrist are extensor carpi radialis longus and extensor carpi ulnaris. Ask the subject to make a fist and

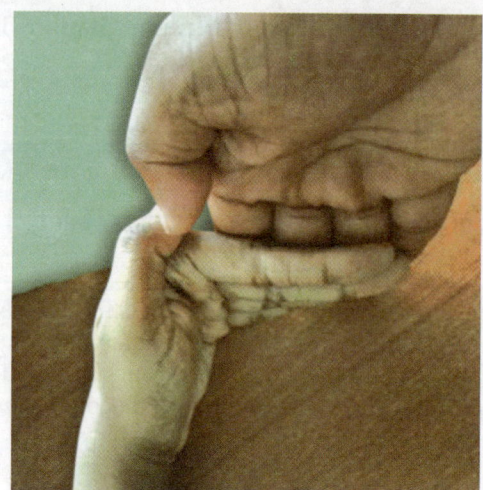

Fig. 27.13: Testing the power of extensors of fingers.

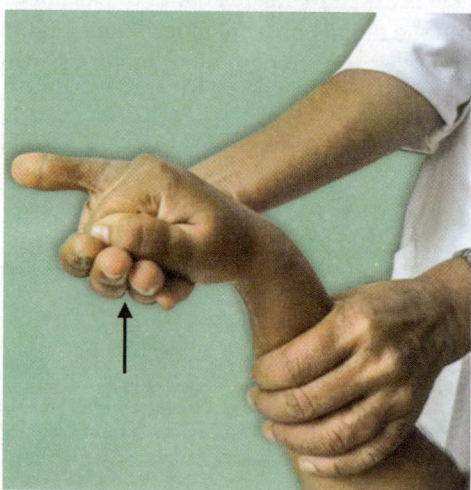

Fig. 27.14: Testing flexors of wrist.

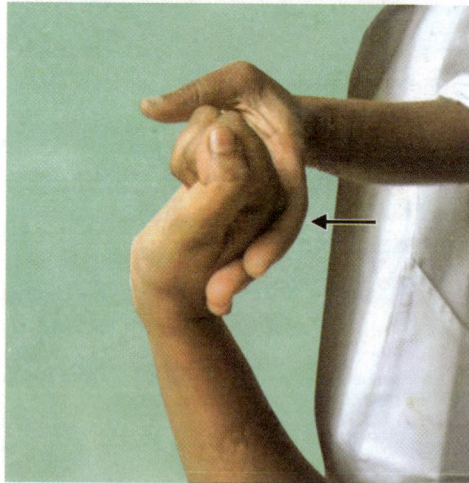

Fig. 27.15: Testing extensors of wrist.

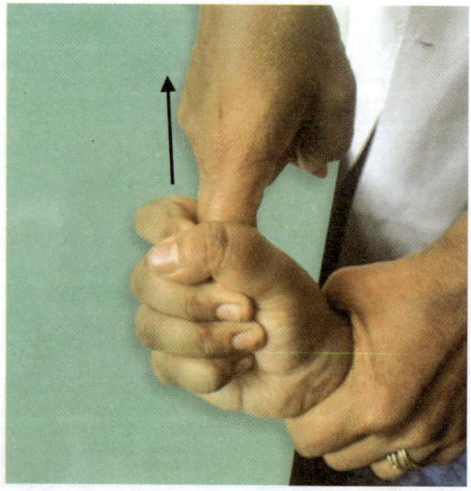

Fig. 27.12: Testing the power of flexors of fingers.

the examiner should try to forcibly flex his wrist against his effort to extend them (**Fig. 27.15**).

Muscles Acting on Elbow Joint Brachioradialis (Radial Nerve; C5, C6)

Action is flexion of elbow with the hand in mid prone position. Keep the subjects arm in the midprone position. Ask him to flex his elbow joint against resistance. The brachioradialis will become very prominent (**Fig. 27.16**).

Biceps (Musculocutaneous Nerve; C5, C6)

Action is flexion of elbow joint. With the hand in the supine position, ask the subject to flex his elbow joint against resistance (**Fig. 27.17**).

Triceps (Radial Nerve; C6, 7, 8)

Causes extension of elbow. With the arm flexed, ask the subject to extend the arm against resistance (**Fig. 27.18**).

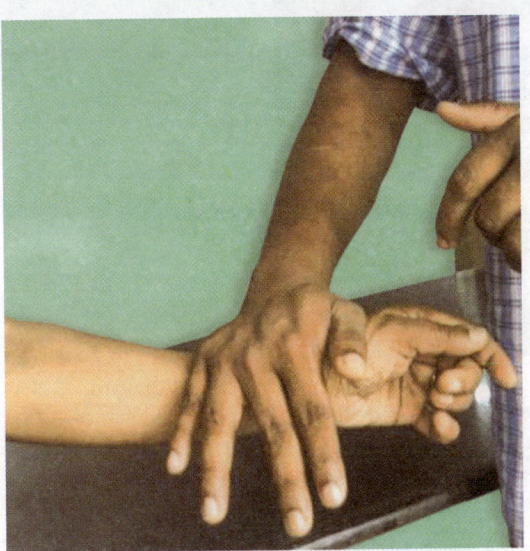

Fig. 27.16: Testing brachioradialis.

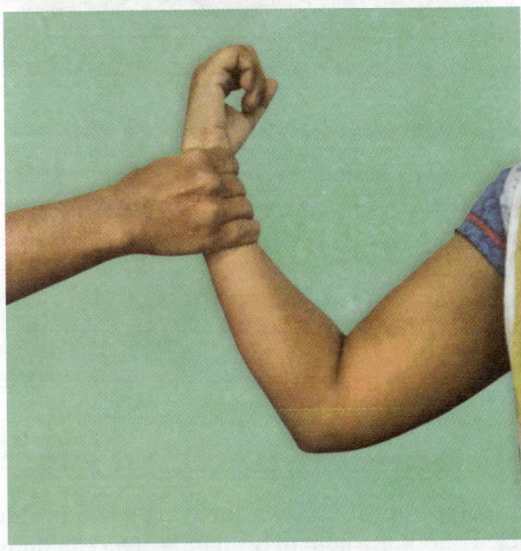

Fig. 27.17: Testing biceps.

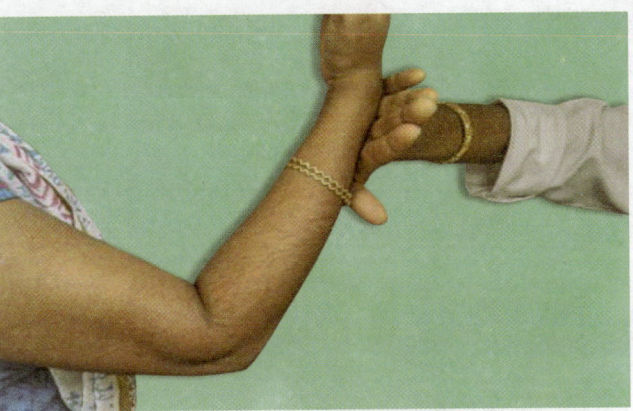

Fig. 27.18: Testing triceps.

MUSCLES OF SHOULDER

Supraspinatus (Suprascapular Nerve; C5, 6)

Action is abduction of shoulder joint. From the adducted position, ask the subject to abduct his arm against resistance. The first 30° of the movement is due to contraction of supraspinatus.

Deltoid (Axillary Nerve; C5, 6)

Action is abduction and extension of upper limb at shoulder joint. The first 30° of abduction is due to contraction of supraspinatus. The remaining 60° of the abduction is due to the action of deltoid. The anterior and posterior fibers help to move the abducted arm forwards and backwards. These movements are tested against resistance (**Figs. 27.19A to C**).

Infraspinatus (Suprascapular Nerve; C5, 6)

Action is external rotation. The subject is asked to hold his elbow to his side with the forearm flexed to right angle. Ask him to rotate the flexed forearm outwards against resistance offered by the examiner (**Fig. 27.20**).

Pectoralis (Lateral and Medial Pectoral Nerves; C5, 6, 7, 8, T1)

Ask the subject to bring his stretched out arms forwards and to clap his hands against resistance.

Serratus Anterior (Long Thoracic Nerve; C5, 6, 7)

Ask him to push against the wall with his extended hands (**Fig. 27.21**). If the muscle is paralyzed, the scapula will project out of the vertebral border, which is referred to as **winging of scapula**.

Latissimus Dorsi (Thoracodorsal Nerve; C6, 7, 8)

The subject is asked to clap his hands behind his back with the examiner applying resistance to the act.

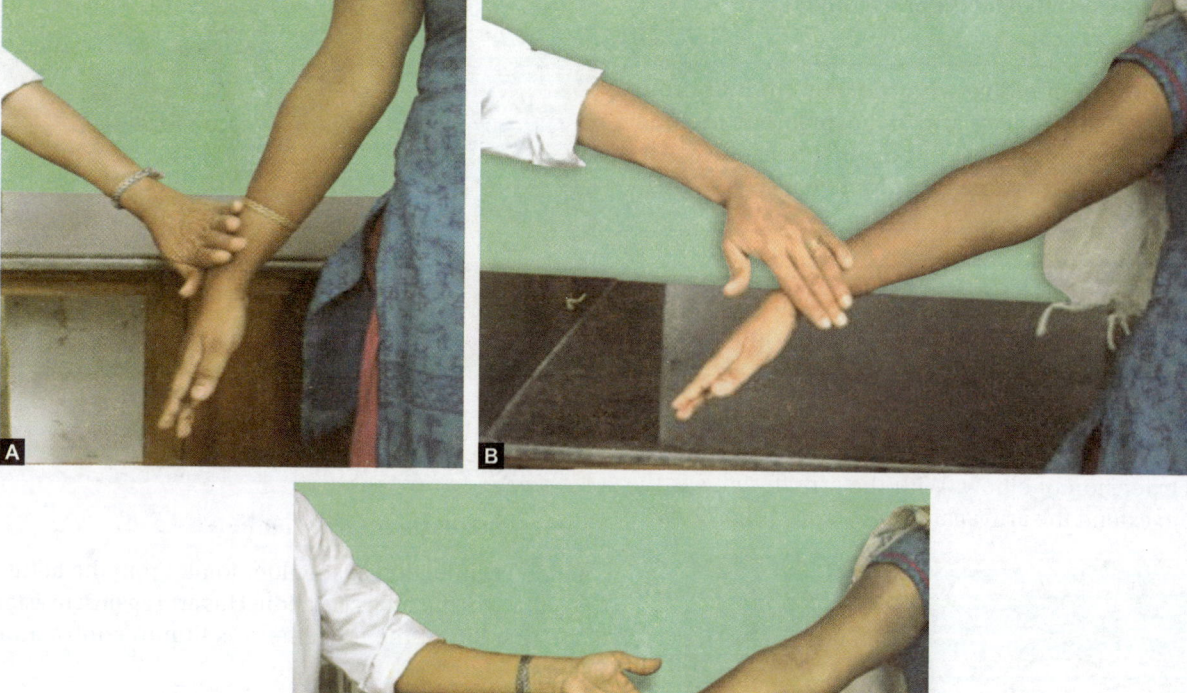

Figs. 27.19A to C: Testing the power of deltoid by asking the subject to abduct the arm from 60° onward (A) testing the anterior (B) and posterior (C) fibers of deltoid.

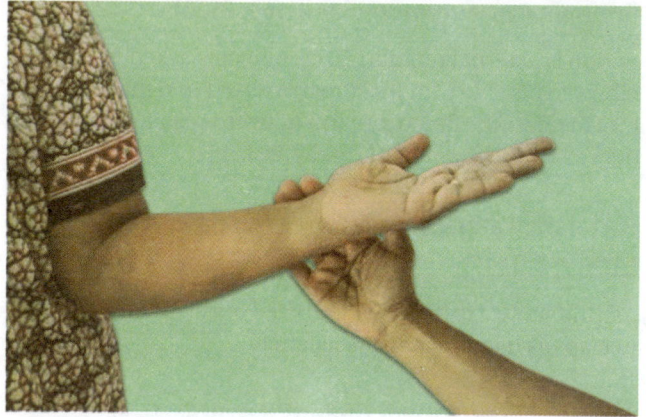

Fig. 27.20: Testing left infraspinatus.

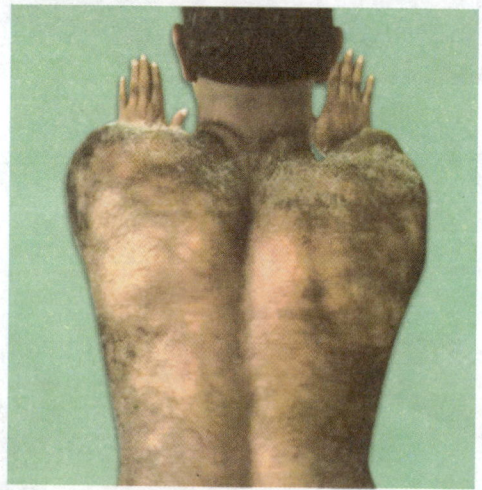

Fig. 27.21: Testing the power of serratus anterior.

MUSCLES OF NECK, ABDOMEN AND BACK

Muscles of Neck (C3, 4, 5)

Test the flexion and extension of the neck against resistance applied to the forehead and occipital region respectively. Testing neck flexion and extension is important in myopathies, in myasthenia gravis and in motor neuron disease.

Muscles of Abdomen (T5 to L1)

Ask the subject to sit up from the lying down posture on his back without the help of his hands. If he can do so, his abdominal muscles have normal strength.

Erector Spinae and Muscles of Back

Ask the subject lying down in the prone position, to raise his head by extending the neck and back. Normally the muscles will stand out prominently during the act.

Trapezius

Asking the subject to shrug his shoulders against resistance tests the upper part of the muscle **(Fig. 27.18)**. To test the lower part, he is asked to approximate the shoulder blades.

Diaphragm (Phrenic Nerve; C3, 4, 5)

Look for paradoxical respiration. Paradoxical movement of the diaphragm is seen in its paralysis during coughing, sneezing, etc. The diaphragm ascends when it should descend and vice versa.

MUSCLES OF LOWER LIMB

Flexors and Extensors of Toes

Dorsiflexion and plantar flexion of toes and foot is done against resistance. Extension of big toe is due to the action of extensor hallucis longus (deep peroneal nerve; L5, S1). Extension of other toes is due to the action of extensor digitorum longus and brevis (deep peroneal nerve). Flexion of toes is due to the action of flexor digitorum longus and flexor hallucis longus (tibial nerve; L5, S1).

Dorsiflexors (Common Peroneal Nerve; L4, 5) and Plantar Flexors (Tibial Nerve; L5, S1) of Ankle

Dorsiflexion of ankle is due to the action of tibialis anterior. Ask the subject to dorsiflex and plantar flex the ankle against resistance.

Extensors of Knee (Femoral Nerve; L3, 4)

Ask the subject to flex his knee. Press the examiner's hand on his shin and ask him to extend his knee against resistance.

Flexors of Knee (Sciatic Nerve; L4, 5)

Ask the supine subject to flex his extended knee against resistance. The examiner should support the raised leg with the left hand on the thigh and right hand on the ankle.

Extensors of Thigh (Inferior Gluteal Nerve; L5, S1)

The subject should lie on his stomach. Lift the subject's foot off the bed and ask him to push the foot down against resistance with the leg extended.

Flexors of Thigh (Femoral Nerve; L1, 2, 3)

The subject should lie on his back. With the leg extended ask the subject to flex his thigh against resistance offered to the thigh.

Adductors of Thigh (Obturator Nerve; L2, 3, 4)

Ask the subject to bring the abducted limb toward midline against resistance.

Abductors of Thigh (Superior Gluteal Nerve; L4, 5, S1, 2)

Place the subject's legs together and ask him to separate them against resistance.

Rotators of Thigh

Ask the subject to roll the extended lower limbs outwards and inwards against resistance on the bed.

GRADING OF POWER OF MUSCLES

Grade 0—Complete paralysis, no contraction
Grade 1—Only flicker or trace of contraction
Grade 2—Active movement eliminating gravity
Grade 3—Active movement against gravity but not against resistance
Grade 4—Active movement against gravity and moderate resistance
Grade 5—Normal power

Abnormalities in Muscle Power

- Hemiplegia is paralysis of one side of the body, i.e., the arm, leg and face (upper motor neuron lesion above the brain stem).
- Crossed hemiplegia is paralysis of arm and leg of one side and cranial nerve palsy of the opposite side (seen when the lesion is in the brainstem).
- Quadriplegia is paralysis of all the four limbs (lesion in the upper cervical segments of spinal cord).
- Paraplegia is paralysis of both legs (in lesions of lower segments of spinal cord).
- Monoplegia is paralysis of one limb.

MOTOR CRANIAL NERVES

Motor cranial nerves (III, IV, VI, XI, XII) should be tested. Motor part of other cranial nerves should also be tested (I, II and VIII are sensory nerves). Refer examination of cranial nerves.

GAIT

The subject's legs and feet should be fully exposed while studying gait. Ask him to walk away from you, to turn around at a given point and then to walk toward you. Abnormalities of gait are usually due to joint problems in the legs or due to neurological disorder. Alcohol intoxication may also cause difficulty in walking. Local causes include painful corn, osteoarthritis of hip, etc. (for details *refer* page 137).

ABNORMAL MOVEMENTS

Look for abnormal movements if any.

- Abnormal involuntary movement is called **dyskinesia**. It is commonly associated with diseases of the motor system. Observe the movements during sleep, rest and voluntary activity.
- **Tremors** are regular, to and fro movements of the extremities produced by alternating contraction of agonist and antagonist. The common tremor disorders include enhanced physiological tremor, parkinsonian tremor, cerebellar tremor, dystonic tremor, drug-induced tremor and psychogenic tremor. It can be fine tremor or coarse tremor. Fine tremor is seen in anxiety states, hyperthyroidism, etc. Coarse tremors are present in neurological conditions like Parkinson's disease, cerebellar disease, etc. Parkinson's disease is due to deficiency of dopamine as a result of lesion of the nigrostriatal pathway. The tremor seen in this disease is absent during sleep but is present at rest (**resting tremor**) and is increased in emotional conditions. It is seen most commonly in the fingers, wrist and forearm. It may also affect lips or foot. They do not increase during voluntary activity. Diseases of the neocerebellum are also associated with coarse tremors. The tremors in these cases are described as '**intention tremors**' because they are present during voluntary movements. They are absent at rest.
- In diseases called **chorea** (dancing movements) and **athetosis**, the caudate nucleus and putamen of basal ganglia are involved. The involuntary movements seen in these diseases are associated with voluntary activity making the movement purposeless.
- **Myoclonus** is sudden shock-like jerks of limbs and trunk. It may be due to cortical or brainstem pathology. Epileptic myoclonus is fairly common.
- **Seizure or fit** is due to the uncontrolled electrical activity in the brain, which may produce a convulsion, thought disturbances, etc. Epilepsy is a pattern of repeated seizures. In epilepsy, the movement is complex and repetitive and affects one part of the body.
- **Tics** are usually fairly small twitchy movements made semivoluntarily. It often affects the face (blinks, grimaces), neck and shoulders.
- **Metabolic flaps** are regular, abrupt movements present in outstretched hands. It is seen in hepatic failure, uremia, and respiratory failure.

REPORT PATTERN

Name:
Age:
Sex:
Occupation and address:

General Examination

- Moderately built and well nourished; no pallor, icterus, cyanosis, edema, dyspnea, club bing or lymphadenopathy.
- Body temperature: 37°C
- Respiratory rate: 16/min, regular, abdominothoracic
- Pulse: 70/min, regular, normal in volume and character, no thickening of vessel wall, no radiofemoral/brachiofemoral delay. All other peripheral pulsations are felt equally on both sides.
- Blood pressure in the right upper limb in supine position:
  Palpatory method—116 mm Hg
  Auscultatory method—120/80 mm Hg

Higher Functions

- **General appearance and behavior:** Normal
- **Level of consciousness:** Conscious
- **Mental and emotional state:** Normal
- **Orientation in time and place:** Well oriented
- **Memory and intelligence:** Normal
- **Sleep:** Normal
- **Gait:** Normal
- **Speech:** Normal
- **Delusions and hallucinations:** Absent

Motor System Examination

I. Bulk of muscle (cm)		
	Right side	Left side
Upper arm		
Forearm		
Thigh		
Leg		

II. Tone of muscle		
	Right	Left
Upper limb		
At small joints	Normal	Normal
At large joints	Normal	Normal
Lower limb		
At small joints	Normal	Normal
At large joints	Normal	Normal

III. Power (strength of muscles)		
	Grade	
1. Muscles of upper limb	Right	Left
Abductor pollicis brevis	5	5
Opponens pollicis	5	5
First dorsal interosseus	5	5
Interossei and lumbricals	5	5
Flexors of fingers	5	5
Flexors of wrist	5	5
Extensors of wrist	5	5
Brachioradialis	5	5
Biceps	5	5
Triceps	5	5
Supraspinatus	5	5
Deltoid	5	5
Infraspinatus	5	5
Pectoralis	5	5
Serratus anterior	5	5
Latissimus dorsi	5	5
2. Muscles of abdomen		5
3. Muscles of back		
Erector spinae	5	5
Trapezius—upper part	5	5
Trapezius—lower part	5	5
4. Diaphragm		
5. Muscles of lower limb		
Dorsiflexors of foot	5	5
Plantar flexors of foot	5	5
Extensors of knee	5	5
Flexors of knee	5	5
Extensors of hip	5	5
Flexors of thigh	5	5
Abductors of thigh	5	5
Adductors of thigh	5	5
Rotators of thigh	5	5

Impression

The motor system of the subject appears to be normal.

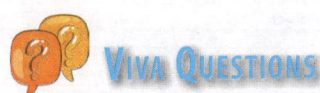

Viva Questions

1. **What is hypertonia? What are the types?**
   Increase in tone is called hypertonia and it is associated with increased gamma neuron discharge. Types of hypertonia are **spasticity and rigidity**.
   In spasticity, the descending inhibitory control of the cortex is lost but the striato-pallido-nigral system remains mostly unaffected. This results in the development of typical spasticity. The spasticity seen in upper motor neuron paralysis (hemiplegia) in man resembles the decerebrate rigidity. An attempt to cause a movement of the spastic limb puts a stretch on the antagonistic group of the muscles. The cortically uninhibited gamma neurons stimulate the intrafusal fibers and cause reflex contraction of the muscle, which opposes the passively imposed movement. This goes on till the externally applied force exceeds the one, which could be induced by a maximum reflex activity. To avoid the injury to the antagonistic muscle, it undergoes reflex relaxation (lengthening reaction) and the limb suddenly yields. This is described as the clasp-knife rigidity of the upper motor neuron paralysis or the lengthening reaction. It is a sign of extrapyramidal involvement. Pure pyramidal lesion in the medullary pyramids produces hypotonia.
   In Parkinson's disease and the related hypokinetic rigid diseases, the striato-pallido-nigral system is damaged and loses its inhibitory influence on the gamma system. The cortically originating influences could be blocked only partially as they find their way along the remaining pathways. The gamma system released from the striato-pallido-nigral system shows excessive activity and enhances the muscle tone. This type of hypertonia is described as the **plastic (cog-wheel or lead-pipe) type of rigidity**.

2. **What is the difference between spasticity and rigidity? Give examples.**
   If hypertonia is confined only to one group of muscles (either flexors or extensors) involved in the movement of a joint, it is referred to as spasticity, e.g., internal capsular lesion. When hypertonia involve both flexors and extensors equally, it is referred to as rigidity, e.g., basal ganglia lesion.

3. **What is the difference between decorticate and decerebrate rigidity?**
   » In lesions of cerebral cortex or internal capsule, the posture will be that of hemiplegia. There will be flexion of upper limbs and extension of lower limbs. This is decorticate rigidity.
   » In superior pontine lesion, there is hyperextension of all limbs with internal rotation of arms and plantar flexion of feet. This is decerebrate rigidity.

4. **What is hypotonia?**
   Hypotonia is diminution of muscle tone. Complete loss of tone is seen in paralysis due to lower motor neuron lesion. Cerebellar diseases are also associated with reduction in tone. In man the neocerebellum is well developed and injury to the neocerebellum produces hypotonia. There will be decreased resistance to passive movements and the range of movements will be increased.

5. **What is a reflex? What is its basic unit?**
   A reflex is defined as an involuntary response to an adequate stimulus. The basic unit of a reflex is the **reflex arc**. A reflex arc consists of a receptor, an afferent nerve and its cell body (in dorsal root ganglion or corresponding cranial nerve ganglia), a center consisting of two or more neurons with synaptic connections, anterior horn cell and a motor efferent nerve and an effector organ that gives the motor response. An injury to any part of the reflex arc abolishes the reflex.

6. **What is hemiplegia?**
   Paralysis of one side of the body is hemiplegia. The lesion may be in the pyramidal tract above the brainstem.

7. **What is crossed hemiplegia?**
   The type of hemiplegia in which there is same-sided cranial nerve palsy and opposite side hemiplegia is called crossed hemiplegia. This is seen when the lesion to the pyramidal tract is in the brainstem where the cranial nerve nuclei are present.

8. **What are the features of cerebellar lesion?**
   » Hypotonia
   » Wide-based ataxic gait
   » Incoordination of voluntary movements
   » Dysdiadochokinesis
   » Intension tremor
   » Pendular knee jerk
   » Nystagmus
   » Dysarthria

28

Examination of the Cranial Nerves

LEARNING OBJECTIVES

- Name the 12 cranial nerves
- Describe the functions of each cranial nerve
- Test the integrity of each cranial nerve
- Effects of lesion to each cranial nerve

PY10.11: Demonstrate the correct clinical examination of the motor system in a normal volunteer or a simulated environment.

INTRODUCTION

There are 12 pairs of cranial nerves, which leave or enter the brain through the foramen at the base of the skull. The cranial nerves supply different structures in the head and neck. The tenth nerve (vagus) also supplies the viscera in the thorax and abdomen. The twelve cranial nerves are numbered in the order of their emergence from the adult brain. They are:

- Olfactory nerve
- Optic nerve
- Oculomotor nerve
- Trochlear nerve
- Trigeminal nerve
- Abducent nerve
- Facial nerve
- Vestibulocochlear nerve
- Glossopharyngeal nerve
- Vagus nerve
- Accessory nerve
- Hypoglossal nerve

The cranial nerves contain one or many of the following types of fibers: special sensory, general sensory, somatic motor and parasympathetic visceral autonomic motor. *The olfactory, optic and vestibulocochlear nerves are purely sensory nerves. The oculomotor, trochlear, abducent, accessory and hypoglossal nerves are purely motor nerves.* Other cranial nerves contain both sensory and motor components. The cranial nerves containing parasympathetic fibers are III, VII, IX and X.

The nuclei of the motor cranial nerves (LMN) receive impulses from the motor cortex through corticonuclear fibers (UMN). Bilateral UMN connections are present for all the motor cranial nerve nuclei except that part of the facial nucleus which supplies the muscles of the lower part of the face and that part of the hypoglossal nucleus which supplies the genioglossus muscle.

The sensory afferents of the cranial nerves are the axons of neurons situated in the ganglia on the nerve trunks or from sensory organs such as nasal mucosa, retina or inner ear. These form the first order neurons. They synapse with the corresponding second order neurons in the brainstem. Their axons cross the midline and synapse with the third order neurons mainly in the thalamus. The axons of the third order neurons terminate in the sensory cortex of cerebrum.

OLFACTORY NERVE

Olfactory nerve is a sensory nerve. Actually there is no olfactory nerve as such. Olfactory receptors cells are bipolar sensory neurons situated under the nasal epithelium. Their central process project in numerous bundles, not as a discrete nerve, up through the cribriform plate of the ethmoid bone of skull into the olfactory bulb on the inferior surface of the frontal lobe. The central process of the cells in the olfactory bulb forms the olfactory tract. On reaching the anterior perforated substance, it divides to form medial and lateral olfactory striae. The medial olfactory stria connects the olfactory bulb of one side with that of the opposite side. The lateral olfactory stria carries the fibers to the primary olfactory cortex situated in the periamygdaloid and prepyriform areas of the temporal lobe. This area projects to secondary olfactory cortex in the parahippocampal gyrus and other parts of brain. These connections are responsible for the emotional and autonomic responses associated with olfactory sensations.

Examination of Olfactory Nerves

Familiar odoriferous substances like camphor, coffee powder, asafoetida, clove oil, etc., are taken in suitable containers and labelled with numbers. The bottles should be covered so that the subject is not able to see the contents. Those substances that cause irritation of the mucous membrane like ammonia should not be used. These substances will also stimulate the trigeminal sensory nerve ending and irritate the nose, even when the sense of smell is absent.

- Each nostril should be tested separately by occluding the other one.
- Ask the subject to clean his nose and to close one of his nostrils. Ask him to close his eyes. Open one of the bottles and bring it near his nose with his eyes and mouth closed. If he smells it at a distance ask him the name of the substance. If he do not get the smell at a distance, ask him to take the bottle near and sniff it. Repeat the whole process with the other nostril. A person with normal sense of smell will be able to identify the smell after sniffing.

Abnormalities

- Local causes which impair the sense of smell include rhinitis, sinusitis, etc.
- Lack of sense of smell is called **anosmia**. Anosmia occurs due to lesions in the olfactory bulb or tract. Subfrontal meningiomas, head injury causing damage to the cribriform plate, idiopathic Parkinsonism, etc., can cause bilateral anosmia. Since the olfactory tracts on both sides are interconnected through the anterior commissure, unilateral lesions of olfactory cortex do not result in anosmia.
- Altered sense of smell is called **parosmia** and it is seen following head injury.
- **Olfactory hallucinations** may be present as an aura of epilepsy.

OPTIC NERVE

The optic nerve is also a purely sensory nerve. Rods and cones in the retina are the visual receptors. Rods mediate dim light vision and cones mediate bright light and color vision. Sensory afferent fibers, which are axons of ganglion cells, form the optic nerve. Fibers from the temporal half of retina (nasal half-field of vision) is placed laterally while those from the nasal retina (temporal visual half-field) are placed medially in the optic nerve. At the optic chiasma, fibers from the nasal half of retina (temporal visual half-field) cross to the contralateral optic tract, while the fibers of temporal half of retina do not cross and join the ipsilateral optic tract. Majority of optic tract fibers pass via the lateral geniculate body of thalamus to the primary visual cortex (area 17 or striate cortex), which lies on either side of the calcarine fissure. The primary visual cortex is connected to the visual association area (area 18, 19), which surrounds it. Visual association area is responsible for visual localization and discrimination, spatial orientation and complex visual perception.

A few optic tract fibers pass via the superior colliculus to the midbrain to form the afferent limb of pupillary light reflex via connections to the Edinger-Westphal nuclei.

Method

To test the optic nerve the following must be examined:
- Acuity of vision
- Field of vision
- Color vision
- Optic fundus

Acuity of Vision

Visual acuity is the resolving power of the eye, both for near and distant objects in the visual field. Each eye should be tested separately by covering the other one (do not close the eye).

If the subject is wearing glasses, vision should be tested both with and without glasses.
- Near vision
- Distant vision

Near vision is tested by using **Jaeger's test chart** (Fig. 28.1). Ask the subject to read (if he is literate) printed matter with letters of various sizes with smallest size at the bottom at a distance of 25 cm from the eye. If he can read without difficulty the last line, he has normal near vision. Each eye should be tested separately.

Distant vision is clinically tested using **Snellen's chart** (Fig. 28.2). It has a series of printed letters of varying sizes, black letters on a white background, arranged in 8 horizontal lines. The top most letter is the largest and it is visible by a normal eye at a distance of 60 meters. The letters in the second line is visible at a distance of 36 meters and the subsequent lines at distances of 24, 18, 12, 9, 6 and 5 meters respectively. The size of the letters are so designed that from the specified distance, the letter as a whole subtends an angle of 5 minutes of arc at the nodal point. Modified

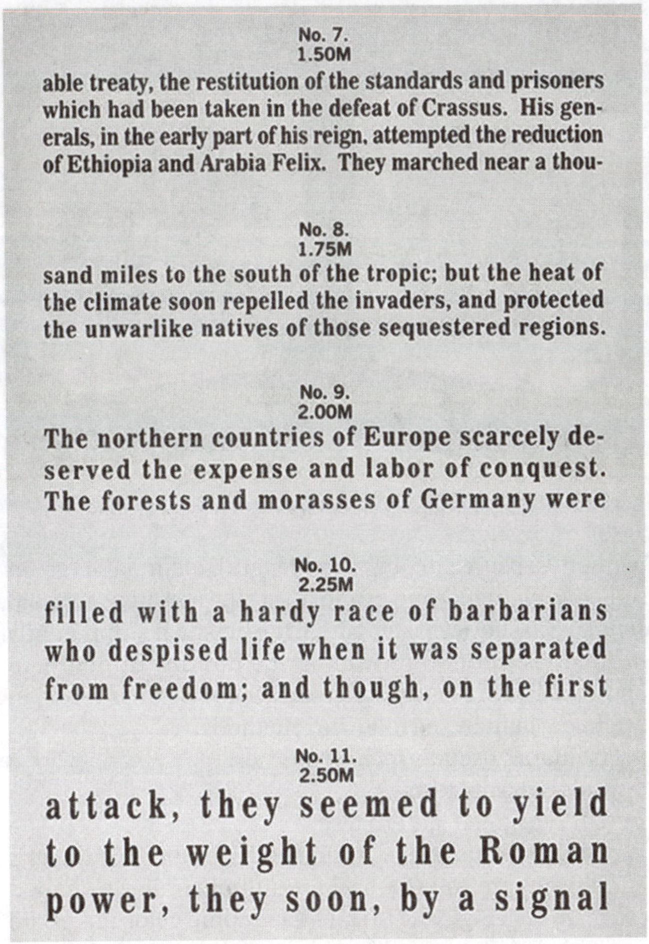

Fig. 28.1: Jaeger's test chart for near vision.

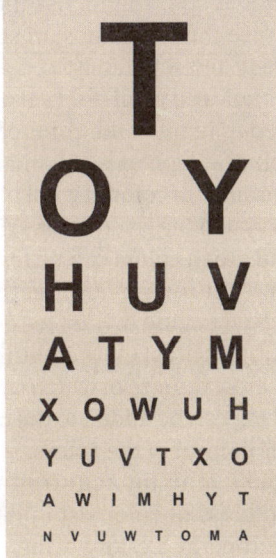

Fig. 28.2: Snellen's chart for testing distant vision.

Snellen's chart contains numbers, symbols or pictures and is used for those who are not able to read English letters.

Method

- The subject is seated at a distance of 6 meters from the chart. At this distance, ocular accommodation does not occur and the light rays will be parallel. Ask him to read the chart from the top to the bottom line or as far as he can read. Each eye should be tested separately.
- The visual acuity is recorded by the formula VA = d/D where 'd' is the distance at which the subject is seated and 'D' is the distance at which a person with normal vision can be read the letter. If he can read the 7th line, his distant vision is normal and is expressed as 6/6. If he can read only the first line at this distance, his vision is 6/60. If he is able to read the 8th line at a distance of 6 meters, his vision is 6/5.
- If he is not able to read the first line, bring him closer to the chart until he can read the top letter. If he can read it at a distance of 5 meters, his vision is 5/60.
- If he is not able to read the first line even at a distance of 1 meter, ask him to close one eye with his hand and to count the examiner's fingers at 6 meters distance. If this is not possible, come close and find out at which distance he is able to count the fingers.
- If this is also not possible, see whether he can perceive hand movements. If not, show him the light of a small torch. Move it in various directions and ask him to point at it. Repeat with the other eye. If he is not able to perceive light, then record it as 'no perception of light' (no PL).
- Visual impairment may be due to local ocular conditions like cataract, glaucoma, and opacities in the media. This should be ruled out.

Field of Vision

Field of vision is defined as that area on a screen, in which objects are visible, while the gaze is fixed on the center. Moving and white colored objects are identified quickly. Field of vision can be tested by **confrontation method** and by **perimetry**.

Confrontation Test

Clinically a gross defect in the peripheral visual field can be found out by this test. When two persons are standing in front of each other the visual fields of their opposite eyes (for example, the right eye of the subject and the left of the examiner) correspond with each other. The examiner assumes that his field of vision is normal and compares the subject's field with his own.

- Ask the subject to sit on a stool.
- The examiner should sit before him at a distance of about one meter, with the eyes in level with the subject's.
- First test binocular visual fields with both eyes open by the subject and the examiner. Ask the subject to look into the examiner's eyes. The examiner then holds up his hands on each side at the face level, with the hands about 1 meter apart. Move the index finger and bring the

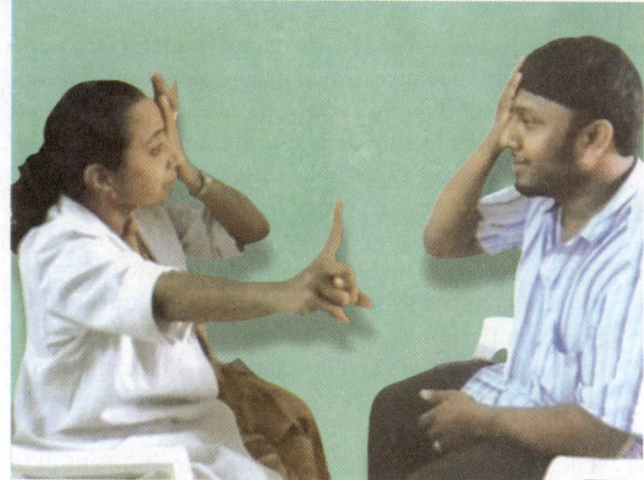

Fig. 28.3: Confrontation method to test the field of vision.

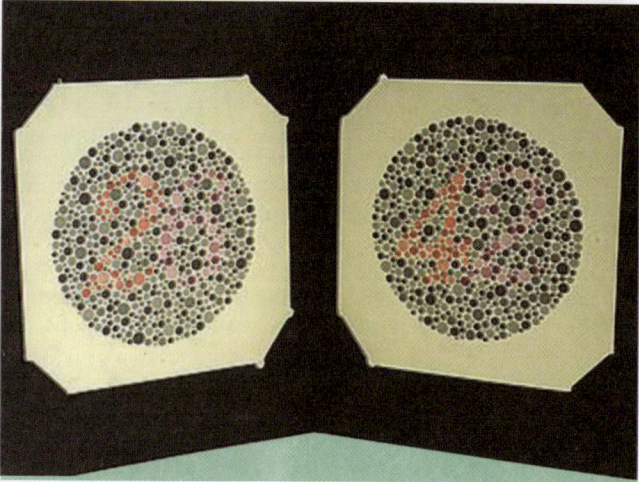

Fig. 28.4: Ishihara's chart for testing color vision.

hands to the center and ask him to say when he sees the finger **(Fig. 28.3)**. Do it from different meridians. If both see the finger movement at the same time the subject's field of vision is assumed to be normal.

- To test monocular visual field, ask the subject to close one eye (say right eye) with his hand.
- Examiner should close his opposite (left) eye.
- Both should look into each other's eye. The examiner should extend his right arm in a plane equidistant from both.
- Move the right index finger and bring the right arm slowly toward the center while keeping it equidistant between subject and examiner.
- Instruct the subject to inform as soon as he sees the finger. Both the examiner and subject should be able to see the finger at the same time, e.g., at the same distance from the center. Then the subject's field of vision is assumed to be normal.
- Repeat the same procedure at least in six meridians.
- Repeat with the other eye. Note down to what extent in each meridian the subject is showing absence of vision as compared to examiner's vision.

Visual field can be accurately tested using a perimeter. (Details are dealt with in the chapter perimetry).

Visual field defects in one eye indicate a retinal or optic nerve disorder. Lesions of the optic chiasma, in the optic tract, optic radiations or occipital cortex give rise to visual field defects affecting both eyes. Visual field defects include anopia, homonymous hemianopia (right or left homonymous hemianopia), heteronymous hemianopia (bitemporal hemianopia and binasal hemianopia), quadrantanopia, etc.

Color Vision

Human eye is sensitive to wavelengths of light ranging from 400 nm to 700 nm, which is the visible part of the electromagnetic spectrum. Cones perceive colors. There are three types of cone pigments, erythrolabe (red sensitive pigment sensitive to long wave length), chlorolabe (green sensitive pigment) and cyanolabe (blue sensitive pigment sensitive to short wavelength). If the person has apparently normal vision inquire whether he has any difficulty in appreciation of the various colors. Color vision is tested in bright daylight by the following methods:

- Ishihara's pseudoisochromatic test
- Colored wool tests
- Edridge green lantern test

Ishihara charts are printed with numbers or designs in colored circles on a background of similarly shaped color circles **(Fig. 28.4)**. The lithographic color plates are available in book form. The figures are intentionally made of colors that are likely to look the same as the background to an individual who is color-blind. Ask the subject to read the numbers or trace the wavy lines on successive plates. Each eye has to be tested separately.

In **Holmgren's colored wool test (yarn matching test)**, the subject is asked to identify the color of wool of various colors. He is given one type of wool and is asked to pick out from a large number of colored wool pieces of different shades, those that match the given color. With Ishihara's test cards, only red and green colors can be tested.

Edridge green lantern is an electrical apparatus used to test would-be engine drivers for evidence of color blindness. The subject is asked to identify the color of a small illuminated area, the size of which can be varied. The effects of rain and fog can be added to the colors by placing appropriate lenses in front of the colors.

Color blindness may be acquired or congenital. Acquired unilateral loss of color vision is a characteristic feature of optic neuropathy. Lesions of the visual cortex may result in color blindness.

Examination of Optic Fundus

Using an ophthalmoscope, the blood vessels and nerves in the fundus can be directly visualized **(Fig. 28.5)**. Examine

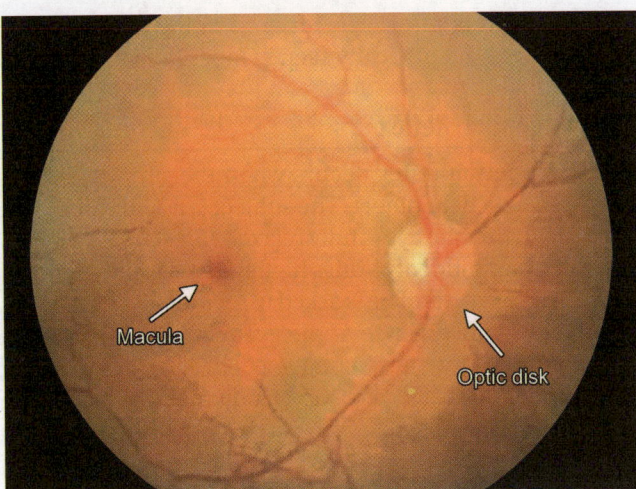

Fig. 28.5: Normal fundus of eye.

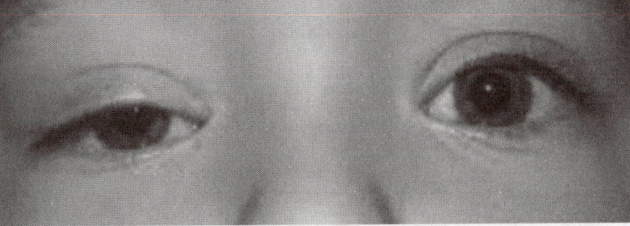

Fig. 28.6: Ptosis of right eye.

the color, contour, shape and margins of the optic disc. Examine the retinal vessels and look for hemorrhages and exudates. Look for macular edema, degeneration, etc.

OCULOMOTOR, TROCHLEAR AND ABDUCENT NERVES (III, IV, VI)

III, IV and VI cranial nerves are tested together because they function as a physiological unit in the control of the smooth and coordinated movements of the eyes. The superior oblique muscle is supplied by the IV cranial nerve and the lateral rectus by the VI nerve. The III nerve supplies all other extra ocular muscles.

Inspection

Look for any abnormalities on inspection of the eyes like:
- Lid retraction
- Ptosis, miosis, enophthalmos, exophthalmos and anhidrosis
- Proptosis
- Squint
- Observe the size, shape and equality of the pupils on both sides.

Oculomotor Nerve (III Cranial Nerve)

Nucleus of the third cranial nerve is in the midbrain. There are two major nuclei (a) main motor nucleus and (b) accessory or parasympathetic nucleus (Edinger-Westphal nucleus). Thus the oculomotor nerve consists of two types of fibers, somatic motor and the parasympathetic motor. In the orbit, the superior ramus of the nerve supplies the superior rectus and levator palpebrae superioris. The inferior ramus supplies the inferior rectus, inferior oblique, and medial rectus. The parasympathetic fibers from the inferior ramus pass to the ciliary ganglion and then to the ciliary muscle and sphincter pupillae. The clinical examination of the integrity of the III includes the following.

- **Test for levator palpebrae superioris**: This voluntary muscle helps to elevate the upper eyelid. Paralysis of the levator palpebrae superioris results in **ptosis**, i.e., drooping of the upper eyelid with consequent narrowing of the palpebral fissure **(Fig. 28.6)**. Voluntary elevation of the upper eyelid is not possible. (Ptosis also occurs in sympathetic palsy, myasthenia gravis and ocular myopathies. Muller's muscles of the eyelids are involuntary muscle supplied by the sympathetic nerves and they are in a state of tonic contraction. Sympathetic paralysis leads to loss of tone of Muller's muscle resulting in partial ptosis).
- See whether there is any squint. If present, ask if there is double vision (diplopia).
- Note the size of the pupils. See whether they are equal in size on both sides, abnormally dilated or constricted.
- Observe the pupillary reaction to light and accommodation.

Pupillary Light Reflexes

- **Direct light reflex:** Each eye is tested separately. A shining torch is brought from the side of the eye and shown into one eye taking care that the light does not fall into both eyes simultaneously **(Fig. 28.7)**. Observation is constriction of that pupil. When the light is switched

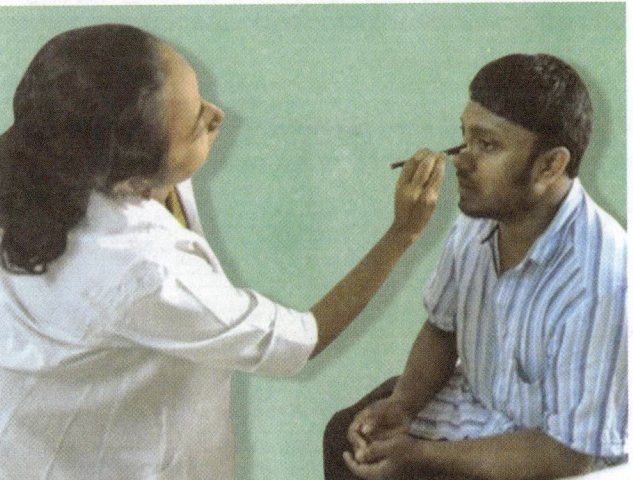

Fig. 28.7: Testing pupillary light reflex (direct) of left eye.

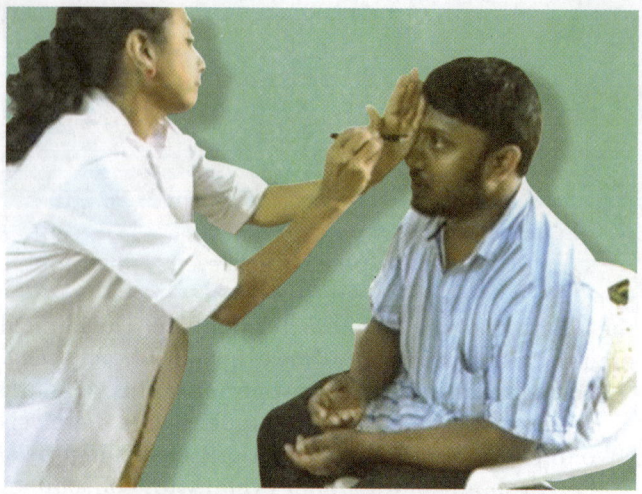

Fig. 28.8: Testing the indirect light reflex.

off the pupil comes to the original size. Afferent for this reflex is the optic nerve, center in the midbrain and the efferent is the oculomotor nerve.

- **Indirect or consensual light reflex:** A hand or a book is placed between the two eyes so that when light is thrown into one eye it does not fall on the opposite eye. Shine a torch into one eye and observe the pupil of the opposite eye **(Fig. 28.8)**. Normally it is seen that the pupil of the opposite eye constricts. This is consensual light reflex. Thus the pupils of both eyes constrict when light is thrown into one eye.

Abnormalities of Light Reflex

- The pupil may not respond to direct and consensual light reflex. This occurs in III nerve palsy.
- The pupil will not constrict in direct light reflex, but constricts in consensual reaction. Lesion is in the optic nerve on the side of abolition of direct light reflex.
- **Argyll-Robertson pupil**: The pupils are small, constricted and do not react to light but react normally to accommodation. The lesion is in the pretectal area and is characteristically seen in tabes dorsalis.

Accommodation Reflex

Accommodation reflex occurs when the subject focuses his vision on a near object. The subject is asked to look at a distance so that the eye is fully relaxed **(Figs. 28.9A and B)**. The examiner suddenly brings his finger vertically in front of the subject's nose and he is asked to look at it. The response observed is convergence of the eyeballs and constriction of the pupils. One more change occur in the eye during accommodation reflex, i.e., increase in the curvature of the anterior surface of lens which can be visualized only with the help of a slit lamp.

IV and VI Cranial Nerves

The IV nerve nucleus lies just caudal to the third nerve nucleus. The nerve fibers of the fourth nerve decussate. Due to decussation of fibers to the opposite side, the right trochlear nucleus innervates the left superior oblique and vice versa. Lesion of IV nerve, leads to paresis of superior oblique. There will be extortion of eye due to unopposed action of inferior oblique and this leads to diplopia.

The sixth cranial nerve nucleus is in the pons. The nerve is long and thin and in the orbit it supplies the lateral rectus. Bilateral sixth cranial nerve lesions are common as a feature of raised intracranial pressure. There will be paresis of lateral rectus and there will be diplopia.

Eye Movements

Horizontal movement of the eye laterally is termed abduction and inwards (medially) is termed adduction. Vertical movement upward is elevation and downward is depression **(Fig. 28.10)**. Convergence refers to adduction of both eyes to fixate on a near object. Conjugate eye movement means both the eyes always move together and

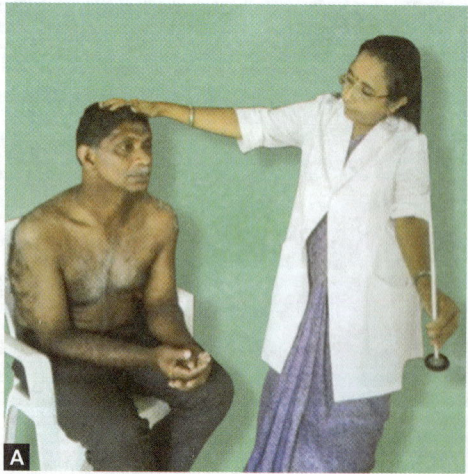
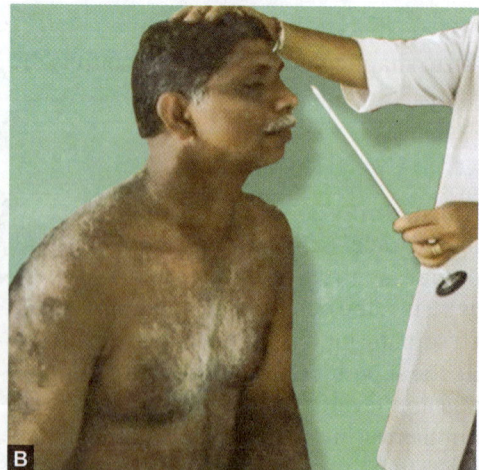

Figs. 28.9A and B: Testing accommodation reflex.

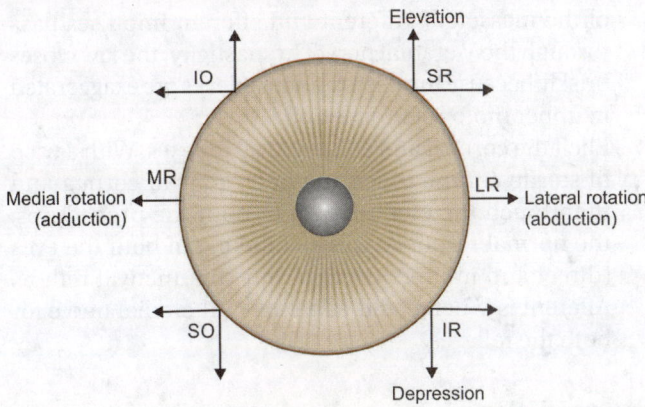

Fig. 28.10: Movements of eyeball. (SR: superior rectus; MR: medial rectus; IR: inferior rectus; IO: inferior oblique; LR: lateral rectus; SO: superior oblique)

to the same extent. The III, IV and VI cranial nerves are involved in eye movements.

Examination of the Extraocular Muscles

- Ask the subject to sit on a stool.
- The examiner should stand in front of him at a distance of about one meter.
- Instruct him to close one eye with his hand.
- Ask the subject to keep his head still or steady it by placing the left hand of the examiner on his head.
- Show him the right index finger held directly in front of his eyes at about half a meter distance. Inquire about double vision. If there is weakness of a muscle, it may lead to diplopia. Look for squint or nystagmus.
- Then ask him to follow the movements of the index finger. See that he does not turn his neck. Move the finger to the right, left, up and down in a large 'H' pattern.
- In case the subject does not turn his eyes, snap the middle finger and the thumb to produce a sound; he will then follow the sound.
- Move the finger to the medial side, e.g., the nasal side and find out how far he can turn the eyeball medially. This is the function of the medial rectus muscle.
- In this medial position raise the finger up. Find out how far the eyeball gets elevated. Moving the eyeball upward in the medially deviated position is the function of the inferior oblique muscle.
- In the same medial position, move the finger down. Find out how much the eyeball gets depressed. This is the function of the superior oblique muscle.
- Bring back the finger in the center move the finger laterally, and then back to the center. This is the function of the lateral rectus muscle.
- From the center move the finger upward, note the range and bring the finger back to the center.
- Now move it downward and note the range and bring it back in the center.
- Moving the eyeball from the center upward and downward is the function of the superior and inferior rectus respectively.
- Now repeat the whole procedure with the other eye.
- Note down the observations.
- Look for nystagmus at about 30° away from the primary position of gaze. When looking for nystagmus, the subject should not be asked to look too far in any direction since at extremes of gaze nystagmus can be normal.

Convergence

Ask the subject to look at the finger suddenly placed about half a meter—in front of him. Both the eyes turn inwards and fix on the finger normally.

TRIGEMINAL NERVE

The trigeminal nerve contains two types of fibers, the general sensory and the somatic motor.

Sensory Component

First order neurons are in the trigeminal ganglion. The three sensory divisions of the trigeminal nerve are **ophthalmic, maxillary and mandibular divisions**. They mediate general sensation from the skin of face, sensation inside the mouth and nose and proprioception. The central processes pass through the trigeminal nerve into the pons. Afferents mediating touch sensation pass to the principal sensory nucleus of the trigeminal nerve in the pons. Pain and temperature afferents go into the spinal tract and pass caudally into the medulla and into the spinal nucleus of trigeminal nerve, which extends down from the medulla as low as the upper cervical spinal cord.

- Test all the sensations of face including pinna of ear. Patients with impaired sensation on one side of the face may have a trigeminal nerve lesion, a trigeminal sensory nucleus lesion or a lesion in the central trigeminal sensory pathways.
- Test the corneal reflex on either side. Ask the subject to look straight with eyes wide open. Using a cotton wisp or a clean tissue paper, touch the cornea, approaching from the side. The normal response is a brisk blink.

Motor Component

From the motor nucleus of trigeminal nerve in the pons, fibers pass through the motor root of the trigeminal nerve and enter the mandibular nerve. These fibers supply the muscles of mastication (masseter, temporalis and lateral pterygoids).

- Note the symmetry of the temporal fossae and the angles of the jaw.
- Look for wasting of temporalis and masseter muscles.

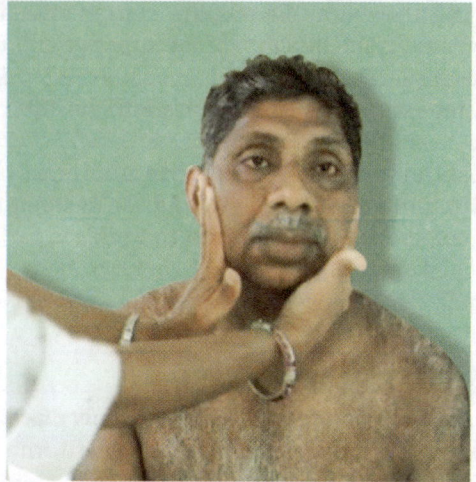

Fig. 28.11: Testing the power of masseter of both sides.

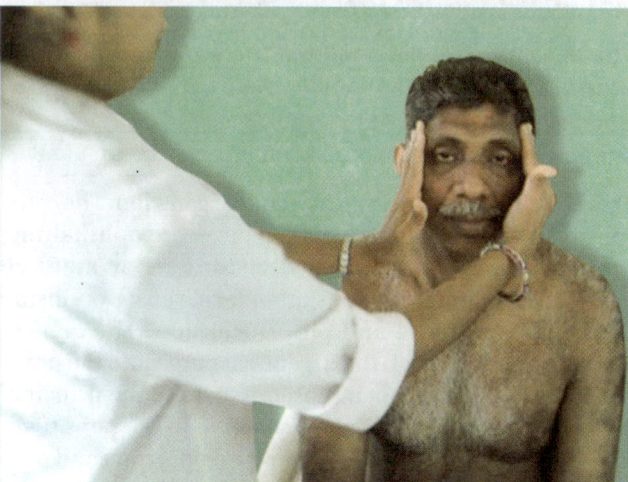

Fig. 28.12: Power of temporalis.

- Ask the subject to clench his teeth. Feel for the contraction of master **(Fig. 28.11)** and temporalis muscles **(Fig. 28.12)**.
- Ask him to push his open jaw sideways against resistance offered by the examiner to test the power of the pterygoid muscles.
- If there is lesion of the trigeminal nerve on one side, there will be deviation of the jaw toward the side of lesion due to weakness of the pterygoid muscle on the affected side.

Reflexes

- Elicit the jaw jerk. Ask the subject to open his mouth slightly, so that the jaw remains relaxed. Place the index finger below the lower lip. Strike it lightly with a percussion hammer in a downward direction (*refer* **Fig. 29.3**). Closure of the mouth is the reflex response, but it is usually not observed in normal subjects. Ask an assistant to feel for the reflex contraction of the masseters. Afferent and efferent impulses pass through the V cranial nerve. In spasticity, the jaw closes briskly because the deep tendon reflexes are exaggerated in upper motor neuron lesion.
- Elicit the corneal and conjunctival reflexes. With a wisp of sterile cotton, touch the outer part of cornea and then touch the conjunctiva. In both the procedures, the normal response will be blinking of both the eyes (direct and indirect corneal and conjunctival reflex). Afferent is V nerve and efferent is VII cranial nerve for both the reflexes.

Sensory Part

Each side of the face is tested separately for pain, light touch and temperature sensations. The ophthalmic division of trigeminal nerve supplies the forehead, upper part of the side of the nose and the scalp anterior to the vertex, maxillary division supplies the malar region and upper lip and the mandibular division of V cranial nerve supplies the chin.

FACIAL NERVE

The facial nerve contains the following four types of fibers:
1. The special sensory for taste
2. The general sensory
3. The somatic motor
4. The parasympathetic motor fibers which are of two types, the secretomotor and the vasomotor.

The nerve cell bodies of the sensory components of the facial nerve are in the geniculate ganglion in the facial canal. Gustatory sensory afferents from the anterior 2/3 of tongue travel in the lingual nerve and then via the chorda tympani nerve join the facial nerve in the facial canal. Central projections reach the medulla via the nervus intermedius.

The facial nerve nucleus is in the caudal pons. It receives upper motor neuron input from both cerebral hemispheres. Axons of the lower motor neurons emerge from the pons and form the facial nerve. It emerges from the skull at the stylomastoid foramen. In the parotid gland, it divides into branches that supply all the muscles of facial expression, the platysma muscle, posterior belly of digastric and stylohyoid on one side. In the facial canal, a branch of the facial nerve supplies the stapedius muscle.

Secretomotor parasympathetic efferents leave the pontomedullary junction in the nervus intermedius, which joins the facial nerve. Some of the parasympathetic fibers leave the facial nerve at the geniculate ganglion and join the greater petrosal nerve to supply the lacrimal glands. Others leave via the chorda tympani nerve to reach the sublingual and submandibular salivary glands.

Facial nerve lesion may be associated with loss of taste, hyperacusis (if stapedius is paralyzed), etc. A lower motor neuron lesion affecting the facial nerve nucleus or the facial nerve as a whole will cause weakness of all the muscles of one side of face. A unilateral upper motor neuron lesion will cause weakness of lower half of the face with sparing of the upper half because there is bilateral representation of the upper half of the face in the motor cortex.

The Sense of Taste (Special Sensory)

Taste receptors are distributed widely over the mucous membrane of tongue, mouth and pharynx. Besides the facial, the glossopharyngeal (posterior two-thirds of tongue), and the vagus (pharynx) contain the sensory fibers for taste. Sweet, sour, salt, bitter and umami are considered as primary taste sensations. Taste buds having peak sensitivity for each of the primary tastes are grouped together in different areas of the mucous membrane of mouth. The receptors could be stimulated only when the substance is applied in the form of a solution. The solution of each substance is tested over different parts separately. Facial nerve carries taste sensation from the anterior 2/3 of tongue.

Method

- Solutions of 1 % sugar, 0.2% tartaric or lactic acid, 0.5% sodium chloride, and 0.002% quinine are taken in labelled containers.
- Cards labelled as 'sweet', 'sour', 'salt' and 'bitter' are made.
- Ask the subject to sit on a stool.
- Instruct him to clean the mouth using water.
- Put the labelled cards before him on the table.
- Ask him to protrude the tongue. Mop the excess of saliva with sterile gauze.
- Dip the applicator in one solution; take it out and drain the excess of the solution.
- Rub it gently on a part of the tongue on one side.
- Ask him to put his finger on the card according to the taste he identifies.
- Mop the solution and the saliva first with wet and then with dry gauze.
- Repeat on different parts of the tongue on each of the right and the left sides.
- Repeat for each of the taste after washing the mouth.
- Record the results showing the various spots in the tongue where different tastes were appreciated.

General Sensory

Facial nerve carries general sensations from the tympanic membrane, the external auditory meatus and tragus of the ear.

Somatic Motor

- Facial nerve supplies the muscles of facial expression (anterior belly of occipitofrontalis, orbicularis oculi, orbicularis oris, buccinators, depressor anguli oris and platysma). It also supplies the stapedius muscle in the middle ear.
- Note the facial symmetry and the nasolabial folds. See whether there is deviation of the angle of the mouth and epiphora.
- **Wrinkling of forehead:** To test the anterior belly of occipitofrontalis, ask him to raise his eyebrows and observe the wrinkles on the fore head. Note whether the wrinkles are equal on both sides **(Fig. 28.13)**.
- **Blinking:** Ask him to blink. The blink rate will be reduced on the affected side in LMN palsy.
- **Forced eye closure:** Ask him to tightly close his eyelids. If he can close, attempt to raise the eyebrows while his eyes are closed **(Fig. 28.14)**. Normally, this is not possible. Mild weakness of orbicularis oculi can be detected. In severe lower motor neuron facial weakness, the patient will not be able to close the affected eye.

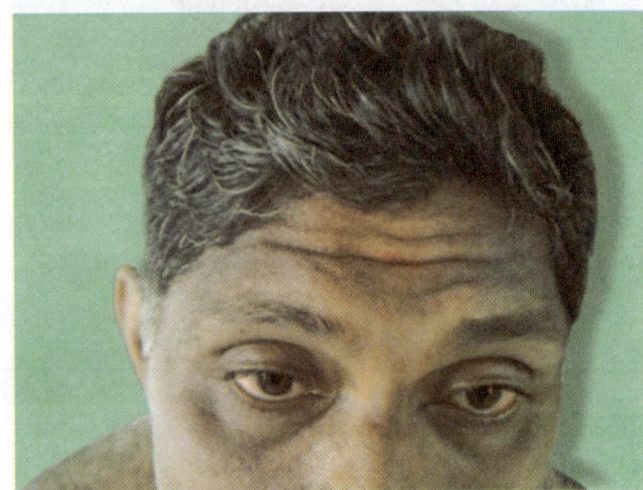

Fig. 28.13: Testing the power of anterior belly of occipitofrontalis.

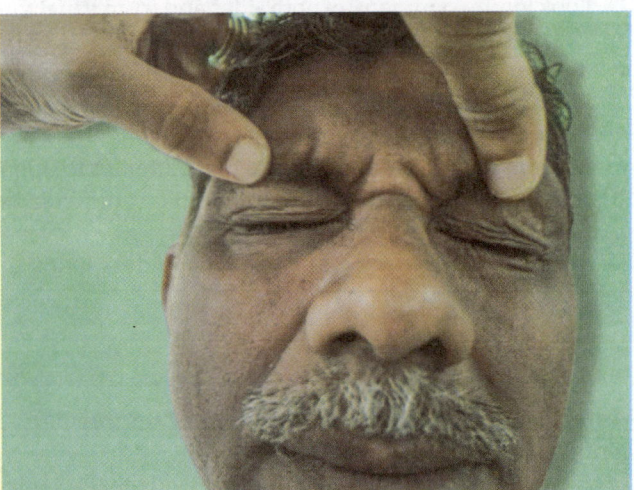

Fig. 28.14: Testing the power of orbicularis oculi.

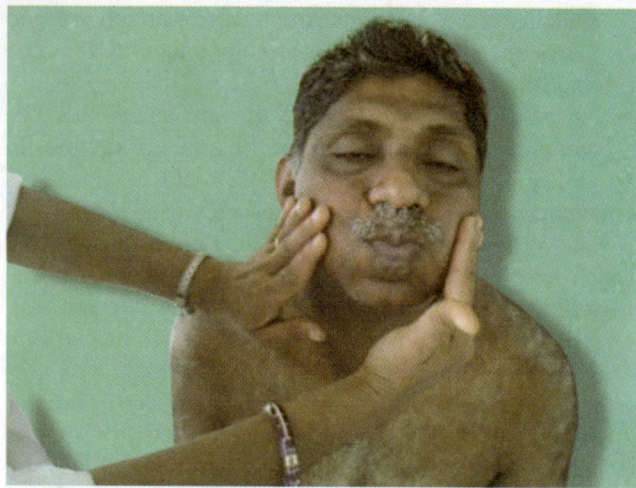

Fig. 28.15: Testing the power of buccinator.

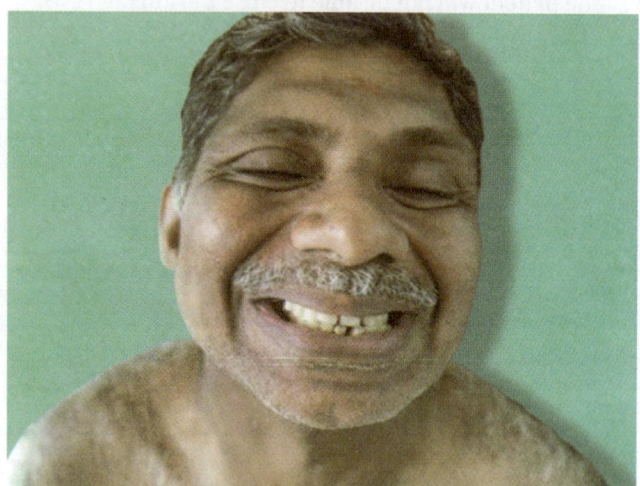

Fig. 28.16: Looking for deviation of angle of mouth by asking him to show his teeth.

- **Blowing the cheek:** Ask him to blow out his cheeks. Look for the symmetry of both sides and try to expel the air by pressing on the buccinator muscle **(Fig. 28.15)**.
- Ask him to show his teeth and then to grimace **(Fig. 28.16)**. The angle of the mouth will deviate to the side opposite to the side of palsy.

Ask him to purse his lips together and attempt to open them using the fingers of the examiner to test orbicularis oris. Ask the subject to whistle.

Ask for hyperacusis. Paralysis of stapedius leads to defective tympanic reflex and hyperacusis.

VESTIBULOCOCHLEAR (ACOUSTIC) NERVE

Vestibulocochlear nerve, which is a purely sensory nerve, contains two types of fibers.
1. Afferent fibers from the cochlea that mediate the sense of hearing.
2. Fibers from the vestibular apparatus that mediate the sense of equilibrium. These fibers reach the vestibular and cochlear nuclei in the brainstem.

Testing the Cochlear Part

First inspect the external auditory canal for excess earwax, discharge or perforation of the tympanic membrane.

Watch Test

Bring the wristwatch near the subject's ear and ask whether he can hear the tick sound.

Rinne's Test

Strike the tuning fork of frequency 512 Hz on a firm surface. Avoid metallic objects, which may dampen the vibrations. Place the vibrating tuning fork over the mastoid process on one side of the subject **(Fig. 28.17A)**. Hold it like that till he fails to hear the vibrating sound. Immediately hold the tuning fork in front of the external auditory meatus of the same side **(Fig. 28.17B)**. A normal person can still hear the sound because air conduction is better than bone conduction. Then Rinne test is said to be positive. Repeat the test on the opposite side.

In conductive deafness, bone conduction will be better than air conduction. In sensory neural deafness, both air conduction and bone conduction are decreased. But still air conduction is better than bone conduction.

Weber's Test

Strike the tuning fork and place its base on the middle of the fore head or on the vertex. Ask him whether he can hear the sound equally in both the ears or is appreciated better in one ear, i.e., lateralized **(Fig. 28.18)**. A normal person can hear the sound equally on both the ears. But in a person with conduction deafness, the sound will be better heard in the diseased ear, i.e., the sound lateralizes to the abnormal ear. This is because bone conduction is better than air conduction in middle ear disease. In sensory-neural deafness, the sound lateralizes to the normal ear.

Schwabach Test

The bone conduction of the subject and the examiner is compared in this test. Apply the base of the vibrating tuning fork to the mastoid process of the side being tested. Once the subject stops hearing the sound, apply the tuning fork to the mastoid process of the examiner provided his bone conduction is normal. If the examiner continues to hear the sound, the subject's bone conduction is defective. Repeat the procedure on the opposite side. **Audiometry** discussed in chapter 50 will help to distinguish between sensorineural deafness and conduction deafness.

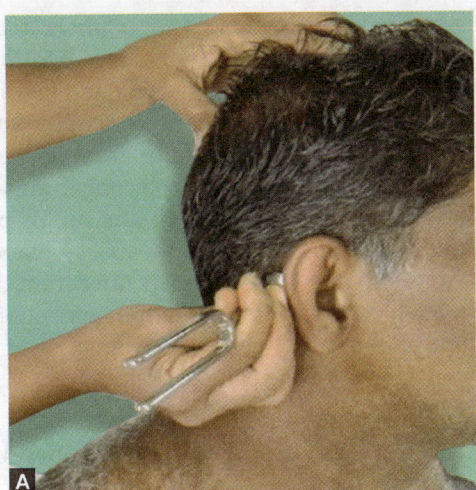
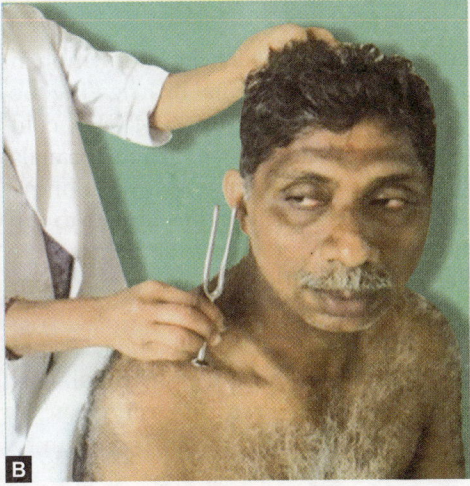

Figs. 28.17A and B: Rinne's test: (A) Bone conduction; (B) Air conduction.

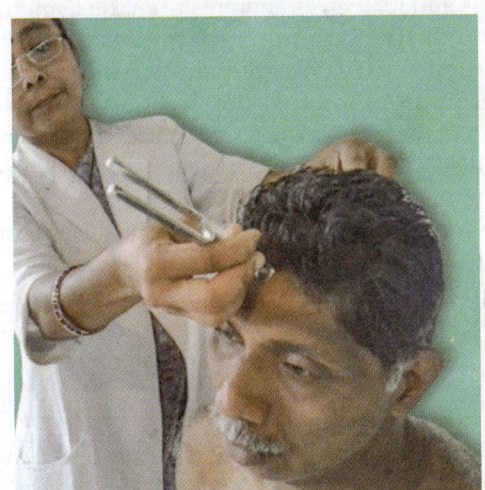

Fig. 28.18: Weber's test.

VESTIBULAR PART

The vestibular part arises from the vestibular apparatus. The vestibular nucleus has connections, through the vestibulospinal tracts, for reflex movements of the limbs and trunk in response to the stimulation of the vestibular organ. It has also connections through the median longitudinal bundle for the control of the conjugate eye movements in relation to the movements of head; and with the cerebellum, to help in the control of the muscle tone in relation to postural adjustments.

Ask the subject whether he has tinnitus or vertigo. Look for nystagmus.

Caloric and Rotational Tests

Caloric and rotational stimuli are used to produce changes in the endolymph current in the semicircular canals and thus test the vestibular apparatus.

Rotation Test (Barany's Test)

The semicircular canals contain receptors, which detect the movement of head in space. In the horizontal plane rotation of head stimulates the horizontal semicircular canals. In the rotation test only the post-rotary effects are observed. In the post-rotary state, the endolymph continues to move in the direction of rotation though the head is now stationary. The result is inhibition of the receptors in one canal and stimulation of the other one.

Method

- Rotating chair with a backrest is used.
- Make the subject sit comfortably in the chair. Adjust the backrest and position the subject so that his head lies in a plane 30° below the horizontal.
- Ask him to close the eyes to prevent the opticokinetic nystagmus.
- Rotate the chair rapidly at a rate of 1 round in 2 seconds for about 30 seconds in the clockwise direction.
- Now stop abruptly.
- Ask him to open the eyes and look for nystagmus.
- Hold the index finger before him and ask him first to touch his nose and then your finger and again his nose with his index finger.
- Ask him to repeat this with his eyes closed.
- Ask him whether he feels any sensation of whirling, nausea and falling down.
- Repeat the past pointing test and confirm that it is a temporary aberration.
- In health post rotary nystagmus is present for about 20 seconds with slow component in the direction of the rotation of the chair. This is called nystagmus to the left as the fast component is toward left. The effect is due to the stimulation of the left canal. Past pointing occurs toward right, e.g., in the direction of rotation.

Caloric Test

Convection currents can be produced in the endolymph in a vertically positioned semicircular canal by irrigating the external auditory meatus with warm (up to 44°C) or cold (from 12°C to 30°C) water. Any one of the semicircular canals can be placed in the vertical plane by properly positioning the head in the space. The effects seen are similar to the post-rotary effects of clockwise rotation to the right.

- Make the subject sit on a stool with a backrest. Confirm that the eardrums are intact.
- Instruct him to sit upright and tilt his head backwards making an angle of about 60° above the horizontal. This brings the horizontal canal in a vertical position.
- Explain him the test; assure him and instruct him to signify the onset of dizziness or nausea.
- The irrigation should be stopped as soon as the onset of dizziness or nausea is noted.
- Hold a kidney tray by the side of one of his ears and slowly irrigate the external auditory canal with about 150 mL of the cool water.
- Immediately examine for nystagmus.
- Carry out the past pointing test.
- While you are prepared to support and hold him, ask him to get up and stand. Find out the side on which he falls.
- In a healthy individual—say if the right ear is irrigated—there occurs horizontal nystagmus with the slow component to the right (this is called as nystagmus to the left), past pointing, e.g., the finger of the subject goes to the right, and falling to the right. Subjective sensation of nausea and dizziness may occur.
- These responses are obtained from the stimulation of the canal in the vertical position. They are decreased or may even be completely absent if there is something wrong with the above-mentioned connections.

Labyrinthitis and acute vestibular neuritis causes vertigo and nystagmus.

GLOSSOPHARYNGEAL NERVE

The glossopharyngeal nerve contains special sensory fibers, general sensory fibers, autonomic parasympathetic fibers and somatic motor fibers. It carries the sense of taste from the posterior 1/3 of tongue. It mediates somatic sensation of the palate and pharynx. The autonomic secretomotor fibers arise from the inferior salivatory nucleus and supply the parotid gland. Motor fibers supply the stylopharyngeus muscle that cannot be tested clinically.

Ask the subject to open the mouth. Using an orange stick touch lightly the posterior pharyngeal wall. **Gag reflex** will be observed if the sensation is normal.

VAGUS NERVE

The vagus nerve contains special sensory taste fibers, general sensory fibers from the viscera, somatic general sensory fibers, somatic motor fibers and large number of parasympathetic motor fibers. Motor efferent fibers supply the muscles of pharynx and larynx. The superior laryngeal nerve supplies the cricopharyngeus muscle of larynx and conveys sensation from larynx. The recurrent laryngeal nerve supplies laryngeal muscles other than cricopharyngeus. Sensory fibers supply pharynx, larynx, trachea, lungs, heart, esophagus, stomach and intestine. Parasympathetic motor fibers arise from the dorsal motor nucleus of vagus in the medulla and supply the thoracic and abdominal viscera. Parasympathetic functions are not considered during clinical examination.

The vagus nerve has three nuclei:

1. **The main motor nucleus** formed by the nucleus ambiguus the efferent fibers of which supply the constrictor muscles of the pharynx and the intrinsic muscles of the larynx.
2. **Parasympathetic nucleus** forms the dorsal nucleus of vagus and it receives afferents from the hypothalamus through the autonomic pathways and from the glossopharyngeal nerve (carotid sinus reflex). The efferent fibers supply the involuntary muscles of bronchi, heart, esophagus, stomach, intestine as far as the distal 1/3 of the transverse colon, liver, spleen and kidney.
3. **The sensory nucleus** of vagus is the lower part of the nucleus of tractus solitaries. It receives taste fibers from the pharynx and soft palate whose cell bodies are located in the inferior ganglion of vagus nerve. The second order fibers end in the ventral posteromedial nucleus of thalamus of same side and the third order neurons end in the postcentral gyrus.

- Usually IX and X cranial nerves are tested together.
- Notice the pitch and quality of the subject's voice. Ask if there is nasal regurgitation of swallowed fluids or history suggestive of aspiration.
- Ask the subject whether he has dysphagia. Bilateral lesions of vagus nerves will invariably be associated with dysphagia. See whether there is dysarthria.
- Look for the position of the uvula. It will be normally central in position, but will be deviated to the normal side in unilateral palsy.
- Ask him to open the mouth widely and look for the symmetry of the palatal arches. Ask him to say 'Ahh'. See whether the arching of the palate is equal on both sides and also see whether there is deviation of uvula. Weakness of elevation of palate on the affected side along with deviation of uvula to the unaffected side is due to unopposed action of palatal muscle of the normal side. It is seen in unilateral X nerve palsy.
- See whether there is dysphonia. Ipsilateral vocal cord paralysis leads to dysphonia.
- Elicit the **palatal reflex**. Ask the subject to open the mouth widely. Touch the soft palate with cotton

tipped small stick. There will be contraction of the palate. The afferent is the V nerve and efferent is X cranial nerve.
- **Pharyngeal (gag) reflex**: Ask the subject to open the mouth and using a tongue depressor push the tongue down. Touch the posterior pharyngeal wall with the cotton tip on each side separately. The subject will gag immediately on touching. This reflex is absent or decreased in LMN lesions and exaggerated in UMN lesions.
- Test the taste sensation from the posterior 1/3 of tongue, both halves separately.

ACCESSORY NERVE

The accessory nerve is a purely somatic motor nerve that is formed by the union of a cranial and a spinal root. **Spinal root** of accessory nerve consists of axons of nerve cells in the spinal nucleus situated in the anterior grey column of cervical spinal cord (C2-6). Instead of leaving the spinal cord in the spinal roots, they pass rostrally up into the medulla through the foramen magnum and emerge as the accessory nerve along with its cranial root through the jugular foramen in the skull. The spinal root separates from the cranial root and forms the spinal accessory nerve and it supplies the sternocleidomastoid and upper part of trapezius muscle.

The cranial root is formed of nerve fibers from the nucleus ambiguus of medulla. It soon leaves the accessory nerve to rejoin their equivalents in the vagus nerve and is distributed in its pharyngeal and recurrent laryngeal branches to the muscles of the soft palate, pharynx and larynx.

Accessory nerve thus brings about movements of the soft palate, pharynx and larynx and controls the movement of sternocleidomastoid and trapezius.

Sternomastoid

- Observe the position of the head. With bilateral sternomastoid weakness, head will fall backwards.
- See the patient getting up from lying down position. Normally the head will leave first from the bed, but with sternomastoid weakness head will lag behind.
- See whether the chin is deviated to one side. In unilateral XI nerve paralysis, the chin will be directed to the side of lesion due to paralysis of sternocleidomastoid. The left sternocleidomastoid helps in the rotation of head to the right and vice versa.
- Ask him to flex his neck against the examiner's resistance to test the power of both the sternocleidomastoids together.
- Ask the subject to turn his head to either side when the examiner offers resistance on the chin. This movement is mediated by the sternomastoid of the opposite side,

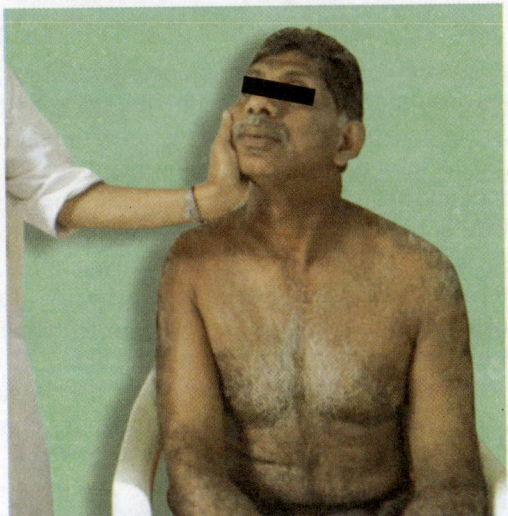

Fig. 28.19: Testing the power of left sternocleidomastoid (note the muscle contracting).

which can be seen to contract actively **(Fig. 28.19)**. Asking the patient to turn his head to the right against resistance offered by the examiner who pushes carefully against the right side of the face therefore assesses weakness of the left sternocleidomastoid.

Trapezius

- Stand behind the subject and observe the bulk and symmetry of the trapezius muscle on both sides.
- Look for the position of the head. In bilateral trapezius weakness, head will fall forward.
- Ask him to shrug the shoulder against resistance applied on his shoulders and compare the strength on both sides **(Fig. 28.20)**.
- Sometimes winging of the scapula can occur with trapezius weakness while abducting the shoulder.

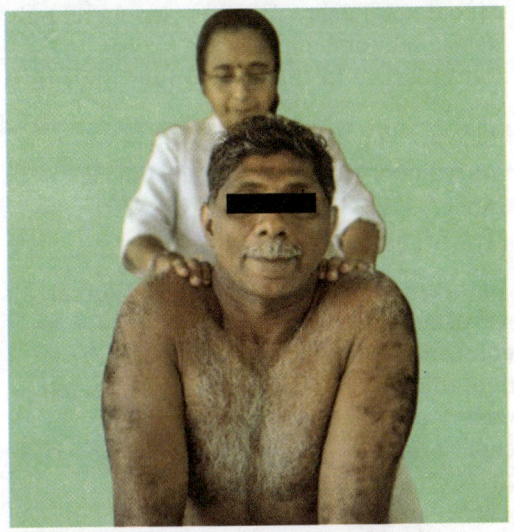

Fig. 28.20: Testing the power of trapezius.

HYPOGLOSSAL NERVE

Hypoglossal nerve is a purely motor nerve, which supplies all the intrinsic muscles of the tongue—the styloglossus, the hypoglossus and the genioglossus muscles of the same side. The hypoglossal nerve controls the movements and shape of the tongue and helps in mastication, deglutition and speech.

- Ask the subject to protrude the tongue and see whether there is any deviation of tongue. In unilateral XII nerve paralysis, the tongue will be deviated to the side of lesion.
- Look for wasting of tongue muscles, fasciculation, etc.
- Ask him to move the tongue in all directions.
- To test the power of the tongue muscles, ask the subject to press on the examiner's finger through his cheek on both sides.
- Palpate the tongue to feel for the tone. It will be spastic in UMN lesions and flaccid in LMN lesions.
- LMN lesions of XII nerve produce weakness, wasting, flaccidity and fasciculation of tongue, whereas UMN lesion produces only weakness and spasticity. Both the conditions produce dysarthria and dysphagia.

Report Pattern of a Normal Subject

Name:
Age:
Sex:
Occupation and address:

General Examination

- Normally built and nourished
- No pallor, icterus, cyanosis, edema, dyspnea, clubbing or lymphadenopathy.
- **Body temperature:** 37°C
- **Respiratory rate:** 16/min, regular, abdominothoracic
- **Pulse:** 70/min, regular, normal in volume and character, no thickening of vessel wall, no radiofemoral/brachiofemoral delay. All other peripheral pulsations are felt equally on both sides.
- Blood pressure in the right upper limb in supine position:
  - Palpatory method—116 mm Hg
  - Auscultatory method—120/80 mm Hg

Higher Functions

- **General appearance and behavior:** Normal
- **Level of consciousness:** Conscious
- **Mental and emotional state:** Normal
- **Orientation in time and place:** Well oriented
- **Memory and intelligence:** Normal
- **Sleep:** Normal
- **Gait:** Normal
- **Speech:** Normal
- **Delusions and hallucinations:** Absent

EXAMINATION OF CRANIAL NERVES

I. OLFACTORY NERVE

Sense of smell
- Right side—normal/absent/altered
- Left side—normal/absent/altered

II. OPTIC NERVE

Visual acuity

Near vision
- Right eye—normal
- Left eye—normal

Distant vision using Snellen's chart
- Right eye 6/6
- Left eye 6/6

Field of vision as tested by confrontation method
- Right eye—normal
- Left eye—normal

Color vision
- Right eye—normal
- Left eye—normal

OCULOMOTOR (III), TROCHLEAR (IV) AND ABDUCENT NERVE (VI)

- No ptosis
- No squint
- No nystagmus
- No diplopia
- Size and shape of pupil—normal
- Eye movements on both sides—normal in all directions

Pupillary Reflexes

Light reflex
- Direct—normal on both eyes
- Indirect or consensual light reflex—normal on both eyes

Accommodation reflex—normal

V. TRIGEMINAL NERVE

- Cutaneous sensation on the face on both sides—normal
- Sensations in the mucous membrane of mouth and nose—normal
- Corneal reflex—normal on both eyes
- Muscles of mastication—normal power on both sides of face
- No deviation of the jaw on opening the mouth

VII. FACIAL NERVE

- Nasolabial folds—normal on both sides
- No deviation of the angle of mouth

- No epiphora
- No hyperacusis
- Power of the muscles of facial expression—normal on both sides
- Tests of taste sensation:

	Anterior 2/3 of tongue	
	Right side	Left side
Sweet	Present	Present
Salt	Present	Present
Sour	Present	Present
Bitter	Present	Present

VIII. VESTIBULOCOCHLEAR NERVE

Tests for Cochlear Function

- Watch test—normally heard on both sides
- Rinne's test—air conduction is greater than bone conduction on both sides
- Weber's test—vibration equally appreciated on both sides

Tests of Vestibular Function

No vertigo or nystagmus
- Barany's test—normal, no nystagmus at the end of rotation
- Caloric test—normal on both sides

IX. GLOSSOPHARYNGEAL NERVE

Taste Sensation

	Posterior 1/3 of tongue	
	Right side	Left side
Sweet	Present	Present
Salt	Present	Present
Sour	Present	Present
Bitter	Present	Present

Palatal reflex
- On right side—normal
- On left side—normal

X. VAGUS NERVE

- No regurgitation of fluid through the nose
- No nasal twang to the voice
- No dysphagia
- Palatal reflex—normal on both sides
- Pharyngeal reflex—normal on both sides

XI. SPINAL ACCESSORY NERVE

- Flexion of the head against resistance—normal (both the sternomastoids become prominent)
- Rotation of the chin to the right against resistance—normal
- Rotation of the chin to the left against resistance—normal
- Shrugging of shoulder against resistance—normal on both sides

XII. HYPOGLOSSAL NERVE

- No deviation of tongue when it is protruded out.
- No fasciculation or wasting of tongue muscles.
- Movement of tongue normal in all directions.
- Power of tongue muscles—normal on both sides.

Impression

The cranial nerves of the subject appears to be normal.

Viva Questions

1. **Name the purely sensory and purely motor cranial nerves.**
   I, II, VIII cranial nerves are sensory nerves and IV, VI, XI and XII are motor nerves.
2. **Name the cranial nerves that contain autonomic parasympathetic fibers.**
   III, VII, IX and X cranial nerves contain parasympathetic fibers.
3. **What are the common errors of refraction? How is it corrected?**
   » Hypermetropia or long-sightedness is corrected using a biconvex glass
   » Myopia or short-sightedness, corrected using biconcave glass
   » Astigmatism, corrected using cylindrical glass
   » Presbyopia corrected with biconvex reading glass
4. **What are the mechanisms of color vision?**
   » Retinal mechanism based on Young-Helmholtz theory. According to this theory, there are three kinds of cones containing three types of pigments sensitive to red, green and blue color. The ganglion cells of retina add or subtract input from one type of cone to the input of another type. Further processing occurs in the lateral geniculate body of thalamus and in the visual cortex.
   » Cortical mechanism states that there are color blobs (clusters of cells) arranged in a mosaic in layer IV of the primary visual cortex (area 17). Fibers from the lateral geniculate body of thalamus project to these color blobs, which along with the visual association area (area 18) are involved in color perception.

5. **What is the significance of testing color vision?**
   » It is part of routine health checkup while joining professional course or jobs.
   » Driving license will be issued only to those who have normal color vision. Otherwise they will not be able to identify the signals.
   » Workers in textile industry require a high degree of color perception.

6. **What is color blindness?**
   Color blindness is the failure to appreciate one or more of the three primary colors. Individuals with normal color vision have three types of cones and are called **trichromats**. In **anomalous trichromats**, there is no complete blindness for any color but one of the cones will be weak and the appreciation of that color will be less. Persons with only two types of cones are called **dichromats** and those with only one type of cone are called **monochromats**.
   As far as color vision is concerned individuals may be trichromats, dichromats and monochromats.
   » Trichromats
      • With normal color vision
      • Protanomaly (red cone weak)
      • Deuteranomaly (green cone weak)
      • Tritanomaly (blue cone weak)
   » Dichromats (one cone absent)
      • Protanopia (red-blind)
      • Deuteranopia (green-blind)
      • Tritanopia (blue-blind)
   » Monochromats have only one type of cone and has only black and white vision
   Deuteranomaly is more common (50% of the total cases of color blindness). It is seen in approximately 5% of male population. The decreasing order of occurrence is deuteranopia, protanopia and least is protanomaly. *Tritanomaly and tritanopia are extremely rare.*

7. **What does conjugate movement of eye mean?**
   Both the eyes always move together and to the same extent. This is called 'conjugate deviation'. The voluntary conjugate deviation is caused by the motor centers located in Brodmann's area 8. The automatic fixation movements are mediated through the sensory centers located in the occipital cortex.

8. **What is squint?**
   In some people each eye when tested separately shows full range of movements; but when both are examined simultaneously one of the eyes may fail to show the optimum range. This is described as squint or strabismus. In squint, the eyes point in different directions. A squint is described as convergent or divergent strabismus, depending on whether the eyes point toward or away from each other. It is not caused because of paralysis of any muscle. It can be due to decreased tone in eye muscles. It is evident only when both the eyes are examined together and hence is described as concomitant. The subject is asked to follow the movements of the index finger medially and laterally. In subjects having concomitant strabismus, one of the eyes may fail to show the optimum range of movements.

9. **What is nystagmus?**
   Nystagmus means involuntary, to and fro movements of the eyeballs. It may occur in any one direction, horizontal or vertical; or it may occur in both the directions. In health the eyeballs move to fix the gaze on objects and there are no such apparent to and fro movements. The to and fro movements seen in nystagmus are usually slow in one direction and fast in the opposite one. They are described as the slow and the fast components. Thus nystagmus to the left means fast component of the movement is toward the left. A disturbance in the central nervous system, which is concerned with maintenance of equilibrium, causes nystagmus.

10. **What is physiological nystagmus or opticokinetic nystagmus?**
    A physiological nystagmus is seen when looking out of the window of a moving train. The visual field is rapidly and successively passing in one direction. While looking out the person fixes his gaze on an object of interest and as the object moves away slowly the eyes also follow the object (the slow component) till it becomes difficult to see the object as it goes out of the visual field. The eyeballs then suddenly move in the opposite direction, i.e., in the direction of the motion of the train to fix the gaze on some other object (the fast component).

11. **What are the effects of lesion of III cranial nerve?**
    » In lesions of the III cranial nerve, there will be weakness of medial rectus, superior rectus, inferior oblique and inferior rectus.
    » In medial rectus paresis, the eye cannot be adducted. It becomes abducted due to unopposed action of lateral rectus and slightly depressed because of the action of superior oblique.
    » There will be paresis of elevation due to weakness of superior rectus and inferior oblique.
    » Paresis of depression due to involvement of inferior rectus.
    » There will be ptosis due to weakness of levator palpebrae superioris.
    » Pupils will be dilated and unreactive due to paralysis of sphincter pupillae muscle.

12. **Trace the pathway for pupillary light reflex.**
    When a beam of light is thrown into one eye, the pupils of both eyes constrict. Constriction on the same eye is direct light reflex and on the opposite side is indirect or consensual light reflex. Afferent impulses from the retina pass through the optic nerve, optic chiasma and optic tract. A small number of fibers without going to the lateral geniculate body separate out and synapse in the neurons in the pretectal nucleus in the midbrain. From here the fibers reach the parasympathetic nuclei of the third cranial nerve (Edinger-Westphal nuclei) of both sides and synapse in the neurons here. The parasympathetic nerve fibers pass through the third cranial nerve to the ciliary ganglion in the orbit. The postganglionic parasympathetic fibers pass through the short ciliary nerves to supply the constrictor pupillae of iris and ciliary muscles. Since the pretectal nucleus has connections with the Edinger-Westphal nuclei of both sides, when light is thrown into one eye, pupils of both eyes constrict (consensual light reflex).

13. **Explain the pathway for accommodation reflex.**
    While looking at a distant object if the subject looks at a near object the eyes converge due to the contraction of both medial recti. The ciliary muscles contract and the anterior curvature of lens increases and thereby its refractive power increases. In addition, both the pupils constrict to restrict the light rays entering the eyes.
    The afferent impulses travel in the visual pathway and reach the visual cortex. From the visual cortex impulses reach the frontal eye fields from where the efferent corticomesencephalic fibers descend through the internal capsule to reach the oculomotor nuclei in midbrain. Some fibers from these nuclei reach the medial recti muscles. Some of the descending fibers synapse with the Edinger-Westphal nuclei on both sides from where fibers reach the constrictor pupillae and ciliary muscles.

14. **Why 3rd, 4th and 6th cranial nerves are tested together?**
    These three nerves innervate the extraocular muscles of the eye which help in the movement of the eyeball within the orbit. By testing the movements of the eyeball like elevation, depression, adduction, abduction and rotatory movement of the eye ball, all these muscles can be tested together. They work together in a coordinated manner normally so that the image falls on the corresponding points in both retinas. So the three nerves are tested together.

15. **Name the muscles of mastication.**
    Masseter, temporalis, internal and external pterygoid and buccinator.

16. **What is Argyll-Robertson pupil?**
    This is a condition where accommodation reflex is present and pupillary reflex absent. This condition is commonly seen in neurosyphilis where the pretectal nucleus is damaged and the pupillary light reflex is abolished.

17. **What are the divisions of the trigeminal nerve? Name the parts supplied by each.**
    Ophthalmic, maxillary and mandibular divisions.
    » **Ophthalmic division** supplies the lacrimal gland, the skin of upper eye lids and its conjunctiva, forehead and the scalp as far as the vertex.
    » **Maxillary division** supplies the skin of cheek, lower eye lid and its conjunctiva, sides of the nose, upper lip and upper teeth. It also supplies the mucous membrane of nose, upper part of pharynx, roof of mouth, soft palate, tonsils and cornea.
    » **Mandibular division** supplies skin of lower part of face, lower lip, ear, tongue and lower teeth. The motor part of trigeminal nerve innervates all the muscles of mastication except buccinator which is supplied by seventh cranial nerve.

18. **What are the abnormalities of olfaction?**
    Anosmia, parosmia and hyposmia develop due to bilateral damage of the olfactory epithelium or the olfactory pathway. Hyperosmia or increased sensitivity to smell is seen in conditions like pregnancy and adrenal insufficiency.

19. **Mention the unique features of olfaction.**
    » Olfactory receptor cell (bipolar neuron) is the only nerve cell that is exposed to the external environment.
    » Olfactory cells are not only receptors but also neurons. Bipolar olfactory sensory neuron function both as receptor and ganglion cell (first order neuron).
    » Olfactory receptor cells (sensory neurons) undergo rapid turnover by proliferation and differentiation of the basal cells of olfactory mucosa (exception to the statement that neurons cannot regenerate).
    » Olfaction has no direct relay in the thalamus.
    » Olfaction has *no direct* neocortical projection.
    » In contrast to all other sensory pathways, the olfactory afferent pathway has only two neurons.

OBJECTIVE STRUCTURED PRACTICAL EXAMINATION

I. Test the VII cranial nerve of the subject
» Explain the procedure to the subject and ask him to sit on a stool
» Observes facial symmetry, palpebral fissure and nasolabial fold
» Ask the subject to wrinkle his forehead
» Ask the subject to close the eyes tightly and the examiner tries to open the eyes
» Ask the subject to show the teeth
» Ask to blow out the cheeks by filling it with air. Examiner presses on the cheeks and see whether air is escaping from the angle of the mouth
» Taste sensation from the anterior 2/3rd is tested

II. Test the 3rd, 4th and 6th cranial nerves
» Ask the subject to sit on a stool and explains the procedure briefly
» Look for ptosis and squint
» Observes the size and shape of pupil
» Tests the eye movements in all directions after fixing the subject's head with the left hand
» Pupillary light reflex both direct and indirect tested
» Accommodation reflex tested

29

Examination of Reflexes

LEARNING OBJECTIVES

- Elicit superficial and deep reflexes
- Discuss the clinical significance of each reflex
- Explain the pathway for each reflex
- What is clonus?

PY10.11: Demonstrate the correct clinical examination of reflexes in a normal volunteer or simulated environment.

INTRODUCTION

Reflexes are elicited in response to a stimulus to test the integrity of the nervous system. A reflex is defined as an involuntary response to an adequate stimulus. The basic unit of the reflex is the reflex arc. It consists of a receptor, a sensory pathway, a center, a link with motor unit and an effector organ (muscle or gland). An injury to any part of the reflex arc will abolish the reflex action.

Spinal cord is the center of all the reflex activities in the limbs. The responses produced by the spinal cord are modified by the influences from other parts of the nervous system. Apparently new reflexes, which appear because of a disease of the nervous system are described as pathological reflexes, e.g., extensor plantar response.

Types of Reflexes

- Deep tendon reflexes or stretch reflexes
- Superficial reflexes
- Visceral reflexes or organic reflexes

Deep Reflexes or Stretch Reflexes

Deep reflexes are monosynaptic reflexes. The stretch reflexes are myotatic reflexes, i.e., the sensory stimulus is the stretch given to the muscle. During stretch of the skeletal muscle, the receptor, which is the muscle spindle get stimulated. The resulting afferent impulses enter the appropriate segment of the spinal cord and bring about the efferent discharge to cause the contraction of the same muscle. If the reflex arc is damaged, the reflex gets abolished. Thus in the lower motor neuron type of paralysis where the a-motor neurons are damaged or in cases of damage to the nerve root these reflexes will be absent.

Injuries in various parts of the nervous system other than the reflex arc itself are capable of modifying the response seen during health. Thus in the upper motor neuron type of paralysis the stretch reflexes change according to the type of the upper motor neuron affected. The extrapyramidal damage is associated with exaggerated reflexes, the pyramidal damage with sluggish or flaccid reflexes and the cerebellar damage with pendular reflexes.

Superficial Reflexes

The superficial reflexes are polysynaptic reflexes. The superficial reflexes are elicited by stimulation of skin or mucous membrane. They are either withdrawal reflexes or their modifications. When an adequate sensory stimulus is applied, the motor response occurs in the form of contraction of an appropriate group of muscles. The severity of contraction depends on the number of the receptors (sensory units) stimulated.

Superficial reflexes will be brisk in anxiety, psychosis, etc. There is a center in the midbrain, which normally inhibit the superficial reflexes. In Parkinson's disease and other extrapyramidal extrapyramidal diseases, this center is involved leading to brisk superficial reflexes.

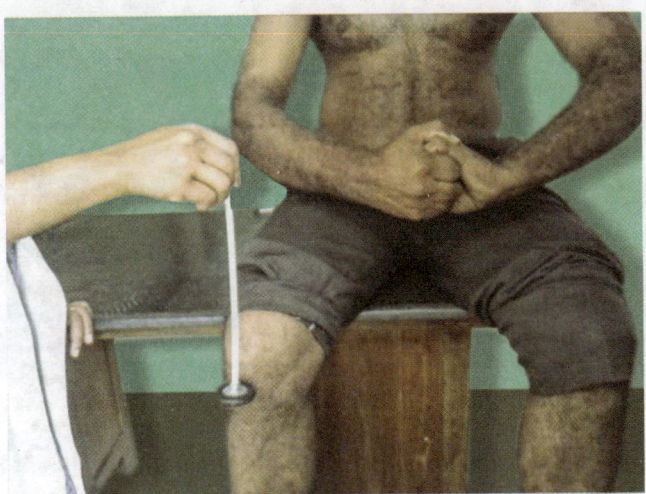

Fig. 29.1: Jendrassik's maneuver to elicit knee jerk.

Reinforcement

It is carried out by the method of Jendrassik if it is difficult to elicit the deep tendon reflexes. This should be done before concluding that the reflex is absent. It consists of hooking the flexed fingers of the two hands of the subject and pulling them apart while the reflex in the lower limbs is being elicited **(Fig. 29.1)**. This effort diverts the subject's attention and thus causes relaxation of the muscles involved in the reflex. Making a fist, grasping firmly the arm of the chair or side of the bed, etc., has also been used to obtain the same results. To reinforce the reflexes in the upper limbs, the subject is asked to clench his jaws tightly while eliciting the reflex. Even after reinforcement if a reflex cannot be elicited, it has pathological significance.

DEEP REFLEXES OR MUSCLE STRETCH REFLEXES (TENDON JERKS)

Precautions while Eliciting the Deep Reflexes

- Instruct the subject to assume the required position and to relax completely.
- After bringing the limb in the proper position, instruct the subject to passively extend and flex the muscle to be examined.
- Feel for the site of the tendon where the stretch stimulus has to be given.
- Optimum amount of tension must be present in the muscle to be examined.
- Place the palm of the examiner on a suitable part of the muscle to feel its contraction during the reflex.
- A brisk, painless and localized stroke can be imparted over the tendon using a knee hammer or percussion hammer **(Figs. 29.2A and B)** to produce the sudden stretch in the tendon or the muscle to be examined.
- The degree of movement if present or absence of movement must be both felt and seen.

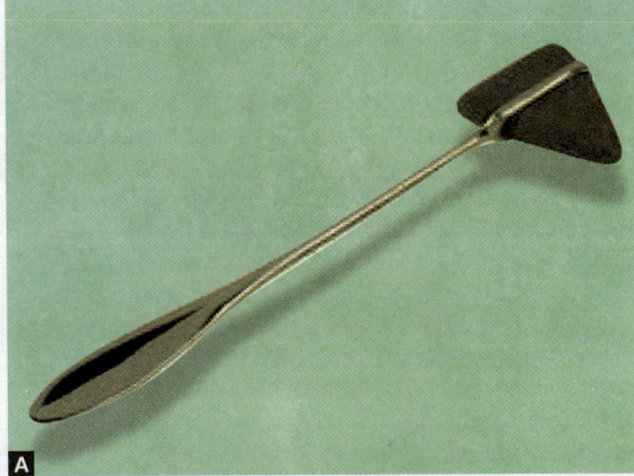
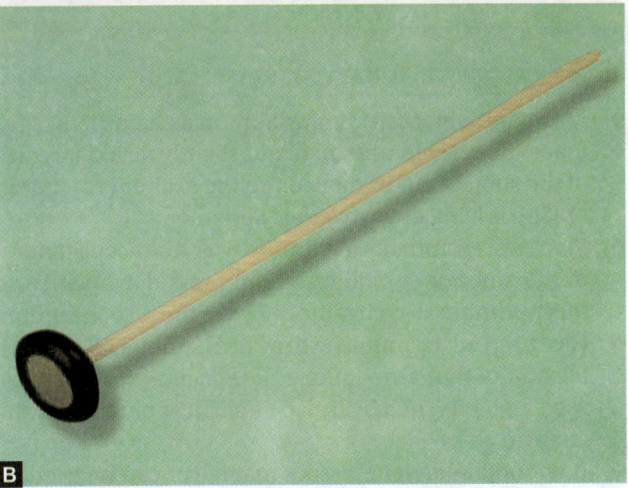

Figs. 29.2A and B: Two types of knee hammers.

- Always examine the same reflex on the opposite side and compare.
- Interpretation of results depends on:
  - Rapidity or the speed with which contraction occurs
  - Amplitude and range of movement
  - Duration of contraction.

Jaw Jerk (Trigeminal Nerve)

- The subject should sit comfortably on a stool and ask him to slightly open his mouth.
- Place the examiners left index finger or thumb firmly on his chin and tap it suddenly with a knee hammer **(Fig. 29.3)**.
- Observation is closure of the mouth. But it is difficult to elicit this reflex in a healthy person. The contraction of the masseter and temporalis can be felt easily.
- Afferent and efferent impulses pass through trigeminal nerve. Center is in the pons.
- Exaggerated jaw jerk occurs in bilateral UMN lesion of fifth cranial nerve. Unilateral UMN lesion does not affect this reflex.

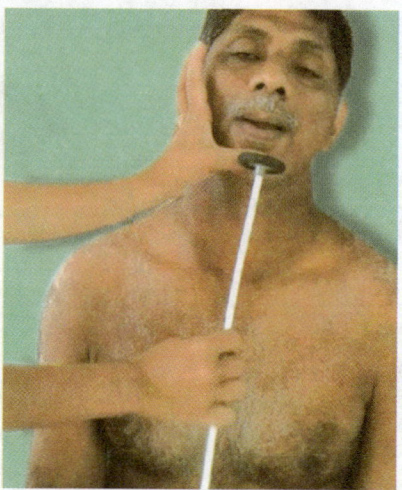

Fig. 29.3: Eliciting jaw-jerk.

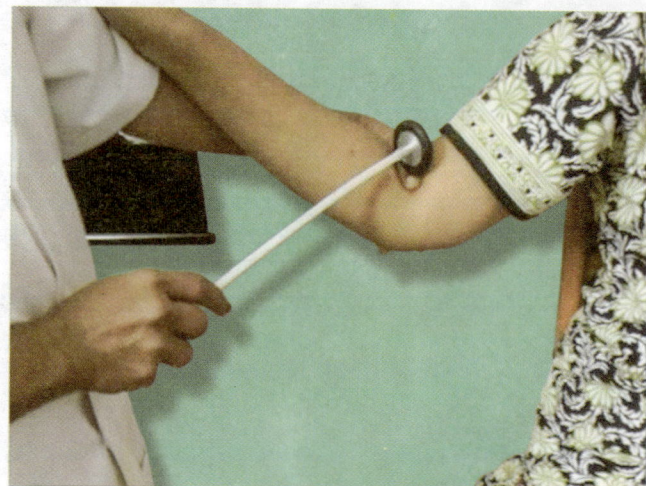

Fig. 29.4: Biceps jerk.

Biceps Jerk (Musculocutaneous Nerve; C5, 6)

- Make the subject sit comfortably on a chair.
- Place the relaxed pronated and slightly flexed forearm of the subject on his thigh or on the examiners left arm or if he is lying down over his abdomen.
- Place the examiner's left thumb over his biceps tendon in the anterior cubital fossa and press downwards, so that optimum stretch is produced in the biceps tendon.
- Give a tap on the thumb with a knee hammer (Fig. 29.4).
- Flexion of that arm at the elbow occurs which can be seen and felt. There will also be slight supination of the forearm.
- If not obtained, Jendrassik's maneuver can be tried by asking the subject to clench his teeth while the reflex is being elicited.
- Before coming to a conclusion make sure that the reflex is absent.
- Repeat the procedure on the opposite arm.
- The reflex will be absent in LMN lesion at C5, 6 spinal segments or roots. It will be exaggerated in UMN lesion above C5 spinal segment.

Triceps Jerk (Radial Nerve; C6, 7 and 8)

- Place the flexed and pronated forearm of the subject on his thigh or with the left hand of the examiner hold the wrist of the subject and pull the forearm slightly toward the midline.
- Give a sudden tap directly on the triceps tendon just above the olecranon process, 5 cm above the elbow (Fig. 29.5).
- Slight extension of the arm is seen. Contraction of triceps is better felt than seen.

Supinator Jerk (Radial Nerve; C5, 6)

- Place the subject's forearm midway between flexion and extension with slight pronation.

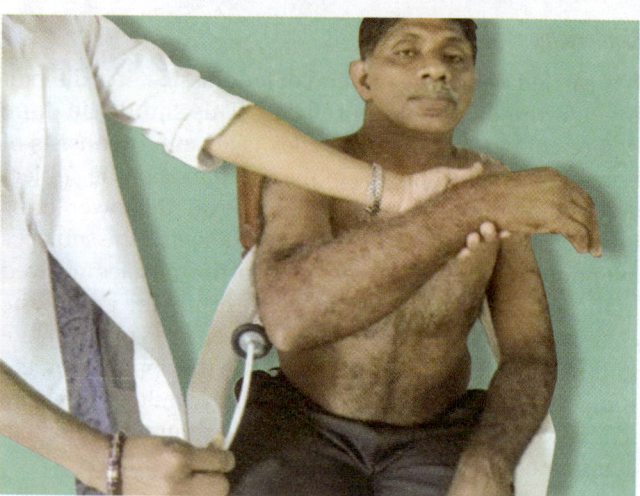

Fig. 29.5: Triceps jerk.

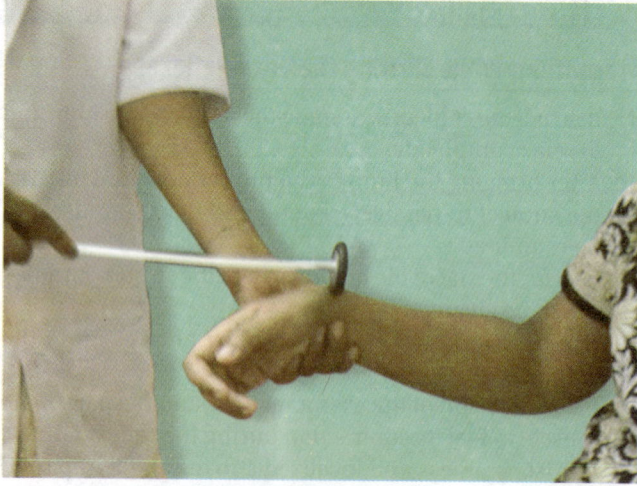

Fig. 29.6: Supinator jerk.

- Tap the brachioradialis tendon over the distal portion of the radius just proximal to the styloid process directly to cause a sudden stretch of the muscle (Fig. 29.6).

- Flexion of forearm at the elbow and supination of the arm is observed normally. The muscle can also be seen contracting.
- In UMN lesion above C5 spinal segment there will be exaggerated flexion and supination of the forearm, along with marked flexion of wrist and fingers and adduction of the thumb.

Knee Jerk or Patellar Jerk (Femoral Nerve; L 2, 3 and 4)

- Knee hammer got its name because knee jerk was the first deep reflex to be clinically tested.
- The subject should be in the sitting posture on a stool with the legs hanging down.
- Ask him to relax the legs and make his thigh bare with his consent so that the contraction of the quadriceps femoris can be observed.
- Feel for the patellar tendon and give a sudden tap on it directly with the knee hammer **(Fig. 29.7)**.
- Effect is seen as extension of the leg at the knee joint.
- Repeat it on the other side.
- Another method is the subject can be made to sit on a chair with one leg crossing over the other and tap the tendon.
- If the subject is in the supine position, place the examiner's left forearm under both the knees of the subject and passively flex them to about 30–45°, so that the quadriceps is slightly stretched. Ask him to relax the limb muscles by allowing his limb to rest completely on the examiner's hand.
- Tap the patellar tendon directly.
- Observation is extension of the leg at the knee (the quadriceps can be seen contracting).
- Absent knee jerk in LMN lesion at L2,3 4 spinal segments or roots. Exaggerated response in UMN lesion is associated with adduction of thigh.
- Pendular knee jerk is seen in cerebellar diseases. This can be elicited only with the leg hanging down.

Ankle Jerk (Tibial Nerve; L5, S1, 2)

- If the subject is lying down, keep the lower limb slightly flexed and externally rotated at the hip, slightly flexed at the knee and the ankle resting on the other leg. Slightly dorsiflex the foot to stretch the Achilles tendon and strike with the knee hammer on the tendon.
- If he is standing, place the flexed knee of the subject on a stool with the foot and the ankle extending unsupported over the edge of the stool. Dorsiflex the ankle and strike the Achilles tendon **(Fig. 29.8)**.
- Observation is plantar flexion of the foot due to contraction of calf muscles.
- Repeat it on the other leg.
- In hypothyroidism the ankle jerk shows delayed relaxation.
- Exaggerated response in UMN lesion above L5. Absent response in LMN lesion at L5 level.

Methods to Elicit Clonus

Clonus denotes a series of rhythmic, involuntary muscle contractions, induced by sudden passive stretch of a muscle. The clonus persists as long as the stretch is maintained. Clonus is associated with exaggerated tendon reflexes and spasticity of muscles in upper motor neuron lesions.

Ankle Clonus

With the subject in the supine position, flex the hip and knee to 90°. Support the calf of the patient on the examiner's left palm and with the right hand suddenly dorsiflex the foot. This causes a sudden stretch of the Achilles tendon and the foot goes into clonic movements as long as the stretch is maintained.

Patellar Clonus

Ask the subject to lie supine in the bed. Keep the lower limb straight and relaxed. The patella of the patient is grasped

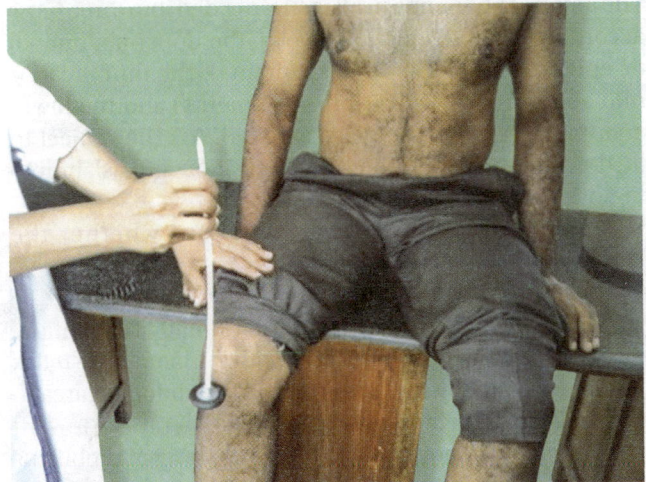

Fig. 29.7: Knee jerk.

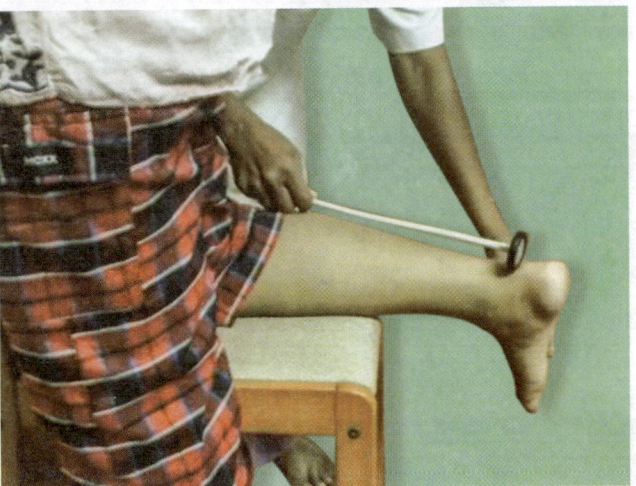

Fig. 29.8: Ankle jerk.

between the index finger and the thumb and suddenly pushed down. This will stretch the quadriceps tendon and the patella goes into clonic contraction as long as the stretch on the tendon is maintained.

SUPERFICIAL REFLEXES

The superficial reflexes are elicited in response to application of a stimulus to either skin or mucous membrane. They are:
- Corneal reflex
- Conjunctival reflex
- Gag/palatal and pharyngeal reflex
- Abdominal reflex
- Cremasteric reflex
- Plantar reflex
- Anal reflex

CORNEAL AND THE CONJUNCTIVAL REFLEXES (V AND VII CRANIAL NERVE)

- Stand on one side of the subject and ask him to look at a far object situated on the opposite side.
- Bring the cotton wisp from the back, so that he does not see it and blink.
- Touch the lateral edge of cornea at its conjunctival margin and observe the response (the center of cornea should not be touched as it carries the risk of corneal ulceration).
- On touching the cornea, there is a bilateral closure of the eyes.
- Touch the conjunctiva of the eye from the side **(Fig. 29.9)**. Bilateral closure of eyes is observed.
- Test both eyes separately.
- For both the reflexes, the afferent impulses travel in the ophthalmic division of the trigeminal nerve and the efferent motor fibers travel in the facial nerve supplying the orbicularis oculi. The center is in the pons.

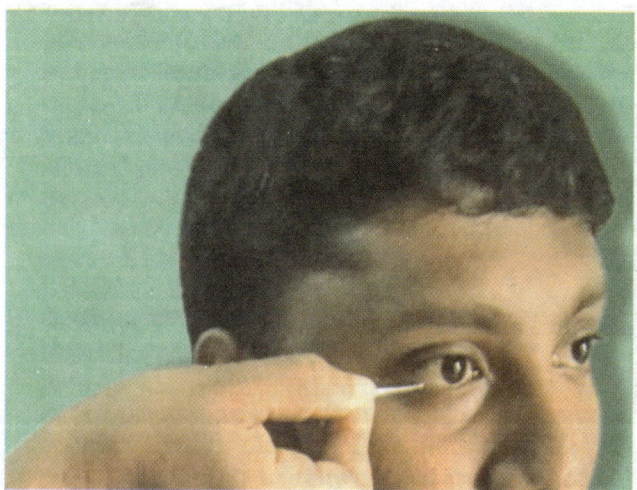

Fig. 29.9: Method of eliciting conjunctival reflex.

PHARYNGEAL AND PALATAL REFLEXES (IX AND X CRANIAL NERVES)

- Ask the subject to sit in front of the examiner and to open the mouth wide.
- Touch the posterior pharyngeal wall with a swab stick.
- Normal observation is elevation and contraction of the pharynx and retraction of the tongue.
- This reflex will be absent on the side of damage of the nerve.
- When the pharyngeal mucosa is stimulated, the afferent impulses pass along the glossopharyngeal nerve to the medulla and the motor impulses travel down along the vagus to the pharyngeal muscles (for details of palatal reflex, *refer* page 170 and 171).

PUPILLARY REFLEXES (II AND III CRANIAL NERVES) (REFER TO PAGE 163)

- **Pupillary light reflex (direct and indirect):** Afferent impulses pass through optic nerve and efferent impulses pass through oculomotor nerve to supply the sphincter pupillae of iris.
- **Accommodation reflex** (afferent and efferent same as that of light reflex).
- **Ciliospinal reflex:** Pinch the skin on the lateral aspect of neck. Observation is pupillary dilatation of the same side. This is due to stimulation of cervical sympathetic fibers, which causes contraction of the radial muscles of iris (dilator pupillae muscle). Ciliospinal reflex is abolished in lesions of the cervical sympathetic nerves and in lesions of cervical and upper thoracic spinal segments.

ABDOMINAL REFLEX (T6 TO T12 SPINAL SEGMENTS)

The anterior abdominal wall is sub-divided into three parts according to the segmental levels—the upper abdominal or epigastric (T6-T9 spinal segments), the umbilical or mid abdominal (T9-T11 spinal segments) and the lower abdominal (T11-T12 spinal segments). Ask the subject to lie down in the bed in the supine position and ask him to remove the cloths covering the abdomen.
- Palpate the abdomen gently to see whether the abdominal muscles are relaxed.
- Ask him to breathe in and out slowly and deeply.
- Stimulation is to be carried out at the end of expiration.
- With the blunt point of a key or with the handle of a reflex hammer, lightly stroke the skin of the abdomen area.
- Stroke the skin horizontally from the lateral side toward the midline, above, at and below the level of umbilicus without crossing over to the other side **(Fig. 29.10)**. Repeat it on the opposite side.

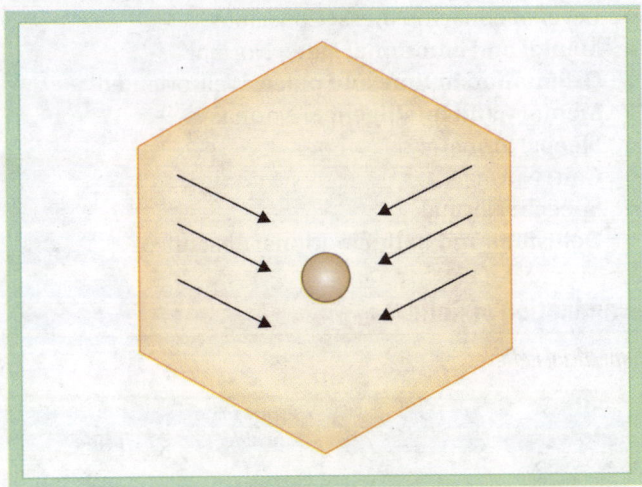

Fig. 29.10: Direction of stroking the skin of abdomen for eliciting abdominal reflex.

- On scratching the skin, the abdominal muscles in the area stimulated contract and cause deviation of the umbilicus towards the area stimulated. In very obese persons, if a blunt instrument does not obtain the reflex, a pointed instrument should be used to scratch and to cause mild pain.
- If the movement of the umbilicus is not visible, the contraction of the abdominal muscles can be palpated if the reflex is present.
- The afferent impulses pass through the posterior roots and efferent impulses pass through the anterior roots of the concerned spinal segments.
- It is difficult to elicit this reflex in obesity, distended abdomen, etc.
- It is exaggerated in anxious and psychoneurotic patients.
- This reflex is lost in UMN lesion above the level of the reflex arc or in LMN lesions affecting the corresponding reflex arc.

CREMASTERIC REFLEX (L1, 2)

- Ask the male subject to lie supine in bed and to remove the garments locally from the genital organ and inner part of the thigh.
- Ask him to abduct the thighs slightly and to expose their medial surfaces and the scrotum.
- Stroke the skin on the inner aspect of the thigh in a downward and inward direction.
- Watch for movement of scrotum and testicle.
- Reflex contraction of the ipsilateral cremasteric muscle occurs and the testicle on the stimulated side gets elevated.
- The afferent impulses pass through femoral nerve and the efferent impulses pass through the genitofemoral nerve. Center is in the 1st and 2nd lumbar segments.
- The reflex is absent in LMN lesion and pyramidal tract lesion. It may also be absent in hydrocele.

PLANTAR REFLEX (L4, 5, S1, 2)

- Ask the subject to lie supine in the bed.
- Distract his attention while eliciting the reflex.
- Scratch the skin on the plantar surface of foot with a key or with the end of a percussion hammer (**Fig. 29.11**). Start from the lateral side of the heel and carry it forwards toward the little toe, and now turn medially across the metatarsals till the base of the great toe is reached (do not cross the big toe). This is Babinski's method.
- On applying the stimulus, all the toes flex and adduct (flexor plantar response: **Fig. 29.12**). The smaller toes flex more than the great toe at the metatarsophalangeal joint. This response is seen in all healthy individuals after 18 months of age. Before this age, there occurs an extension of the great toe.
- Afferent and efferent impulses pass through tibial nerve. The center for this reflex is the 4th and 5th lumbar and the 1st and 2nd sacral segments.

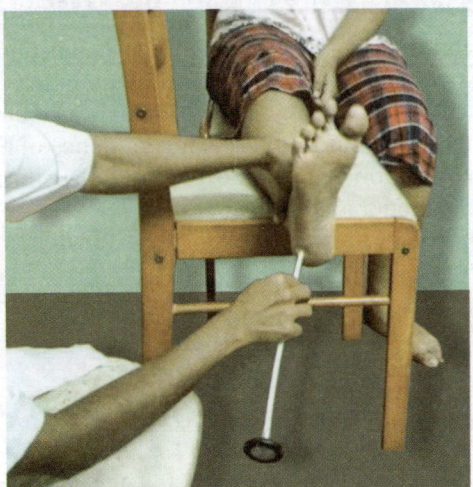

Fig. 29.11: Eliciting plantar reflex.

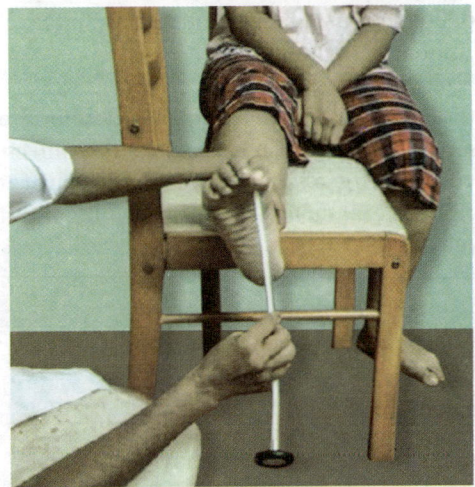

Fig. 29.12: Normal plantar response.

- Babinski's sign and other similar variations are pathological reflexes. In upper motor neuron lesion, the observation while eliciting plantar reflex is dorsiflexion of great toe and fanning out of other toes (extensor plantar response). Sometimes there will be dorsiflexion of foot and flexion at knee and hip and withdrawal of the limb. This is referred to as **Babinski's sign**. This is seen in upper motor neuron lesion above L5 spinal segment.

ANAL REFLEX (PUDENDAL NERVE; S3, 4, 5)

Stimulation of the perianal skin causes contraction of the external anal sphincter. This is combined with per rectal examination. The index finger of the gloved hand of the examiner is inserted into the anal canal of the subject in the lateral decubitus position and lightly scratches the perianal skin. Feel for the reflex contraction of the external anal sphincter. Afferent and efferent impulses pass through pudendal nerve.

VISCERAL REFLEXES OR ORGANIC REFLEXES

The visceral reflexes are deglutition, defecation, micturition and sexual reflexes. In clinical examination these reflexes are not tested. Inquire the subject about these reflexes. Ask him whether he has dysphagia, incontinence of bowel or bladder, retention or urgency of micturition, abnormalities in sexual functions, etc.

Report Pattern

Name:
Age:
Sex:
Occupation and address:

General Examination

- Normally built and nourished
- No pallor, icterus, cyanosis, edema, dyspnea, clubbing or lymphadenopathy.
- Body temperature: 37°C
- Respiratory rate: 16/min, regular, abdominothoracic
- Pulse: 70/min, regular, normal in volume and character, no thickening of vessel wall, no radiofemoral/brachiofemoral delay. All other peripheral pulsations are felt equally on both sides.
- *Blood pressure in the right upper limb in supine position*:
    - Palpatory method—116 mm Hg
    - Auscultatory method—120/80 mm Hg

Higher Functions

- **General appearance and behavior:** Normal
- **Level of consciousness:** Conscious
- **Mental and emotional state:** Normal
- **Orientation in time and place:** Well-oriented
- **Memory and intelligence:** Normal
- **Sleep:** Normal
- **Gait:** Normal
- **Speech:** Normal
- **Delusions and hallucinations:** Absent

Examination of Reflexes

Superficial Reflexes

Reflex	Response on right side	Left side
Conjunctival	Normal	Normal
Corneal	Normal	Normal
Palatal	Normal	Normal
Pharyngeal	Normal	Normal
Abdominal	Normal	Normal
Cremasteric (male subject)	Normal	Normal
Plantar	Normal	Normal
Pupillary reflexes		
Direct light reflex	Normal	Normal
Indirect (consensual) light reflex	Normal	Normal
Accommodation reflex	Normal	
Ciliospinal reflex	Normal	Normal

Deep Tendon Reflexes

Reflex	Right side	Left side
Jaw jerk	Normal (++)	
Biceps jerk	Normal (++)	Normal (++)
Triceps jerk	Normal (++)	Normal (++)
Supinator jerk	Normal (++)	Normal (++)
Knee jerk	Normal (++)	Normal (++)
Ankle jerk	Normal (++)	Normal (++)

Visceral Reflexes (from History)

Reflex	
Micturition reflex	Normal
Defecation reflex	Normal
Swallowing reflex	Normal
Sexual functions	Normal

Impression: The reflexes of the subject appear to be normal.

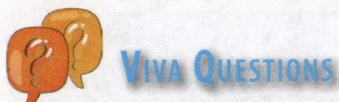

Viva Questions

1. **What are the components of a reflex arc?**
   A reflex arc consists of a receptor, an afferent nerve and its neuron (in dorsal root ganglion or corresponding cranial nerve ganglion), a center consisting of two or more neurons with synaptic connections, anterior horn cell or motor neuron in the cranial nerve nuclei and its motor efferent nerve fiber and an effector organ, which produces the motor response.

2. **What is stretch reflex?**
   When a skeletal muscle with intact nerve supply is stretched suddenly, it reflexly contracts. The receptor involved is muscle spindle. It is a monosynaptic reflex and it plays a very important role in the maintenance of muscle tone and posture.

3. **What is the physiological basis of reinforcement or Jendrassik's maneuver?**
   During reinforcement, there is increased gamma efferent discharge and this increases the sensitivity of muscle spindle primary sensory endings to stretch. This procedure also increases the sensitivity of alpha motor neurons.

4. **How will you grade reflexes?**
   » Grade 0 (–): Reflex absent, no contraction of muscle even on reinforcement
   » Grade 1 (+): Diminished (sluggish) reflex
   » Grade 2 (++): Normal contraction and quick relaxation
   » Grade 3 (+++): Exaggerated—rapidity, amplitude and duration of contraction increased
   » Grade 4 (++++): Exaggerated and associated with clonus (repetitive muscular contraction following sudden sustained stretch)

5. **Give the conditions where Babinski sign is positive. Why plantar reflex is up going in infants?**
   It is positive in infants, during deep sleep, UMN lesion, and severe hypoxia. In infants, the pyramidal tract is not fully developed and myelination of pyramidal tract occurs only after the child starts walking.

6. **What are the abnormal superficial and deep reflexes seen?**
   » Reflexes may be absent in lower motor neuron lesion, during deep sleep, etc.
   » Deep reflexes become exaggerated in nervousness, upper motor neuron lesion, thyrotoxicosis, etc.
   » Pendular reflex is seen in cerebellar lesions.
   » Some of the superficial reflexes are altered in UMN lesion, e.g., up going plantar (positive Babinski sign). Most of the superficial reflexes are absent in UMN lesion.

7. **What is the reason for pendular knee jerk?**
   It is seen in cerebellar lesion where there is hypotonia of muscles on the affected side. Hypotonia and lack of braking action are the reasons for pendular knee jerk.

8. **What is the reason for the absence of abdominal and cremasteric reflex in pyramidal tract lesion (UMN lesion)?**
   Superficial reflexes are polysynaptic reflexes. In addition to the spinal reflex arc, these reflexes have a cortical pathway. The afferent impulses travel up in the spinal cord up to the parietal cortex and the efferent fibers descend to the anterior horn cells of spinal cord through the pyramidal tract. A lesion in the pyramidal tract will also involve these fibers leading to abolition of these reflexes.

9. **What is clonus?**
   Regular, rhythmic contraction of a skeletal muscle when it is subjected to sudden, maintained stretch is called clonus. It is a feature of hypertonia and is due to increased gamma efferent discharge to the muscle spindles of the hypertonic muscle. Here, stretch reflex and inverse stretch reflex alternate.
   For example, ankle clonus is a neurological sign elicited in the gastrocnemius muscle in hypertonia. When the stretch is removed, clonus stops.

10. **What are the properties of reflexes?**
    One-way conduction, reaction time and central delay, summation, after-discharge, reciprocal inhibition, irradiation and recruitment, fractionation and occlusion, summation of subliminal fringe, post-tetanic potentiation, fatigue, habituation and sensitization.

11. **Mention a few conditions where deep tendon reflexes are diminished or absent.**
    » Tendon reflexes are absent in the stage of spinal shock in spinal cord injury
    » In lesions of the anterior or posterior nerve root, the reflex arc is disrupted and deep reflexes will be lost. In tabes dorsalis where the posterior root is affected, deep reflexes will be lost.
    » In poliomyelitis there is damage to the anterior horn cells and deep reflexes will be lost.
    » In coma reflexes will be absent.
    » In some normal individuals, it will be difficult to elicit deep reflexes. Jendrassik's maneuver will be useful.

12. **Give examples where deep tendon reflexes are exaggerated.**
    » Upper motor neuron lesion (in spasticity)
    » Hyperthyroidism where the neurons become hyperexcitable
    » Anxiety

OBJECTIVE STRUCTURED PRACTICAL EXAMINATION

I. Elicit the knee jerk in the subject
- » Ask the subject to sit on a tall stool so that the legs hang freely
- » Explain the procedure to the subject and ask him to relax and expose the right leg
- » Place the left hand on the subject's right thigh
- » Feel for the patellar tendon and with the knee hammer strikes the tendon
- » Feels the contraction of quadriceps muscle and watches the forward movement of the leg
- » Repeats the same procedure on the left leg

II. Elicit the plantar reflex of right leg on the subject provided
- » Explains the procedure to the subject
- » Ask him to lie on the cot in the supine position
- » Fix the ankle joint with the left hand
- » With a key or the pointed end of the knee hammer, give a firm scratch along the lateral aspect of the sole starting from the heel towards the little toe and then medially along the base of the toes up to the big toe
- » Watch for the response

Section 3: Experimental Physiology (Amphibian Experiments)

30. Common Appliances Used in the Experimental Physiology Laboratory
31. Pithing of Frog and Dissection of Muscle Nerve Preparation
32. Mounting the Muscle-Nerve Preparation
33. Simple Muscle Twitch
34. Effects of Two Successive Stimuli on Muscle Contraction
35. Genesis of Tetanus
36. Effect of Afterload and Freeload in Skeletal Muscle Contraction
37. Effect of Continuous Stimulation of a Muscle (Study of Fatigue and Recovery)
38. Effects of Temperature on Muscle Contraction
39. Velocity of Nerve Impulses
40. Normal Cardiogram of Frog
41. Effect of Temperature on Frog's Heart
42. Stannius Ligatures
43. Extrasystole and Compensatory Pause
44. Effect of Vagal Stimulation on Frog's Heart
45. Effect of Drugs and Ions on Isolated Frog's Heart

Chapter 30

Common Appliances Used in the Experimental Physiology Laboratory

LEARNING OBJECTIVES

- Identify and name the different instruments used in the experimental physiology laboratory
- Describe the uses of each of them
- Explain the various types of stimuli used for animal experiments
- What are the advantages of electrical stimuli
- Explain the circuit diagram for induced current, faradic current and galvanic current

PY3.18: Observe with computer assisted learning—(i) Amphibian nerve-muscle experiments and (ii) amphibian cardiac experiments.

STUDY OF INSTRUMENTS USED

The instruments are classified into two groups:
1. Electrical equipments
2. Mechanical equipments

ELECTRICAL EQUIPMENTS

Low Voltage Unit

In the experiments, a low voltage direct current is used to stimulate the tissues. It is less injurious to the tissues. The intensity and duration of the current can be easily controlled. The current can be obtained from storage batteries or from the low voltage unit.

The low voltage unit, which is fixed on the wall, is a step down transformer in which the high voltage current (220 Volts) is stepped down to about 2.5–5 volts. A rectifier converts alternating current (AC) to direct current (DC). This low voltage direct current is supplied to each seat through two terminals one positive and the other one negative. Positive terminal is colored red and negative black (see **Fig. 30.8**).

DuBois-Reymond Inductorium

This instrument works on the principle of electromagnetic induction. An induction coil is a device, which transforms

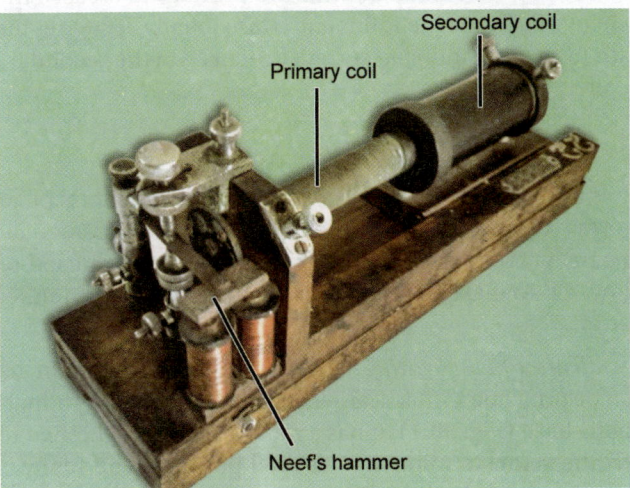

Fig. 30.1: DuBois-Reymond inductorium.

direct current into induced current. It is based on the principle that any change in the magnetic field around a coil induces an electric current in it. The type of the apparatus used is called DuBois-Reymond induction coil (**Fig. 30.1**). It consists of a primary coil fixed on a frame and a movable secondary coil covering the primary coil but having no connection with it.

Parts of Inductorium

Fixed primary coil: It is made of 300 turns of thick copper wire wound around a soft iron core. Its two ends are connected to the two terminals on the top of the vertical plate of the frame. The low voltage terminal, primary coil and the simple key are connected in series to form the primary circuit. When the circuit is complete, a constant current flows through it.

Sliding secondary coil: It is made of 5000 turns of thin copper wire. It can slide on two horizontal metal slide rods. There are two terminals in the secondary coil, which are connected to the stimulating electrodes through a short-circuiting key. The secondary coil and the stimulating electrodes form the secondary circuit. At every make and break of the circuit in the primary coil, an induced current is generated in the secondary coil. Break shock is stronger than make shock.

Base

It may be in the form of a wooden plate or two heavy metallic bars. It gives stability. It is grooved and the secondary coil slides over it. It carries a scale to measure the distance of the secondary coil from the primary coil. If the base is wooden, it has a hinge on which it can be folded to half **(Fig. 30.1)**. If the base is in the form of metal bars, there is an arrangement for turning the secondary coil at a right angle with the primary coil.

Moving the secondary coil away from the primary or turning it at an angle with the primary decreases the change in the magnetic flux and consequently decreases the strength of the induced current produced in the secondary coil.

Electromagnet

It is in series with the primary coil. The central brass pillar forms its other terminal. The upper end of the brass pillar bears a screw and a contact point that can be raised or lowered to make or to break the contact with the hammer strip.

A tall brass pillar bearing the Neef's hammer: It works on the same principle as that of an electric bell. It has two terminals at its base **(Fig. 30.1)**. It has a nut that can be tightened to fix the screw terminal in a desired position. The screw is placed on a metal base that makes a contact with the other end of the primary coil. The lower end of the screw offers a contact with the hammer strip. When the Neef's hammer is introduced in the primary circuit, the alternate make and break stimuli are rapidly repeated at a rate of about 40/sec. This produces repeated induced current in the secondary circuit.

Induced Current

A current is induced in the secondary coil only when there is a change in the strength of the magnetic field of the primary coil. As current is passed through the primary coil, there occurs a change in the magnetic field in the surrounding space. This change produces a momentary current in the secondary coil. Thus starting, stopping or altering the strength of the current in the primary circuit induces a current of momentary duration in the secondary coil. When the strength of current passing through the primary coil is constant, no current is induced in the secondary coil. Changes in the strength of the magnetic field occur only at the make and break of the current. The induced current is always of short duration. The strength of the induced current can be increased or decreased by changing the distance between the primary and secondary coils.

The change in the magnetic field occurring during break is, therefore, greater as compared to the one occurring during make. The induced current developed in the secondary coil, being proportional to the change in the magnetic field, is stronger during the break in the primary circuit than the one induced during the make (in the primary circuit).

Vibrating Interrupter

The reed is a metal strip. It can he mounted on a stand. It has a pin contact point at one end and a screw contact point at the other end. Fixing the reed in the stirrup at the desired distance can vary the vibrating length of the reed **(Fig. 30.2)**.

The metal contact point dips in a mercury cup from which a wire is taken to complete the circuit. The vibrating reed is thus a device for giving a desired number of shocks per second. Usually it is designed to give 5 to 30 shocks per second.

Stimulating Electrodes

Stimulating electrodes are used for delivering the electrical stimulus to the tissues. It consists of two copper wires held together by a piece of plastic.

Simple Key

Simple spring key is used to make or break the circuit. The simple key consists of two terminals for electric connections and a knob attached to the tip of the metal piece and a metal contact at which knob makes contact **(Fig. 30.3)**. When the

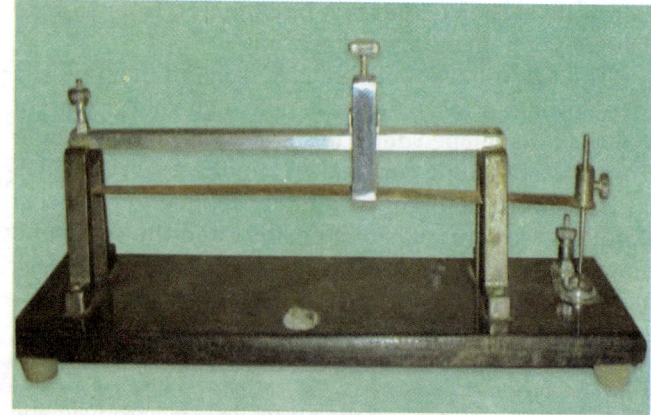

Fig. 30.2: Vibrating interrupter.

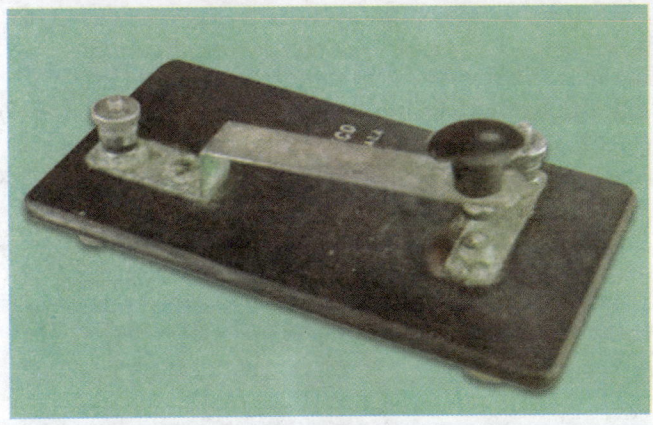

Fig. 30.3: Simple key.

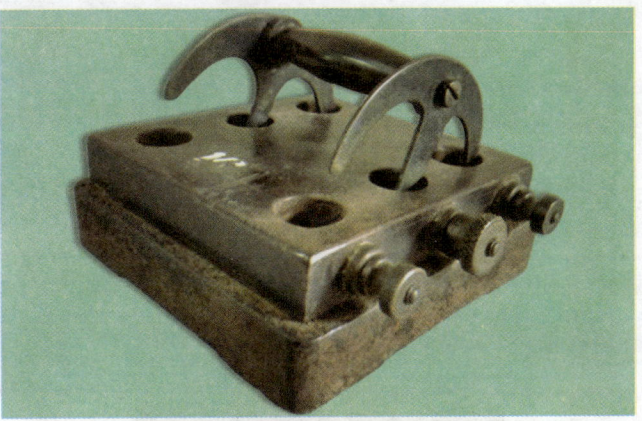

Fig. 30.5: Mercury commutator.

key is pressed, the knob touches the metal contact and the circuit becomes complete. When it is released, the spring goes back and the circuit is broken. Simple key is connected in the primary circuit.

Short-Circuiting Key

This key is included in the secondary circuit. There are two metal blocks fixed on either side of a rectangular base. Each metal block carries two terminals for electric connection. Attached to one block is another metal piece with a handle **(Fig. 30.4)**. This metal block can be raised or lowered. When it is in the horizontal position, it connects the two metal pieces. One of the two terminals in each block is connected to the secondary coil and the remaining two terminals are connected to the electrodes. The short-circuiting key is used to short circuit the induced current obtained from the secondary coil. When the key is closed, current from the secondary coil is short circuited as the thick metal piece offers much less resistance than the wires of the electrodes. So current will not pass through the electrodes. Only when the key is open, current passes through the electrode. Thus the short-circuiting key prevents unnecessary stimulation of the tissues by closing the handle.

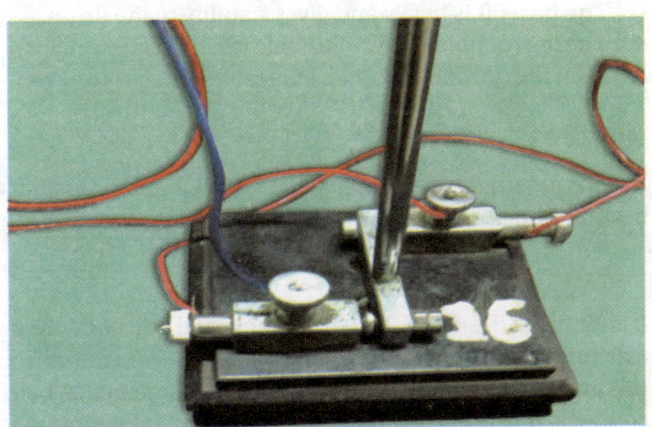

Fig. 30.4: Short-circuiting key with the handle closed.

Mercury Commutator

The mercury commutator is an instrument, which is used to change the direction of flow of current. It consists of 4 depressions that contain mercury and 6 terminals for electrical connections. There is a bridge in the center, which can be moved to either side to direct the current to flow to one pair of electrodes at a time **(Fig. 30.5)**. The two pairs of electrodes are connected to two pairs of terminals on either side of the bridge. The remaining two terminals are connected to the short-circuiting key. Mercury commutator is used in the lab for calculating the velocity of conduction of nerve impulse in the sciatic nerve of frog.

Muscle Bath or Luca's Trough

The original pattern devised by Lucas was a chamber with all glass walls and was named after him. It has the following features:
- A trough made out of some non-conducting material. It can be mounted on a stand.
- The bottom has two holes closed with corks. One of them is used to fix the tissue with a pin. The other can be used for draining the fluid that has an independent outlet with rubber tubing and a clamp for drainage of fluid. It is usually used to study the effect of temperature and different ions on muscle contraction.

Time Tracer (Fig. 30.6)

A time scale should always be taken at the base of every record. It can be done with a tuning fork of known frequency. A tuning fork of frequency 100 vibrations per second is taken so that one vibration will correspond to 0.01 second **(Fig. 30.6)**. Connect the low voltage terminals, the simple key and the terminals of the time tracer. Adjust the writing point of the tuning fork just below or above the base line and then press the simple key and switch on the drum. Stop the drum immediately after the time tracing is recorded.

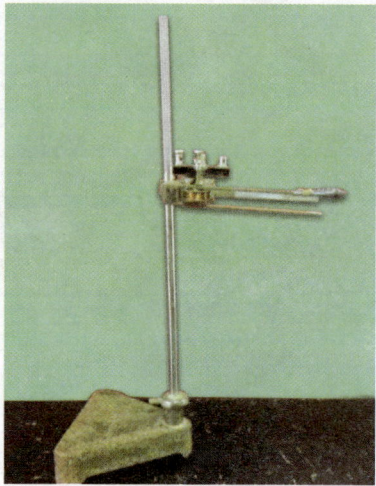

Fig. 30.6: Arrangement for taking the time tracing.

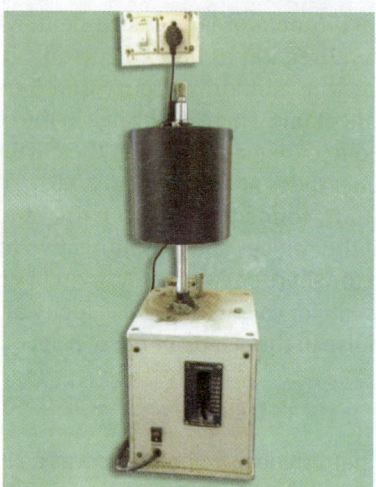

Fig. 30.7: Electric kymograph.

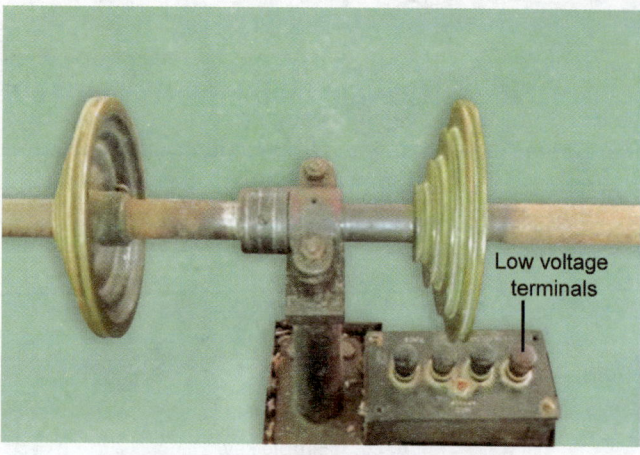

Fig. 30.8: Central shaft with pulleys.

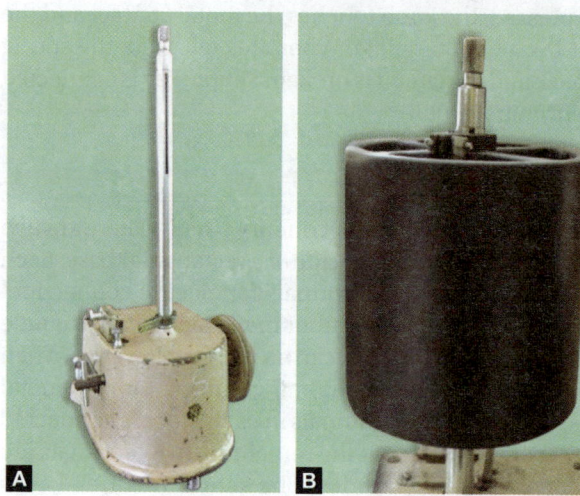

Figs. 30.9A and B: (A) Mechanical kymograph; (B) Drum mounted on the shaft of the kymograph.

Electrically Driven Kymograph

Electric kymographs are available. Each kymograph is a separate unit with the built-in gear system and with a slow and fast speed arrangement. No separate overhead pulley system is necessary. This type of kymograph is directly connected to the power supply (**Fig. 30.7**). The different combinations of gears provided can obtain varying speeds of rotation.

MECHANICAL EQUIPMENTS

Power Shaft and Pulleys

A horizontal power shaft driven by an electric motor is provided on the table. The cone-pulleys with four grooves are fixed to the power shaft at each seat (**Fig. 30.8**). When the central shaft rotates, the pulleys also rotate. Identical pulleys are present in the mechanical kymograph also. The pulley of the kymograph is connected to the pulley in the central shaft by means of a leather belt.

Pulley Driven Kymograph or Sherrington-Starling Recording Drum

Kymograph is a device that moves smoothly at an even speed. It consists of a metal gearbox to which a vertical rotating shaft is connected (**Figs. 30.9A and B**). Its parts are:

- **The base:** It is heavy and gives stability to the drum.
- **The legs** or hoofs with adjustable leveling screws help to keep the drum horizontal if the table surface is uneven.

Side Hoof

It helps to turn the drum on its side so that the spindle shaft becomes horizontal.

Shaft

It is for fixing the drum. The shaft is powered by a horizontal axis running through the metal case of the kymograph. To this axis, on one side, a series of pulleys are attached. A belt connects one of these pulleys to one of the pulleys on the power shaft. The drum or the cylinder rotates with the shaft.

The shaft has a screw in its center at the top and a groove on one side. A small rectangular plug mounted on the screw inside the shaft butts out through the groove. It can be raised or lowered by rotating the top screw. A groove on the inner side of the ring inside the cylinder allows the mounting of the cylinder on the shaft. This arrangement avoids the possibility of rotation of the cylinder independent of the shaft when it is moving.

Contact Arms or Strikers

There are two horizontal contact arms that project from the lower end of the vertical shaft. It consists of two parts, which can be drawn apart to form any desired angle between them. They are fitted stiffly enough on the shaft to rotate with it and strike past the contact button.

The tips of the arms make contact with a spring or contact button on the superior surface of the base at the left side. The insulated carrier of the spring is adjustable and is clamped by a screw.

There are two terminals for electrical connection; one is attached to the insulated spring or contact button and the other to the metal case of the gearbox. By means of these terminals, the insulated carrier along with the spring can be made to act as a key in the primary circuit. The circuit is made or broken when the tip of the contact arms makes and breaks its contact with the spring.

Gear and Pulley Arrangement

The kymograph is provided with fast, slow and neutral gears and its catch. The drum can be started or stopped by turning a clutch on the left side of the metal gearbox. The clutch when turned vertical causes movement of the shaft and when horizontal stops the movement of the shaft. Wheel on the right side is provided with four pulley grooves. A similar wheel is seen on the shaft above the table.

In each gear, the drum can be made to rotate at different speeds by connecting different-sized pulleys of the kymograph and the power shaft.

A screw with a nut is attached to the base of the kymograph at the right posterior corner of superior surface. A wire can be fixed to it to convey the current through the base and the drum itself.

Myograph Stand, X-Block and Femur Clamp

Myograph stand has a heavy triangular base that gives stability to the stand **(Fig. 30.10)**. The shaft carries a sliding plate with a groove and a handle. A screw can fix the handle in any position. With the use of the sliding handle the writing lever can be taken away from the recording surface when a record is not being taken and brought back again to the same position when desired. Appliances like X-block carrying the femur clamp, frog board, time tracer, etc., can be fixed on this stand.

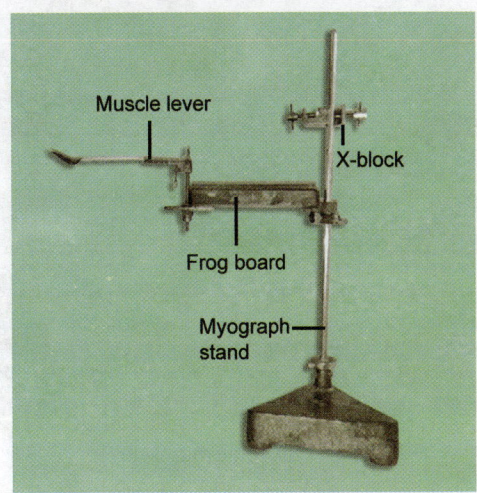

Fig. 30.10: Frog board and X-block fixed on the myograph stand.

X-block is used to fix other instruments like heart lever, femur clamp and other clamps on the myograph stand. It has two grooves each at right angles to each other. One groove accommodates the rod of the myograph stand and the other groove holds other instruments. Screws provided can tighten both grooves **(Fig. 30.10)**.

Femur clamp or muscle grip is used to hold the femur of the muscle-nerve preparation. It can also be used to hold the electrode in position.

Frog Board or Myograph Board

The frog board is used for placing the preparation for the experiment. It has a holder and a screw by which it can be fixed on the central rod of the myograph stand at any desired level **(Fig. 30.10)**. The board has a lower wooden board on which a layer of cork is fixed.

Writing Lever

It writes and magnifies the mechanical movements. It should be light so that there is very little inertia. Its pointer should write without twisting. The lever is made of Aluminum. The pointer is prepared from cut X-ray film paper. The line written by the pointer on the paper is called trace and the varnished paper with the trace record is called the tracing or graph.

Muscle Lever

Isotonic Muscle Lever

It is used to record isotonic contractions of muscles. It can be attached to the frog board. The muscle lever has a long arm, a fulcrum and a short arm **(Fig. 30.11)**. The long arm should be long enough so that it describes an arc of a large circle. Then only the record will represent the original movement.

The horizontal bar constitutes the fulcrum. The long arm of the lever has two to three holes in its metal strip. Weight

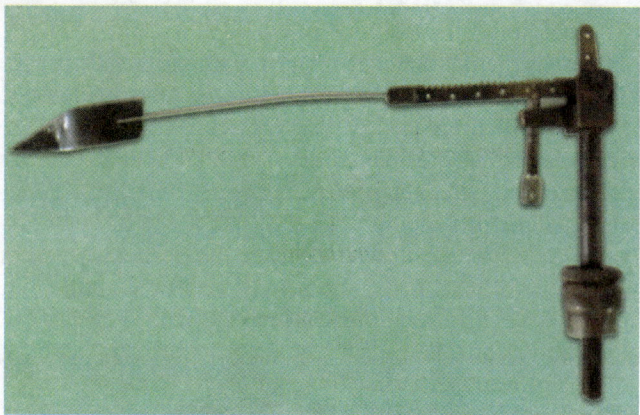

Fig. 30.11: Isotonic muscle lever.

hook can be attached to one of the holes. There is a screw called after load screw near the fulcrum of the lever that can limit the downward movement of the fulcrum to the desired level. The afterload screw can be adjusted to keep the lever horizontal. For the recording of muscle contractions, the muscle is tied to the hole in the short vertical piece of the lever. When the muscle contracts, the vertical piece is pulled resulting in the upward movement of the lever, which records the contraction on the writing surface. The afterload screw checks the downward movement of the lever.

Isometric Muscle Lever

It is used to record isometric skeletal muscle contractions. It records change in the tension developed in the muscle during contraction while the muscle length is kept constant.

Heart Lever

The contractions of heart are weaker than that of skeletal muscle. So a sensitive writing lever is used to record the contractions of frog's heart. It is lighter than the muscle lever **(Fig. 30.12)**.

Weight Hook

Weight hook is a metal piece weighing 10 g having a hook at one end. The hook can be introduced into one of the holes in the isotonic muscle lever. This gives a smooth recording and also helps in bringing the lever to the base line. It can also be used to hold weight while doing load and after load experiment.

Recording Surface

A glazed paper is rolled round the drum and is pasted at the cut ends in such a way that the paper is fixed tightly. It should not move round the cylinder. The gum should be allowed to dry well before smoking is undertaken; otherwise the heating, which occurs while smoking, creates folds at the gummed junction. Instead of gum, the snugly rolled paper can be fixed by applying pieces of cellophane tape at the junction.

Smoking

The cylinder is passed over a rod, which is fixed, in a smoking rack. Below it is placed a special sooty flame. A sooty flame can be prepared by burning a wick in kerosene oil lamp with deficient air. A mixture of benzene and kerosene in the ratio of 1:9 also gives a satisfactory sooty flame.

The drum is then rolled uniformly at an optimum speed. This ensures a uniform deposit of soot on the glazed surface. Smoking is continued till an even brown surface is produced. When done properly, it gives a velvety chocolate-brown color. Never cease rotating while the flame is below the paper; never allow it to get overheated else it gets charred, becomes brittle and gets torn by the writing lever.

Varnishing

After the record is taken the paper is cut at the proper place to get a continuous trace. Varnishing is done to make the record permanent. It is done by dipping the paper in a solution of resin in methylated spirit. One hundred and fifty grams of resin is dissolved in two liters of spirit. Other solution recommended is a saturated solution of gum mastic or white shellac in spirit. Shellac may alternatively be dissolved in petrol. A small quantity of caster oil or liquid paraffin may be added to prevent the varnish from setting too hard.

The paper is slowly passed through the solution and then is allowed to drain and dry. From time to time, spirit should be added to the solution as it gets evaporated.

The cylinder surface is usually made to rotate from right to left, i.e., in the clockwise direction. The writing lever should be always horizontal and the position of the myograph with the frog board should be so adjusted on the stand that the movements over all the range of the pointer are recorded on the paper.

Electrical Connections

❖ Arrange the low voltage terminals, simple key and inductorium in series to form the primary circuit. Put a short-circuiting key in between the electrodes and the

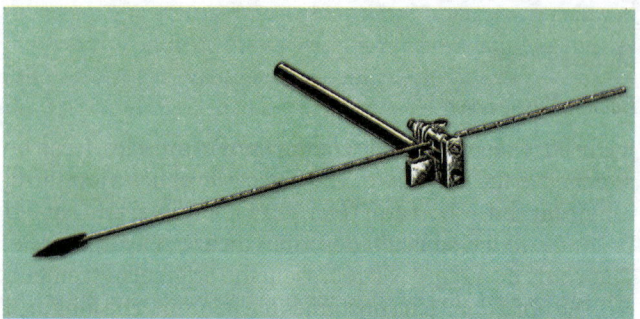

Fig. 30.12: Heart lever.

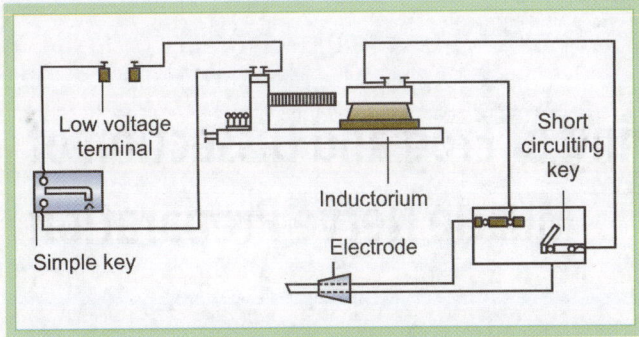

Fig. 30.13: Circuit diagram for obtaining induced current.

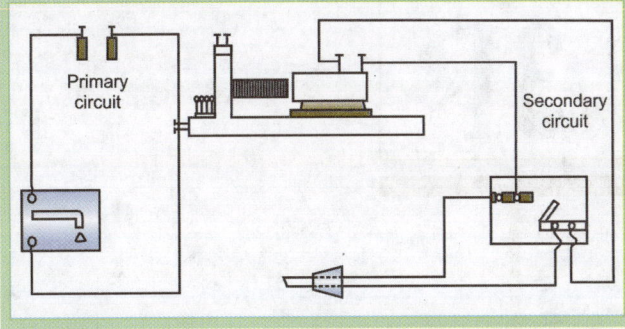

Fig. 30.14: Circuit diagram for continuous stimulation of tissue (Faradic current).

secondary coil of the secondary circuit **(Fig. 30.13)**. This is called a **simple circuit for induced current**.

- Low voltage terminal or battery, simple key, inductorium and drum are connected in series to form the primary circuit. The secondary circuit is made as before. This is described as **drum in circuit**. The simple key is included in the circuit to avoid unnecessary stimulation of the muscle if the drum goes on rotating.
- Low voltage terminals, simple key, Neef's hammer and inductorium are connected in series to form the primary circuit. The secondary circuit is made as before. This provides **faradic current** and is done to demonstrate the phenomenon of tetanus **(Fig. 30.14)**.
- Low voltage terminal, simple key, inductorium and vibrating interrupter are connected in series to form the primary circuit. Secondary circuit is made as before. This connection is made to give shocks to the muscle at a rate of 5–30 per second to show the effect of successive stimuli on muscle contraction.

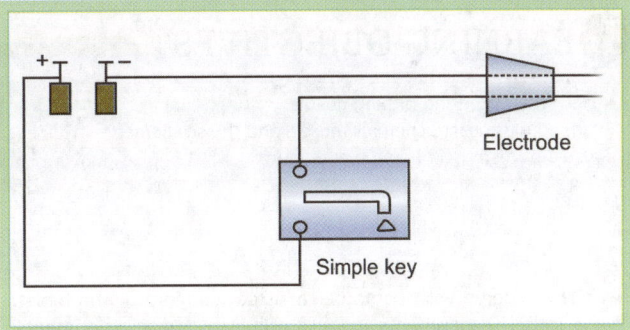

Fig. 30.15: Circuit diagram for direct stimulation of muscle (Galvanic current)

- For directly stimulating the muscle, **galvanic current** can be used. Connect the low voltage terminals, the simple key and the electrodes to form the circuit **(Fig. 30.15)**. Place the electrode over the muscle and press the simple key and then release it.

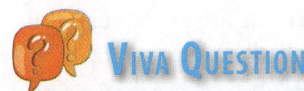

Viva Questions

1. **What are the factors that affect the strength of induced current?**
   - The distance between the primary and the secondary coil, when the distance increases the strength of the stimulating current decreases and vice versa
   - Number of turns in the coil
   - The strength of the direct current coming to the primary coil
2. **What are the different types of stimuli used in the laboratory?**
   Chemical, thermal, osmotic, mechanical and electrical

Chapter 31

Pithing of Frog and Dissection of Muscle Nerve Preparation

LEARNING OBJECTIVES

- Pith the frog using pithing needle
- Identify the gastrocnemius muscle and the sciatic nerve
- Isolate the muscle nerve preparation

PY3.18: Observe with computer assisted learning (i) Amphibian nerve-muscle experiments and (ii) amphibian cardiac experiments.

PITHING OF FROG

Pithing is the process of destroying the central nervous system. The organized animal no more exists on pithing; but the individual organs continue to maintain the vitality for some time. Their activity can only be elicited on direct stimulation. In all the physiological experiments on the tissues of the frog, pithing is preferred to anesthesia because the latter is likely to affect the various systems, vitiating the observations.

Materials

Pithing needle, a piece of cotton cloth, frog.

Procedure

- Wrap the frog with the cloth and hold it with its dorsal side facing you, in the fist of the left hand with the index finger free.
- Bend the head of the frog ventrally with the free index finger till the skin on the dorsum of the frog is stretched.
- Feel for the depression at the joint of the skull with the vertebral column, with the pithing needle in the right hand.
- Pierce the skin deeply with the pithing needle through the depression **(Fig. 31.1)**. As the needle pierces through the resistant ligaments to reach the spinal canal the initial feeling of resistance will disappear.

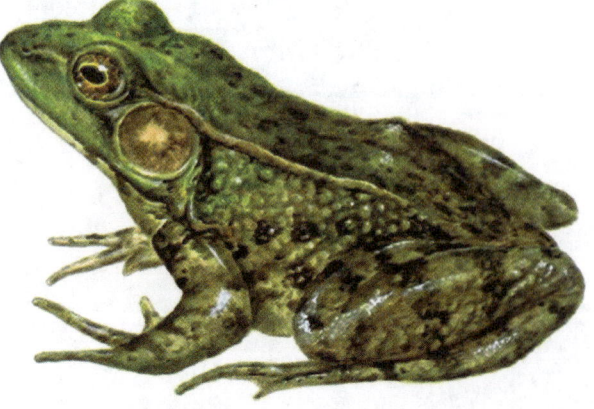

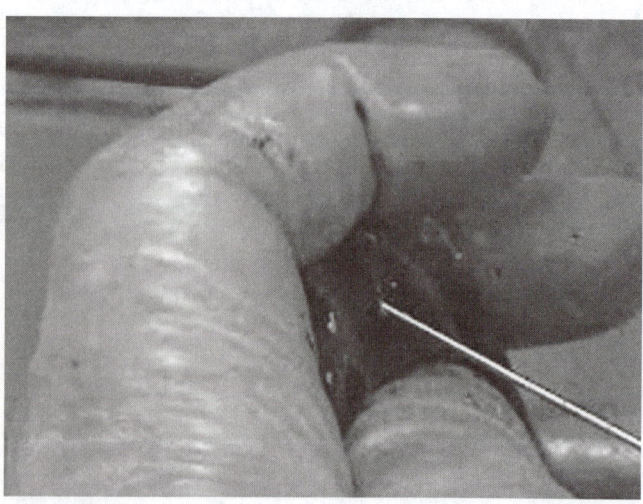

Fig. 31.1: Pithing of frog.

- Move the needle from side to side, thus separating the brain from the spinal cord.
- Pass it upwards and rotate it to destroy the upper part of the brain.
- Withdraw the needle and pass it downwards and rotate it. Push it up and down two or three times ensuring complete destruction of the cord. While the cord is being destroyed violent movements of the limbs occur often accompanied by micturition.

DISSECTION OF THE NERVE-MUSCLE PREPARATION

Apparatus: A pair of forceps, a pair of scissors, frog-board, pins for fixing the tissue, a pair of bone-cutting forceps, cotton, isotonic saline (0.65% NaCl), two bowls, thick thread, glass hook.

Procedure

- Start the dissection immediately after pithing the frog.
- Lay the pithed frog on the board with its dorsum upwards, i.e., with the belly down
- Stretch out the limbs.
- With the forceps catch the skin on the back in the midline and with the scissors in the right hand make a midline incision on the dorsum of the body and also on the back of both the thighs
- Cut the fibers attaching the skin with the fascia below and reflect the flaps. Completely remove the skin round the knee and leg up to the foot.
- Identify the tendon of gastrocnemius muscle just above its attachment to the bone and separate it from the tissue below **(Fig. 31.2)**.
- Pass a ligature with the help of an aneurysm needle between the bone and the tendon and tie it at the lowest level round the tendon.
- Cut the tendon below this ligature to separate it from its bony attachment.

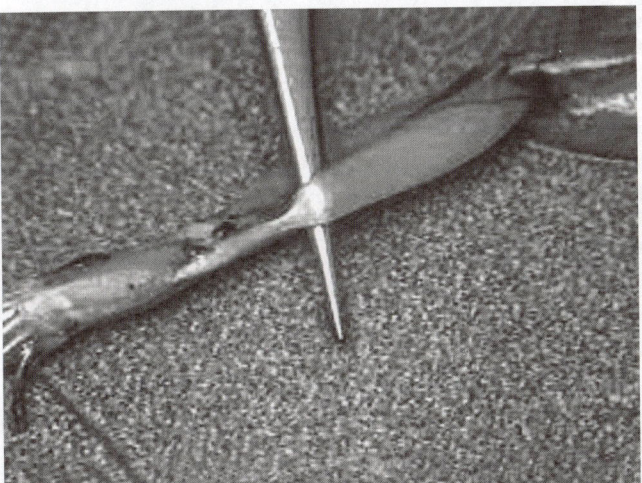

Fig. 31.2: Separating the tendon of gastrocnemius muscle.

- If during dissection cutaneous stimulation causes reflex movements of the limbs, the conclusion is that the cord is not destroyed completely.
- Hold the end of the ligature and tear off the muscle from the bones so that it is now separated up to the knee joint.
- Cut the tibia and fibula nearest to the knee joint.
- Separate the joint and the muscle from any remaining attachment.
- Now look for a shining line that separates the biceps on the lateral side and the semimembranosus on the medial side.
- Push the sharp end of the scissors in between the two muscle masses to pierce through the fascia and levering the end of the scissors upwards cut the fascia along the shining line.
- Deeply lie the adductors medially and the vasti muscles laterally.
- Retract forcefully the two muscles by your two thumbs and placed in the groove between them will be seen a big nerve. This is the sciatic nerve. During dissection the nerve should never be caught or teased with the scissors or forceps.
- Trace the nerve up to the iliopubic line and down to the knee joint as far as possible cleaning it with the closed end of scissors.
- Now hold the tip of the urostyle (the cartilaginous prolongation of the vertebral column) with the forceps and lift it up. Snip off its muscular attachments at the lower end.
- Make two parallel incisions on either side of the urostyle 1 cm away from it and parallel to it, in its muscular attachments.
- Lift it up and look inside the abdominal cavity.
- A network of nerves is seen emerging out of the vertebral column. This is the sciatic plexus. It usually consists of the 7th, 8th, and 9th spinal nerves. If you cannot see the nerves, continue your dissection towards the upper end.
- Extend the incision lateral to the plexus upwards through the muscles to reach beyond the origin of the plexus, cutting the transverse process of the 9th or sacral vertebra **(Fig. 31.3)**.
- Identify and separate the thick sciatic nerve in the plexus and clean it from the mesh of the blood vessels seen there. A glass hook can be used for handling the nerve.
- With the help of the bone cutting forceps, cut the vertebral column above the 7th and below the 9th vertebrae transversely without injuring the nerves.
- Cut with the bone cutting forceps the piece of the vertebral column in its mid-line.
- Hold the half piece of the vertebral column with the fingers and put the sciatic nerve on a slight stretch and go on cleaning it down into the thigh. At the junction of the thigh and the abdomen the nerve goes deep below the pyriformis and the iliococcygeus muscles

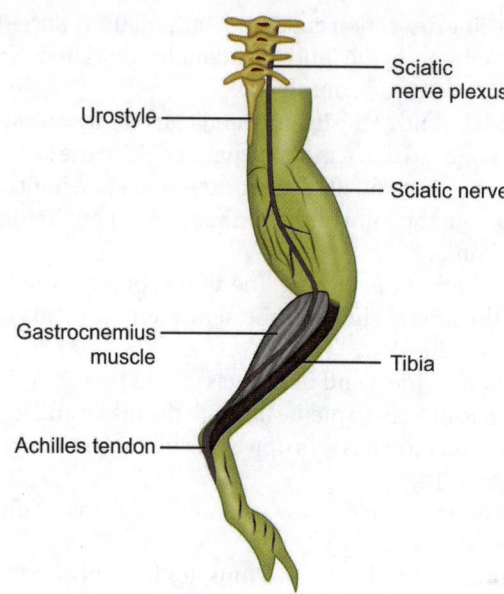

Fig. 31.3: Exposure of sciatic nerve of frog.

and its course is not clearly seen. You must be careful in cleaning and exposing it at this site.

- Sharp snips must cut branches going to the muscles of the thigh along the course of the nerve with the scissors. (While cutting these branches the muscles supplied by them will contract.) Thus clean the nerve up to the knee joint.
- Cut all the muscles round the thigh just above the knee joint. Cut the femur with the bone cutting forceps first and finally complete the separation with the scissors. Take care not to injure the nerve during this operation. As far as possible the nerve should not be allowed to come in contact with the freshly cut tissues.
- Moisten the tissues with saline and separate the body of the frog by cutting any attachments the knee joint.
- Thus the gastrocnemius muscle—sciatic nerve preparation (with the knee joint) is now ready.

A piece of the vertebral column is retained because:
- During dissection it could be easily held and the nerve can be dissected without touching it.
- Maximum length of the nerve is obtained.
- When kept across the electrodes the nerve does not slip down because of the weight of the bone.
- If the nerve is cut, slight stimuli can stimulate the injured surface and cause the muscle to contract irregularly.

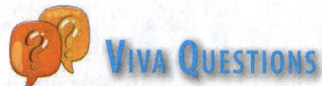

Viva Questions

1. **What are the advantages of using frogs as experimental animals?**
   » Frog is easily available
   » It is harmless and less expensive
   » It is easy to dissect the frog
   » Extra oxygen supply is not needed during the experiment because frog's tissues can directly absorb O_2 from the atmosphere
   » The tissue preparation can be maintained for longer duration if kept moist with Ringer solution
   » Adjustment of temperature is not needed to keep the tissues alive since frogs are cold blooded animals.

2. **What are the advantages of using sciatic nerve-gastrocnemius muscle preparation?**
   » It is easy to dissect out this preparation
   » The sciatic nerve is long and large enough to place the electrodes below it
   » The gastrocnemius muscle is large and hence on contraction records a graph of adequate amplitude
   » Since the muscle is a slow muscle, it is not fatigued easily.

3. **Name another muscle which can be used for study purpose.**
   The sartorius muscle of a frog can be used, but the force generated by its contraction may not be sufficient to move the lever during recording.

Chapter 32

Mounting the Muscle-Nerve Preparation

LEARNING OBJECTIVES

- Mount the muscle-nerve preparation properly on the myograph stand
- Discuss the composition and functions of Ringer's fluid

PY3.18: Observe with computer assisted learning (i) Amphibian nerve-muscle experiments and (ii) amphibian cardiac experiments.

PROCEDURE

- Pass a pin through the capsule of the knee joint and fix it firmly in the cork of the muscle board.
- Tie the ligature on the tendon of gastrocnemius muscle to the short arm of the muscle lever.
- Pour sufficient quantity of normal saline to keep the muscle and nerve moist.
- Place the nerve over the electrodes.
- Attach a load of 10 g to the hole nearer the fulcrum of the lever. This mechanically brings the phase of relaxation to completion.
- Adjust the lever to fix it in such a position that the long arm of the lever becomes horizontal.
- Place the myograph stand near the drum so that the lever points to the left. Make sure that the drum moves from right to the left. If the drum is moving in the opposite direction, the belt connecting the central shaft pulley on the table and the pulley on the drum can be kept twisted.
- The lever should lie tangential to the drum, i.e., it should make a right angle with the radius of the drum.
- Make sure that the electrodes do not touch each other, and also see that the nerve is touching both the electrodes.

Electric Connections

- Electric connections should be done at the beginning of the experiment.
- Arrange the circuit based on the type of current (induced or faradic) that is needed for the experiment.
- Always place a short-circuiting key between the electrodes and the secondary coil to avoid unnecessary stimulation of the tissue.
- Run the drum and confirm that a spark is obtained when the contact break.
- Adjust the strength of the stimulus as required for the experiment by moving the secondary coil.

Adjustments in the Kymograph

Arrange the gear and the pulleys as directed in the experiment. The drum will not move when it is in the neutral gear. The combinations of the various pulleys give fast, medium and slow speeds. To study the various phases in detail, a fast gear and fast speed is selected. Fast speed is obtained by connecting the largest pulley on the table shaft and the smallest one on the drum with the belt. If a series of contractions are to be obtained, a slow speed and a slow gear must be used. Slow speed is obtained by connecting the smallest pulley on the table shaft with the largest pulley on the drum. Medium speed is obtained by connecting the pulleys of same sizes on the central shaft and the drum.

The kymograph must be in the horizontal level. Adjusting the screws at the bottom of the kymograph can do this. When the kymograph is not in level, the writing lever will not mark a complete graph on the smoked paper.

Mounting the Cylinder

- Mount the cylinder with the black-sooted paper on the axle shaft of the kymograph at the desired level.

- Make sure that the cylinder fits firmly on the axle of the drum properly.
- Mount the cylinder in such a way that the desired surface faces the lever when the striker touches the contact knob to complete the circuit.
- Make sure that the record is not taken on the joint where the paper is pasted. This helps in cutting the paper properly before varnishing.

Mounting the Preparation

- A suitable weight is attached to the writing lever to keep it taut. The weight also brings the process of relaxation to completion mechanically and the lever touches the base line. To reduce inertia, the weight should always be applied as near to the fulcrum as is possible.
- The lever must always lie in the horizontal level.
- After load screw should be adjusted so that the lever is horizontal (**Fig. 32.1**).
- Whenever recording is not being done, the nerve should be removed from the electrodes and kept soaked in saline. This serves two purposes. No unwanted stimuli are imparted to the nerve; and the nerve does not get dried up.

Adjustments of the Myograph and the Lever

- The lever should be adjusted so as to write on the smoked paper at the desired level.
- The writing point of the lever should touch the surface of the paper lightly and should not press upon it heavily.
- The direction of the lever should be tangential to the surface of the drum.
- Never change the position of the myograph stand once the experiment has started. The recording of the points

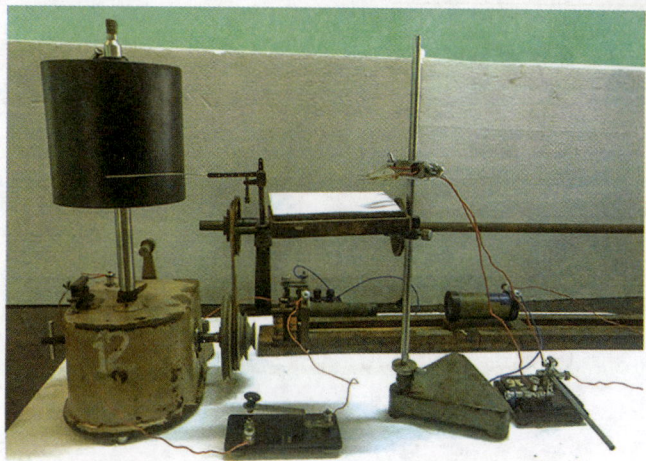

Fig. 32.1: Arrangement of the apparatus for recording frog's skeletal muscle graphs.

which denote time on the graph, depend upon the fixed position of the lever, relative to the recording surface. Use the handle at the base of the stand to adjust the lever.

Precautions

- Always draw a base line before recording the graph.
- Record a suitable time trace whenever the periods are to be measured and compared.
- Always mark the various points like point of stimulation, point of contraction, etc.
- After the graph is recorded, the myograph should be immediately taken away from the paper by turning the handle at the base. Otherwise unnecessary lines will be marked on the paper accidentally.

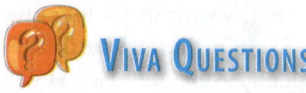 **VIVA QUESTIONS**

1. **What is the composition of Ringer's solution?**
    » Sodium chloride—0.6 g
    » Calcium chloride—0.01 g
    » Potassium chloride—0.0075 g
    » Sodium bicarbonate—0.01 g
    » Distilled water—up to 100 mL
2. **What are the functions of each component?**
    » Sodium chloride makes the solution isotonic with the frog's tissues
    » Calcium chloride maintains the excitability of the tissues
    » Potassium chloride is necessary for maintaining the resting membrane potential
    » Sodium bicarbonate maintains the pH of the solution.

Chapter 33

Simple Muscle Twitch

LEARNING OBJECTIVES

- Dissect out frog's muscle nerve preparation
- Draw the circuit diagram for induced current
- Record the response of the muscle to a single stimulus
- Explain the simple muscle twitch recorded
- Discuss the causes of latent period in the graph

PY3.18: Observe with computer assisted learning amphibian nerve-muscle experiments.

INTRODUCTION

When a skeletal muscle is stimulated, it contracts after a latent period and this is immediately followed by relaxation, this is called simple muscle twitch. Here, a single stimulus produces a single contraction and it can be recorded as a simple muscle curve. This is recorded from the gastrocnemius muscle of frog. The simple muscle twitch has a total duration of approximately 0.1 second.

MATERIALS

Frog, isotonic saline (0.65% NaCl), tuning fork of frequency 100 Hz (vibrations per second), isotonic muscle lever, myograph stand, frog board, electrode, kymograph with drum, pins, thread.

PROCEDURE

Connections for Electric Circuit

- Arrange the primary circuit with low voltage terminals, primary coil, key and drum in series.
- From the secondary coil take the current to the electrode through the short-circuiting key.
- Adjust the strength of current to a submaximal break shock.

Adjustments of Kymograph

- **Pulley and gear:** Connect the largest pulley wheel on the table shaft with the smallest pulley on the drum for fast speed.
- Adjust the drum in fast gear.
- Bring the two limbs of the striker at the base of the shaft in alignment with each other.

Mounting the Preparation and Recording the Graph

- Pith the frog and prepare the gastrocnemius muscle-nerve preparation.
- Mount the preparation in the muscle board.
- Raise the afterload screw just enough to support the lever horizontally. Attach a suitable weight. For a muscle of moderate size, 10 g applied to the hole nearest to the fulcrum is sufficient.
- Take the lever away from the drum by rotating the axle of the stand with the handle at its base.
- After that never change the position of the stand and the drum till the experiment is over.
- Adjust the distance between the primary and the secondary coil so that the break shock acts as a submaximal stimulus of highest intensity (the make shock should not cause the muscle to contract).
- To activate the stimulus, turn the axle of the drum so that the strikers touch the contact button and the circuit gets completed.
- Open the short-circuiting key in the secondary circuit. Give a make and then a break shock, and confirm that the curve is properly recorded on the paper.

- Draw a base line by starting the drum and making the lever to write upon it. The short-circuiting key must be closed and the lever should be brought near the paper to write upon it by adjusting the handle at the base of the stand.
- Turn the lever away and stop the drum.
- Draw a time tracing with a tuning fork of frequency 100 vibrations per second.
- Fixing the tuning fork in an X-block on a stand and vibrating it can record the time tracing below the base line.
- Start the drum and touch the vibrating writing point lightly on the moving surface till the circle is completed. Stop the drum. A time trace is drawn.
- Now bring the myograph in position so as to write on the cylinder.
- See that the writing point is level with the base line and touches the drum lightly enough as not to exert any pressure but firmly enough to draw a good trace.
- Open the key in the secondary circuit.
- Place the right hand on the key in the primary circuit and the left on the clutch of the drum and watch the lever.
- Start the drum.
- Watch the moving surface of the cylinder and note the area that comes in front of the lever when the strikers strike the contact point.
- Just before the desired surface of the paper comes in front of the writing point, close the primary circuit.
- The muscle will contract and as soon as it contracts, open the key and stop the drum.
- Close the key in the secondary circuit.
- Withdraw the lever from the paper, with the help of the handle at the base.
- Put the drum in the neutral gear.
- Hold the axle of the drum and rotate it so that the strikers and the knob come in alignment to make a contact. At this moment the nerve was stimulated.
- Bring the lever back in the original position to write on the surface of the paper.
- Stimulate the nerve again.
- The muscle will contract and will draw a vertical arc, denoting the point of stimulation.
- Hold the short arm of the lever and move it so that the line drawn by the writing point cuts the base line and the time trace.
- Withdraw the myograph.
- Label this point as PS (point of stimulation).
- Holding its axle, rotate the drum to the left, so that the point of beginning of contraction comes opposite to the writing point.
- Turn the myograph back, so that the writing lever comes near the paper. Adjust the position of the cylinder, so that the writing point touches exactly the point of contraction.
- Draw a vertical line passing through this point of contraction and cutting the base line and the time trace by moving the short arm of the lever with the fingers.
- Name the point as PC (point of contraction).
- Similarly draw vertical arcs at the points of maximum contraction (PMC) and at the end of relaxation (PR), i.e., the point where the curve touches the baseline again. Do not draw a perpendicular from the point of maximum contraction to the base line. It should be an arc of the same circle. Otherwise it will cut the time trace at a wrong point.
- Name the points as 'PMC' and 'PR' (**Fig. 33.1**).

OBSERVATION

A simple muscle twitch has the following components (**Fig. 33.1**):
- Latent period
- Contraction period
- Relaxation period

Latent Period (LP)

Latent period is defined as the time, which is required by the muscle to respond to a stimulus. Latent period of a skeletal muscle is 0.01 second. It extends from the point of stimulation (PS) to the point of contraction (PC).

Contraction Period (CP)

It extends from the point of contraction to the point of maximum contraction (PMC). It lasts for about 0.04 seconds. It is the time during which contraction in the muscle fibers occur due to entry of sodium ions through the ion channels,

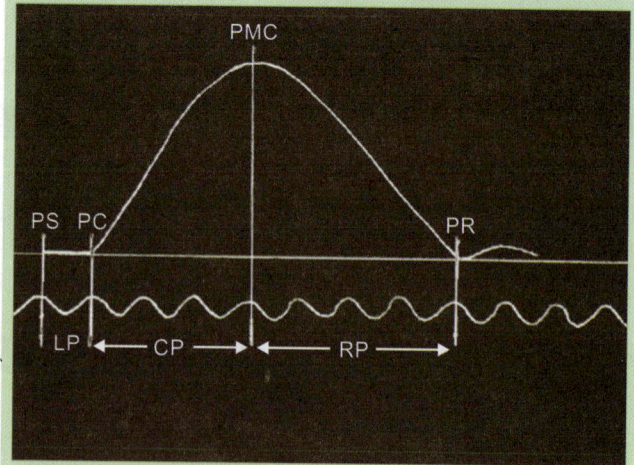

Fig. 33.1: Simple muscle twitch (PS: Point of stimulation; PC: Point of contraction; PMC: Point of maximum contraction; PR: Point of relaxation; LP: Latent period; CP: Contraction period; RP: Relaxation period) one wave in the time tracing corresponds to 0.01 second.

causing depolarization of the muscle cell membrane and release of calcium ions from the sarcoplasmic reticulum. This is responsible for sliding of actin and myosin resulting in muscle contraction. The height of the contraction indicates the degree of shortening of the muscle.

Relaxation Period (RP)

It extends from the PMC to the point of relaxation (PR). It has duration of 0.05 seconds and it is longer than the contraction period. The ratio of contraction phase and the relaxation phase is constant in all fibers.

Precautions

- ❖ Handle the nerve with the glass hook only
- ❖ Keep the muscle-nerve preparation always moist with normal saline or Ringer's solution
- ❖ Unnecessary repeated stimulation of the muscle will lead to fatigue
- ❖ While rotating the drum manually, keep the kymograph in neutral gear
- ❖ Never change the position of the myograph stand till the whole experiment is over
- ❖ Level the drum before starting the experiment.

VIVA QUESTIONS

1. **What is a simple muscle twitch?**
   When a single threshold stimulus is applied to a muscle it contracts and this is called simple muscle twitch.

2. **What is the total duration of SMT?**
   Normal duration is 0.1 second. It is longer when the muscle is fatigued.

3. **What is latent period and give its duration?**
   Latent period is defined as the time, which is required by the muscle to respond to a stimulus. It extends from the point of application of stimulus to the point of contraction in the graph. Latent period of a skeletal muscle is 0.01 second.

4. **What is the reason for relaxation period and how much is its duration?**
   It is the period during which calcium ions are pumped back into the sarcoplasmic reticulum causing decreased calcium concentration in the sarcoplasm. This results in muscle relaxation. It has duration of 0.05 seconds.

5. **What are the causes of latent period?**
   - » Time taken by the nerve impulse to reach the myoneural junction, i.e., conduction time along the nerve, about 0.002 seconds.
   - » The delay at the neuromuscular junction, about 0.005 seconds.
   - » Time taken for the release of neurotransmitter and the neurotransmitter to reach the motor end plate and generate action potential (excitation-contraction coupling).
   - » Calcium ions to be released from sarcoplasmic reticulum for muscle contraction.
   - » Time taken to overcome the inertia of the lever.

6. **What is physiological curve?**
   After the relaxation period in the simple muscle twitch graph, few small curves are obtained which is referred to as physiological curves. It is due to inertia of the lever.

7. **Why is a weight suspended from the lever while the graph is being recorded?**
   - » The load reduces the height of the graph so that it will not go beyond the drum.
   - » It helps to keep the lever horizontal.
   - » It exerts a slight stretch on the gastrocnemius muscle so that the muscle responds to the stimulus more effectively.

8. **What are the advantages of induced current?**
   The strength of the current can be adjusted by changing the distance between the primary coil and the secondary coil. Thus minimum strength can be used to stimulate the nerve. It is of very short duration and therefore will not damage the tissue.

9. **Which speed and gear is used to record simple muscle twitch?**
   SMT is recorded with fast speed and fast gear.

10. **Correlate the mechanical and electrical events of simple muscle twitch.**
    The electrical event will be completed at the start of the contraction phase of the mechanical event **(Fig. 33.2)**.

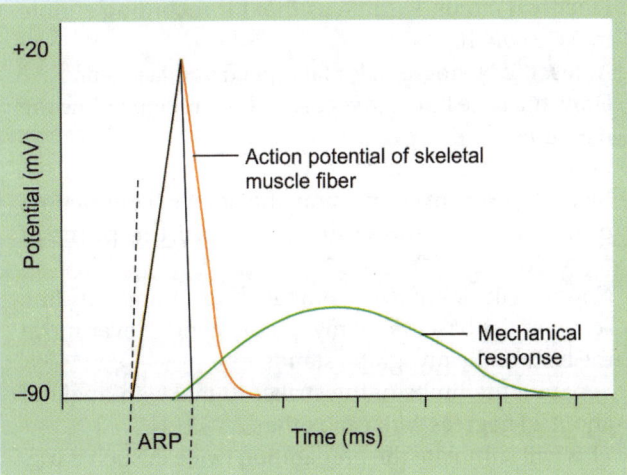

Fig. 33.2: Correlation between electrical and mechanical events in skeletal muscle.

Chapter 34

Effects of Two Successive Stimuli on Muscle Contraction

LEARNING OBJECTIVES

- Demonstrate the effect of two successive stimuli on muscle contraction.
- Define refractory period. What are the differences between absolute and relative refractory period?

PY3.18: Observe with computer assisted learning amphibian nerve-muscle experiments.

REQUIREMENTS

Frog, isotonic saline (0.65% NaCl), tuning fork of frequency 100 Hz (vibrations per second), isotonic muscle lever, myograph stand, frog board, electrode, kymograph with drum, pins, thread.

METHOD

- Electrical circuit is same as that for recording simple muscle twitch.
- Adjust the kymograph for fast speed and fast gear.
- Draw the base line and record a time tracing below the base line.
- Record a simple muscle curve.
- Mark the point of stimulation, the point of contraction, point of maximum contraction and the point of relaxation.
- Now turn the lever away from the drum by adjusting the screw at the base of the myograph stand. Never move the base of the myograph stand.
- Separate the limbs of the striker to make an angle of about 20 degrees with each other.
- This will stimulate the preparation twice in such a way that the second stimulus will probably fall after the relaxation phase of the previous contraction.
- Rotate the cylinder by manipulating the axle so that a fresh part of the smoked paper faces the lever, as the first limb touches the contact knob.
- Bring the lever in position so as to write on the paper on the same base line. If the lever does not touch the level of the base line, adjust the level of the cylinder.
- Open the key in the secondary circuit. Start the drum, close the key in the primary circuit till the two limbs of the strikers strike past the contact point and open the key immediately.
- Stop the drum and close the key in the secondary circuit.
- Two curves are recorded on the drum.
- Mark the point of stimulation, the point of contraction, and end of relaxation of both the curves. See that the lines denoting them cut the time trace.
- Turn the lever away from the writing surface.
- Reduce the angle between the two limbs of the striker to about 12°. This will most probably give the second stimulus during the relaxation phase of the first contraction.
- Rotate the drum round its axle in the same horizontal plane so that the lever writes on a fresh area of the paper as the first limb of the strikers touches the contact knob.
- Repeat all the procedures required to draw the curves.
- Mark the various points.
- Obtain on successive fresh areas of paper keeping the angle at 8° so that the second stimulus falls during the contraction period.
- Adjust the angle between the strikers to 2° so that the second stimulus falls during the latent period.
- If the second stimulus does not fall in the desired phase of the first contraction the angle between the two limbs of the striker must be varied accordingly to obtain the desired result. It is better to try trial and error method.

OBSERVATIONS

- When the second stimulus falls immediately after the first contraction, the height of the second contraction will be greater than the first curve **(Fig. 34.1)**. This is because of beneficial effect of the previous contraction. **Latent period is shortened** and the graph will be wider in the second contraction.
- When the second stimulus is given in the relaxation phase of the first contraction, the second contraction starts before the completion of the previous relaxation **(Fig. 34.2)**. The graph is described as **superposition**.
- When the second stimulus is given in the contraction phase, the muscle starts contracting vigorously at a speed, faster than the previous one. The curve obtained will be taller and wider than the simple muscle twitch **(Fig. 34.3)**. Here there is **summation** of two contractions or summation of two waves or summation of the mechanical events.
- When the second stimulus is given in the latent period of first contraction only a simple muscle curve is obtained. The height of this curve and that of the one obtained in the beginning of the experiment by the single stimulus are equal. The second stimulus here has no effect at all. If the second stimulus falls in the absolute refractory

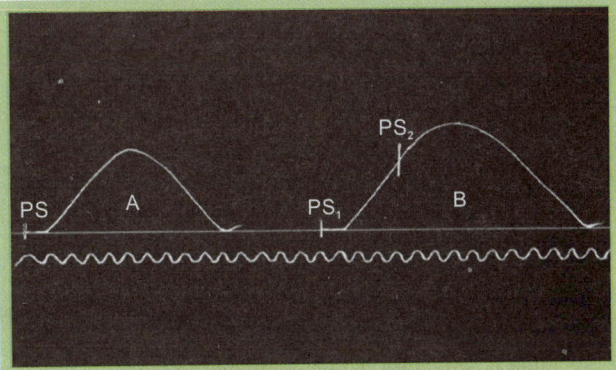

Fig. 34.3: Effect of two successive stimuli with the second stimulus falling in the contraction period of previous contraction. The first graph A is a simple muscle twitch. The second one B is summation curve. Compare the two curves and observe that the summation curve is taller and wider than the simple muscle twitch.

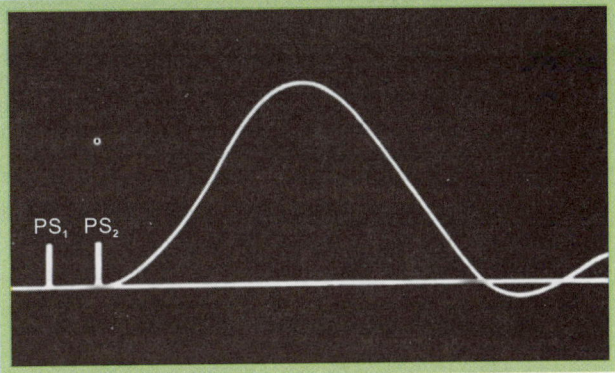

Fig. 34.4: Effect of two successive stimuli on skeletal muscle contraction with the second stimulus falling during the latent period of previous contraction PS1—first point of stimulation and PS2 is second point of stimulation (see **Fig. 34.5** also).

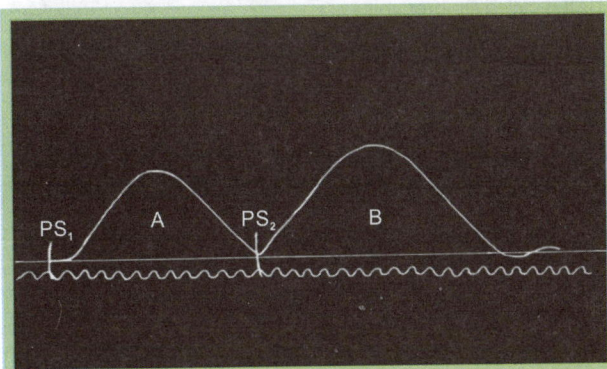

Fig. 34.1: Beneficial effect (graph B is taller and wider due to beneficial effect).

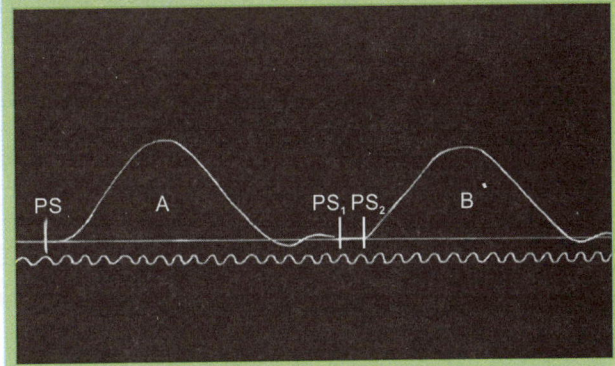

Fig. 34.5: Comparison of simple muscle twitch and two successive stimuli with the second stimulus falling in the latent period of previous contraction. (A) Simple muscle twitch; (B) Effect of two successive stimuli on muscle contraction when the second stimulus falls in the latent period of previous contraction. Both the curves are similar because there is no effect for the second stimulus.

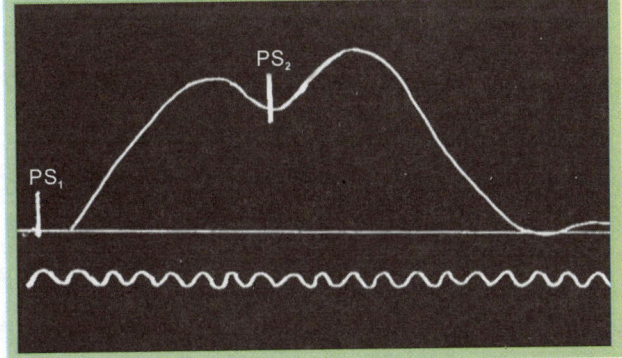

Fig. 34.2: Effect of two successive stimuli on muscle contraction. The second stimulus falls in the relaxation period of previous contraction (superposition graph).

period of the first stimulus, there will be no effect **(Figs. 34.4 and 34.5)**. The absolute refractory period is during the latent period of first contraction.

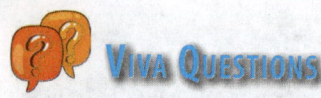

1. **What are the causes of beneficial effect? Why is it called so?**
   » Accumulation of calcium in the sarcoplasm
   » Increase in temperature
   » Increase in elasticity
   » Decrease in viscosity
   The second contraction is benefitted by the first contraction, so the graph is called beneficial effect.

2. **Is superposition possible in cardiac muscle?**
   Yes, cardiac muscle is in the relative refractory period after 1/3rd of diastole. So if a second stimulus falls during this period, heart responds by producing an extra beat or extrasystole.

3. **What is refractory period. Mention the types.**
   Refractory period is the period during which the excitability of an excitable tissue is decreased. It is divided into absolute refractory period and relative refractory period.

4. **Give the differences between simple muscle twitch and summation.**
   » Summation has two points of stimulation
   » Summation is taller and wider than SMT.

5. **What are the types of summation?**
   » Wave summation or temporal summation
   » Quantal summation or multifiber summation.
   In wave summation, two successive waves of contractions are fused and hence the name. The second stimulus is applied in the contraction period of the previous contraction. Same strength of current is used for the two stimuli.
   In quantal summation, if the strength of the stimulus is increased, a taller and wider contraction will be obtained. This is because, more and more motor neurons get stimulated with stronger stimuli. That is, more and more motor units are recruited for contraction. To demonstrate this, first apply a threshold stimulus and record the effect. After 20 seconds (to avoid beneficial effect), increase the strength of the current and give the stimulus. A larger contraction will be obtained due to quantal summation.

6. **What is a motor unit?**
   A motor neuron with all its branches and the muscle fibers supplied by it is called a motor unit.

7. **What are the factors that increase the strength of muscle contraction?**
   » Intensity of current
   » Frequency of stimuli
   » Initial length of muscle fiber
   » Temperature
   » Type of muscle fiber.

8. **Why there is no effect, if the second stimulus falls in the latent period?**
   The whole of absolute refractory period of action potential falls during the latent period.

Chapter 35

Genesis of Tetanus

LEARNING OBJECTIVES

- Demonstrate the effect of repetitive stimuli on muscle contraction
- Explain the difference between clonus and tetanus

PY3.18: Observe with computer assisted learning amphibian nerve-muscle experiments.

INTRODUCTION

Tetanus is defined as the continuous state of contraction of muscle resulting from multiple successive stimuli. It is a fusion of contractions and the entire muscle fibers contract maximally.

APPARATUS

Vibrating interrupter that consists of a reed and a mercury cup, kymograph, smoked cylinders, mercury.

Electric Connections

Connect the vibrating interrupter, the induction coil and the key in series in the primary circuit. Note that the drum is not included in the circuit. Short-circuiting key is included in the secondary circuit.

PROCEDURE

- Adjust the kymograph for fast gear and medium speed.
- Adjust the vibrating length of the reed so as to give five stimuli per second.
- Mount the gastrocnemius muscle-nerve preparation as for simple muscle twitch.
- Take the lever away from the paper with the help of the handle at the base of the stand.
- Adjust the strength of the current for break shock.
- Adjust the myograph stand to touch the paper at a tangent.
- Start the drum and draw a base line on the smoked paper. Then stop the drum.
- Adjust the tip of the vibrating reed so that the contact is just above the mercury cup and is not touching the mercury.
- Open the short-circuiting key in the secondary circuit and close the simple key in the primary circuit.
- Start the drum and allow the reed to vibrate with a sudden upward jerk. It will start vibrate with (at its adjusted frequency of five per second). The nerve will be stimulated at each break shock.
- Allow the lever to record a few contractions.
- Open the key in primary circuit and stop the drum. Now turn the myograph away from the drum making sure that the base of the myograph stand is not moving.
- Label the graph and write down 5 stimuli per second.
- Fix the length of the reed to give about ten stimuli per second (the number of stimuli is written on the reed).
- Repeat and obtain another record on the adjacent surface of the paper and label it.
- Similarly obtain records for fifteen, twenty, twenty-five and thirty stimuli per second. Label all the recordings (**Figs. 35.1 and 35.2**).
- Now remove the vibrating interrupter from the primary circuit and include the Neef's hammer instead.
- Obtain a record with a high frequency of stimulation, i.e., about 100 stimuli per sec. Label it as faradic current.

OBSERVATION

Refer **Figures 35.1 and 35.2**.

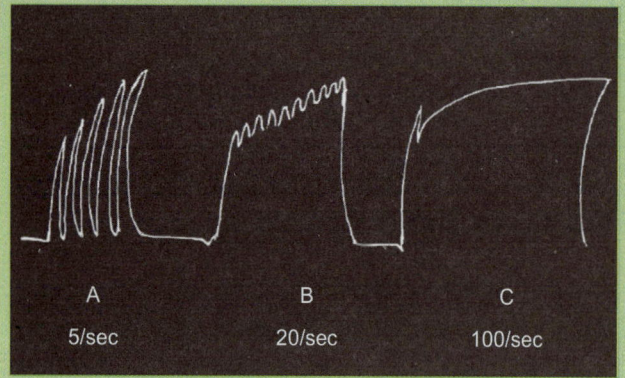

Figs. 35.1A to C: Effect of successive stimuli on muscle contraction. (A) frequency 5 stimuli/sec, the successive stimulus falls after complete relaxation of previous contraction. So individual graphs are obtained, (B) frequency 20 stimuli/sec, the successive stimulus falls in the relaxation period of previous contraction. So there is incomplete fusion of mechanical events, which is referred to as clonus, (C) frequency 100/sec, the successive stimulus falls in the contraction period of previous contractions and so there is complete fusion of mechanical events, which is referred to as tetanus.

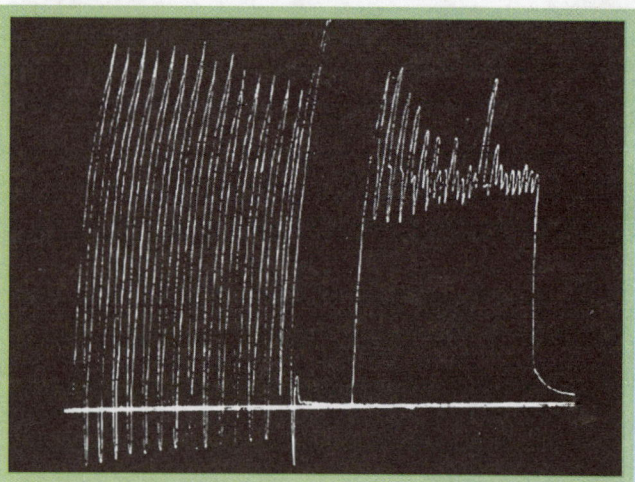

Fig. 35.2: First graph is recorded with a frequency of 10 impulses per second and the second graph is obtained with a frequency of 25 per sec. Note that when the frequency is 10/sec, individual contractions are obtained. When it is increased to 25/sec, there is incomplete fusion of the mechanical events, which is referred to as clonus or incomplete tetanus.

 Viva Questions

1. **What is clonus? Is it possible in heart?**
   Clonus is incomplete tetanus. When the successive stimuli fall during the relaxation period of previous contraction, there will be incomplete fusion of mechanical events. This is referred to as clonus. It is not possible in cardiac muscle. This is because, when the successive stimuli fall, the muscle will be in the refractory period.

2. **Do tetanic contractions occur normally in the body?**
   Yes. In the body, most of the muscles especially those maintaining a particular posture are in a state of continuous contraction. This state of contraction is almost similar to tetanus. The difference is that all the muscle fibers in the muscle are not contracting at the same time. While some are contracting, others will be relaxing. This prevents fatigue of the muscles. If all the fibers contract at the same time, as in violent muscular efforts, such a state can last only for a very short duration.

3. **Cardiac muscle cannot be tetanized. Give reason.**
   The absolute refractory period is very long for cardiac muscle. It extends throughout the contraction period and extends to one third of the relaxation phase. For every successive stimulus to be effective, it must fall after the refractory period. In case of the cardiac muscle, whole of the contraction period falls during the refractory period. So, a second stimulus falling during the contraction period has no effect on cardiac muscle. So, cardiac muscle cannot be tetanized.

4. **What is critical fusion frequency?**
   The minimum frequency of stimuli at which tetanus occurs is called critical fusion frequency. It is decreased when the muscle is fatigued. It is inversely proportional to the contraction period.

   $$CCF \propto \frac{1}{CP}$$

5. **What are the factors affecting the genesis of tetanus?**
   » *Type of muscles*: Muscles can be classified as fast and slow according to the majority of the fast or slow fibers in them. In fast muscles, tetanus occurs with higher frequencies when compared to slow muscles. Contraction period is more for slow muscles.
   » *Temperature*: Fall in temperature decreases the velocity of shortening. Tetanus can therefore be produced with lower frequencies at lower temperature.
   » *Refractory period*: Voluntary muscles have very short refractory periods as compared to their contraction periods. But in case of cardiac muscle, the refractory period is very long. So, cardiac muscle cannot be tetanized.
   » *Fatigue*: A muscle that is fatigued contracts slowly and so it goes into tetanus at lower frequencies as compared to the normal muscle.

6. **Why there is fusion of mechanical events when the frequency of stimuli is more than 10/sec?**
   Normal twitch duration is 0.1 sec. So, when the rate of impulse is increased above this limit, there will be fusion of mechanical events. Depending on the rate, the succeeding stimuli may fall in the relaxation or contraction period of previous contraction. If it falls in the relaxation period, there will be incomplete fusion of contractions and clonus results. If it falls in the contraction period, there will be complete fusion of mechanical events and tetanus results.

7. **Will the electrical events fuse during tetanus? If the mechanical and electrical events are simultaneously recorded with a frequency of stimulation of 15/sec, how many action potentials will be recorded?**
   No, the electrical events do not fuse. Separate action potentials will be recorded with a frequency of 15/sec. But there will be partial fusion of mechanical events resulting in clonus.

8. **Distinguish this tetanus from other terminologies.**
   » Tetanus caused by the bacterial toxin from *Clostridium tetani*. Here there is sustained contraction of both agonists and antagonists in the body.
   » Tetany due to hypoparathyroidism where there is decrease in the ionic calcium level. Here due to increased excitability of nerve and muscle, there will be spasm of muscles.

36

Effect of Afterload and Freeload in Skeletal Muscle Contraction

LEARNING OBJECTIVES

- Demonstrate the effect of load and afterload on muscle contraction
- Calculate the work done during freeloading and afterloading
- Discuss the difference between preload and afterload
- Explain Frank-Starling law with the help of the graph obtained

PY3.18: Observe with computer assisted learning amphibian nerve-muscle experiments.

INTRODUCTION

A muscle while lifting a load does external work. If the load acts on the muscle only when it starts contracting is called afterloading. If the load acts on the muscle in the relaxed state by stretching it and determines the initial resting length of the muscle, it is called freeloading. Both affect the performance of the muscle. In the freeloaded condition, the work done by the muscle increases and in the afterloaded condition the efficiency of the muscle decreases.

PRINCIPLE

The amplitude of muscle contraction is observed when the load is applied to the muscle before it starts contraction (freeloaded) and also when it is applied to the muscle after it starts contracting (afterloaded). The work done by the muscle for each contraction is calculated and the optimum weight for maximum work done can be found out. This experiment is done to prove Starling's law of muscle contraction.

REQUIREMENTS

10 g weight, frog, isotonic saline (0.65% NaCl) or Ringer's solution, isotonic muscle lever, myograph stand, frog board, electrode, kymograph with drum, pins, thread, graduated scale.

Afterloading

Procedure

- Arrange the primary circuit with key, induction coil and drum in series. Place the short-circuiting key in the secondary circuit.
- Adjust the kymograph for fast speed and fast gear as for simple muscle twitch.
- Mount the nerve-muscle preparation without attaching a load.
- Arrange for a submaximal break shock.
- Adjust the afterloading screw so that it just supports the arm of the lever.
- Adjust the myograph to write on the drum paper at a suitable place.
- Draw a base line.
- Take a time tracing.
- Attach a load of 10 g in the second hole of the lever from the fulcrum.
- Record a simple muscle curve with this load.
- Mark the point of stimulation and the periods of contraction and relaxation.
- Label the curve as 10 g.
- Attach an additional weight of 10 g and record another curve with the same point of stimulation and the same strength of stimulus. Wait for one minute after each addition of weight.
- Label it as 20 g.
- Similarly obtain records for successive increase in the load attached, with the same point of stimulation and same strength of stimulus and label each curve with its load.

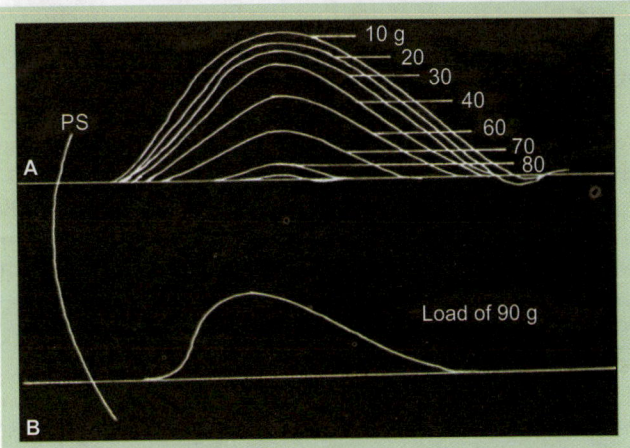

Figs. 36.1A and B: Effect of afterload (A) and freeload (B) on muscle contraction. In the lower graph, 80 g weight is acting as freeload.

- Continue till the muscle is not able to lift the load (**Fig. 36.1A**).

Observation

With increase in load:
- The latent period increases (due to inertia of lever)
- The height of contraction decreases progressively (since the muscle has to lift more load)
- The contraction period decreases (as the duration of active state decreases)
- The relaxation period decreases significantly
- The twitch duration decreases.

Freeloading

Aim

To study the effect of load on contracting gastrocnemius muscle when it is freeloaded.
- Release the afterload screw so that the weight that was unable by the muscle to lift up earlier now acts on the muscle at rest. This weight will stretch the muscle and the resting length of the muscle increases. This condition is known as freeloaded.
- As soon as the screw is made loose, the writing point comes down drawing an arc on the paper. Draw a base line at this level.
- Now stimulate the muscle with the same strength of current that was used previously.

Observation

- It is seen that the muscle contracts isotonically lifting up the lever and a trace is recorded on the drum (**Fig. 36.1B**).
- The force of contraction of a muscle is directly proportional to the initial length of the muscle within physiological limits. This is Starling's law.

- So the height of contraction increases with increase in load within physiological limits (after a limit the amplitude of contraction decreases).

Afterload recording: The first recording is the afterload graph. In this graph, the latent period increases with increasing load. The height of contraction decreases with increasing load. With 90 g weight acting as afterload the muscle is unable to lift this load (**Fig. 36.1A**).

Freeload recording: The second graph seen below is recorded with a load of 90 g after releasing the afterload screw. The weight now acts as freeload and the muscle lifts this load and records a larger curve when it is stimulated (**Fig. 36.1B**).

Recording of Afterloaded and Freeloaded Contractions on a Stationary Drum

- Exclude the kymograph from the primary circuit.
- Adjust the lever for afterloading.
- Record the muscle contraction on a stationary drum after pressing and releasing the simple key once.
- After each contraction rotate the kymograph manually for about 1 cm and add 10 g weights in steps.
- Record the contractions at distances 1cm apart till the muscle is unable to lift the weight.
- Label the weights used under each contraction as 10 g, 20 g, 30 g, etc., and label the recording afterloaded.
- Repeat the same procedure after releasing the afterload screw so that the weight acts on the muscle before it starts contracting.
- The lever comes to lower and lower positions as the load increases.
- Label the weights used under each contraction.
- Label the record as freeloaded.

Calculation of Work Done by the Muscle for Each Contraction (Fig. 36.2)

The following formula is used for calculating the work done:

$$W = w \times h$$

'W' is the work done in g cm, 'w' is the weight lifted in grams, and 'h' is the actual height to which the weight has been lifted by the muscle in cm.

$h = l/L \times H$ ('l' is the distance between the fulcrum and the point of attachment of load, 'L' is the distance between the fulcrum and the writing point of the lever, 'H' is the height of the contraction in cm obtained for a particular weight).

Therefore, $W = w \times l/L \times H$ g.cm

Work done for each weight can be calculated in the afterloaded and freeloaded condition. It is seen that the work done is more in the freeloaded condition. Starling's

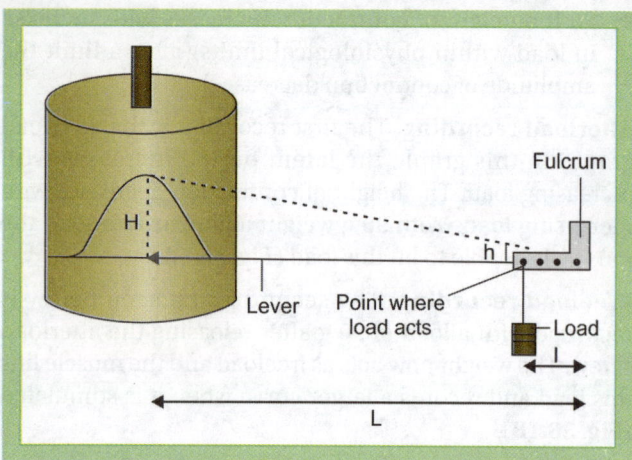

Fig. 36.2: Calculation of work done for a particular load.

law explains this. It states that the force of contraction is directly proportional to the initial length of the muscle fiber within physiological limits.

Enter the results in a tabular column. After tabulating the results, plot a graph showing weight (load) in grams along the X-axis and work done in g cm along the Y-axis.

It is seen from the graph that the work done rapidly increases for the first one or two additions in load after which it declines with each further addition of load. Find out from the graph the optimum load for maximum work done. Optimum load is that load at which maximum work is done.

Also find out the optimum load for the maximum height of contraction, i.e., the load at which the height of contraction is maximal.

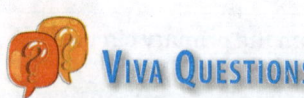

Viva Questions

1. **What is freeloading and afterloading?**
   If the load acts on the muscle only when it starts contracting is called afterloading. If the load acts on the muscle in the relaxed state by stretching it and determines the initial resting length of the muscle, it is called freeloading.

2. **What is Starling's law?**
   Starling's law states that the force of contraction of a muscle is directly proportional to the initial length of its muscle fibers within physiological limit.

3. **State Frank-Starling's law.**
   Frank-Starling's law states that the force of contraction of the heart is directly proportional to the end diastolic volume within physiological limits. When the EDV is increased, force of contraction and the stroke volume increases. If the EDV is increased beyond a limit it leads to heart failure.

4. **Give examples of freeloading and afterloading in the heart.**
   End diastolic volume is the freeload acting on the heart and peripheral resistance and aortic impedance are the afterloads acting on the heart.

5. **Give examples of load and afterload in everyday life.**
   a. Lifting a bucket of water from the ground is afterload.
   b. In short put, since the weight is already in the hand acting on the muscle, it is load.
   c. In weight lifting, the first lift of the weight from the ground is afterload and the second lift above the head is load.

37 Effect of Continuous Stimulation of a Muscle (Study of Fatigue and Recovery)

LEARNING OBJECTIVES

- Demonstrate the phenomenon of fatigue and recovery in the nerve-muscle preparation provided
- Define fatigue and its causes
- Explain the cause of contraction remainder
- Explain the mechanism of recovery after fatigue

PY3.18: Observe with computer assisted learning amphibian nerve-muscle experiments.

INTRODUCTION

Reduced performance or its absence resulting from prolonged and continuous activity is described as fatigue. No permanent functional or structural damage occurs during fatigue; hence it is reversible.

In the intact animal the central nervous system gets fatigued first followed by synapse and finally neuromuscular junction. Nerves are said to be unfatiguable. In the isolated nerve muscle preparation, neuromuscular junction is the first site of fatigue.

PRINCIPLE

In this experiment a muscle is stimulated repeatedly and continuously and the phenomenon of fatigue is demonstrated. After giving rest and nourishment to the fatigued muscle, it is again stimulated and the effect of recovery is also demonstrated.

REQUIREMENTS

Same as that of simple muscle twitch.

ELECTRICAL CONNECTIONS

Arrange the drum, key and the primary coil in series to form the primary circuit. Include the secondary coil, short circuiting key and electrodes in the secondary circuit.

PROCEDURE

- Adjust the kymograph for fast speed and fast gear.
- Dissect and mount the nerve-muscle preparation.
- Draw a base line and take a time trace.
- Record a simple muscle curve.
- After that allow the drum to rotate continuously so that the nerve-muscle preparation is stimulated with each turn of the drum.
- Now turn away the myograph by rotating the handle at its base so as to avoid a continuous recording of all the contractions. This prevents overlapping of contractions.
- Record every third contraction for the first 2 minutes by bringing the myograph near the paper to write upon it.
- Movement of the myograph is to be carried out by the movement of the axle of the stand, with the help of the handle at its base.
- Then record every tenth contraction.
- Continue till the muscle fails to record any contraction **(Fig. 37.1A)**.
- Open the key and stop the stimulation.
- Stop the drum.
- Change the point of stimulus by rotating the drum to record a muscle contraction on the same base line at a different place.
- Stimulate the fatigued muscle directly and record the effect.

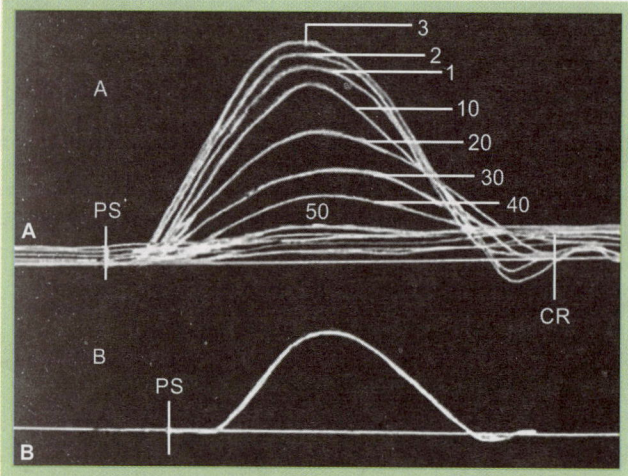

Figs. 37.1A and B: Demonstration of fatigue and recovery on frog's muscle nerve preparation. (A) Fatigue curve (the numbers denote the contractions due to repeated stimulation of the muscle). Note the contraction remainder (CR) at the end of the graph; (B) Recovery curve recorded after a period of rest following fatigue and washing the preparation with saline).

- Wash the muscle-nerve preparation with fresh saline or Ringer solution for sometime
- Bring a fresh surface of the paper in front of the writing lever.
- Wait for three to five minutes to give rest to the preparation and continue washing the preparation with fresh solution.
- Again change the point of stimulation in such a way that the next recording will be adjacent to the previous recording (**Fig. 37.1B**).
- Stimulate the nerve-muscle preparation again and record a contraction on the fresh surface.

OBSERVATIONS

- Due to beneficial effect the first few consecutive contractions will be taller than the first contraction (**Fig. 37.1A**).
- During this period of beneficial effect the latent period is reduced.
- As the beneficial effect passes away the height of contraction continuously decreases.
- The period of relaxation continuously increases.
- When the muscle fails to contract, it is said to be fatigued.
- The fatigued muscle cannot relax completely. So the curve remains above the base line. This phenomenon is described as contraction remainder (**Fig. 37.1A**).
- When the muscle is directly stimulated following fatigue it will contract. On direct stimulation, the muscle responds, even though fatigued through stimulation of its nerve. A nerve is unfatiguable, so the site of fatigue can be at the neuromuscular junction.
- The fatigued muscle, after giving rest and changing the fluid in which it is bathed, can be made to contract again. Rest allows the fatigue to wear off. This curve that is recorded after rest is called recovery curve (**Fig. 37.1B**).

PRECAUTIONS

- All the contractions produced by stimulation of the nerve should be recorded on the same baseline and same point of stimulation.
- The muscle should be directly stimulated immediately after taking the fatigue curve on the same baseline but at a different point of stimulus.
- Give at least 5 minutes after fatigue to record the recovery curve.

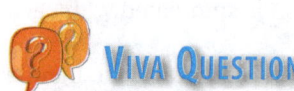

VIVA QUESTIONS

1. **How can you prove that the neuromuscular junction is the site of fatigue in the isolated muscle-nerve preparation?**
   After fatigue, when the muscle is directly stimulated it contracts and records a curve. This shows that the muscle is not fatigued. Nerve is unfatiguable. So, the probable site of fatigue in the isolated preparation is the neuromuscular junction.
2. **What are the causes of fatigue?**
   » Depletion of acetylcholine (neurotransmitter) at the neuromuscular junction
   » Accumulation of metabolites like lactic acid, K^+, etc., in the muscle
   » Decrease in ATP content. So that calcium ions cannot be pumped back into the sarcoplasmic reticulum. Since it is an active process.
3. **What is the reason for the recovery curve?**
   » When rest is given and washed with fresh Ringer solution there will be resynthesis of neurotransmitters at the nerve ending
   » When the muscle is washed with Ringer solution the metabolites get washed off
   » Resynthesis of high-energy phosphate compounds like ATP
4. **What happens when the muscle is directly stimulated continuously?**
   The muscle becomes fatigued due to depletion of glycogen and there will be no energy for muscle contraction. There will be no recovery after giving rest and washing the preparation with Ringer solution. This is because the utilized glycogen cannot be replaced.
5. **What is contraction remainder?**
   An early sign of fatigue is prolongation of relaxation period. When the muscle becomes fatigued the relaxation become incomplete and the muscle remains in a state of partial contraction. In the record the last few curves do not touch the base line. This is called contraction remainder.
6. **Which is the first site of fatigue in the intact body?**
   Central nervous system. Synapses in the brain, then the neuromuscular junction and finally muscle gets fatigued in the intact body.

Chapter 38

Effects of Temperature on Muscle Contraction

LEARNING OBJECTIVES

- Demonstrate the effect of temperature on skeletal muscle contraction
- Explain the changes in the simple muscle twitch with changes in temperature

PY3.18: Observe with computer assisted learning amphibian nerve-muscle experiments.

PRINCIPLE

All the chemical reactions occurring in the body or in living tissues are enzymatic reactions. It is seen that within limits, all the enzymatic reactions and activities in the living tissues are accelerated with a rise in temperature and are slowed down with a fall in temperature. In this experiment the effect of heat and cold on muscle contraction is studied. Increase in the surrounding temperature increases the efficiency of skeletal muscle contraction. This is useful during exercise when the body temperature increases.

REQUIREMENTS

Thermometer, hot Ringer solution (about 40°C), cold ringer solution (10–15°C), gastrocnemius muscle-nerve preparation of frog, Lucas chamber or muscle trough (instead of frog board) and all other equipment needed to record simple muscle twitch.

PROCEDURE

- Arrange the apparatus, electrical connections and pulley combination as for simple muscle twitch (fast gear and fast speed). Use Lucas chamber instead of frog board. Adjust the current for maximal stimulus.
- Note the temperature of the Ringer solution used at room temperature.
- Take two bowls one containing hot Ringer solution and the other containing cold Ringer solution.
- Record a time trace.
- Then record a simple muscle twitch after pouring Ringer solution at room temperature into the muscle trough. Mark the point of stimulation and the points of contraction and relaxation. Label the curve by denoting the temperature of the saline.
- Drain off the Ringer solution from the muscle trough.
- Fill the trough with hot Ringer solution at a temperature 5°C more than the room temperature and record a simple muscle curve. Label it.
- Then again drain the solution from the trough and fill it with Ringer solution at room temperature. Drain it after 2–5 minutes and the muscle will regain room temperature.
- Replace it with the cold Ringer solution having a temperature 10–15°C less than the room temperature. Wait for 2–5 minutes. The muscle will get cooled. Record a simple muscle twitch. Label it.
- Drain the solution from the trough and fill it with Ringer solution at a temperature of 42°C. See the effect.
- Instead of Ringer solution, amphibian normal saline (0.65% NaCl) can also be used.
- Calculate the latent period, contraction period and relaxation period of the muscle contraction with different temperatures.

PRECAUTIONS

- The muscle should be fully immersed in the Ringer solution at different temperatures for at least 5 minutes before taking a record.
- The temperature of the solution should not exceed 42°C because it will cause denaturation of muscle proteins.
- The temperature of the cold solution should not be less than 4°C. Very low temperature will cause coagulation of muscle proteins and the muscle fails to contract.
- The temperature of the solution should be noted accurately immediately after the muscle contraction.
- The effects of warm solution should be recorded before recording the effects of cold Ringer solution. This is because cold solution inhibits all enzymatic activities and it is difficult to revive the muscle activities to normal for a long time.
- In all the tracings taken, the point of stimulation, strength of current and the baseline should remain unchanged.

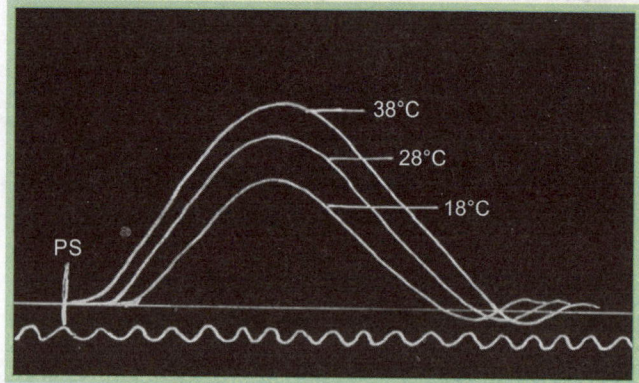

Fig. 38.1: Effect of temperature on muscle contraction (obtained curve) room temperature is 28°C.

OBSERVATION

Change in the amplitude of contraction, duration of latent period, contraction period and relaxation period are noted with change in temperature (Fig. 38.1).

- With rise in temperature, the latent period is reduced, the amplitude of contraction is increased, and the contraction and relaxation periods are decreased.
- Cooling of the muscle has reverse effects, i.e., all the processes become slower and prolonged and the height of contraction decreases.
- These are the observations for ideal curves.
- In the obtained curves, when the muscle is warmed the contraction and relaxation periods are prolonged and when the muscle is cooled, all the periods are decreased.
- At a temperature above 40°C, the muscle may contract without being stimulated because spontaneous chemical reactions occur.

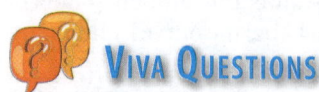 **VIVA QUESTIONS**

1. **What is the effect seen on muscle contraction when the muscle temperature is increased? Give reasons.**
   Hot Ringer decreases the duration of all the phases of muscle contraction and increases the height of contraction. When the temperature of the muscle is increased with in limits, the metabolic activities are accelerated and the viscosity decreases. The muscle ATPase activity increases and the force of contraction increases. Thus, higher amplitude of the curve is obtained. Depolarization and repolarization become fast and an accelerated response is obtained. Faster contraction and relaxation occur leading to reduction in the contraction and relaxation periods.

2. **What are the reasons for the decrease in latent period when the muscle is warmed?**
   » Increase in the velocity of conduction in the nerve
   » Increased rate of neuromuscular transmission
   » Inertia of lever is overcome faster because of decrease in viscosity

3. **What is the reason for the response obtained when the muscle is cooled?**
   When the muscle is cooled, the enzymatic and metabolic activities are slowed down and the viscosity increases. Depolarization and repolarization become slow and a delayed response is obtained. The height of the curve is less because the force of contraction is decreased by cold temperature. If the temperature is reduced to 0°C, the excitability of the tissue will be lost.

4. **Why the ideal curves are not obtained when the kymograph and smoked drum are used for the experiment?**
   When we record the curves at different temperatures using the kymograph the obtained curves are different from the ideal curves. In warm solution, the curve is taller and it takes more time for the lever to come back to the base line. So, the relaxation period is prolonged in the obtained curve. Whereas with cold solution, the height of contraction is less and so the lever reaches the base line earlier. The relaxation period is decreased (ideal curve is shown in **Figure 38.2**).

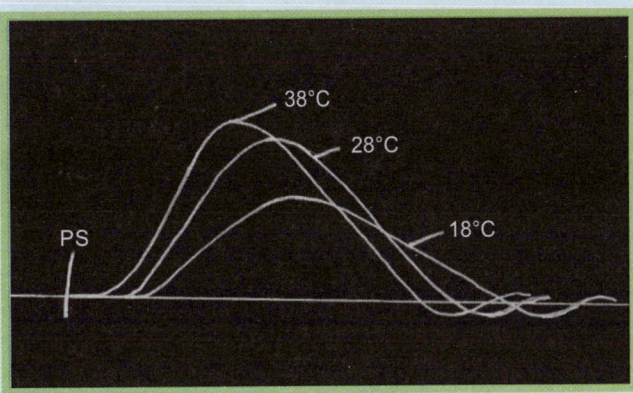

Fig. 38.2: Effect of temperature on muscle contraction (ideal curve). (PS: point of stimulation)

5. **Why is it said that the temperature of the Ringer solution should not exceed 42°C?**
   This is because at higher temperatures there will be denaturation of muscle proteins and the muscle will remain in a state of contraction called **heat rigor**. It is seen when the temperature exceeds 45°C.

6. **What is induced hypothermia? Mention its significance.**
   The body temperature can be reduced to about 25°C by artificially cooling the body during cardiac and brain surgery. This is induced hypothermia. It decreases blood loss during surgery by producing vasoconstriction. Therapeutic hypothermia is also used in times of head injury since it reduces bleeding and has neuroprotective effects. Neuroprotective effect is due to reduced cerebral metabolism and decreased free radical formation. Hypothermia also prevents cerebral reperfusion injury.

Chapter 39

Velocity of Nerve Impulses

LEARNING OBJECTIVES

- Calculate the velocity of conduction in the muscle nerve preparation provided
- Discuss the factors affecting velocity of conduction in a nerve

PY3.18: Observe with computer assisted learning amphibian nerve-muscle experiments.

PRINCIPLE

The sciatic nerve of the frog is a mixed nerve and the maximum velocity is measured by stimulating (with a supramaximal stimulus) all the nerve fibers present in it.

REQUIREMENTS

- Same as that for simple muscle twitch
- Graduated Scale for measuring the distance

PROCEDURE

- Arrange the primary electric circuit by connecting the low voltage terminal, primary coil, and simple key, back to terminal. In the secondary circuit, arrange the secondary coil, short-circuiting key two wires from each terminal to each of the electrodes.
- Adjust the kymograph for fast speed and fast gear.
- Dissect and mount the nerve-muscle preparation. Mount the nerve on both the pairs of the electrodes on the frog board.
- Adjust the position of the electrodes in such a way that one pair is near the muscle, while the other is at the vertebral end.
- Open one of the short-circuiting keys, give the make and the break shocks and find out the maximal stimulus.
- Bring the secondary coil 1 or 2 cm closer to the primary coil, so that the stimulus given is supramaximal.
- Wait for 1 minute, so that the effects of the previous stimulation wane out.
- Adjust the drum, lever, etc., to write on the smoked surface.
- Draw a base line and take a time tracing of 100 vibrations per second below the baseline.
- Stimulate the preparation by stimulating through the electrodes placed near the muscle end.
- Mark the point of contraction. Label it as A.
- Wait for 1 minute. Do not change the position of any instrument.
- After 1 minute stimulate the nerve through the electrodes placed at the vertebral end of the nerve and record the curve.
- Mark the point of contraction and extend it down on the time tracing. Label it as B.
- Mark the point of stimulation. The point of stimulation for both the curves is the same (**Fig. 39.1**).
- From the time tracing, measure the time difference between the two curves in milliseconds.
- Measure the length of the nerve between the central points of the two pairs of the electrodes let it be 'L' cm.
- Deduct the latent period of the first recording (stimulation of muscular end) from the latent period of the second recording (stimulation of vertebral end). The difference in the latent period of the two recordings in milliseconds is taken as time let it be 't' ms.

CALCULATIONS

In t ms the impulse travels through L cm length. Find out the distance it would travel in 1 second (i.e., 1,000 ms).

From the observations determine the velocity of nerve impulse in the sciatic nerve of frog. Velocity = L/t (cm/s)

Express the result in m/s.

The normal conduction velocity in frog's sciatic nerve is about 20–40 m/s.

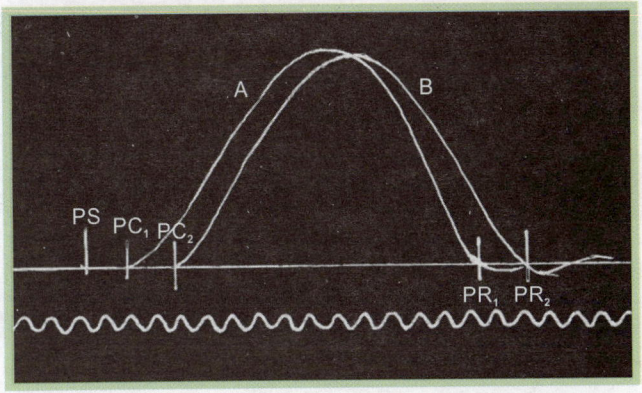

Fig. 39.1: Record for calculating the conduction velocity of the sciatic nerve of frog. (A) the curve obtained when the nerve is stimulated at its muscle end; (B) the record obtained when the nerve is stimulated at its vertebral end.

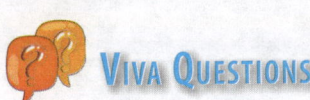

VIVA QUESTIONS

1. **Define an action potential or impulse.**
   An impulse is a self-propagating electrochemical change traveling along the surface of the cell membrane of an excitable cell.
2. **What is the velocity of conduction in frog's sciatic nerve?**
   Around 40 m/s.
3. **What are the factors that affect the velocity of conduction of nerve impulse?**
   » The diameter of the nerve fiber, the velocity increases with diameter
   » Depends on whether the nerve is myelinated or not. It is more in the myelinated nerve than in the nerves without myelin sheath. In the myelinated nerve the impulse travels by saltatory conduction.
   » The pH of the surrounding fluid—within physiological limits, acidosis decreases and alkalosis increases the velocity of conduction.
   » Temperature—within limits increase in temperature increases and hypothermia decreases the velocity of conduction of nerve impulse.
4. **What is the clinical significance of determining the conduction velocity of nerve in humans?**
   Nerve conduction study is used as a medical diagnostic test to evaluate the ability of motor and sensory nerves for conduction of nerve impulses. It helps to detect nerve damage and is also used for the evaluation of diseases of nerve and muscle like myopathy, Lambert-Eaton syndrome, myasthenia gravis, etc.
5. **What is the velocity of conduction of human sciatic nerve?**
   120 m/s.
6. **Give a few conditions where the velocity of nerve conduction is decreased in humans.**
   Diabetic neuropathy, traumatic injury to nerve, Guillain-Barré syndrome, carpal tunnel syndrome and in all peripheral neuropathies velocity of nerve conduction is decreased.

Chapter 40

Normal Cardiogram of Frog

LEARNING OBJECTIVES

- Record a normal cardiogram
- Describe the causes of different waves in the record
- Enumerate the differences between mammalian and amphibian heart

PY3.18: Observe with computer assisted learning amphibian cardiac experiments.

ANATOMY OF THE FROG'S HEART

The frog's heart has only three chambers, two atria (auricles) and one ventricle. The venous blood in the sinus venosus enters the right atrium. From the right atrium it enters the ventricle, where it gets partially mixed up with the arterial blood coming from the left atrium. As the ventricle contracts the blood enters the truncus arteriosus. The blood passes through the pulmonary arteries and the aorta. The blood after getting oxygenated in the lungs is brought to the left atrium through the pulmonary veins. It drains into the ventricle. Normal heart rate in frog is 60 beats/min.

PROCEDURE

- Pith the frog.
- Lay the frog on the dissection board on its back (dorsal surface).
- Fix the upper limbs on the sides with pins.
- Cut the skin in the midline from the jaw to the abdomen with a pair of scissors.
- Take a transverse incision in the skin at the level of the fore limbs.
- Separate the four flaps from the muscles below and reflect them outwards.
- Hold the xiphisternum with forceps and lift it up.
- Cut the muscles of the abdominal wall at the end of the sternum and carefully insert the blunt end of the scissors inside and make a V-shaped incision round its lower end. Take care not to injure the heart.
- Cut along the side of the cartilage upwards till you come across the hard structures of the shoulder girdle.
- With a bone cutting forceps cut the shoulder girdle on either side.
- Separate the sternal piece, totally cutting off all its attachments.
- Observe the heart beating inside the thin pericardium.
- Catch a fold of pericardium at its apex with a small forceps and put a nick on it with a pair of scissors.
- Cut the pericardium up to the base of the heart, taking care not to injure the heart.
- Separate the pericardium completely from the heart so that the heart can be seen beating freely.
- Study the different parts of the heart.

The following structures can be seen:
- The right and left auricles
- The truncus arteriosus which divides into two: the aortic and pulmonary trunks
- The atrioventricular groove

Now invert the heart upwards and identify the following:
- The sinus venosus to which two superior vena cavae and one inferior vena cava opens
- A white transverse crescentic line, where the sinus venosus joins the atria is the site where the autonomic

parasympathetic ganglia (Remak's ganglia) are located.

Measure the rate per minute. It is between 40–60 beats per minute in frog.

The cardiac impulse originates in the sinus venosus and spreads over the atria and the ventricle. The impulse travels along the cardiac muscle fibers and there is no specialized conducting tissue in the frog's heart. The various chambers of the heart contract cyclically in the order of sinus venosus, atria, ventricle and truncus arteriosus.

REQUIREMENTS

Frog, kymograph with smoked drum, Starling's heart lever, myograph stand, frog board, Ringer's solution, forceps, scissors, thread, bent pin, etc.

RECORDING OF THE NORMAL CARDIOGRAM

- Fix the Starling lever on the myograph stand with a frog board. Fix it at such a level that when horizontal, the writing point writes at a desired level on the paper.
- Tie the bent pin to one end of a piece of thread.
- Place the dissected frog with the heart exposed on the frog board attached to the stand, with the head near the rod of the stand, so that the heart comes directly below the lever.
- Fix the frog on the board with pins.
- Fix the pericardium through the base of the heart to the frog board with a pin.
- Hold the ventricle of the frog in between the fingers and the thumb of the left hand and pass the bent pin through the apex of the ventricle. See that the pin does not pass through the cavity of the ventricle.
- Tie the other end of the thread to the heart lever. Keep the thread vertical and taut enough to transmit the myocardial contraction to the writing point of the lever.
- Keep the writing arm of the lever horizontal.
- The lever will now move with each systole and diastole of the heart.
- Put the drum in slow gear and slow speed.
- Adjust the stand so that the lever writes on the paper and obtain a record of about 10 cm long.
- To show the different components of the cardiogram, take recordings at medium and fast speeds.
- Take a time tracing below the record.

OBSERVATION

The upstroke is due to systole and the downstroke is due to diastole or relaxation of cardiac muscle. Each cycle consists

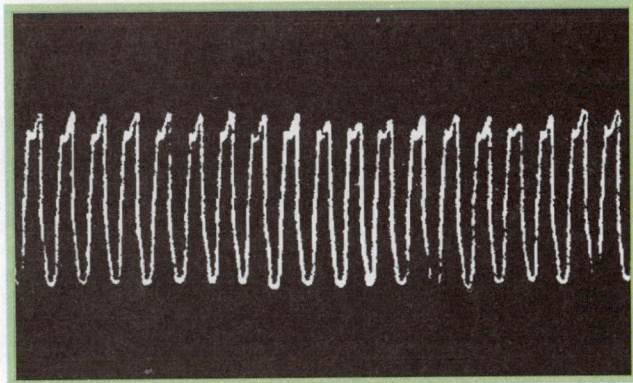

Fig. 40.1: Normal cardiogram of frog recorded at medium speed.

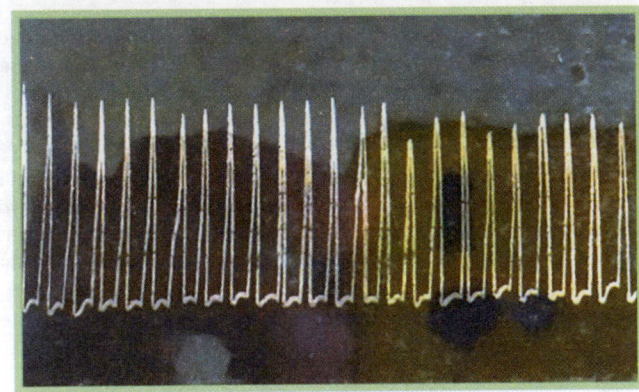

Fig. 40.2: Cardiogram recorded at slow speed.

of a small atrial contraction, which is immediately followed by a large ventricular contraction **(Figs. 40.1 and 40.2)**. This is followed by a small pause. Usually a very small sinus venosus contraction is found to precede the atrial curve and a truncus arteriosus contraction following the ventricular contraction. All these phases can be clearly observed in the record taken on a fast gear and fast speed.

PRECAUTIONS

- While cutting the sternum and the pericardium, care should be taken not to injure the heart.
- The pin should be hooked at the apex through the ventricular musculature. It should not pierce the cavity.
- The thread should be kept vertically and the lever should be placed horizontally.
- The base of the heart should be fixed in order to increase the amplitude of contraction.
- Pour ringer solution over the heart frequently to prevent it from drying.

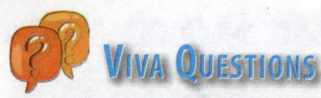

Viva Questions

1. **What are the main differences between amphibian and mammalian hearts?**

Amphibian heart	Mammalian heart
Three chambered—two auricles and one ventricle	Four chambered—two atria and two ventricles
Sinus venosus present	Absent
O_2 and nutrients reach the myocardium by diffusion from the contained blood	Myocardium is supplied by well-developed coronary arteries
Mixed blood is present in the ventricle	Right ventricle contain venous blood and left ventricle contain arterial (oxygenated) blood
Sinus venosus is the pacemaker	SA node is the pacemaker
White crescentic line present in between auricles and sinus venosus	No white crescentic line

2. **Which are the waves seen in the ideal curve and obtained cardiogram?**
   In the ideal curve, four waves are present: A small 's' wave due to contraction of sinus venosus, followed by an 'a' wave due to atrial contraction, a large 'v' wave due to ventricular contraction and a very small insignificant 't' wave due to contraction of truncus arteriosus. In the obtained cardiogram only two waves are seen at slower speeds, the 'a' wave and the 'v' wave, i.e., the atrial and the ventricular components.

3. **Which are the properties of heart that are demonstrated in this experiment?**
   Automaticity, rhythmicity and contractility are demonstrated in this experiment. Automaticity means spontaneous generation of impulses in the heart leading to automatic beating of the heart. This can be clearly demonstrated by cutting the nerve supply of the heart.
   Rhythmicity is demonstrated by noting the rhythmical beating of the heart. Contractility is demonstrated by recording the systole and diastole in the tracings.

4. **Name the ganglia present in the frog's heart.**
   Bidder's, Ludwig's and Remak's ganglia.

5. **Where is the pacemaker of frog's heart located?**
   Sinus venosus is the pacemaker of frog's heart because it generates the maximum rate of impulses.

6. **What is the significance of the white crescentic line?**
   It denotes the junction between auricles and sinus venosus. The parasympathetic ganglia are located here.

7. **While pithing, the spinal cord alone should be destroyed while doing heart experiments. Why?**
   Cardiovascular centers are present in the brain. If they are destroyed there will be alteration in cardiac function.

8. **Name the waves seen in the cardiogram obtained.**
   Atrial (a wave) and ventricular (v wave) components are seen.

9. **What is the normal heart rate of a frog?**
   60 beats/min

Chapter 41

Effect of Temperature on Frog's Heart

LEARNING OBJECTIVES

- Demonstrate the effect of heat and cold on frog's heart
- Explain the changes observed in the recording with changes in temperature and its physiological basis

PY3.18: Observe with computer assisted learning amphibian cardiac experiments.

INTRODUCTION

The effect of heat and cold on sinus venosus and ventricles are studied by applying heat and cold in these areas. There will be a change in the heart rate and amplitude of contraction when heat and cold are applied on sinus venosus. When these are applied on ventricles, there will be no change in the rate but there will be a change in the amplitude of contraction. This proves that sinus venosus is the pace maker of frog's heart.

REQUIREMENTS

All requirements for recording normal cardiogram, spirit lamp, glass blower, small ice pieces.

PROCEDURE

- Expose the heart of a pithed frog and record a normal cardiogram for 10 seconds.
- Heat the glass blower over a flame gently. Blow out air over the back of the hand. See that it is not too hot.
- Now blow the warm air on the sinus venosus and record the effect for 10 seconds.
- Then pour Ringer solution at room temperature over the heart for some time.
- Again take a normal cardiogram.
- Then apply a small piece of ice over the sinus venosus and record the effect.
- Again wash the heart with Ringer solution at room temperature.
- After sometime blow warm air over the ventricle and record the effect.
- Repeat washing with Ringer solution.
- Now apply a small piece of ice over the ventricle on its ventral aspect, i.e., the side opposite to the sinus venosus. This is to prevent melted ice from flowing over the sinus venosus. Record the effect.
- Take a normal cardiogram at room temperature.

(Instead of warm air and ice, warm and cold Ringer solutions can be used. But care should be taken to prevent the solutions from flowing over the sinus venosus while heating and cooling the ventricle).

OBSERVATION

Warmth on sinus venosus increased heart rate but decreased the amplitude of contraction. Cold on sinus venosus decreased the heart rate but increase the force of cardiac contraction **(Fig. 41.1A)**. Change in heart rate is the primary effect. Change in amplitude is only a secondary effect.

Application of warmth on ventricle increased the amplitude of contraction but the heart rate remained unchanged. Cold on ventricle decreased the force of contraction and the heart rate remained unchanged **(Fig. 41.1B)**.

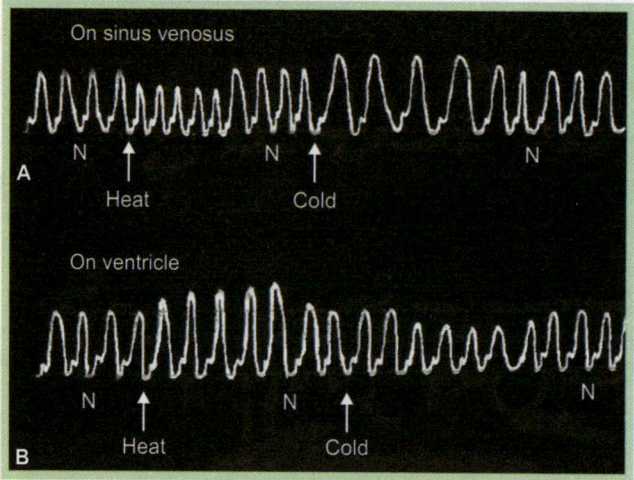

Figs. 41.1A and B: Effect of heat and cold on frog's heart: (A) Effect of heat and cold on sinus venosus; (B) Effect of heat and cold on ventricle.

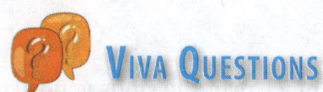 VIVA QUESTIONS

1. **Explain the effect of heat and cold on sinus venosus.**
   Sinus venosus is the pacemaker of frog's heart. So it determines the heart rate. When heat is applied to it, all biological activities are speeded up. So there is increase in heart rate. When heart rate increases, diastolic period is shortened and end-diastolic volume decrease. So the force of contraction decreases obeying Frank-Starling's law. The opposite occurs when cold is applied on sinus venosus.

2. **Explain Frank-Starling's law of heart.**
   The force of contraction of the heart is directly proportional to the end diastolic volume within physiological limits.

3. **What is the effect of heat and cold on ventricle?**
   Ventricle is not the pacemaker. So there is no change in heart rate. When heat is applied, due to increase in metabolism, there is increase in the amplitude of contraction. With cold the amplitude decreases.

Chapter 42

Stannius Ligatures

LEARNING OBJECTIVES

- Demonstrate the effect of first and second stannius ligatures on frog's heart
- Explain the observations seen in the graph obtained

PY3.18: Observe with computer assisted learning amphibian cardiac experiments.

INTRODUCTION

All the parts of the heart can initiate its own impulse. To demonstrate this property of automaticity, this experiment of stannius ligatures is carried out.

Normally the impulse is initiated at the sinus venosus and is conducted to the atria and then to the ventricle. This conduction of the impulse can be blocked by mechanical pressure. Tying thread knots or stannius ligatures at various sites exerts the mechanical pressure.

The first stannius ligature is tied between the sinus venosus and the atria. On tying the ligature, the impulse from sinus venosus is prevented from reaching at the atria. The sinus continues to beat and the atria with the ventricle lie quiescent. After sometime, the atria start initiating their own impulse and the impulse reaches the ventricle and the atria and ventricle start beating independent of the sinus rhythm. The rate of the atrioventricular beat is slower than the sinus rhythm, i.e., they beat at the atrial rhythm.

The second stannius ligature is tied between the atria and the ventricle around the atrioventricular groove. On tying the second ligature the impulse from the atria is prevented from reaching the ventricle. The atria continue to beat while the ventricle lies quiescent. After a short period, the ventricle initiates its own impulse and starts beating independent of the atria. The rate of the ventricular beat is slower than the atrial rhythm, and is described as idioventricular rhythm. Failure of conduction of impulse from one part of the heart to another is described as heart block.

REQUIREMENTS

Cotton thread, cotton wool, Ringer's solution.

PROCEDURE

- Place the drum in slow gear and slow speed.
- Dissect the frog and expose the heart.
- Remove the pericardium completely.
- Lift up the atria and the ventricle with the thumb and two fingers of the left hand.
- Pass the needle with the thread beneath the sinus venosus carefully. Move the thread up and down. It should move freely.
- Remove the needle. Hold the two ends of the thread on either side and bring the thread till it comes behind the junction of the sinus venosus and the atria, i.e., beneath the white crescentic line.
- Tie a loose single knot and leave it.
- Mount the preparation on the board and record a cardiogram for about 10 cm length.
- Now while the record continues, tighten the knot. The Starling lever might move and record a mechanical movement. The heart may show an extra contraction and then the atria and the ventricle will stop.
- This ligature is described as the **first stannius ligature**.
- Obtain a record of about 10 cm length. Only very weak transferred movements of the sinus are recorded. Wait for sometime.
- After an interval of about 5 minutes, the atria will start contracting and then the ventricle will follow this rhythm.
- Obtain a strip of at least 10 cm length.

- Stop the drum. Take the stand with board and the lever away from the cylinder.
- Now pass a piece of thread round the heart just below the ventricle and tie a loose knot around the atrioventricular groove.
- Place the myograph stand with the board and lever in position to write on the paper. Start the drum.
- Take the recording and tighten the knot in the groove between the atria and the ventricle. Mechanical movements of the lever and an extra contraction of the ventricle will be recorded. Then the ventricle will stop. The atria will keep on beating. This ligature is called the **second stannius ligature**.
- Obtain a record of 10 cm length.
- Stop the drum.
- After an interval the ventricle will start beating.
- Start the drum and record the ventricular contractions.
- Obtain a strip of about 10 cm length
- Stop the drum and move the myograph stand away.

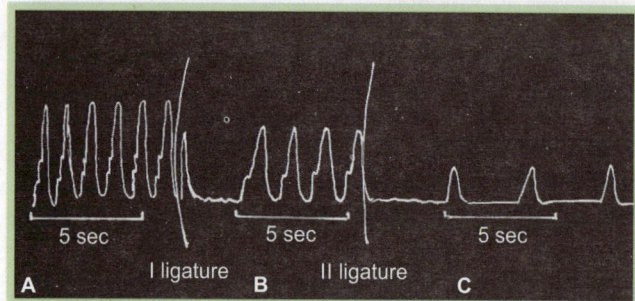

Figs. 42.1A to C: Effect of stannius ligature on frog's heart: (A) Normal cardiogram with a rate of 60/min (sinus rhythm); (B) After applying I ligature between sinus venosus and atria, rate has decreased to 36/min (atrial rhythm); (C) After applying the second ligature between atria and ventricle the rate is only 24/min (idioventricular rhythm).

OBSERVATION (FIGS. 42.1A TO C)

- The record shows that on tying the first stannius ligature the atria and the ventricle stopped contracting. This shows that normally the sinus venosus initiates the rhythm and the atria and the ventricle follow it.
- The atria take sometime before they can initiate their own rhythm. This is due to **override suppression**. The rate of the atrial rhythm is 40 per minute; while the rate of the sinus rhythm is 60 per minute. Thus the atrial rate was slower than the sinus rate.
- On tying the second stannius ligature, the ventricle stopped beating. After sometime ventricle starts beating at its own rhythm.
- The ventricular rate is 15 per minute. It is much slower than the sinus rate. This beat is described as the idioventricular rhythm **(Fig. 42.2)**.

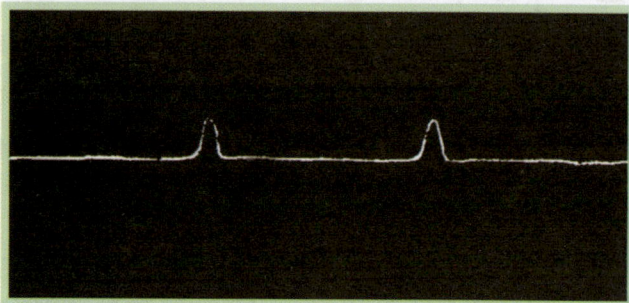

Fig. 42.2: Idioventricular rhythm.

Inference

- Sinus venosus initiates the rhythm and the atria and ventricle follow it. Hence, sinus venosus is called the pacemaker of frog's heart.
- The impulse is initiated at the sinus venosus at a rate more rapid than the one initiated by atria and ventricle.
- Exerting mechanical pressure (by tying the knot) on the heart tissue can stop the conduction of the impulse to the other chambers. This is called heart block.

VIVA QUESTIONS

1. **What is the reason for the quiescent period following the ligatures? Explain the graph obtained.**
   This is due to overdrive suppression. Normally, sinus venosus is the pacemaker and it drives the next chamber, i.e., atria into contraction. After putting the first ligature, the atria and ventricle do not receive any impulse from the pacemaker. So these chambers do not contract. After some time, the atria which is next in hierarchy (order of rhythmicity), start producing impulse of its own. This drives the ventricle also to contract. Atrial and ventricular components are obtained in the cardiogram. But the rate will be slower.
   When the second ligature is applied, the impulse from atria stop suddenly and the heart stop beating producing the second quiescent period. After some time, the ventricle start contracting at its own rhythm called the idioventricular rhythm. Here the cardiogram shows only the ventricular component **(Fig. 42.2)**.

2. **Can the stannius ligatures be applied on mammalian heart?**
   No, first ligature cannot be applied because the sinoatrial node which is the pacemaker is located in the right atrial wall. Second ligature, if applied will occlude the coronary arteries and the heart will not beat due to ischemia. So the desired effect is not obtained.

43

Extrasystole and Compensatory Pause

LEARNING OBJECTIVES

- Demonstrate extrasystole and compensatory pause in frog's heart
- Explain refractory period in frog's heart
- Discuss the reason why cardiac muscle cannot be tetanized

PY3.18: Observe with computer assisted learning amphibian cardiac experiments.

INTRODUCTION

Normally, the ventricle contracts as a result of an impulse coming to it from the atria. But if an artificial extra stimulus is given, it can respond to this extra stimulus depending on whether the stimulus falls in the contraction period or relaxation period. If it falls in the middle third of the relaxation period, the heart responds by an extra contraction called *extrasystole*. The next normal impulse (coming from sinus to the ventricle) then usually falls in the refractory period of the extrasystole. The ventricle, therefore, does not respond to it and remains quiet till the second normal impulse reaches it. This period of inactivity is described as *compensatory pause*. Extrasystole is similar to superposition in skeletal muscle.

Apparatus

Kymograph, myograph stand, frog board, heart lever, connections for induced current, time tracer.

Procedure

- The drum is adjusted for slow gear and fast speed.
- Make electrical connections for induced current. Do not include the kymograph in the primary circuit. Adjust for a break shock.
- Expose the heart, remove the pericardium and mount it on the frog board. Fix the base of the heart and attach its apex to the Starling heart lever.
- Adjust the lever on writing points to write on the paper.
- Fix the electrode on the myograph stand using X-block and femur clamp at the level of the heart.
- Adjust the wires of the electrodes to just touch the sides of the ventricle without hindering the normal beating of the heart.
- Adjust the myograph stand so that the lever writes on the paper.
- Start the drum and record a normal cardiogram.
- Open the short-circuiting key in the secondary circuit, and then give a break shock during the earlier part of the diastole (i.e., during the downstroke of the lever) by pressing and releasing the simple key and record the result.
- Similarly give break shock during the systole (i.e., during the upward movement of the lever).
- Stop the drum.

Observations

- There is a pause following the extra contraction.
- After the pause, the heart has started contracting again in a normal way.
- The duration of the extra contraction and the pause together is equal to one normal cycle (**Fig. 43.1**).

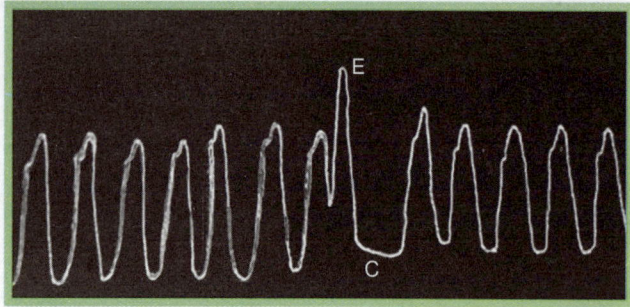

Fig. 43.1: Extrasystole and compensatory pause in frog's heart when an extra stimulus of higher strength is applied to the heart after 1/3 of diastole. E: Extrasystole; C: Compensatory pause.

CONCLUSIONS

The heart can respond to extraneous stimulation. The stimulus has to be given during diastole. The additional contraction is described as extrasystole or premature beat.

The pause following the extrasystole is called *compensatory pause*. This pause is because, when the next normal impulse reaches the heart, it will be in the absolute refractory period of the extrasystole. So, it will not respond. After the pause, the heart picks up its own rhythm.

The beat following the compensatory pause will be of higher amplitude. This is called *post-extrasystolic potentiation*. The cause for this is increased availability of Ca^{2+} in the sarcoplasm due to the extra beat.

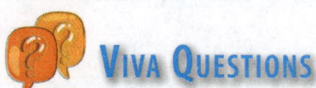

Viva Questions

1. **What is extrasystole?**
   When the ventricle is stimulated by a stronger stimulus than normal after 1/3rd of diastole (relaxation), it responds by an extra contraction. This is called extrasystole or premature contraction. This is followed by a period of rest called compensatory pause.

2. **What is the reason for the compensatory pause? Give its advantage.**
   During extrasystole, when the normal cardiac impulse from the pacemaker reaches the heart, it will be in the absolute refractory period of the previous contraction. So the normal impulse cannot produce an effect. The ventricle has to wait for the next normal impulse to arrive before it can contract. This brief pause is referred to as compensatory pause.
   The duration from the beginning of the beat in which the extrasystole is present to the beginning of the next normal beat is equal to two cardiac cycles.
   Compensatory pause is advantageous to the myocardium because it gets a period of rest during which ventricular filling occurs.

3. **The beat following the compensatory pause will be of greater amplitude. Give the reason.**
   It is due to post-extrasystolic potentiation. The availability of calcium ions will be more in the next beat after extrasystole.

Chapter 44

Effect of Vagal Stimulation on Frog's Heart

LEARNING OBJECTIVES

- Dissect and expose the vagosympathetic trunk on the right side of frog
- Demonstrate the effect of vagal stimulation on heart
- Explain the physiological basis of vagal inhibition and vagal escape

PY3.18: Observe with computer assisted learning amphibian cardiac experiments.

INTRODUCTION

The sympathetic and parasympathetic divisions of the autonomic nervous system supply the heart. The preganglionic parasympathetic fibers arise from the vagal nucleus in the medulla. They travel in the vagus nerve and reach the heart through its cardiac branches. These fibers relay in the postganglionic nerve plexuses containing nerve cells within the heart.

The plexuses are two in number in the frog's heart. One is at the junction of the sinus venosus and the atria, which is called *Remak's ganglion*. It is identified as a whitish crescentic area. The other plexus is at the atrioventricular junction and is named *Bidder's ganglion*. The postganglionic parasympathetic fibers arise from these cells and supply the sinus venosus, the atria and the proximal part of the ventricle. The parasympathetic nerve fibers are inhibitory to the heart.

The sympathetic nerve fibers are excitatory. The preganglionic fibers arise from the intermediolateral horn cells in the spinal cord. These fibers come out with the spinal nerves. They separate from the spinal nerve as white rami communicantes and reach the paravertebral sympathetic ganglia. Postganglionic fibers come out as grey rami communicantes. They join the spinal nerves again. These postganglionic fibers again leave the spinal nerves to join the blood vessels and reach the heart. The cardiac postganglionic sympathetic fibers arising from the upper one or two paravertebral sympathetic ganglia join the vagus nerve after leaving the cranial cavity.

The vagus nerve is a mixed nerve containing both sympathetic and parasympathetic fibers and is referred to as the vagosympathetic trunk. It contains the vagal preganglionic and the sympathetic postganglionic fibers. On mild stimulation of the vagus nerve, only the para sympathetic inhibitory vagal effects are seen. The sympathetic influence is minimal.

Procedure

Exposure of Vagosympathetic Trunk

- Pith the frog and expose the heart
- Remove the thin sheet of muscle tissue together with connective tissue covering the area at the base of the heart.
- Two thin and flat muscles are then exposed, the omohyoid and the sternohyoid muscle. Remove them.
- Stretch out the upper limbs laterally. A triangular mass of muscle with a shining tendon is seen deep in this area, running from above downwards and laterally. It is the inferior levator scapulae muscle.
- Crossing across the muscle is a branch of the carotid artery. After crossing the muscle, it runs along the lower border of the petrohyoid muscle. Along the upper border of this artery runs the laryngeal nerve while the vagus nerve runs along its lower border. Both are thin nerves.
- Isolate the vagus nerve carefully by means of a thin glass hook and pass a thread beneath the nerve. Handle the nerve with great care.

- Keep the area moist by pouring Ringer solution over the nerve.
- Lift up the nerve with the thread and separate it over a length as long as possible.
- Introduce a glass rod behind the nerve and place it in such a way that the nerve alone can be stimulated without stimulating other structures.

Stimulation of Vagosympathetic Trunk

- Adjust the kymograph for slow gear and slow speed. Include the Neef's hammer in the primary circuit.
- Mount the frog on the stand and attach the heart lever to it. Obtain a normal cardiogram.
- Place the electrodes connected to the secondary coil below the right vagus nerve in such a way that both the electrodes touch the nerve.
- Place a fold of dry filter paper below the electrodes so that they do not touch any other tissue. This will prevent unnecessary stimulation of other tissues.
- Adjust the myograph stand to write on the drum.
- Start the drum and record a normal cardiogram.
- While the record is being obtained open the short-circuiting key and close the simple key in the primary circuit to start the stimulation of vagus.
- Stimulate the right vagus with different strengths of current through the Neef's hammer while the cardiogram is being recorded.
- Label the point of stimulation on the paper. Note the time.
- Stimulate with strong current.
- The heart will stop suddenly in diastole. Continue the stimulation and the trace obtained will show a straight line.
- After a period varying from 15 seconds to few minutes, the heart resumes its activity in spite of continuation of the stimulation. Note the time.
- Continue to record till the trace shows some rhythmic activity of the heart.
- Stop stimulation and record a normal cardiogram.
- It is better to repeat the procedure using the left vagus also.

Observations

- With weak stimulation of vagus nerve, the heart rate and the force of contraction progressively decreases. Acetylcholine released at the nerve ending reduces the heart rate, slows the velocity of conduction and diminishes the force of contraction of the heart.
- On continued stimulation of the vagus with strong current, the heart stops in diastole.
- After some time, despite continued vagal stimulation, the heart resumes its activity. This is called *vagal escape* (Fig. 44.1). The usual time for vagal escape varies from 1/2 to 5 minutes.

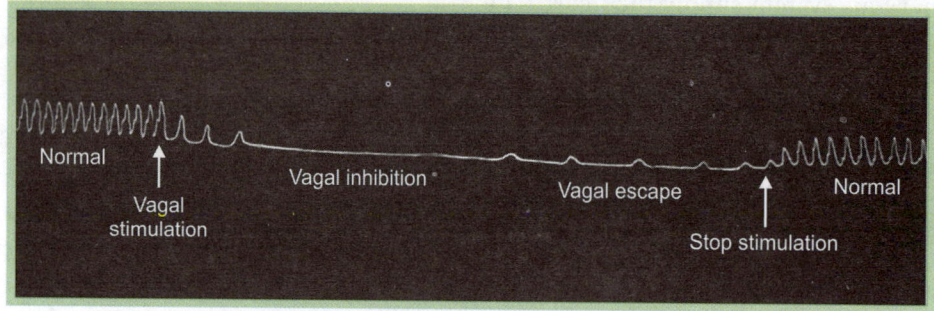

Fig. 44.1: Effect of vagal stimulation on frog's heart.

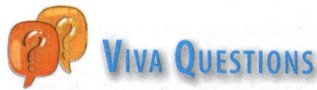 VIVA QUESTIONS

1. **What is vagal inhibition and vagal escape?**
   When the vagus nerve is stimulated continuously, the heart stops for some time. This is vagal inhibition. The acetylcholine liberated at the vagal endings inhibits the heart. When the stimulation is continued, after some time it starts beating at a slower rate. This is *vagal escape*.
2. **What are the causes of vagal escape?**
   » Exhaustion of stored acetylcholine in the nerve.
   » Increased destruction of acetylcholine by the heart tissue.
   » Liberation of adrenaline by simultaneous stimulation of the sympathetic fibers and the effect of acetylcholine being antagonized by adrenaline.
   » Ventricle starts producing impulse of its own (idioventricular rhythm) since it is devoid of vagal supply.

3. **Name the parasympathetic ganglia in the frog's heart.**
   Remak's ganglia, Ludwig's ganglia and Bidder's ganglia.
4. **What is the significance of the white crescentic line in frog's heart?**
   The parasympathetic ganglia are located in the white crescentic line. Stimulation of this part produces effects similar to that of vagal stimulation.
5. **What is meant by vagal tone in humans?**
   The slow stream of impulses passing through the vagus nerve continuously to the heart is known as *vagal tone*. It is responsible for maintaining the heart rate at the normal level, i.e., at about 70–80 beats per minute. After cutting the vagal supply to the heart, the heart rate increases to 160–180 beats/min. The difference between the resting heart rate before and after vagotomy gives a measure of the degree of vagal tone.
6. **What will be the heart rate if both the sympathetic and parasympathetic supply to the heart are blocked?**
   Heart rate increases to about 100 beats/min.
7. **Give the innervation of human heart.**
   Sympathetic and parasympathetic divisions of autonomic nervous system (ANS) innervate heart. Sympathetic division coming from the intermediolateral horn cells of T1 to T5 segments of spinal cord supply all parts of the heart. Parasympathetic supply is through the vagus nerves, which supply the atria and the nodal tissue. Right vagus supplies the SA (sinoatrial) node and left vagus supply the AV (atrioventricular) node. Ventricle is devoid of parasympathetic supply.
8. **What are the effects of stimulation of the nerves to the heart?**
   Sympathetic stimulation increases heart rate (positive chronotropic effect), force of contraction (positive inotropic effect), velocity of conduction of impulse (positive dromotropic effect), and excitability of the myocardium (positive bathmotropic effect). Parasympathetic stimulation produces the opposite effects.
9. **Why do you choose the right vagus for stimulation?**
   Right vagus supplies the pacemaker.

Chapter 45

Effect of Drugs and Ions on Isolated Frog's Heart

LEARNING OBJECTIVES

- Demonstrate the effect of adrenaline and acetyl choline on frog's heart
- Demonstrate the effect of ions on frog's heart
- Explain the physiological basis of the effects obtained

PY3.18: Observe with computer assisted learning amphibian cardiac experiments.

PRINCIPLE

The effect of ions and drugs can be studied by perfusing the isolated frog's heart with the desired solution. There will be changes in the heart rate and force of contraction of heart. There is no need to supply O_2 to the frog's heart because the O_2 dissolved in the perfusion fluid is sufficient to keep the heart alive during the experiment.

REQUIREMENTS

All apparatus for recording normal cardiogram, Ringer's solution, perfusion funnel, Syme's cannula, solutions of 1% $CaCl_2$, 1% KCl, 1% NaCl, 1:10,000 adrenaline and 1:100,000 acetylcholine.

The perfusion funnel has a side tube and a tail fitted with a three-way tap. The solution in the funnel can be directed to the side tube or to the tail to drain it or can be closed in both ways. The side tube is connected to the side tube of the cannula by means of a rubber tube.

The Syme's cannula is a glass cannula with a side tube and a nozzle. The nozzle has a tip and bulbous portion and neck. The side tube of the cannula is connected to the side tube of the funnel by means of a rubber tube (**Fig. 45.1**).

PROCEDURE

- Fix two burette clamps on the myograph stand. To the lower clamp, fix the perfusion funnel. The upper one is for fixing the cannula.

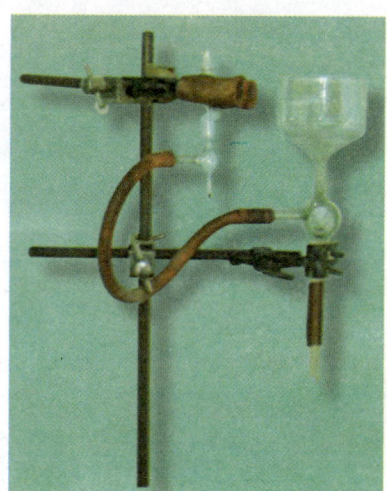

Fig. 45.1: Syme's cannula and perfusion funnel.

- Connect the side tubes of the funnel and cannula by rubber tube.
- Close the funnel using the three-way tap in such a way that no fluid enters into the side tube or tail of the funnel.
- Fill the funnel with Ringer's solution.
- Adjust the drum for slow gear and medium speed.
- Pith the frog and expose the heart. Remove the pericardium.
- Lift the heart up and pass a fine thread with the help of a needle behind the sinus venosus.
- With the help of small sharp scissors, make a small nick in the sinus venosus as low as possible.
- Fill the cannula with Ringer's solution.
- Introduce the tip of the Syme's cannula through the slit into the sinus venosus in a direction towards the heart.

- Tie the thread just over the constriction in the nozzle and tighten it.
- Cut the tissues around the heart and take the heart out along with the cannula.
- Connect the cannula with the perfusion funnel containing Ringer's solution.
- Open the three-way tap to allow Ringer's solution to flow into the cannula.
- Fix the cannula in the burette clamp and adjust the height of the solution in the cannula to about 2 cm by lowering or raising the perfusion funnel for maintaining a constant perfusion pressure.
- Connect the hook of the heart lever to the apex of the heart.
- Perfuse the heart and record a normal cardiogram.
- Now study the effect of ions and drugs on frog's heart.
- The agents should be introduced into the cannula, one agent at a time.
- After adding one agent, record the effect on the drum, wait for some time so that the heart resumes to normal.
- Then add the next agent and so on.

Agents introduced are:
- 1–2 mL of 1% NaCl
- 1 mL of 1% KCl
- 1 mL of 1% $CaCl_2$
- 0.5 mL of 1 in 100,000 solutions of adrenaline
- 0.5 mL of 1 in 1,000,000 acetylcholine solution.

Record the effects of all these agents, label carefully and write down the observations in a tabular column.

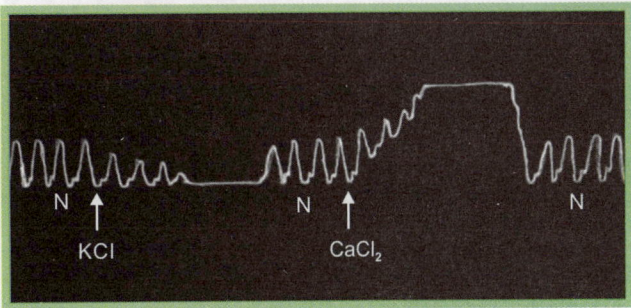

Fig. 45.2: Effect of KCl and $CaCl_2$ on frog's heart.

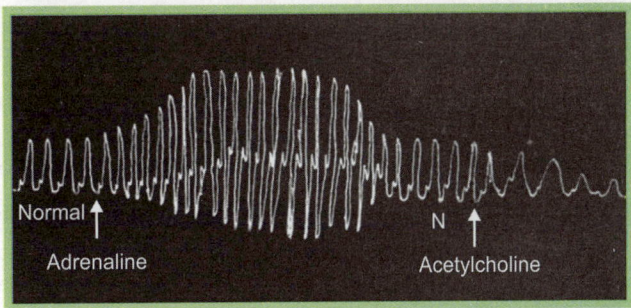

Fig. 45.3: Effect of drugs on frog's heart. Effect of adrenaline (note the increase in the heart rate and amplitude of contraction), acetylcholine (note the decrease in rate and amplitude) N: Normal cardiogram.

Agents	Effects
$CaCl_2$	No effect on heart rate. The amplitude of contraction increases and finally the heart stops in systole **(Fig. 45.2)**
KCl	Heart rate decreases and finally heart stops in diastole **(Fig. 45.2)**
NaCl	No change in heart rate. Amplitude of contraction decreases
Adrenaline	Increase in heart rate and force of contraction **(Fig. 45.3)**
Acetylcholine	Decrease in heart rate and force of contraction **(Fig. 45.3)**.

PRECAUTIONS

- Before introducing the cannula into the sinus venosus, gently squeeze the ventricle to remove blood from the chambers. Otherwise blood clot may obstruct the flow through the nozzle.
- The height of the solution in the cannula should be adjusted to about 2 cm throughout the experiment.
- Isolation of heart and perfusion should be done quickly.

VIVA QUESTIONS

1. **What are the effects of Ca, K, Na, adrenaline and acetylcholine on frog's heart?**
   Refer the above table.
2. **Name a drug that block the action of acetylcholine on heart.**
   Atropine.

Section 4: Biophysics Experiments

46. Cathode Ray Oscilloscope
47. Electrocardiography
48. Spirometry
49. Stethography
50. Perimetry
51. Electromyography
52. Audiometry
53. Ergography
54. Peak Expiratory Flow Rate
55. Ophthalmoscopy
56. Harvard Step Test
57. Cardiovascular Autonomic Function Tests

Chapter 46

Cathode Ray Oscilloscope

INTRODUCTION

The cathode ray oscilloscope (CRO) is an electronic recording device which provides visual display of electrical signals **(Fig. 46.1)**.

CRO consists of a special type of evacuated tube with a narrow end and a broad end **(Fig. 46.2)**. At the narrow end is a cathode, usually a Tungsten filament. In front of the cathode, there are two anodes. Cathode and anode are connected to a power supply of high voltage (2 KV). When high voltage is applied, cathode is heated and emits electrons by thermionic emission.

Electrons emitted are collimated, focused and brought to a narrow beam by anode. This beam is accelerated towards the fluorescent screen at the broad end of the tube by **accelerating anode** placed behind the screen. When electrons strike the screen, it is seen as a visible spot of light on the screen. The intensity of the spot of light can be varied by means of a **control grid** placed in front of the cathode. As the beam moves forward, there is a set of **X plates**, one on either side of the beam. These plates are connected to a sweep generator, which produces a **saw-toothed voltage**.

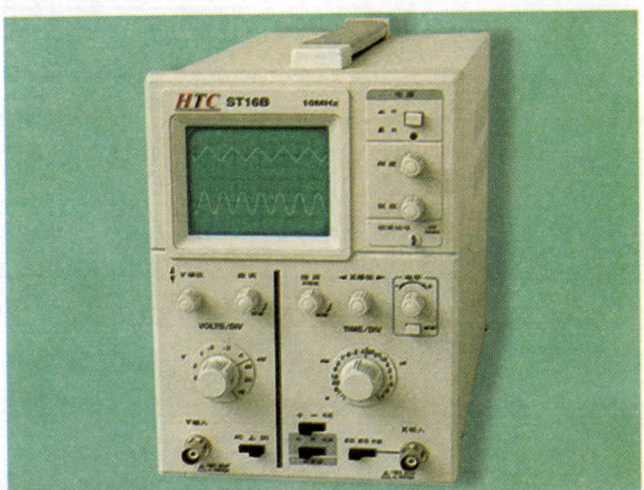

Fig. 46.1: Cathode ray oscilloscope.

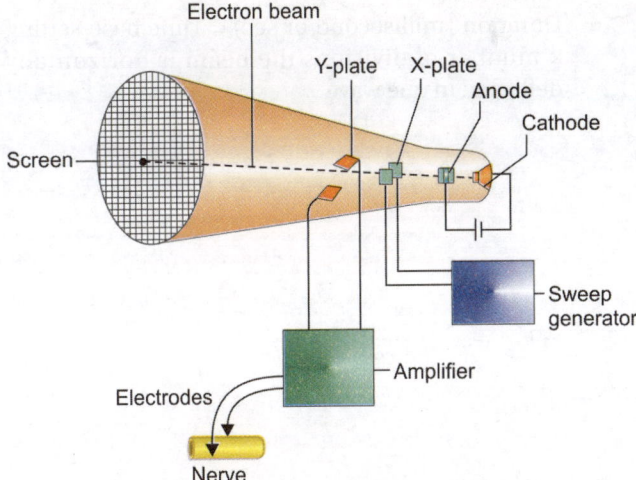

Fig. 46.2: Cathode ray oscilloscope (inner details).

The plates are made alternatively positive so that the beam sweeps in the horizontal direction across the screen. In front of X plates, there are two **Y plates** placed above and below the electron beam and this is connected to the amplifier. The amplifier is connected to the electrodes. If the upper plate is positive, the beam moves in the upward direction and *vice versa*. Any changes in the potential occurring are recorded as vertical deflections of the beam, as it moves across the tube. The screen is graduated in the X and Y-axes. X-axis represents time and Y-axis represents the amplitude of the signal.

Controls on the Panel

- Power switch to switch on or off the instrument.
- Intensity adjustment to adjust the intensity of the electron beam.
- Focus to vary the size of the spot of light.
- Position control which consists of two knobs, one for adjusting the circuital position and the other for horizontal position.
- Vertical gain to select the sensitivity of the amplifier, i.e., the amplitude of movement of the electron beam for a

particular potential can be adjusted. As the vertical gain, adjustment can be done for a wide range of potentials, CRO can be used to record even weak action potentials.
- Input knob is used to feed the signal, which can be visualized in the CRO.
- Time base knob is used to select the sweep speed. The range available is from 0.5 ms/div to 0.2 ms/div. If the time base knob is set at 0.2 ms/div, it means that the beam will take 0.2 second to travel across one division on the screen. From the display of the bioelectrical potentials on the screen, we can calculate the amplitude, duration and frequency of the action potential.
  - Amplitude (V or mv) = Vertical gain setting × number of divisions the beam is vertically deflected in one wave
  - Duration (millisecond or sec) = Time base setting × number of divisions the beam is horizontally deflected in one wave
  - Frequency = Time base setting × number of complete pulse visualized on the screen.

Precautions

Keep the intensity of the beam at the minimal level. The spot of light should not be allowed to remain stationary for long periods as it can damage the screen.

Uses of Cathode Ray Oscilloscope

- Helps to display bioelectrical potentials like nerve action potential, electromyogram, electrocardiogram, electroencephalogram, electroretinogram, etc.
- Used to calibrate electronic instruments.
- Used as cardiac monitors in intensive coronary care unit.
- Used in plotting strength-duration curve to study the excitability of a tissue.

47

Electrocardiography

LEARNING OBJECTIVES

- Record the ECG of the subject provided and analyze it
- Explain the physiological basis of the waves, segments and intervals in the record obtained
- Determine the heart rate from the ECG
- Discuss the significance of PR interval

PY5.13: Record and interpret normal ECG in a volunteer or simulated environment.

INTRODUCTION

Electrocardiography is the technique of recording the electrical activity of the heart during the different phases of cardiac cycle by placing electrodes on the surface of the body. The record obtained is called electrocardiogram.

ELECTROCARDIOGRAPH

Electrocardiograph is the instrument used to record the electrical activity of heart and the record obtained is **electrocardiogram**. Electrodes are placed on the surface of the body since the electrical activity from the heart spreads to the tissues and body fluids and will be conducted to the surface of the body.

Modern instrument has three parts **(Fig. 47.1)**:
1. Electrodes
2. Amplifier
3. An instrument to run the recording paper at the desired speed in paper recording

Electrodes

Electrodes, which conduct electric current, are fixed on suitable body surfaces. Leads are a combination of electrodes, which can pick up electrical activity from the surface of the body.

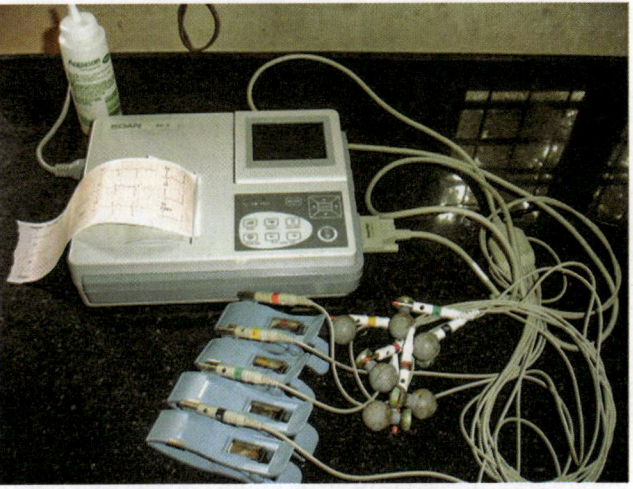

Fig. 47.1: Electrocardiograph showing the limb leads and the chest leads.

There are two types of leads:
1. Bipolar leads
2. Unipolar leads

Bipolar Leads

Here, both the electrodes pick up electrical activity, and potential difference between the two electrodes is recorded. Absence of any deflection indicates that the two electrodes are equipotential. Any recorded deflection indicates a difference in the electric potential between the two electrodes.

Bipolar Limb Leads

They are also known as **standard limb leads**. Einthoven used these leads and he selected three points in the body.
1. Junction between right arm and trunk
2. Junction between left arm and trunk
3. Junction between left foot and trunk

When the above three points are joined together, an equilateral triangle is obtained. Heart is supposed to be in the center of this triangle. This is known as Einthoven's triangle. There are three standard limb leads: lead I, lead II and lead III.
- Lead I connect right arm and left arm with the negative terminal on right arm.
- Lead II is between right arm and left foot with negative terminal on RA.
- Lead III is between left arm and left foot with left arm negative.

The leads are so arranged that positive deflections are obtained in all the leads. Maximum amplitude is obtained in lead II (LII) and it is the sum of the potential obtained in LI and LIII. Einthoven made another postulate stating that the recording of potential is same if the leads are placed in the distal part of extremities as they are extensions from the body and the electrical activity will be conducted to the distal parts (*see* **Fig. 47.3**).

Unipolar Leads

One electrode is kept at **zero potential** and the other electrode is the **active electrode**. Electrode at zero potential is called **indifferent electrode** and the active electrode is called **exploring electrode**. The **active electrode** when placed on a surface of the body, records the changes of potential in this area as compared to the constant potential of the indifferent electrode. An upward deflection in the records obtained indicates a zone of negativity under the exploring electrode.

Unipolar recording is better than bipolar recording. An upward deflection is obtained when the active electrode becomes positive relative to the indifferent electrode and a downward deflection is obtained when the active electrode becomes negative.

Depending on whether the lead is placed on the chest or limb, it is divided into:
- Unipolar limb leads
- Unipolar chest leads

Unipolar Limb Leads

One electrode is placed on distal part of one limb and the other electrode should be at zero potential. Exploring electrode or active electrode is placed in the right arm, left arm or left foot.

Indifferent electrode is designated as V. So, the leads are VR, VL and VF. Indifferent electrode is made by connecting the three limbs, i.e., right arm, left arm and left foot each through a non-inductive high resistance of 5,000 Ω to a common terminal. The indifferent electrode is connected to the negative terminal and the active electrode to the positive terminal of the electrocardiograph.

Augmented unipolar limb leads: Nowadays, modified form of unipolar limb lead is used called **augmented unipolar limb lead** (aV), which gives magnified amplitude. E Goldberger introduced this technique. Here, the limb in which exploring electrode is connected is not connected to indifferent electrode. When such a method is used the record is designated by a prefix 'a' standing for the word augmented. Thus aVR, aVL and aVF records are obtained by disconnecting the right forearm, left forearm and the left foot each time from the central terminus and placing the exploring electrode on each of them in turn respectively. It denotes the potentials picked up at the right arm, left arm and left foot (*see* **Fig. 47.3**).

In augmented unipolar limb leads, the magnification is one and a half times. For example,

aVR = 3/2 VR.

Unipolar Chest Leads

Chest lead gives a greater magnitude of potential as the electrode is near the heart. Exploring electrode is placed on the chest and indifferent electrode is formed by connecting right arm (RA), LA and LF each through a high resistance of 5,000 Ω. Depending on the position of the exploring electrode on the chest, there are 6 unipolar chest leads: V1 to V6. V1 means a record obtained by using the unipolar method while the active electrode is placed on the precordium at the fourth right intercostal space on the sternal border (*see* **Fig. 47.3**).
- V1 at the fourth right intercostal space (RICS) on the lateral sternal border
- V2 at the 4th LICS on the left sternal border
- V3 midway between V2 and V4
- V4 on the 5th LICS in the midclavicular line
- V5 on the 5th LICS in the anterior axillary line
- V6 on the 5th LICS in the midaxillary line

12 leads are used clinically. They are leads I, II, III, aVR, aVL, aVF, V1, V2, V3, V4, V5 and V6.

Other leads used in diseased conditions are **esophageal lead** and **intracardiac lead**.

Amplifier

The amplifier present inside the instrument is a **differential amplifier**, i.e., it amplifies only biological signals. Output from the amplifier goes to the recording device.

Recording Device

The different types of recording devices are:
- Cathode ray oscilloscope (CRO)
- Paper recording
- Tape recording
- Telemetry

Recording in CRO

Cathode ray oscilloscope is the ideal instrument for the measurement of the strength and direction of the current because of absence of inertia. But amplification of the current is essential before a satisfactory record is obtained. A biological amplifier is used which magnifies only biological signals. The signal from the amplifier is connected to the Y plate of CRO. This type of recording is used in the **intensive coronary care unit** in cardiac monitors where continuous recording of ECG is shown in the CRO. A positive or upward deflection means that the depolarization wave is moving toward the electrode concerned and vice versa.

Paper Recording

Heated Stylus Method

This is the most commonly used method. The signal from the amplifier passes through a coil suspended between the two poles of a powerful electromagnet. When the signal passes through the coil, the coil will deflect depending on the nature of the signal. These deflections are written on a paper by means of a stylus attached to the coil. The paper is continuously moving by means of a motor at a speed of 25 mm/s. This method is called heated stylus method as the stylus gets heated when current passes through it. The paper is a **thermosensitive** paper which is actually a black paper over which a white thermosensitive coating is applied. When the heated stylus moves over the paper, the white coating is removed and at these regions a black recording is obtained on a white background.

ECG Paper

ECG is recorded on a special type of paper, which is graduated in the X-axis and in the Y-axis. **X-axis** denotes time in seconds and **Y-axis** denotes amplitude in mV. In X-axis, 1 second is divided into five big squares and each big square is divided into five small divisions. In the X-axis, as the paper moves at a speed of 25 mm/s, in every second the stylus moves through 25 small divisions or five large squares. Thus in the X-axis, one smallest division represents 1/25th of a second or 0.04 sec.

Y-axis represents amplitude of the signal and it is calibrated in such a way that one large square represents 0.5 mV. One large square is divided into five small divisions so that the smallest division in the Y-axis represents 0.1 mV (Fig. 47.2).

Standardization

Standardization is the technique of adjusting the sensitivity of the stylus to give a vertical deflection of 10 small divisions in the ECG paper on application of a voltage of 1 mV. Thus one small division in the Y-axis represents 0.1 mV. The recording is arranged in such a way that a potential difference of 1 mV draws a height of 1 cm on the Y-axis

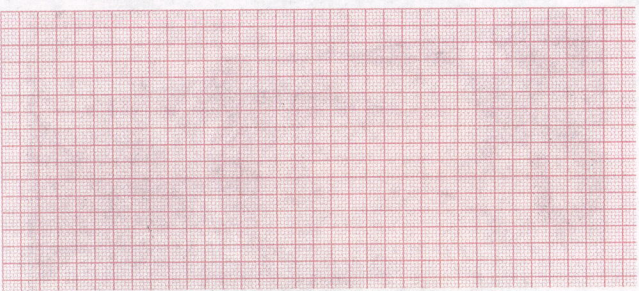

Fig. 47.2: ECG paper [one smallest division (1 mm) in the X-axis denotes 0.04 seconds and one smallest division (1 mm) in the Y-axis denotes 0.1 mV].

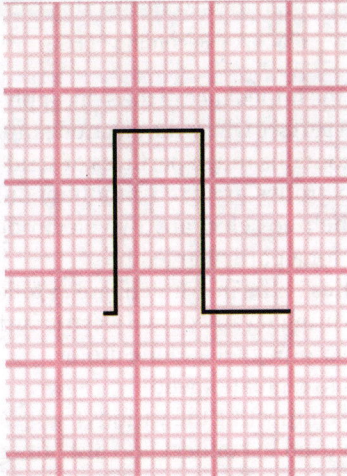

Fig. 47.3: Standardization in the ECG paper so that one small division on the Y-axis represents 0.1 mV.

(Fig. 47.3). Every instrument before use should be checked and adjusted to give this proportion. This is described as calibrating the instrument. Standardization helps in calculating the amplitude of different waves in the ECG.

Tape Recorder Recording

Tape recorder recording of ECG is also called **Holter technique** in which the patient can do his daily activities with simultaneous recording of ECG. The signals are stored in a magnetic tape and can be analyzed at a later date. The effect of exercise can also be recorded by this method.

Telemetry

In telemetry, ECG can be recorded through telephone wires and can be displayed in a computer at a distance. Arrhythmias and other cardiac abnormalities can be assessed in this technique.

METHOD

Paper Recording

- Recording of ECG is done with the subject in the supine position.

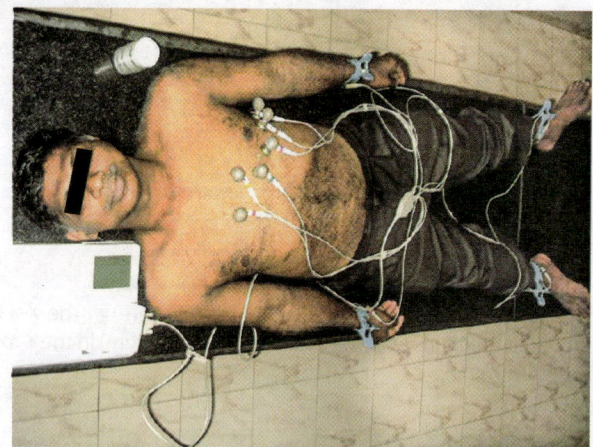

Fig. 47.4: Recording of ECG.

- To reduce the impedance of the skin, apply a special jelly on the skin surface where the electrodes are to be placed. The jelly contains rough particles of sand or glass.
- All the electrodes are fixed simultaneously. Switches or knobs help to select any two electrodes, which are necessary for a particular lead.
- The switches in the instrument are as follows:
  - Switch bringing an external electric current to supply the electromagnet and the motor
  - Switch to regulate speed
  - Switch connecting the various leads
  - Switch used to connect and disconnect the subject from the recording apparatus
  - Switch is used to standardize the instrument.
- Tie the electrodes on the right arm, left arm and left leg. The chest lead is placed over the precordium. *Earthing is done on the right leg* **(Fig. 47.4)**.
- Confirm that the subject is under complete physical and mental rest.
- Confirm that all the lead electrodes are making good electrical contacts with the body surface.
- Calibrate the machine before obtaining the lead records and obtain a record of calibration first.
- Using the lead selector knob in the instrument, the 12 different leads can be selected while recording ECG.
- After obtaining the record, note down the name, age, sex of the subject and also the date.
- Calculate the duration in seconds and the amplitude in millivolt for each wave of ECG. Also calculate the duration of the various segments and intervals. Compare it with normal and see whether there is any abnormality. The heart rate can be calculated from the R-R interval if the heart rate is regular.
- If there is an abnormality in the rhythm, a long strip of lead II can be taken.

Observation

Refer **Figures 47.5 to 47.7.**

Normal Electrocardiogram

The method of naming the various waves is the same in the record obtained at the standard bipolar limb leads and in the unipolar leads. The letters denote the waves associated with the activity of the various parts of the heart tissue during each cardiac cycle P, Q, R, S, T and U.

The first wave *whether positive or negative* is called the 'P' wave. It is due to the activity of the atria. QRS complex follows the P wave. The *first positive* wave following the P wave is called the 'R' wave. The *negative wave*, which precedes 'R', is labelled as 'Q' and the *negative wave*, which follows the R wave, is labelled as 'S'. *All the three waves of QRS complex need not be present in every record.* Only one or any two of the waves from the complex can be present. The complex is due to ventricular activity.

The wave following the QRS complex whether positive or negative is labelled as 'T' and the one following T is labelled as 'U'.

The record runs at isoelectric levels between P, QRS complex, T and U.

The normal pattern of ECG varies with the various leads used. In the standard limb leads, the pattern is almost similar except for the amplitude of the potential. The amplitude is maximal for lead II and is taken as the typical ECG of a cardiac cycle **(Fig. 47.6)**.

In augmented unipolar limb leads, the deflections vary in amplitude and direction according to the position of the exploring electrode. In aVR, the deflections are negative because the depolarizing and the repolarizing waves travel away from the exploring electrode **(Fig. 47.5)**. In aVL and aVF, the deflections are predominantly positive.

In the precordial leads (V1 to V6), the configuration of the complexes in the ECG is determined largely by the spatial position of the heart in relation to the three limb lead positions **(Fig. 47.7)**.

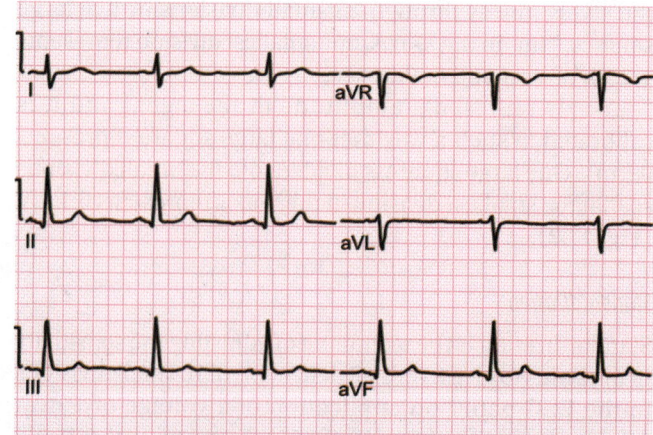

Fig. 47.5: Normal ECG in limb leads (LI, LII, LIII, aVR, aVL and aVF). Note that the waves are negative in aVR.

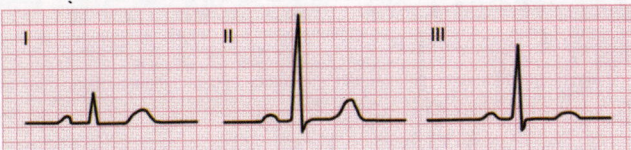

Fig. 47.6: Normal pattern of ECG in the standard limb leads (LI, LII and LIII). Note that the amplitude of the wave is maximal in LII.

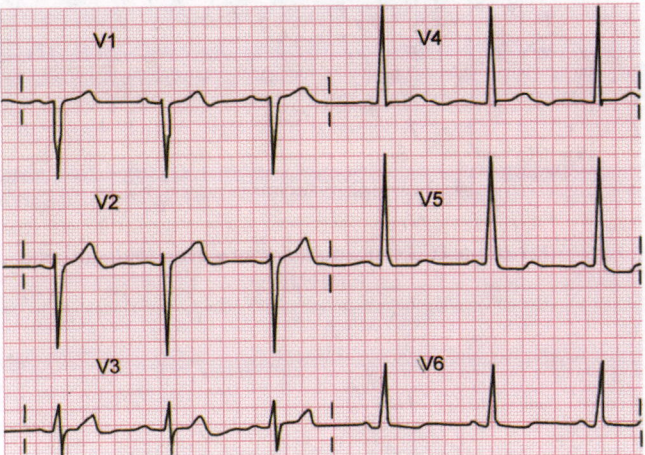

Fig. 47.7: Normal ECG in chest leads (V1–V6).

P Wave

- The cardiac impulse arises at the sinoatrial node and spreads through the atrial muscle fibers to reach the atrioventricular node. The electrical activity during this part of the cardiac cycle is represented by the P wave.
- It is always positive in leads I and II and is usually tallest in lead II. It may be biphasic in lead III and is always inverted in aVR.
- In leads I and II it lasts for 0.08 to 0.1 second and has a maximum height of 0.5 cm, i.e., a magnitude of 0.5 mV. This magnitude indicates the functional activity of the atria.
- The beginning of the P wave indicates that the impulse has started in the atria and the end of the deflection indicates that the atria have come back to a resting state. The impulse reaches the AV node at the peak of the P wave.

P-R Interval

- At the end of the P wave the record runs along an isoelectric line for a very short interval (about 0.08 seconds). It then shows the QRS complex.
- PR interval is calculated from the beginning of the P to the beginning of R (or beginning of the Q wave when it is present).
- In health the PR interval varies between 0.13 and 0.16 seconds and should never exceed 0.2 seconds.

QRS Complex

- The Q wave is the negative wave preceding the positive R wave. It indicates the commencement of the activation of the ventricles. It is small in lead I but may be wider and deeper in lead III, more deep during expiration than during inspiration. Q wave may be present in the left ventricular leads V5 and V6.
- **R wave:** The Q wave is followed by a prominent and sharp upward deflection, which is designated as R wave. It is due to the activation process suddenly starting in both the ventricles. The height of the R wave is a guide of the functional activity of the ventricles. It is tallest in lead II and smallest in lead III. In aVR it is again insignificant. Whenever R is small and insignificant the following S wave becomes comparatively prominent. R wave is smallest in V1 and gradually increases in size from V1 to V6 (**Fig. 47.6**).
- **S wave:** The S wave is prominent in lead III. It is always prominent in aVR. S wave is deepest in V1 and V2 and diminishes progressively from V3 to V6. R and S are of equal amplitude in V3 and V4 (**Fig. 47.6**). In any normal ECG, the amplitude of R and S waves together should be less than 45 mm.
- The QRS complex represents ventricular depolarization and last for 0.08 seconds. It should never exceed 0.12 seconds in health. Its height varies from 1.5 to 2 cm (i.e., 1.5 mV to 2 mV).

ST Segment

At the end of the S wave the record runs on the isoelectric level for a short interval of 0.08 seconds and then shows the T wave. The ST segment is recorded while both the ventricles are in a contracted state.

T Wave

The T wave occurs at the end of the ventricular systole and is associated with the repolarization of ventricles. It is always in the same direction as that of the major deflection of the QRS complex. The wave is thus always positive in leads I and II and always negative in aVR. Its duration is 0.24 seconds. Its voltage is slightly more than that of the P wave. T wave is positive in all the precordial leads normally.

U Wave

The U wave follows the T wave after another isoelectric interval of 0.08 seconds and lasts for a period of 0.08 seconds. It has always the same polarity as that of the T wave. It indicates a state of increased excitability of the heart tissue and slow repolarization of papillary muscles. Its voltage is about 0.02 mV. U wave is usually not present in the normal ECG.

Waves of ECG in lead II (Fig. 47.8)

Waves	Causes	Duration (sec)	Amplitude (mV)
P wave	Atrial depolarization	0.08–0.1	0.1–0.3
QRS complex	Ventricular depolarization	0.08–0.1	1–3
T wave	Ventricular repolarization	0.25–0.35	0.2–0.3

Segments and intervals in a normal ECG in lead II

Segments	Causes	Duration (sec)
PR segment	AV nodal delay	0.04–0.1
ST segment	Interval between ventricular depolarization and repolarization	0.05–0.1

Intervals		
PQ/PR interval	Atrial depolarization + AV nodal delay	0.12–0.2 (0.16)
ST interval	Ventricular repolarization + ST segment	0.3–0.45

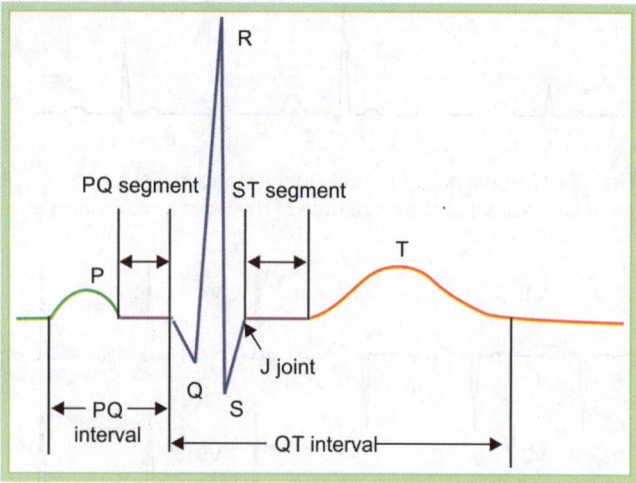

Fig. 47.8: Normal ECG showing different waves, segments and intervals.

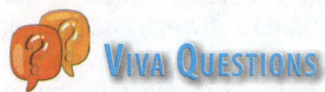
VIVA QUESTIONS

1. **How can you assess the mean electrical axis by seeing the ECG in leads I and III?**
   The mean electrical axis can be determined from the values of the QRS complex above and below the isoelectric line in leads I and III. High values above the base line in lead I (i.e., prominent R wave in lead I) and below the base line in lead III (i.e., prominent S wave in lead III) indicates left axis deviation. In right axis deviation it is vice versa.

2. **How can you determine the heart rate from the ECG? Give the normal value.**
   Heart rate = 60/R-R interval if heart rate is regular:
   » Normal heart rate = 60–90/min
   » Tachycardia—above 100/min
   » Bradycardia—below 60/min

3. **What is respiratory sinus arrhythmia?**
   Change in the heart rate during different phases of respiration is called **respiratory sinus arrhythmia**. Heart rate is increased during inspiration and decreased during expiration.

4. **What are the abnormalities in the rhythm of the heart?**
   Extrasystole or ectopic beats **(Fig. 47.9)**, paroxysmal atrial tachycardia (PAT), atrial flutter, atrial fibrillation **(Fig. 47.10)**, ventricular fibrillation and paroxysmal ventricular tachycardia (PVT), and heart blocks are the usual abnormalities in rhythm.

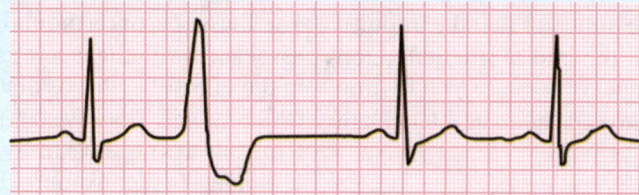

Fig. 47.9: ECG showing ventricular ectopic beat followed by compensatory pause.

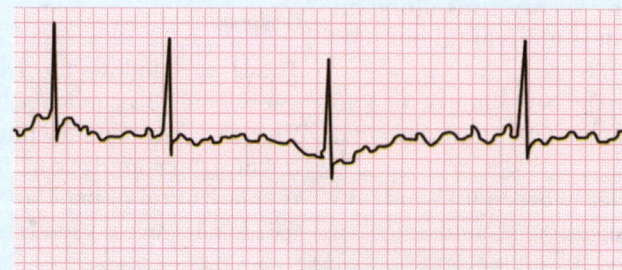

Fig. 47.10: ECG showing atrial fibrillation.

5. **What is mean electrical axis of heart?**
   Mean electrical axis is the mean electromotive force that acts in an average direction during any period of electrical activity, i.e., ventricular depolarization or repolarization. Ventricle is taken because electrical activity changes in the ventricle from time to time. Ventricular depolarization phase is taken for calculating mean electrical axis. QRS complex is taken from bipolar standard limb leads.

   The mean electrical axis is represented by an arrow, the length of the arrow representing **magnitude** of vector, the spatial position of arrow representing the **direction** and the head of the arrow representing **polarity**, i.e., positivity or negativity.
   Normal values of MEA:
   » In infants: +130°
   » In children: +52°
   » At puberty: +67°
   » In adults: +58°

   In diseases of the heart there will be a deviation of mean electrical axis either to the right or to the left. Shift of the axis to more than +110° denotes **right axis deviation** in adults and deviation to more than −20° denote **left axis deviation**.

6. **What is vector cardiography?**
   Vector cardiography is the recording of the instantaneous mean electrical axis of heart by means of an electronic device. Different loop patterns are obtained for atrial depolarization (P-loop), ventricular depolarization (QRS-loop) and ventricular repolarization (T-loop) on the screen of CRO.

7. **Mention some abnormalities in the different waves and segments of ECG.**
   P Wave Abnormalities
   » P wave is a positive wave in all leads except aVR.
   » Larger P waves indicate atrial enlargement as in mitral stenosis and tricuspid stenosis.
   » P wave is inverted when there is an ectopic focus of impulse production in the atrium.
   » When the atrial rate is >300/min it is **atrial fibrillation**. Here a definite P wave is not seen (*refer* **Fig 47.9**).

   PR Interval Abnormalities
   If the duration of PR interval is >0.2 seconds, it indicates delay in AV nodal conduction. This is known as heart block. Depending on the extent, different degrees of heart block can be classified.
   » Partial heart block or **first-degree heart block**: Here, all atrial impulses reach the ventricles but the PR interval is prolonged (>0.2 seconds).
   » **Second-degree block**: All atrial impulses are not conducted to the ventricle and depending on the severity it may be 2:1 block or 3:1 block. In 2:1 block, two P waves will be followed by a QRS complex **(Fig. 47.11)** and in 3:1 block, three P waves will be followed by one QRS complex. Normal AV node has a long refractory period and in adults cannot conduct impulses more than about 230 impulses/min.

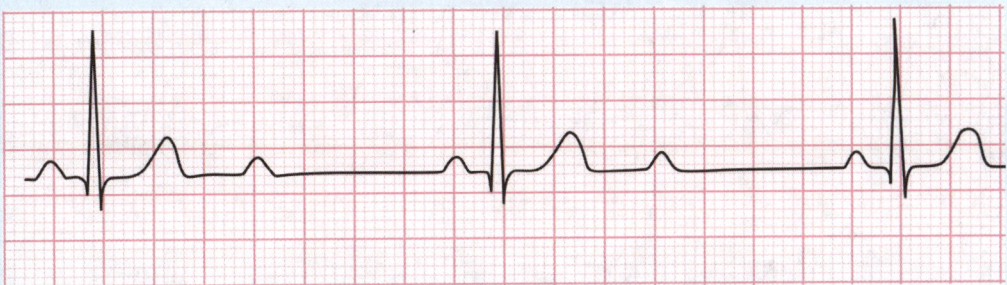

Fig. 47.11: Second degree heart block showing 2:1 block; Two P waves are followed by a QRS complex.

In **Wenckebach's phenomenon**, there is progressive prolongation of PR interval with every successive beat and then one QRS complex is dropped (dropped beat), then again normal pattern with prolongation of P-R interval observed **(Fig. 47.12)**. The cycle is repeated.

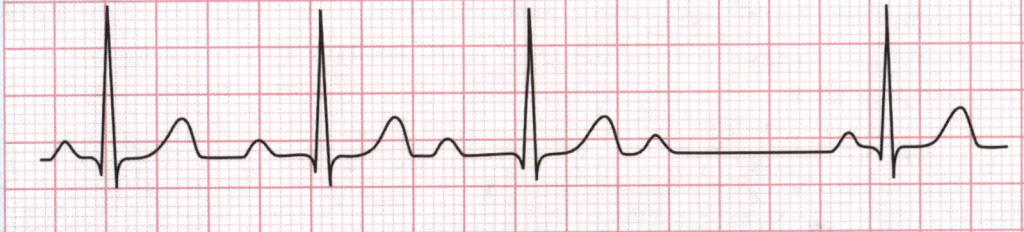

Fig. 47.12: Wenckebach phenomenon. Note the progressive prolongation of PR interval which is followed by a dropped QRS complex (two P waves can be seen).

» **Complete heart block or third-degree heart block**: When the conduction of impulse from the atria to the ventricles is completely interrupted, the atria and the ventricles beat at different rates. This may be due to diseases of AV node or block in the bundle branch (infranodal block). This produces **third-degree heart block (Fig. 47.13)**. Ventricular rate becomes 15–20/min (idioventricular rhythm) and this leads to inefficient pumping of heart and fainting attacks due to cerebral ischemia called **Stokes-Adams syndrome**. The condition is treated with artificial pacemakers.

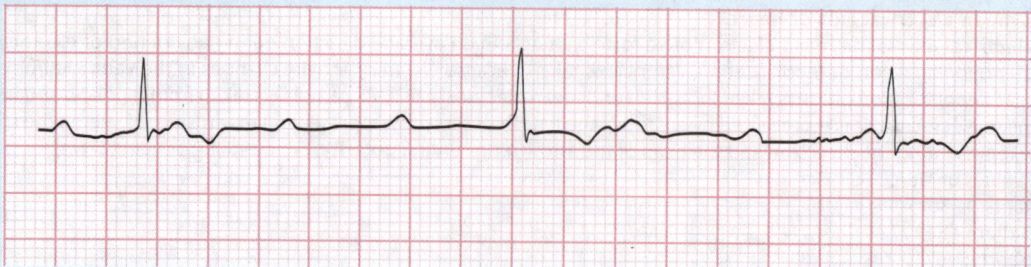

Fig. 47.13: ECG pattern in complete heart block.

Abnormalities in QRS Complex
» When the duration of QRS complex is greater than 0.1 second, the complex will be deformed. This is due to ventricular hypertrophy or bundle branch block.
» Changes in the amplitude of QRS complex are also seen. For example, in right axis deviation, S wave is greater than R wave in lead I. In left axis deviation, S wave is greater than R wave in lead III.
» Ventricular ectopic beat arises from an ectopic focus in the ventricle and produces a **bizarre-shaped** QRS complex followed by a compensatory pause before the next normal beat. When the normal impulse reaches the ventricle the ventricle will be in the absolute refractory period of the premature beat. This is the cause for the compensatory pause (*refer* **Fig. 47.10**).
» Enlarged Q wave is seen in myocardial infarction.

QT Interval Abnormalities
QT interval may be lengthened in myocardial damage, coronary ischemia, or conduction defects.

Abnormalities in ST Segment
» In myocardial infarction, there will be elevation of ST segment in leads overlying infracted area **(Fig. 47.14A)**.
» In leads placed 180° from the area of infarction there will be depression of ST segment **(Fig. 47.14B)**.
» ST depression is also seen in hypokalemia and hypoglycemia.

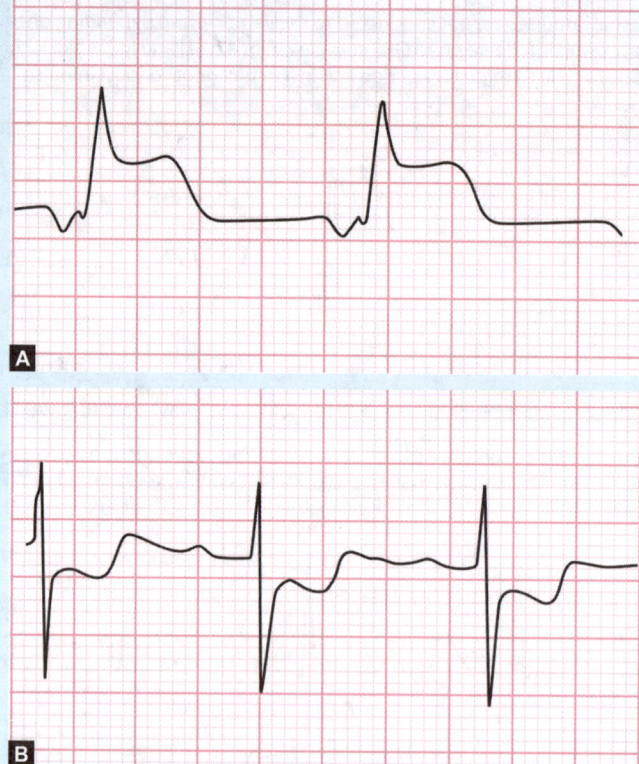

Figs. 47.14A and B: Abnormalities in ST segment: (A) ST elevation; (B) ST depression.

Changes in T Wave

T wave inversion (Fig. 47.15A) is seen in the following cases:
» Normally seen in aVR
» Excessive smoking
» Few hours after myocardial infarction
» Hypokalemia

Tall T wave (Fig. 47.15B) is seen in the following conditions:
» Immediately following myocardial infarction
» Hyperkalemia

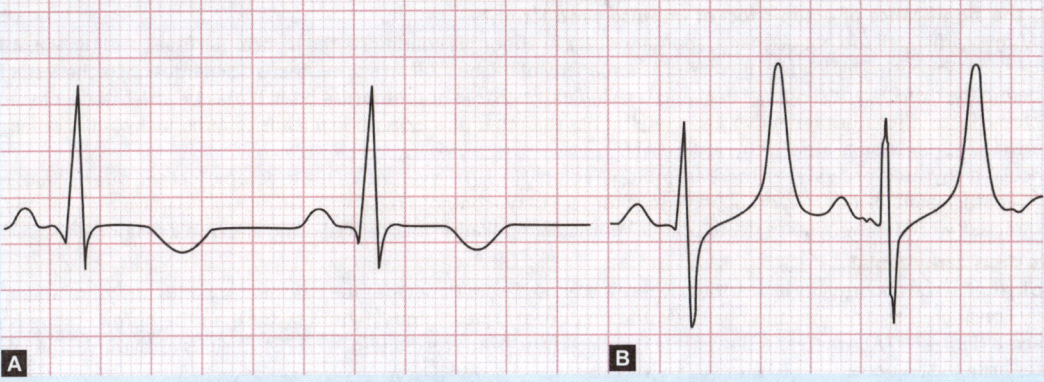

Figs. 47.15A and B: ECG showing changes in T wave: (A) T wave inversion; (B) Tall T wave.

8. **What are the ECG changes in myocardial infarction?**
   Myocardial infarction occurs due to obstruction of coronary arteries as a result of thrombosis or embolism. Depending on the site of infarction, changes are seen in Q wave, ST segment and T wave. Q wave becomes prominent. ST elevation occurs in all the leads within hours and T inversion occurs within days. Both these changes return to normal in a few weeks' time. But the Q wave changes are permanent **(Figs. 47.16A to E)**.
   » Normal ECG pattern
   » ST elevation in acute myocardial infarction
   » Prominent Q wave, ST elevation and T wave inversion after a few days of MI
   » Prominent Q wave and T wave inversion. ST segment comes to isoelectric level after a few weeks
   » ST segment and T wave came back to normal but Q wave remains prominent even after recovery.

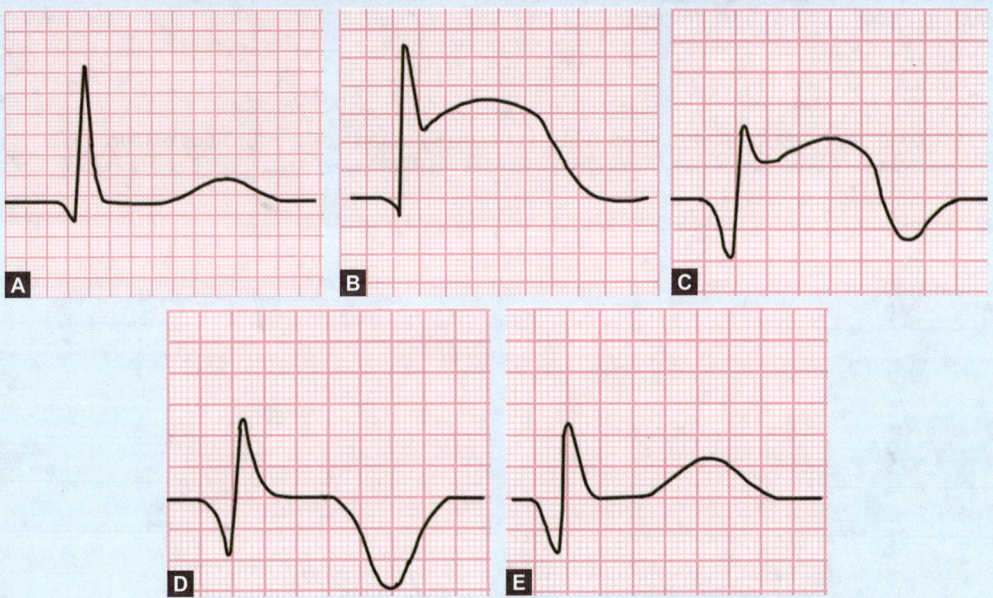

Figs. 47.16A to E: ECG changes in myocardial infarction.

9. **What is the significance of PR interval?**
   PR interval = P wave + PR segment
   Due to atrial depolarization and AV nodal delay, ventricular depolarization occurs about 0.16 seconds after atrial depolarization. Determination of PR interval is important clinically because it gives an idea about AV nodal delay. **Ventricular activation time (VAT)** corresponds to AV nodal delay. If it exceeds 0.2 seconds, it denotes some abnormality in the conduction of impulse.

10. **What are the causes of AV nodal delay?**
    » AV node is made up of small diameter fibers, which have a low conduction velocity.
    » There are multiple branching systems in AV node.
    » Number of gap junctions is less between successive cells in the conducting pathway. So, velocity of conduction is reduced.

11. **What is the significance of ectopic foci of impulse production?**
    Normally, myocardial cells do not discharge spontaneously. In abnormal conditions, the myocardial fibers and the Purkinje fibers may discharge spontaneously. This leads to increased automaticity of the heart. If an ectopic focus discharges once, the result is a beat that occurs before the expected next normal beat and is called **extrasystole** or **premature beat**. It may be atrial, nodal or ventricular beat. If the ectopic focus discharges repetitively at a rate higher than that of the SA node it leads to rapid tachycardia called **paroxysmal tachycardia**, e.g., paroxysmal atrial tachycardia (PAT).
    Ventricular tachycardia occurs when there are multiple ectopic foci in the ventricle. Due to ectopic foci and due to circus movement of impulses, ventricular fibrillation may occur because of the lack of synchronous contraction of different parts of the ventricle. If fibrillation is not corrected, within a few minutes death occurs. Ventricular fibrillation is corrected using electronic defibrillators.

12. **What is sinus arrhythmia?**
    Sinus arrhythmia is an abnormality in heartbeat where it is either fast or slow. One type is respiratory sinus arrhythmia. Sinus arrhythmia is usually considered as a normal and healthy variation in heart rate. A sinus rhythm faster than the normal range is called **sinus tachycardia (Fig. 47.17A)**, whereas a slower rate is called **sinus bradycardia (Fig. 47.17B)**. In sinus arrhythmia, the impulse always originates from the SA node.

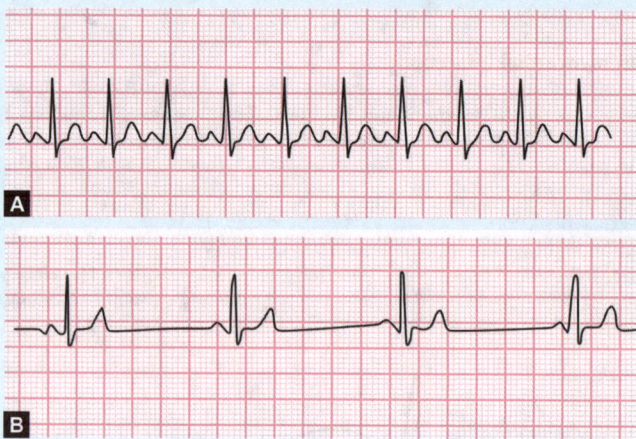

Figs. 47.17A and B: Abnormalities in heart rate: (A) Sinus tachycardia; (B) Sinus bradycardia.

Chapter 48: Spirometry

LEARNING OBJECTIVES

- Record spirogram of the given subject
- Interpret the record obtained
- Define various lung volumes and capacities
- Explain timed vital capacity and its significance

PY6.8: Demonstrate the correct technique to perform and interpret spirometry.

INTRODUCTION

Spirometry is the technique of measurement of various lung volumes and capacities of air breathed in and out.

SPIROMETER

A wet type spirometer consists of specially designed water sealed inner and outer chambers. The space between the two chambers is filled with water. A vessel is placed inverted like bell in between these two chambers immersed in water. The spirometric bell is attached to a chain running over two pulleys balances the weight of the bell. Loss in weight caused by immersion of the bell in water should be balanced by the weight of the extra length of chain. A counterweight attached to the chain balances the bell in position (Fig. 48.1). A wide air passage going through the center of the spirometer communicates with the cavity of the bell. The other end of the passage is connected through corrugated rubber tubing to a disposable mouthpiece. This tube is provided with a two-way breathing valve, which allows the subject to breath room air or spirometric air.

At the top of the bell is placed soda lime to remove CO_2 from the expired air. The instrument is also provided with two stopcocks, one for draining water and the other for introducing O_2 into the bell.

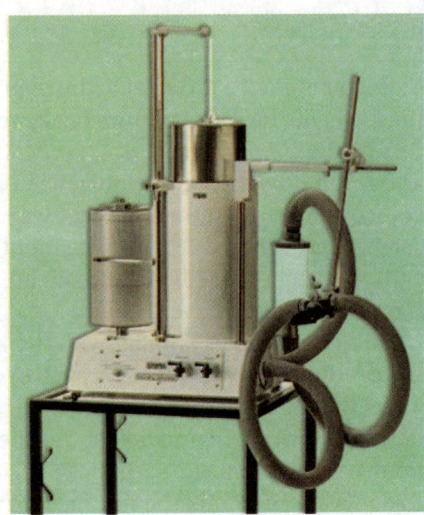

Fig. 48.1: Spirometer (wet type).

The bell moves up and down as air moves in and out of the chambers. This causes movement of the counterweight, which in turn is attached to a recording pen. An electrically driven kymograph to which is pasted a special chart paper provides the recording surface. The record obtained is known as spirogram.

The kymograph can be moved at two speeds, 60 mm/min and 1,200 mm/min with the help of the knob provided in the kymograph. The graduated chart paper provided is 10 meters long and 30 cm wide. One small division vertically is equal to 30 mL. When the speed of the kymograph

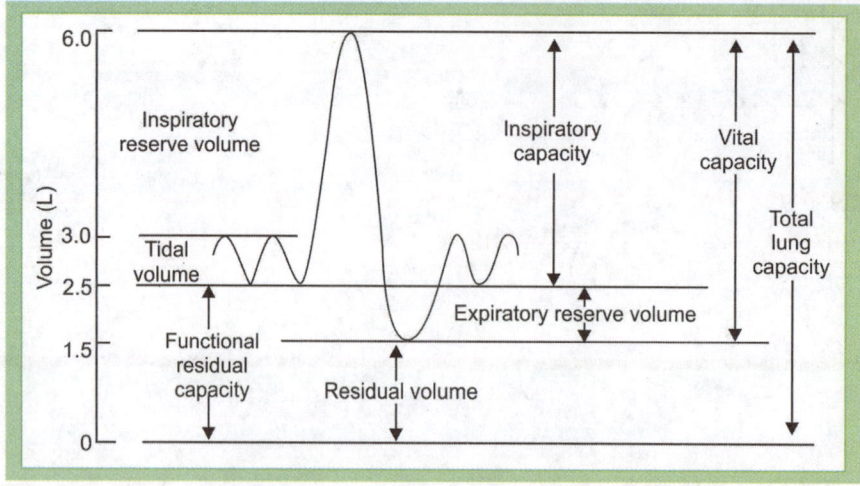

Fig. 48.2: Normal lung volumes and capacities.

is adjusted at 60 mm/min, 60 small divisions move horizontally in one minute. When the speed is adjusted at 1200 mm/min, 1200 small divisions move horizontally in one minute. A nose clip is also provided with the instrument.

Procedure

- The spirometer is filled with water to the required level.
- Raise and lower the bell and confirm that it moves freely over the full range.
- Count the respiratory rate of the subject.
- The subject should be seated facing away from the spirometer. Apply the nose clip and the mouthpiece.
- Instruct the subject to breathe in and out atmospheric air with normal resting rate and depth.
- After the subject becomes familiar with the apparatus and the procedure, adjust the two-way valve so that, the subject breathes air from the spirometer.
- Switch on the instrument and adjust the speed of the kymograph at 60 mm/min.
- The subject is asked to breathe normally through the mouthpiece connected to the spirometer and the volume of air that is taken in or given out with each normal breath is recorded on the graduated paper provided in the spirometer. This gives the tidal volume.
- The subject is then asked to inhale maximally and then to exhale rapidly and completely into the mouthpiece. This gives the measurement of vital capacity (**Fig. 48.2**). It should be taken care that the subject's nose is clipped properly so that he breathes only through the mouthpiece.
- Then ask the subject to breathe in and out of the spirometer as rapidly and as deeply as possible for 15 seconds. The movements are simultaneously recorded. This help to calculate the maximum breathing capacity (**Fig. 48.3**).

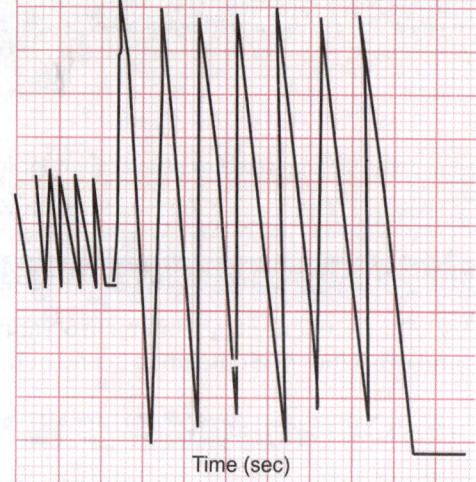

Fig. 48.3: Maximum voluntary ventilation (one smallest division in the Y-axis is equal to 30 mL and 10 small divisions in the X-axis is equal to 5 seconds).

- Now adjust the speed of the kymograph to 1,200 mm/min. Ask the subject to take a deep inspiration and to forcefully and rapidly expire into the spirometer. The procedure can be repeated to get a better record. From the record, the forced vital capacity or timed vital capacity can be calculated (**Fig. 48.4**).
- Reliable and accurate results cannot be obtained if the subject is not co-operative.

Using spirometer, we can determine the volume of air taken in and given out at various stages of respiration. A graph is recorded on a graph paper with time on the X-axis and volume in mL on the Y-axis. During inspiration, an upstroke is recorded, and *during expiration, a down stroke is recorded* (**Fig. 48.2**).

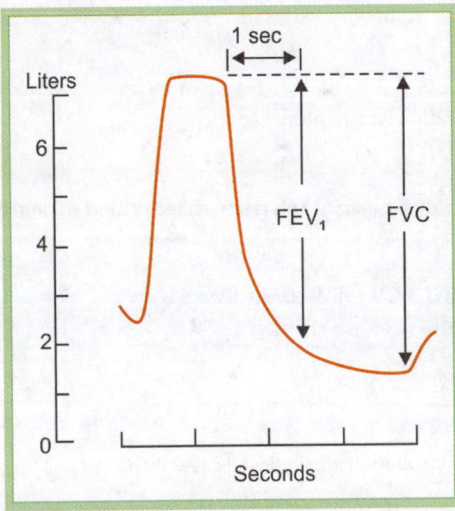

Fig. 48.4: Forced expiratory volume (FEV).

Weight in kg:
Height in cm:
Lung volumes and capacities
Tidal volume = ... mL
Vital capacity = ...mL
  Respiratory minute volume or pulmonary ventilation = (tidal volume) × (respiratory rate) = mL/min
  Maximum voluntary ventilation = (volume of one graph) × (number of graphs in 15 sec) × (4) = mL/min

Timed vital capacity (TVC_1% or FEV_1%)

$$= \frac{\text{Volume of air expired in the first sec} \times 100}{\text{Vital capacity}}$$

Volume of air expired in the first second is calculated from the graph obtained while recording vital capacity at the kymograph speed of 1,200 mm/min.
  The vital capacity forms about 75% of the total lung capacity (TLC). The average inspiratory capacity is about 60% of TLC while the average expiratory reserve volume is about 20% of TLC. Residual volume is about 20–35% of the total lung capacity. It is more in the aged.

Report

Name:
Age:
Sex:

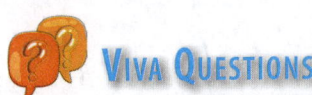

VIVA QUESTIONS

1. **What is minimal air? What is its medicolegal importance?**
   On opening the thorax, the lungs collapse because of the elastic recoil of the fibers and most of the air in the lungs is driven out. Even then some air remains trapped in its parenchymatous substance. This air is called the minimal air. This air cannot be driven out even after squeezing the lung physically. This lung tissue, therefore, always floats in water. The lung tissue of a newly born child, which has not taken its first breath, is solid and it sinks in water. The floating of the lung is thus a very important test for finding out the occurrence of death prior to or after taking the first breath.

2. **Which are the lung volumes and capacities that remain more or less constant?**
   Total lung capacity (TLC), residual volume and functional residual capacity (FRC).

3. **What is the significance of functional residual capacity (FRC)?**
   FRC is the amount of air remaining in the lungs at the end of a normal expiration. It is therefore the sum of the residual air and the expiratory reserve volume.
   » FRC acts as a buffer to aerate the pulmonary capillary blood in between breaths.
   » It keeps the alveolar gas composition relatively constant.

4. **Define the different static lung volumes and capacities and give their normal values.**
   Tidal Volume
   Volume of air inspired or expired during each normal breath is tidal volume. Normal values:
   Newborn   –   15–20 mL
   Males   –   600 mL
   Females   –   450 mL

   Inspiratory Reserve Volume
   Extra volume of air that can be inspired over and above the normal tidal volume is inspiratory reserve volume.
   Normal value—3–3.2 L

   Expiratory Reserve Volume
   Extra volume of air that can be expired by forceful expiration after the end of a normal expiration is expiratory reserve volume.
   Normal value—1.1 L

   Residual Volume (RV)
   The volume of air remaining in the lungs even after the most forceful expiration is residual volume. This volume cannot be measured by spirometry.
   Normal value—1.2 L
   It is much greater in emphysema.

Lung Capacities
Lung capacities are combinations of specific lung volumes.

Inspiratory Capacity
The volume of air that can be inspired by a forceful effort after a normal expiration is inspiratory capacity.
IC = TV + IRV = 0.5 + 3 = 3.5 L

Functional Residual Capacity
Volume of air remaining in the lungs after a normal expiration is functional residual capacity. This is also called resting volume of lungs.
FRC = ERV + RV = 1.1 + 1.2 = 2.3 L

Total Lung Capacity
Volume of air in the lungs after a maximum inspiration is total lung capacity. TLC = TV + IRV + ERV + RV = 6 L
Total lung capacity is decreased in:
» Pulmonary edema
» Pneumothorax
» Lung tumors

Vital Capacity
The volume of air that can be expired rapidly and forcefully after a maximum inspiration is called vital capacity.
VC = IRV + TV + ERV = 3 + 0.5 + 1.1 = 4.6 L

5. **What are the factors affecting vital capacity?**
   » Age—vital capacity is maximal in young adults.
   » Sex—VC is more in males than in females.
   » Build and physical training—VC will be more in well-built individuals and in athletes.
   » Height—VC varies with height.
     - In males—height in cm × 25 mL.
     - In females—height in cm × 20 mL.
     - Athletes—height in cm × 29 mL.
   » Body surface area—VC can be calculated from body surface area.
     - In males—2.6 L/m^2 body surface area
     - In females—2.1 L/m^2 body surface area

6. **What is vital index?**
   Vital capacity related to the body surface area is called vital index.

   $$\text{Vital index} = \frac{\text{Vital capacity}}{\text{Body surface area}}$$

   $$= \frac{4.8 \text{ L}}{1.7 \text{ m}^2} = 2.6 \text{ L/m}^2 \text{ body surface area}$$

7. **Give the variations in vital capacity.**
   Physiological Decrease:
   » In pregnancy due to inability of diaphragm to move down satisfactorily, there will be a reduction in VC.

   Pathological Decrease:
   » Neurological diseases affecting muscles of respiration like neuritis, poliomyelitis, etc.
   » Diseases of muscles like myasthenia gravis.
   » Deformities of thoracic cage, like kyphosis, scoliosis, etc.
   » Diseases of lung like emphysema, fibrosis, pneumonia, tuberculosis, etc.
   » Diseases of pleura, like pleural effusion, pneumothorax, etc.
   » Diseases of heart like congestive cardiac failure (CCF), pericardial effusion, etc.
   » Diseases of abdominal cavity like ascites, large tumors, etc. Ascites is collection of fluid in the peritoneal cavity.

8. **What is the importance of measuring vital capacity?**
   » VC has prognostic value during treatment of a respiratory problem. If the vital capacity increases with treatment it means that the patient is responding to the treatment.
   » We can assess the progress of a chronic disease like emphysema. If there is a rapid reduction in vital capacity it means that the disease is rapidly progressing and the mortality is higher.
   » VC is used for assessing physical fitness.

9. **Which are the lung volumes and capacities that cannot be measured using spirometer?**
   TLC, FRC and RV cannot be measured using an ordinary spirometer since RV cannot be expelled out.

Chapter 49

Stethography

LEARNING OBJECTIVES

- Record the movements of breathing using stethograph
- Demonstrate the effect of hyperventilation and breath-holding on respiration
- Explain the mechanism of respiration

INTRODUCTION

Stethography is the process of recording the respiratory movements in man. The instrument used is called **stethograph** and the record obtained is called **stethogram**. Respiratory movements can also be recorded using physiograph **(Fig. 49.1)**.

AIM

Record the normal respiratory movements of the given subject and to study the changes seen with voluntary hyperventilation, deglutition, breath holding and exercise.

APPARATUS

- Electric kymograph, recording drum
- Stethograph
- Marey's tambour.

Stethograph

It consists of a corrugated canvas rubber tube (60 cm long and 2 cm in diameter) with side clips **(Fig. 49.2)**. One end of the tube is closed and the other end can be connected to the Marey's tambour through pressure tubing.

There is a metallic chain with a hook at its tip attached to the closed end of the stethograph for tying the instrument

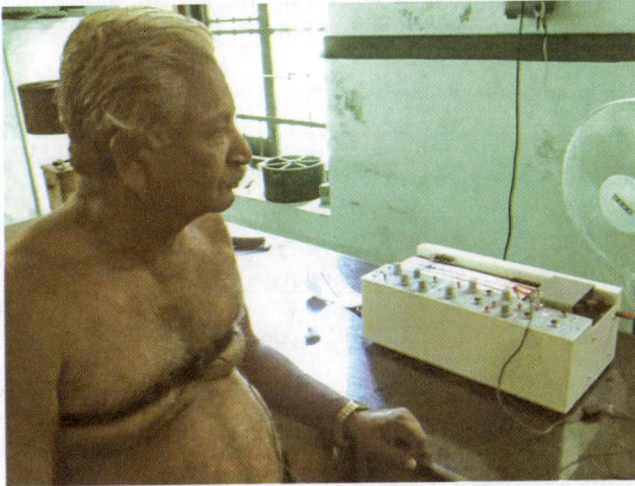

Fig. 49.1: Stethographic recording using physiograph.

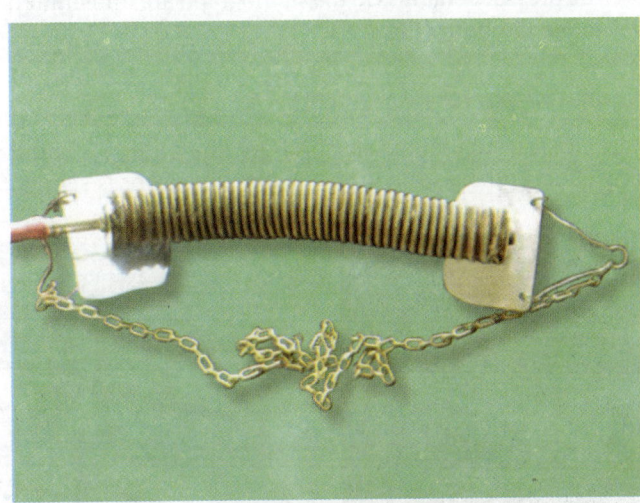

Fig. 49.2: Stethograph.

around the chest. When tied tightly around the chest, the stethograph is stretched out during each inspiration without significant decrease in the diameter. The volume of the interior space increases with each expansion occurring during inspiration; and the space being closed on all sides, the pressure decreases. The membrane of the tambour thus gets depressed and its lever records a down stroke.

Marey's Tambour

It consists of a writing lever, metal tube to which the stethograph is connected and a diaphragm which is attached to the end of the metal tube. The diaphragm consists of a metallic cup with a thin rubber membrane tied tightly around its mouth. The writing lever is placed in contact with the rubber membrane by means of a metal disc **(Fig. 49.3)**.

PROCEDURE

- Arrange the recording apparatus on a table.
- Adjust the kymograph for slow gear and slow speed.
- Mount the Marey's tambour on a stand and adjust it, so as to record the movement of the lever on the smoked paper.
- Ask the subject to sit comfortably on a stool in front of the apparatus facing away from the apparatus.
- Tie the stethograph tightly around the chest just above the nipples (at the level of fourth intercostal space) where chest movements are maximal. See that the subject is comfortable with the stethograph tied in position. Also see that it does not slip out by ordinary movements.
- Explain the whole procedure to the subject. Ask him to do the whole procedure without recording, so that he becomes familiar to it.
- Connect the stethograph to the Marey's tambour so that the pressure changes in the stethograph are transmitted to the tambour **(Fig. 49.4)**.

Normal Respiratory Movements

Instruct the subject to relax and breathe quietly without any effort and start the drum. The writing lever is seen to

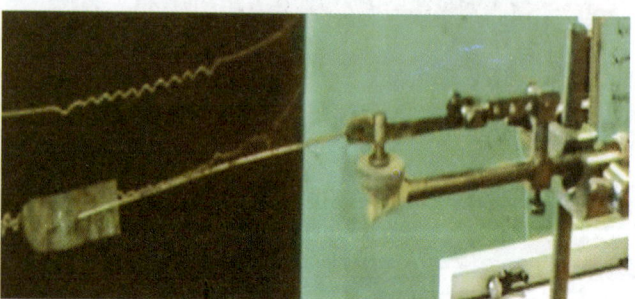

Fig. 49.3: Marey's tambour.

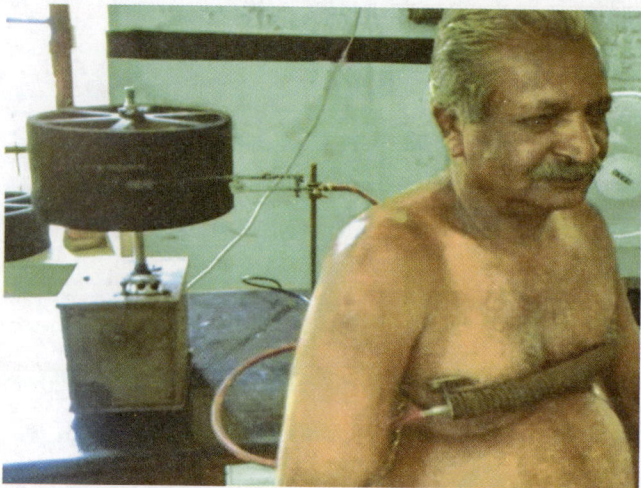

Fig. 49.4: Recording of respiratory movements using stethograph.

move with movements of the chest. Bring the writing lever in contact with the recording surface at a tangent. Keep the stethograph sufficiently taut so that the recordings are about an inch in height. Record the movements of the chest over a length of 10 cm strip of the smoked paper. Stop the drum.

Voluntary Hyperventilation

Ask the subject to breathe as deeply and rapidly as he can. Record the movements continuously till normal respiration is resumed.

Effect of Swallowing

While normal respiratory movements are being recorded, ask the subject to drink water from a cup and record the effect.

Effect of Breath Holding

Ask the subject to hold his breath at the end of normal inspiration and also at the end of deep inspiration. Note the difference in the breath holding time.

Effect of Exercise

Ask the subject to do moderate exercise like jogging for 2–3 minutes and record the respiratory movements, till the normal pattern is resumed after stopping exercise.

Write the title of the experiment and label the various events recorded in the smoked paper.

OBSERVATION (FIG. 49.5)

- During inspiration the chest expands and the stethograph is stretched. The pressure inside the stethograph decreases, this fall in pressure is being transmitted to the Marey's tambour. The rubber diaphragm is therefore pulled down causing a downward movement of the

Chapter 49: Stethography

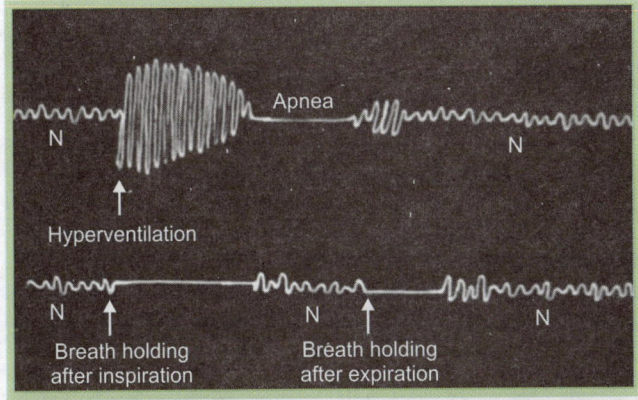

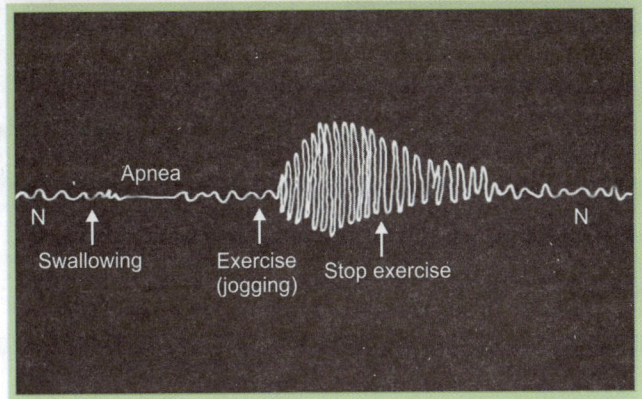

Fig. 49.5: Stethographic recording in kymograph during different maneuvers.

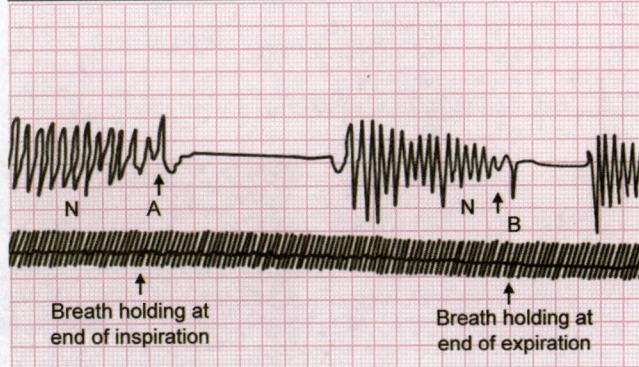

Fig. 49.6: Respiratory movements recorded during different maneuvers in a physiograph. (Lower graph is the time tracing; one impulse corresponds to one second).

writing lever. During expiration, recoil of the stethograph causes the reverse changes and therefore an upward movement of the writing lever occurs. Thus, down stroke in the tracing represent inspiration and upstroke, expiration.

* From the graph, calculate the respiratory rate based on the speed of the kymograph.
* The height of the strokes give a measure of the extent of expansion of the chest and the volume of the air breathed.
* During voluntary hyperventilation, there is an increase in the rate and depth of respiration. Eventually, a state of fatigue sets in which is followed by a temporary cessation of breathing (apnea), after which breathing returns back to normal **(Fig. 49.6)**.

* The act of deglutition is preceded by a deep inspiration and is accompanied by an apnea (temporary stoppage of breathing). This is called **deglutition apnea** and is followed by normal breathing.
* At the end of the breath holding period, deep inspiratory and expiratory movements occur. The subject can hold his breath for a longer time after the end of deep inspiration.
* During exercise, respiration becomes deep and rapid. Hyperventilation in exercise is not followed by apnea. This is because, the pCO_2 is high during exercise and so there is no depression of respiratory center. Even after stopping exercise during the recovery period, ventilation is high for sometime to wash out the excess CO_2 and to pay for the O_2 debt.

PRECAUTIONS

* Stethograph should be tied at the level of fourth intercostal space.
* The subject should sit comfortably facing away from the instrument.
* The drum should move at slow speed (2.5 mm/sec).
* Before and after taking the recordings for each maneuver, normal recordings should be taken.
* Breath holding time should be taken after quiet inspiration and expiration and after deep inspiration and expiration.

VIVA QUESTIONS

1. **What is Cheyne-Stokes respiration? What are the conditions and where it is recorded?**
   Cheyne-Stokes respiration is a type of periodic breathing seen in both physiological and pathological conditions **(Fig. 49.7)**. In this type, regular alternating periods of hyperventilation and apnea are seen. The change over from one to the other occurs gradually.
   Physiological conditions are:
   » Deep sleep
   » Infants
   » High altitude.

Pathological conditions are:
» Congestive cardiac failure (CCF)
» Morphine poisoning
» Raised intracranial tension
» Uremia.

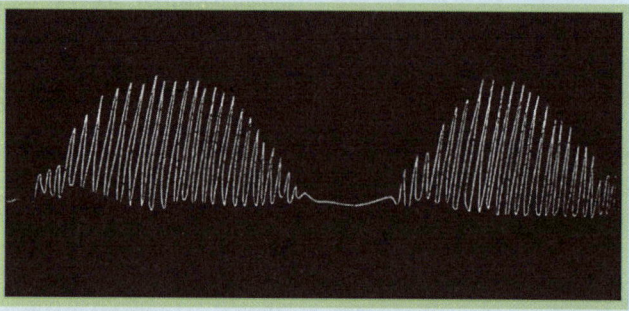

Fig. 49.7: Cheyne-Stokes breathing recorded in stethograph.

2. **What is the reason for apnea following voluntary hyperventilation?**
   During hyperventilation, more of CO_2 is washed off and pCO_2 falls. Carbon dioxide (CO_2) is the most potent stimulus for respiration. Reduction is pCO_2 inhibits the respiratory center leading to apnea. During apnea, there will be accumulation of CO_2 and this regains respiration.

Chapter 50

Perimetry

LEARNING OBJECTIVES

- Chart the field of vision in the given subject using perimeter
- Explain physiological blind spot and give its physiological basis
- Trace the visual pathway

PY10.20: Demonstrate testing of field of vision.

INTRODUCTION

Technique of charting out the field of vision is called **perimetry**. The instrument which is used in perimetry is **perimeter (Fig. 50.1)**. It measures the boundaries of the field of vision. Visual field is defined as the area on a screen in which objects are visible, while gaze is fixed on an object. In clinical practice, perimetry is carried out to decide the site of lesion along the visual pathway, to detect tumors like pituitary tumor, retinal diseases like retinitis pigmentosa and to detect glaucoma.

PERIMETER (FIG. 50.1)

Perimeter is an instrument with which the visual field is recorded. Parts of perimeter are:
- An arc of a circle made of some rigid material
- A stand to support the arc
- A chin rest attached to the stand.

The stand gives stability to the instrument. It has a vertical limb upon which the arc is pivoted. The vertical limb is broad and helps to screen the activities of the examiner from the subject. It bears a circular scale to read the meridian in which the arc is brought.

The chin rest is adjustable. A knob helps to adjust the level of the chin rest so that the visual axis is brought in the axis of the rotation of the arc.

The arc, which is rigid and broad, is the most important part of the perimeter **(Fig. 50.1)**. Its concavity faces the

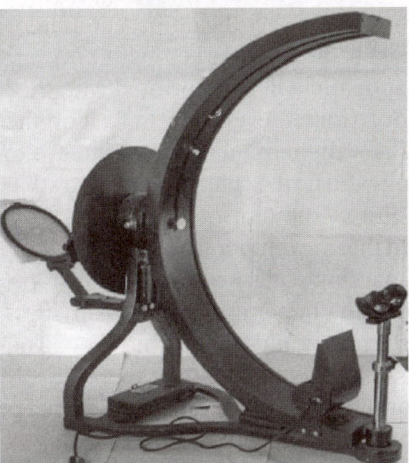

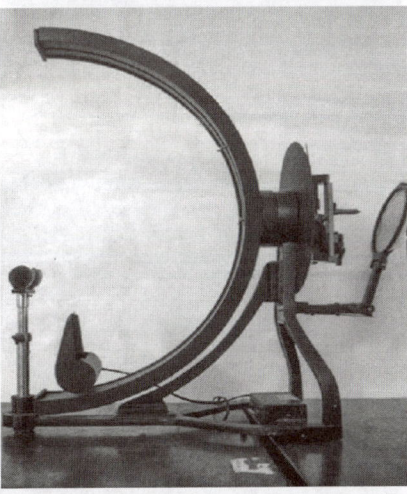

Fig. 50.1: Perimeter (view from two different angles).

subject and it is pivoted on the vertical limb of the stand just in front of the chin rest. When rotated it describes a hollow hemisphere. In whatever meridian it is placed, all the points on it are equidistant from the retina. It usually extends from 90° on one side to 30° on the other. Its surface is matt black. The arc is graduated in degrees and the scale is marked on the convex surface. The radius of the arc, i.e., the distance between the test object and the eye varies between 250 and 330 mm. There is a sliding holder in the metal arc, which holds the test object. This holder can be moved towards the center or to the periphery.

The fixation object occupies the point of pivot. The subject is asked to fix his gaze on it, while the visual field is demarcated. The fixation object should be large enough (about 5 mm in diameter). During the test, the subject should not move his eyes.

The chart is attached to the back of the perimeter and it rotates with the arc **(Fig. 50.1)**. There is a pricking point moving on the fixation chart, along a scale. It marks the distance in degrees from the central fixation point. There is a test object that can be moved from periphery to the center of the perimeter.

A point is marked on the chart paper with the pricking tip when the subject sees the object at different positions.

The chart is already marked with normal visual field and blind spot and will be imprinted with the letter R (for right eye) or L (for left eye). Now to fix it on the perimeter, turn the arc on the temporal side of the eye to which the chart belongs and fix the chart in such a way that the central fixation point of the chart corresponds to the point of rotation and that the temporal meridian on the chart comes under the marking scale. Fix it in this position.

Field of vision depends on the sensitivity of the retina, the size of the object and color of the object. The visual field for colored objects is smaller than the white objects and is different for different colors. The field decreases in size in the order of yellow, blue, red and green.

APPARATUS

Perimeter charts, test objects of various sizes and colors.

Perimeter Chart

Field of vision is marked on a special type of chart. The central point of the chart corresponds with the visual axis. The chart paper shows two types of markings, concentric circles around the central point and radial longitudinal lines. The concentric circles denote the angular distance (in degrees) away from the point of fixation **(Fig. 50.2)**. The longitudinal lines show the degrees through which the metal arc is rotated.

In each eye field in the chart, the temporal field is shown on its lateral side, i.e., on the left side for the left eye and on the right side for the right eye. The horizontal and vertical meridians passing through the center of the chart divide it into four quadrants. For a 10 mm white object at 330 mm and with optimum illumination, the field extends to about 50° upwards, 60° nasally, 70° downwards and more than 90° temporally.

The field for blue and yellow is roughly >10° in each direction than that for the white and for red and green another >10°.

The blind spot represents the projection of that area of retina where the optic nerve leaves the retina. It is oval in shape with a long vertical axis. Objects are invisible in this part of the field.

PROCEDURE

- Ask the subject to sit comfortably on a stool.
- There should be good illumination with the light coming from behind the subject.
- Ask the subject to place his chin on the chin rest and adjust the chin rest at such a level that the visual axis and the axis of rotation of the arc coincide.

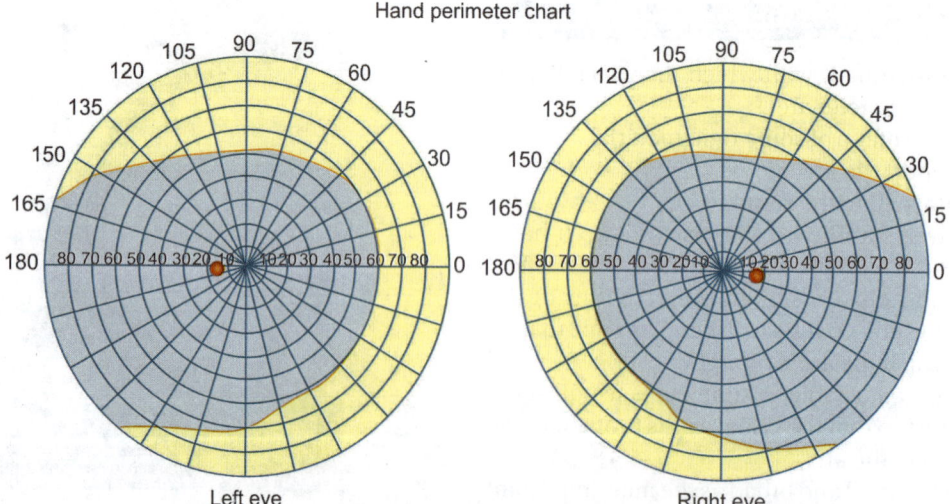

Fig. 50.2: Perimeter chart showing the normal field of vision in the left and right eyes. The dark spot is the blind spot.

- Mount the chart paper on the perimeter.
- The field of vision of each eye should be plotted separately.
- The subject is asked to close his opposite eye with his hand.
- Stand in front of the subject, behind the perimeter on the side of the closed eye, so that the subject does not see the examiner.
- Ask the subject to fix his eye that is being tested on the central point of the metal arc (point of fixation).
- Start with a white object 5 mm in diameter.
- Start from the periphery and come to the center.
- Instruct the subject to respond as soon as he sees the object.
- This point is marked on the chart paper by making a perforation with the sharp pointer provided at the back.
- The procedure is repeated at different positions achieved by rotating the metal arc by 10–15° through a full circle.
- Start from the lower lateral quadrant and mark the blind spot.
- The markings or perforations are joined on the chart and we get the visual field of that eye.
- The procedure can be repeated with objects of different sizes and colors.
- Mark the visual field of the other eye similarly.
- To identify scotomas, it is not just sufficient to delineate the boundaries of the visual field. It is necessary to scan the whole field completely and to eliminate any area where vision is absent. So, continue moving the object towards the center in all meridians and mark the points where he cannot see the object and this helps to identify scotomas.

OBSERVATIONS AND INFERENCES

- See whether the visual field of the subject charted, corresponds to the normal field shown in the chart. Mild variations are normal and may be due to technical error.
- Area within the visual field where vision is absent is called a **scotoma**. Blind spot is a physiological scotoma.
- Loss of vision is called **anopia**.
- **Hemianopia** is loss of half of the visual field.
- **Quadrantanopia** is loss of one-fourth field of vision.
- Bilateral hemianopia is loss of half of the field of vision on either side, in which similar, i.e., corresponding halves (e.g., temporal halves of both sides) of the field of vision is lost, is called **heteronymous hemianopia**. Thus, the heteronymous hemianopia may be binasal or bitemporal.
- **Homonymous hemianopia** means loss of opposite halves of the field of vision, i.e., loss of temporal side of one eye and the nasal side of the other eye. It is either of the right or the left side. In the right side homonymous hemianopia, the temporal half of the right and the nasal half of the left side is lost. In the left side homonymous hemianopia, the temporal half of the left side and the nasal half of the right side is lost. The lesion is on the opposite side. Lesions along the visual pathway beyond optic nerve cause hemianopia.

PRECAUTIONS

- The test object must be moved from periphery to the center so that no blind area in the field will be missed.
- The visual field should be mapped first with white test object of diameter 5 mm.
- If any blind spot is detected, its limit should be mapped out. If the scotoma is small, use smaller test object to determine the limit.

DISCUSSION

As the test object moves from periphery to center, it disappears and then appears again. The disappearance is due to **blind spot** (physiological scotoma). It is obtained 15° lateral to the central point on the chart. This is because the photoreceptors are absent at the region of optic disc. Occasionally, blind spots are found in portions of the field of vision other than the optic disc area. Such blind spots are called **scotomas or scotomata (Fig. 50.3)**. It may be due to allergic reactions in retina, lead poisoning, excessive use of tobacco, etc. It can also be due to damage of optic nerve fibers as a result of glaucoma.

In tubular field of vision, the field of vision is narrowed to a tubular shape. It is seen in advanced glaucoma and in retinitis pigmentosa. Loss of vision first occurs in the peripheral portion of retina leading to tubular vision and gradually it spreads to the center leading to complete loss of vision.

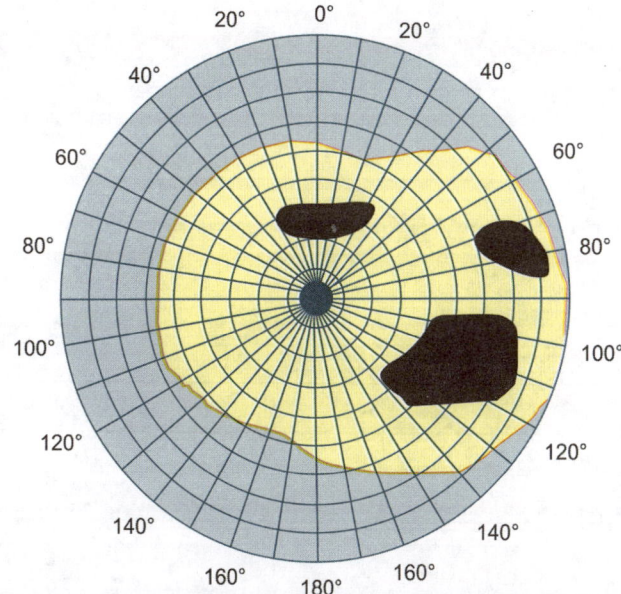

Fig. 50.3: Perimetry showing scotomas of right eye.

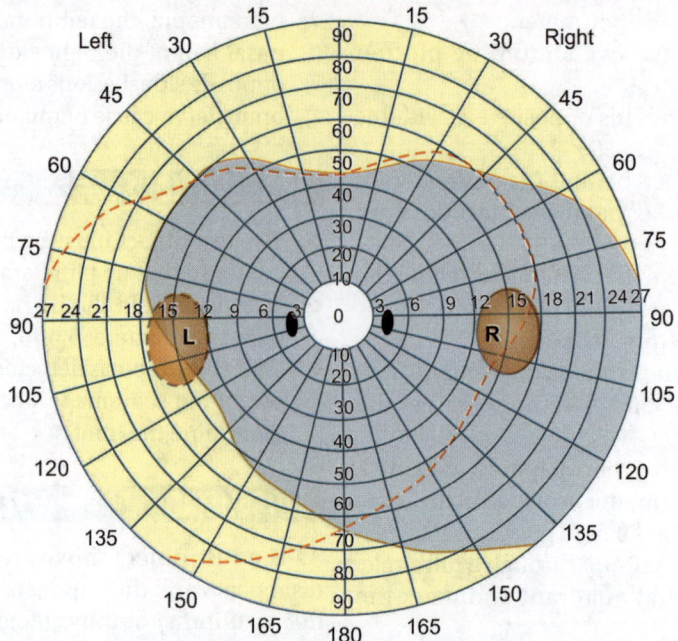

Fig. 50.4: Perimeter chart showing binocular field of vision (the fields of vision of both eyes can be charted in the same sheet).

Binocular Vision

If the field of vision of both eyes is charted in the same sheet, there will be overlap of visual fields **(Fig. 50.4)**. This is called **binocular vision**. Binocular field is the combination of the right and the left uniocular fields. Depth perception is possible due to binocular vision. The ability to determine distance is called **depth perception**.

Chapter 51

Electromyography

LEARNING OBJECTIVES

- Define electromyography and name the type of electrodes used.
- Demonstrate the phenomenon of recruitment of motor units using electromyograph.
- Abnormalities recorded in EMG.

Electromyography is the technique of recording the electrical activity of skeletal muscles at rest or during activity. The instrument is called **electromyograph** and the record obtained is called **electromyogram (EMG)**. It helps to detect the nature and location of motor unit lesions, the extent of lesion, reflex responses, etc.

PRINCIPLE

When the muscle is in the relaxed state, no potentials are recorded, as it is electrically silent. When an action potential moves through the muscle fibers, some amount of energy is transmitted to the skin. When large number of muscle fibers contract, a summated effect can be recorded from the skin and potential with greater amplitude is obtained. In EMG, both visual and audio display of electrical activity is obtained.

APPARATUS

Electromyograph, which consists of electrodes, amplifiers, cathode ray oscilloscope, frequency modulated tape recorder, audio amplifier, photographic device and electronic stimulator.

ELECTRODES

Electrodes are used to pick up the electrical activity from the muscle. Two types of electrodes are used:
1. Surface disk electrodes
2. Needle electrodes

Surface disk electrode is placed on the skin and summated potentials from groups of muscle fibers or from a muscle can be recorded **(Fig. 51.1)**. **Needle electrodes** are very fine needles, or a thin platinum wire passed through the core of a hypodermic needle **(Fig. 51.2)**. It can be

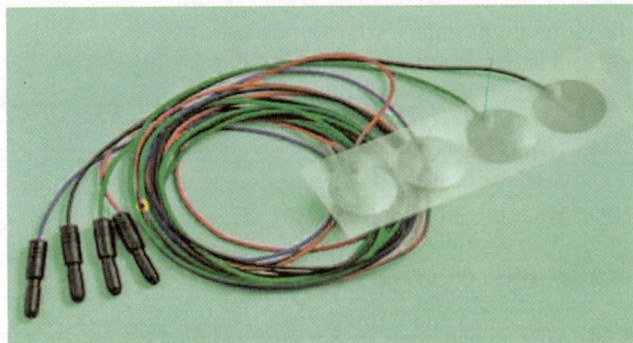

Fig. 51.1: Surface disk electrodes.

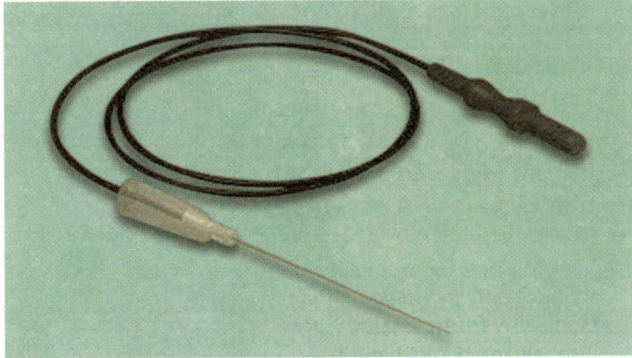

Fig. 51.2: Needle electrode.

introduced into a single fiber or between two or three fibers. The record obtained depends on the number of muscle fibers involved. Thus, the recording can be monophasic, biphasic and polyphasic.

- ❖ **Amplifier** is a biological or differential amplifier, which picks up only biological signals.
- ❖ **Loudspeaker** makes the sounds associated with muscular contractions audible.
- ❖ **Frequency modulated** tape recorder helps to store the signals. It helps to redisplay the signals later to assess the prognosis of the disease.
- ❖ **Photographic** device takes photographs from the oscilloscope and stores it.
- ❖ **Electronic stimulators** incorporated in the electromyograph are used to provide single, double or a series of pulses. The amplitude, duration and frequency of the pulses can be adjusted.

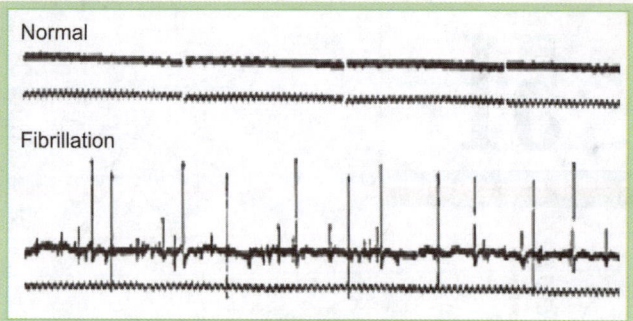

Fig. 51.3: EMG at rest showing normal pattern (above) and fibrillation potentials (below).

Uses of EMG

- ❖ Helps in the diagnosis of neuromuscular disorders.
- ❖ Neuropathy can be distinguished from myopathy.
- ❖ Helps to distinguish between diseases of central nervous system and peripheral nervous system.
- ❖ Helps to assess the prognosis of neuromuscular diseases, i.e., to check whether the patient is responding to treatment.
- ❖ Helps in nerve conduction studies. Conduction velocity is decreased in peripheral neuropathy.
- ❖ Normally at rest no spontaneous electrical activity is recorded from the muscle. Following denervation of muscle due to spinal cord lesions, abnormal spontaneous activities like fibrillation potentials **(Fig. 51.3)** and fasciculation potentials can be recorded during the resting phase.

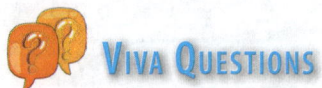

VIVA QUESTIONS

1. **Define electromyography.**
   Refer page 259.
2. **What is the principle of EMG?**
   Refer page 259.
3. **Mention the uses of EMG.**
   Refer page 260.
4. **Why no potentials are not recorded from the muscle during rest?**
   This is because there is no discharge of impulses from the motor neuron.
5. **Name one condition where there is recording of spontaneous electrical activity at rest.**
   In spinal cord lesions where there is denervation of muscle, fibrillation potentials will be recorded.

Chapter 52

Audiometry

LEARNING OBJECTIVES

- Describe the principle of audiometry
- Differentiate between conduction deafness and nerve deafness
- Trace the auditory pathway

PY10.20: Demonstrate test of hearing by audiometry.

INTRODUCTION

Audiometry means the measurement of the ability of hearing. It helps to assess the degree of hearing loss and to chart the audibility curve. It is determined by finding out the lowest intensities of various tones (or frequencies) heard by the subject. The graph showing the frequencies against the intensity is called the **audiogram**. The curve plotted is called the **audibility curve**. The instrument used to produce the various sounds is called **audiometer**. There are different types of audiometric tests like pure tone audiometry and speech audiometry.

Pure tone audiometry is a hearing test used to determine the presence or absence of hearing loss. If hearing loss is present, it will help to assess both the type and the degree of hearing loss. A pure-tone hearing test determines the faintest tones a person can hear at selected frequencies from low to high. Pure tone air conduction test and pure tone bone conduction tests are used to differentiate between conduction deafness and sensorineural deafness. Pure tone bone conduction testing can measure the response of the inner ear (cochlea) to sound independently of the middle and outer ear.

APPARATUS

Pure Tone Audiometer (Fig. 52.1)

The pure tone audiometer consists of an earphone connected to an electronic oscillator that can provide pure

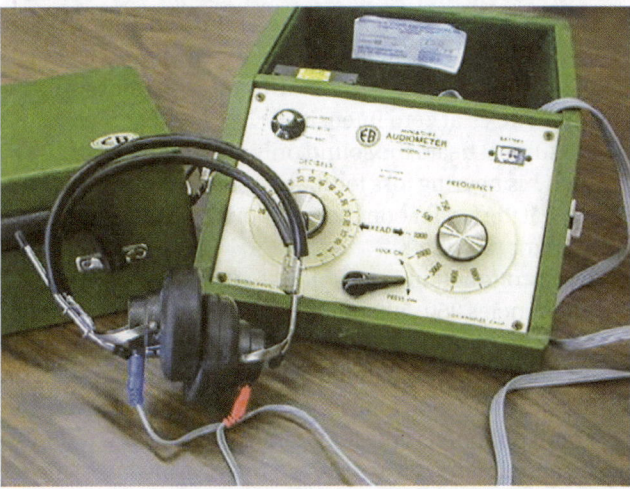

Fig. 52.1: A pure tone audiometer.

tones from low to high frequencies. It is also provided with two controls, a mechanical vibrator, a power switch, a lamp, a signal lamp and an interrupter.

Out of the two controls, one gives the frequency of the pure tones in hertz and the other is for adjusting the intensity or loudness of the pure tone in decibels **(Fig. 52.1)**. Normally, the instrument is calibrated in such a way that, at zero decibels, a normal person can hear all frequency tones.

The audiometer, in addition to being equipped with an earphone for testing air conduction by the ear, is equipped with a mechanical vibrator for testing bone conduction from the mastoid process of the skull into the cochlea.

The subject will be provided with a signal lamp to be switched on when he hears the sound.

The interrupter helps to detect whether the subject is malingering or not.

PROCEDURE

- The test should be performed in a soundproof room. While one ear is being tested, the opposite ear must be masked to exclude it from the test.
- Keep the earphones in position and make the subject familiar with the sound.
- Choose different frequencies and detect the point of loudness at which he first hears the sound, by increasing the intensity gradually from the lowest level.
- Usually, air conduction thresholds are measured for tones of frequencies 125, 250, 500, 1,000, 2,000 and 4,000 Hz.
- For each frequency, a series of tone pips (short high-pitched sounds) are delivered at increasing intensities (beginning from subthreshold) and the subject is instructed to signal every time he hears a sound. Each frequency is tested in the intensity range of 0–100 dB.
- The subject can respond to the sound by raising a finger or hand, or by switching on the signal lamp.
- A normal person will be able to appreciate all the frequencies at zero intensity.
- If a subject hears the sound only at an intensity of 20 dB, then his hearing loss for that frequency sound is 20 dB.
- Repeat the test for bone conduction using the mechanical vibrator provided.
- Bone conduction thresholds are measured for tones of frequencies 250, 500, 1,000, 2,000 and 4,000 Hz.
- Graphs can be plotted with frequency of sound in Hertz on the X-axis and hearing loss in decibels on the Y-axis for air conduction and bone conduction separately. The graph obtained is the audiogram.
- By audiometry, we can assess the hearing loss if any at different frequencies of sound.

OBSERVATION

- The instrument is calibrated in such a way that a normal person can hear all the frequencies at zero intensity (Fig. 52.2).
- The curve will be a straight line parallel to the X-axis in a person with normal hearing.
- In cases of deviation from normal, the audibility curve obtained helps to differentiate between nerve deafness and conduction deafness.

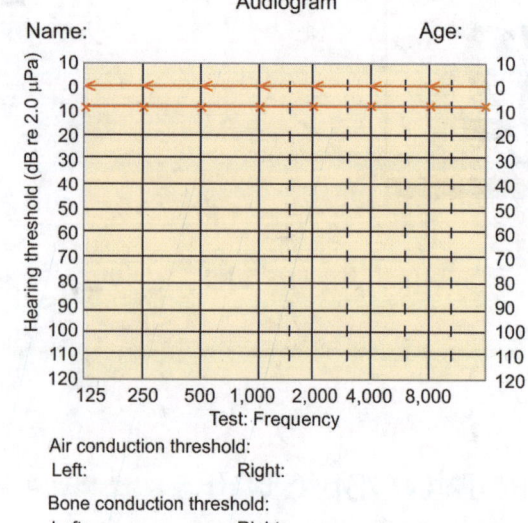

Fig. 52.2: Normal audiogram recorded from the left ear: <—bone conduction (unmasked); X—air conduction (unmasked).

- In nerve deafness, both air conduction and bone conduction are affected and the hearing loss is more for higher frequencies (Fig. 52.3A).
- In conduction deafness, bone conduction is normal and air conduction is impaired and the hearing loss is more for lower frequencies (Fig. 52.3B).

DISCUSSION

Audiometry can be made use of *to distinguish between conduction deafness and nerve deafness (sensorineural deafness)*. Here, graphs for air conduction and bone conduction are plotted separately.

In normal audiogram, the threshold for hearing through air conduction is 0 dB and the threshold for bone conduction is slightly higher may be about 5 dB which means that air conduction is slightly better than bone conduction. The threshold of bone conduction is a measure of cochlear function.

In **conduction deafness**, air conduction is impaired but bone conduction is normal (Fig. 52.3B). The threshold for air conduction is higher than bone conduction here and there is a wide air-bone gap.

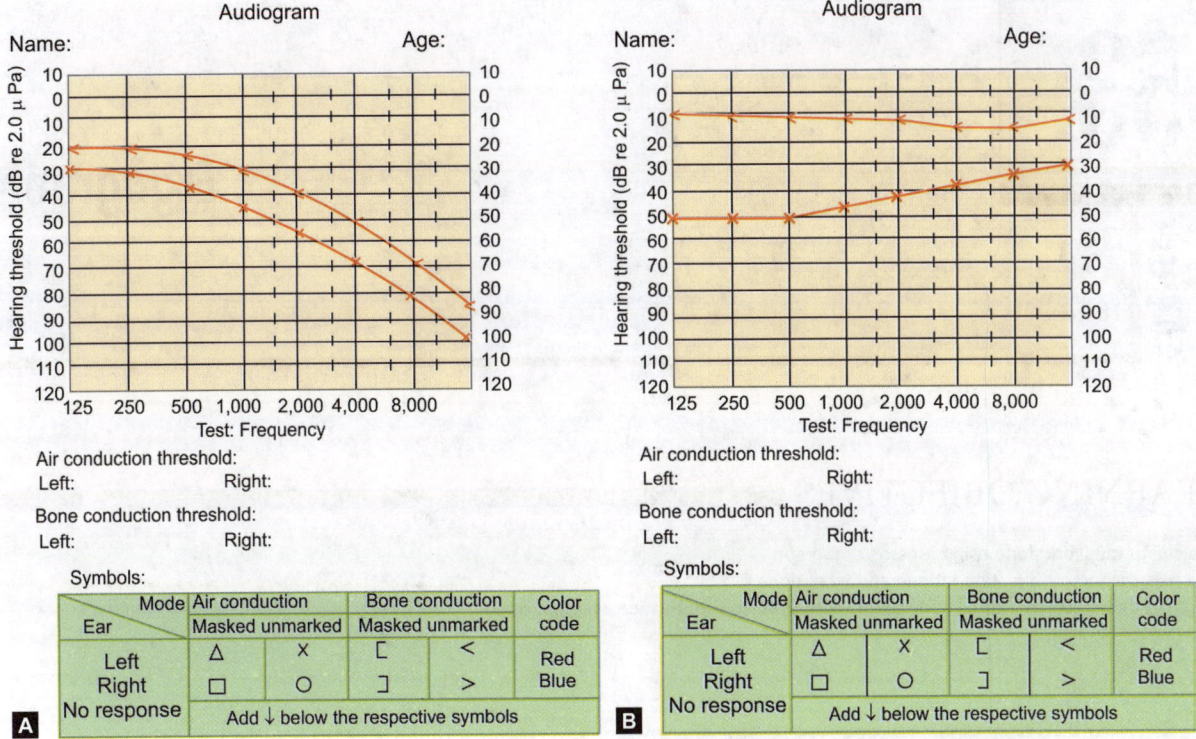

Figs. 52.3A and B: Audiogram showing sensorineural deafness (A) and conductive deafness (B) recorded from the left ear. Note that in sensorineural deafness, both air and bone conduction are equally affected and hearing loss is more for higher frequencies. In conductive deafness, bone conduction is normal and the hearing loss for air conduction is about 50 dB at frequency 500 Hz; whereas at higher frequencies, the hearing loss is less.

Difference in the thresholds of air and bone conduction (air-bone gap) is a measure of the degree of conduction deafness. In sensorineural deafness, both air conduction and bone conduction are impaired with equal severity. The threshold for bone conduction remains slightly higher than air conduction **(Fig. 52.3A)** and the air-bone gap are normal. Thus, an audiogram provides an objective measurement of the degree of deafness. The tonal range most affected can also be determined.

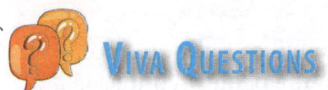

Viva Questions

1. **What are the types of deafness?**
   Conduction deafness and sensorineural deafness.
2. **How will you differentiate between conduction deafness and neural deafness?**
   Refer page 262 and 263.
3. **What are the causes of conduction deafness?**
   Impacted wax or foreign body in the external ear, damage to the tympanic membrane and ear ossicles, otosclerosis, etc.
4. **Mention the causes of nerve deafness.**
   Congenital deafness, damage to the hair cells or VIII cranial nerve, prolonged use of drugs like streptomycin, lesion of the auditory pathway.

Chapter 53

Ergography

LEARNING OBJECTIVES

- Calculate the work done using Mosso's ergograph
- Discuss the factors affecting fatigue and work done
- Explain the effects of arterial and venous occlusion, and motivation on work done

INTRODUCTION

Ergograph (**Fig. 53.1**) is the instrument with which a record of work performed is obtained. Erg is the unit of work. Ergography is the technique of recording the work performed.

The original ergograph was constructed by Mosso. In the ergograph, there is an arrangement for fixing the hand and the fingers in appropriate holders. A weight attached to a cord is made to hang over a pulley. The other end of the cord is attached to a sliding plate, which moves to and fro. The plate carries a lever system to record its movements. The other end of the plate is connected through a sling to the middle finger of the hand. The lever is made to write on a kymograph. In some models, a pencil placed in the sliding plate is made to write on a paper which is made to slide with the to and fro motion of the plate itself.

PROCEDURE

- Place the ergograph on one side of the table

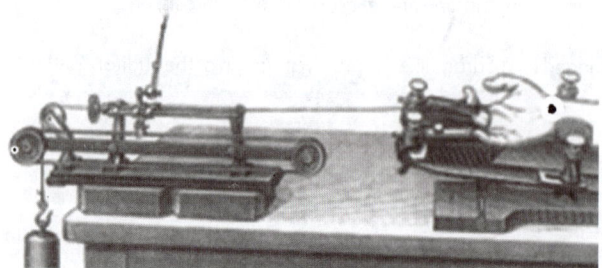

Fig. 53.1: Ergograph.

- Attach a weight of 3 kg to the cord. See that the cord carrying the load hangs freely over the pulley. Remove the weight.
- Ask the subject to sit in such a way that he can place his arm in the instrument with ease and comfort.
- Tie a blood pressure cuff round his arm.
- Wind the metronome key. Adjust the metronome to give a bell sound in every 2 seconds, i.e., at a frequency 30/min. Instruct the subject to pull the load maximally with the middle finger without moving the shoulder when he hear each bell and to leave it immediately after pulling.
- Arrange the kymograph and its drum with its axis in a horizontal plane. Adjust the position to allow the to and fro moving lever to write on the slow moving drum paper.
- Alternately, arrange a pencil or ballpoint pen in the ergograph and a paper on the platform underneath.
- Open the holders, which fix the forearm. Instruct the subject to insert the forearm in the prone position.
- Insert the index and the ring fingers in the tubes provided for them and leave the middle finger free.
- Pass the string attached to the sliding plate over the middle finger and suspend a weight of 3 kg to the other end.
- Adjust the position of the subject, the ergograph and the length of the cord carrying the weight in such a way as to allow free movements of the middle finger with the load attached to it.
- Close the holders and fix the forearm.
- Note the time. Instruct the subject to commence the exercise at the bell of the metronome. Start the stopwatch and the metronome.

- Obtain a record until complete fatigue, i.e., the weight can no longer be moved. Stop the stopwatch and note the duration.
- Now cheer up the subject, if the encouragement is proper the subject is now able to perform work for a longer time. Continue till he is fatigued again.
- Now if necessary allow the subject to take the hand and the arm out of the instrument.
- After sufficient rest (say of 10 minutes) repeat the experiment to obtain again a full fatigue graph; but this time obstruct the venous blood flow by raising the pressure in the cuff to 40 mm Hg. Release the cuff pressure as soon as the fatigue is established.
- After rest for 10 minutes inflate the cuff to systolic blood pressure, i.e., to about 120 mm Hg to produce arterial as well as venous occlusion.
- Again after sufficient rest ask the subject to carry out work now for 30 seconds and then rest for 30 seconds and so on. Find out how long this can be carried out.

Observations and Inferences

- The graph of fatigue is very similar to the one obtained from the isolated muscle of the frog. The phenomenon of beneficial effect in the form of staircase can be seen.
- After the beneficial effect the graph shows a period of steady state. During this period the height of contraction is maximum and is maintained at a constant level.
- The steady state is then replaced by the onset of fatigue. The height of contraction slowly declines. The contractions then become irregular. Mistakes occur in keeping the time and later the contractions stop.
- Proper encouragement can overcome the fatigue at least temporarily. It indicates that the fatigue does possess a cortical component. The actual duration of work is decided more by the psychological set up of the subject. Interest in the experiment may prolong the period especially of the steady state.

Calculation of the Work Done

Roughly the graph can be divided into two portions, first part a rectangle and the adjacent one a triangle (**Fig. 53.2**).

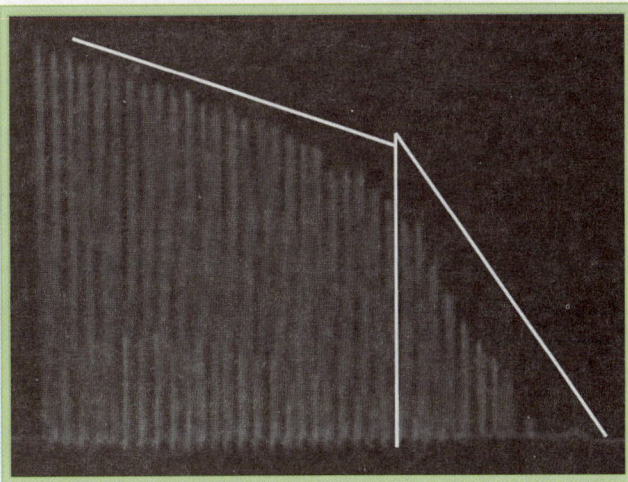

Fig. 53.2: Record obtained.

Draw these two figures on the graph. Find out the area of each figure, add them up, and then divide the total area by the length of the baseline. The resulting number gives the average height of each contraction.

Calculate the number of contractions from the duration and the speed at which the contractions were carried out.

Work done in gm cm = 3,000 g × No. of contractions × Average height in cm through which the load is lifted.

Calculate the work done in the following situations:
- At one stretch
- At one stretch while the blood supply was obstructed
- With alternate periods of rest and activity.

Cessation of blood supply results in production of less amount of work and is accompanied by pain and cramps.

The total amount of work done by alternate periods of rest and activity is more than the work that was carried out in one stretch.

Using Bicycle Ergometer the quantitative study of the work done, energy intake, mechanical efficiency and oxygen debt can be carried out.

Viva Questions

1. **Define ergography.**
   Page 264.
2. **How can you produce venous and arterial obstruction?**
   Refer page 265.
3. **Why is middle finger selected for lifting the weight?**
   It is the longest and strongest finger.
4. **What is the reason for improvement of physical performance by motivation?**
   Fatigue possess a cortical component (refer page 265).

Chapter 54

Peak Expiratory Flow Rate

LEARNING OBJECTIVES

- Define peak expiratory flow rate and give the normal value
- Explain the significance of doing peak expiratory flow rate

PY6.8: Demonstrate the correct technique to find out PEFR.

AIM

To determine the peak expiratory flow rate.

APPARATUS

- **Wright's peak flow meter (Fig. 54.1):** The measurement of peak expiratory flow was pioneered by **Martin Wright** who produced the first meter specifically designed to measure this index of lung function in the late 1950s.
- **Mini Wright's peak flow meter (Fig. 54.2):** Wright's peak flow meter is a simple device used for the measurement of ventilatory function of lungs. A mini version of the flow meter is a short cylinder made of plastic. An indicator moves in a slot alongside a scale with numbers on it which indicates liters/minute. There is a handle provided near the mouthpiece. The end opposite to the mouthpiece has holes in it for allowing air to exit the apparatus.

PROCEDURE

- Ask the subject to hold the peak flow meter by its handle making sure that the fingers are clear off the scale and the slot, and are not obstructing the holes at the end of the apparatus.

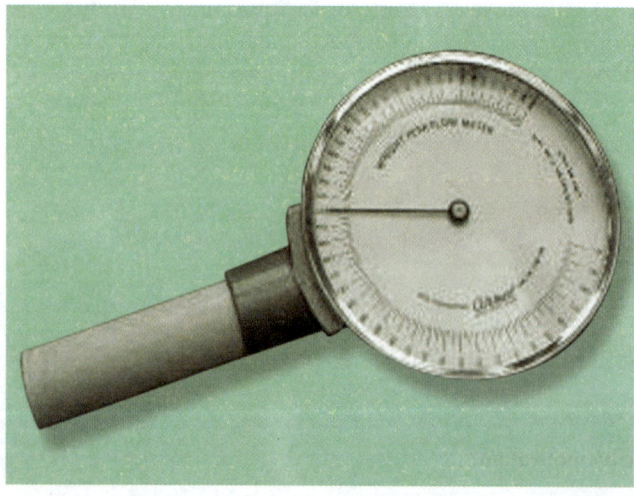

Fig. 54.1: Wright's peak flow meter.

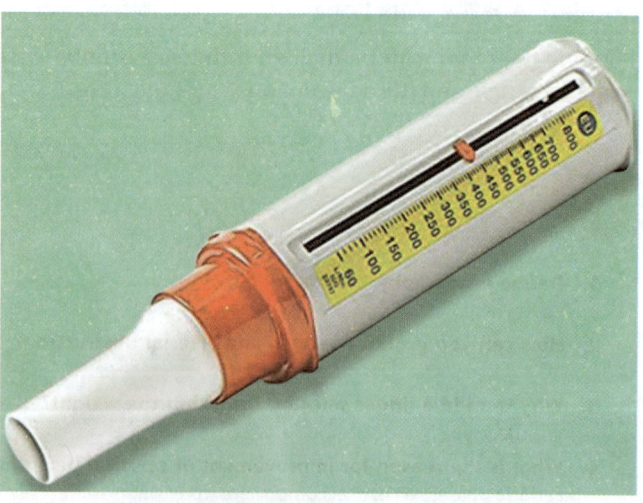

Fig. 54.2: Mini Wright's peak flow meter.

- Ask the subject to take a deep breath, place the mouthpiece firmly between the teeth and lips and then to blow out with a short sharp blast. Not the reading on the scale. Bring the indicator back to zero.
- Take 6 readings at intervals of 1 minute and select the maximum value for the report.
  Normal range of PEFR: 350–600 liters/minute

DISCUSSION

Peak expiratory flow rate (**PEFR**) is the maximum flow rate or peak flow rate of air during a single forced expiration. This value is useful in distinguishing between reversible and irreversible pulmonary diseases. The peak flow meter is a small, hand-held device used to monitor a person's ability to breathe out air. It measures the airflow through the bronchi and thus the degree of obstruction in the airways. Peak expiratory flow is typically measured in units of liters per minute (L/min).

It is of special importance in cases of asthma, where the effectiveness of treatment with a bronchodilator can be quickly evaluated. But the instrument is not useful for assessing the degree of disability of the patients with lung fibrosis and other restrictive conditions because they may have normal expiratory flow rates. The major factor that limits expiratory flow rate during maximal forced expiration is the narrowing of small airways. Thus the flow rate is a function of lung volume rather than the effort exerted. This is called **effort independent flow**.

Peak flow readings are higher when patients are feeling well and lower when the airways are constricted. The normal expected value depends on the patient's sex, age, and height. It is classically reduced in obstructive lung disorders such as asthma. Due to the wide range of 'normal' values and the high degree of variability, peak flow is not the recommended test to identify asthma. From changes in recorded values, one can determine lung functionality, the severity of asthma symptoms, and treatment. A small portion of people with asthma may be benefitted from regular peak flow monitoring. When peak flow is being monitored regularly, the results may be recorded on a peak flow chart (**Fig. 54.3**). It is important to use the same peak flow meter every time.

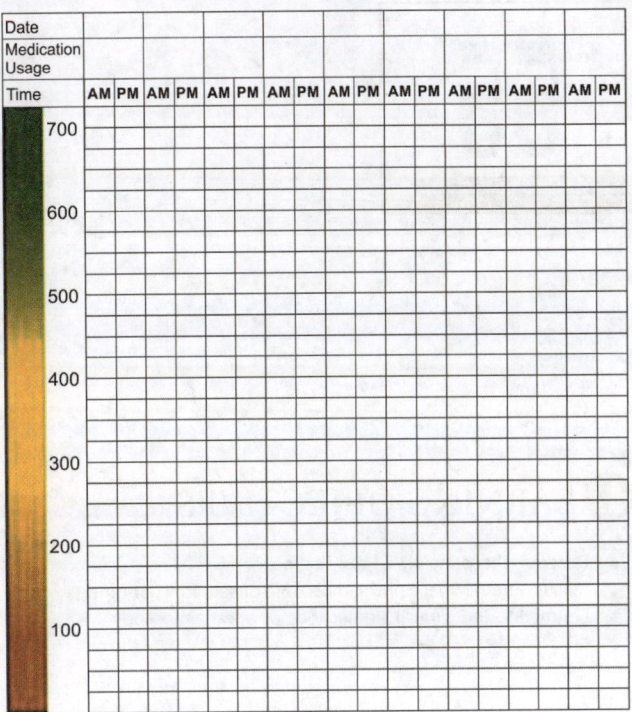

Fig. 54.3: Peak flow meter chart showing the green, yellow and red zones.

Peak flow readings are often classified into three zones of measurement according to the **American Lung Association**; green, yellow, and red. Asthma management can be planned based on the green-yellow-red zones.

Zone	Reading	Inference
Green zone	80–100% of the usual or normal peak flow readings	A peak flow reading in the green zone indicates that the asthma is under good control.
Yellow zone	50–79% of the usual or normal peak flow readings	Indicates caution. It may mean respiratory airways are narrowing and additional medication may be required.
Red zone	Less than 50% of the usual or normal peak flow readings	Indicates a medical emergency. Severe airway narrowing may be occurring and immediate action needs to be taken.

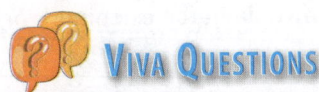

VIVA QUESTIONS

1. **Define peak expiratory flow rate. Give the normal value.**
   It is the maximum velocity or rate with which air is forced out of the lungs in a single forced expiration. Expressed in liter/minute. Normal value 350–400 L/min.

2. **What is the significance of PEFR?**
   - It helps to detect large airway diseases.
   - Helps to distinguish between reversible like asthma and irreversible like emphysema respiratory conditions. In asthma, after taking bronchodilator there will be a marked increase in the value of PEFR.
   - It is also useful to study the effect of training in athletes.

Chapter 55

Ophthalmoscopy

LEARNING OBJECTIVES

- Describe the principle of ophthalmoscopy
- Discuss the normal ophthalmoscopic observation of fundus of eye
- Enumerate the clinical significance of ophthalmoscopy

PY10.17: Describe and discuss the functional anatomy of eye.

AIM

To view the fundus of the eye.

APPARATUS

Ophthalmoscope was invented by Helmholtz in 1851.

Ophthalmoscopy is of two major types:
1. **Direct ophthalmoscopy** is one that produces an upright image of approximately 15 times magnification **(Fig. 55.1)**.
2. **Indirect ophthalmoscopy** is one that produces an inverted, or reversed, image of 2–5 times magnification. The *direct ophthalmoscope* is an instrument about the size of a small flashlight (torch) with several lenses that can magnify up to about 15 times. This type of ophthalmoscope is most commonly used during a routine physical examination.

PRINCIPLE

A parallel beam of light from a battery operated lamp is deflected through right angles by an angled mirror located at the top of the instrument. The observer looks through a hole in the mirror along the path of the light through the pupil. So that structures of the eye including the fundus are illuminated and can be inspected.

Lenses of graded focal length may be placed behind the hold on the mirror and are moved by a milled wheel, conveniently placed so that it can be controlled by the index finger of the hand holding the ophthalmoscope. There is a series of lenses marked '+' which are convex lenses and an array of lenses marked '–' which are concave. Each lens also bears a number which corresponds to its focal length of half a meter and twenty diopters to one-twentieth of a meter. These lenses are used to compensate for refractive errors like hypermetropia or myopia in the examiner's or patient's eyes.

PROCEDURE

❖ During routine examination, the fundus may be inspected through the untreated pupil. But for a thorough fundal examination, the pupils must be dilated with a short acting mydriatic like tropicamide or cyclopentolate drops 0.5–1%. After examination,

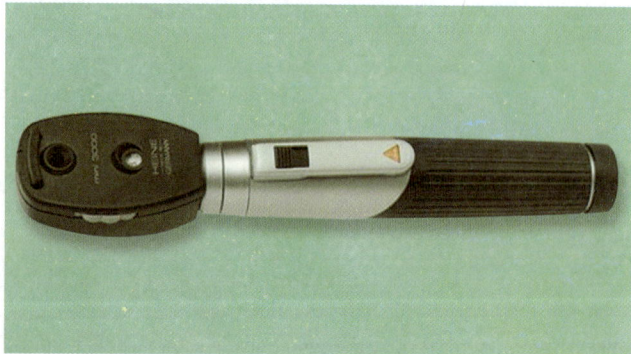

Fig. 55.1: Direct ophthalmoscope.

pupils can be constricted using miotics like 2% eserine or pilocarpine drops.
- The subject should be examined in the dark room if possible.
- The ophthalmoscope should be held in the right hand and the right eye should be used to examine the patient's right eye.
- The subject should be asked to look straight ahead to keep an eye fixed on a selected distant object and to keep both eyes open.
- Vision in the eye which is not being examined should not be obstructed by the examiner's head; otherwise the patient's gaze tends to wander.
- The examiner's eye should be placed as close as possible to the ophthalmoscope. This enables greater area to be visualized through the sight hole, as when we look through a key hole. The ophthalmoscope should be held steadily by pressing it against the side of the nose and against the superior orbital margin.
- It is helpful to rest the ulnar border of the examiner's free hand above the patient's superior orbital margin.
- The examination should begin with the ophthalmoscope held 20–30 cm away from the patient's eye with the light directed into the pupil. The pupil will then appear to glow uniformly red in normal circumstances. This is the red reflex. The ophthalmoscope and the examiner's head are moved closer to the patient's eye and the ophthalmoscope should come as close as possible to the patients eye, without touching the eyelashes or cornea and the fundus is studied.

DISCUSSION

Ophthalmoscopy is done as part of a routine physical or complete eye examination. It is used to detect and evaluate symptoms of various retinal vascular diseases or eye diseases such as glaucoma.

The arteries, arterioles and veins in the superficial layers of retina near its vitreous surface can be seen clearly using ophthalmoscope. **Fundus** of the eye is the interior surface of the eye opposite to the lens. It includes the retina, optic disk, macula and fovea. Retina is the only place in the body where arterioles are readily visible. The optic disk can also be seen clearly by ophthalmoscopy **(Fig. 55.2)**. The ophthalmoscopic observations in a normal eye are as follows:
- Optic disk is creamy pink and the center of the disk is pale and hollowed out.
- Retina is pinkish red.
- Blood vessels consist of 4 main arteries and their accompanying veins.
- Macula appears slightly darker than the surrounding retina.

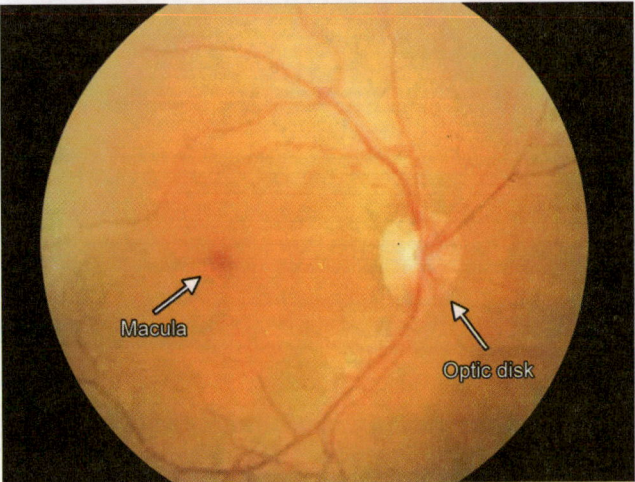

Fig. 55.2: Appearance of normal fundus of eye.

Clinical Importance

Ophthalmoscopic examination helps not only in the diagnosis of eye diseases like retinitis pigmentosa, papilledema, etc., but also in detecting systemic disorders which affect the blood vessels of the eye leading to retinopathy. Thus, diseases affecting blood vessels like diabetes mellitus, hypertension, etc., can be evaluated by ophthalmoscopic examination.

- Cerebrospinal fluid (CSF) pressure can be indirectly assessed by ophthalmoscopy, where there will be **papilledema** in the optic disc. Optic disk is bulged in raised intracranial tension. Papilledema is due to compression of the retinal vein as it crosses the extension of the subarachnoid space to enter the optic nerve.
- In patients with headache, the finding of swollen optic disc (papilledema) on ophthalmoscopy indicates raised intracranial pressure **(Fig. 55.3)**. It may be due to hydrocephalus, brain tumor, etc.
- Cupped optic discs **(Fig. 55.4)** are seen in glaucoma (ocular hypertension).
- In patients with diabetes mellitus, abnormal growth of blood vessels, exudates, hemorrhages, aneurysms, etc., are seen in the fundus. Regular ophthalmoscopic eye examinations (once every 6 months to 1 year) are important to screen for diabetic retinopathy **(Fig. 55.5)**. Thus visual loss due to diabetes can be prevented by retinal laser treatment if retinopathy is diagnosed early.
- In arterial hypertension, hypertensive changes of the retina include arteriolar constriction, twisting and kinking of tiny retinal blood vessels, flame-shaped hemorrhages, cotton wool spots, yellow hard exudates and papilledema **(Fig. 55.6)**. These changes known as hypertensive retinopathy closely mimic those in the brain and may predict cerebrovascular accidents (strokes).

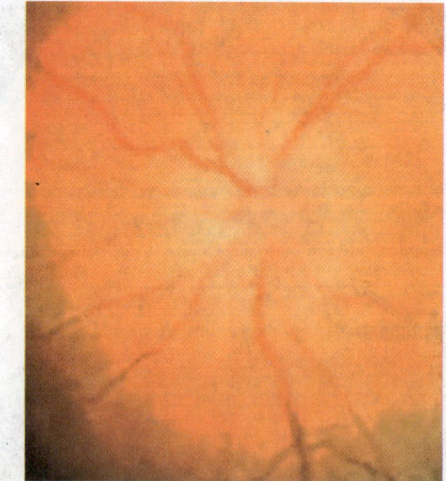

Fig. 55.3: Papilledema.

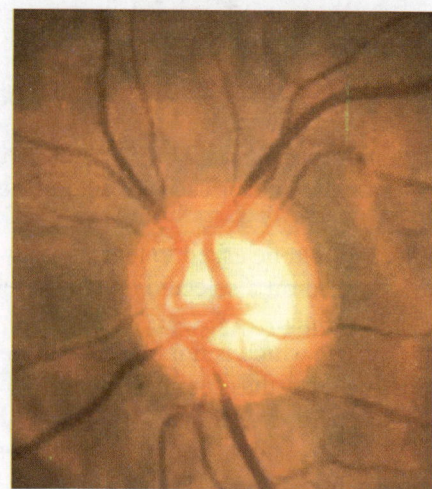

Fig. 55.4: Cupping of optic disc.

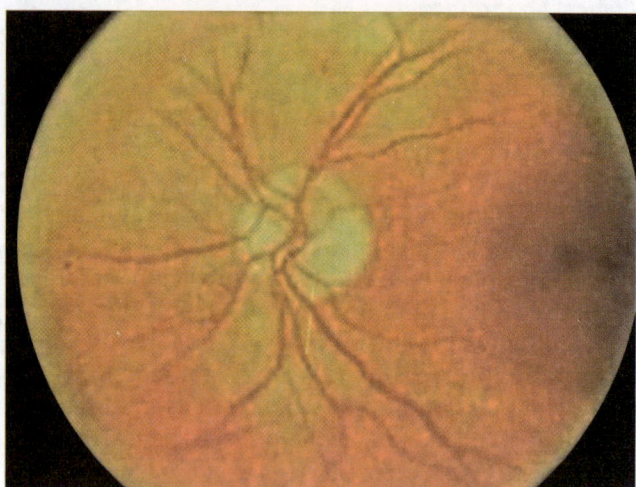

Fig. 55.5: Diabetic retinopathy.

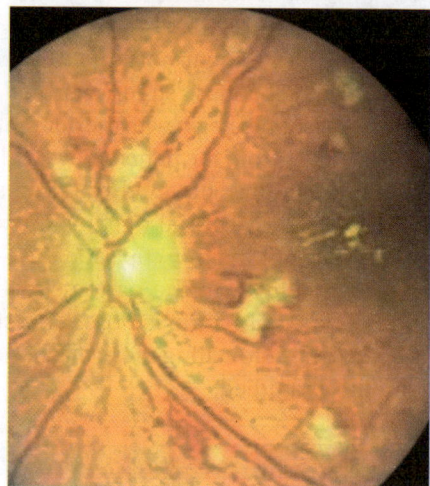

Fig. 55.6: Hypertensive changes in the retina.

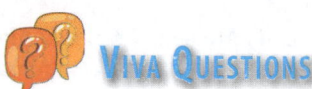

VIVA QUESTIONS

1. **What are the parts of the ophthalmoscope?**
   Handle with a rechargeable battery and a head that contains a bulb, a set of apertures for the light source and a set of lenses.
2. **Describe the appearance of normal fundus of eye?**
   Refer page 269.
3. **Enumerate the clinical significance of ophthalmoscopy.**
   Refer page 269.
4. **Name a few conditions that can be diagnosed by ophthalmoscopy.**
   Refer page 269.

Chapter 56

Harvard Step Test

LEARNING OBJECTIVES

- Calculate cardiac efficiency index
- Grading of efficiency index

PY3.15: Demonstrate the effect of exercise and record changes in cardiorespiratory parameters.

AIM

To study the response of the cardiovascular system to standardized exercise.

This test also referred to as exercise tolerance test or stress testing is done as a test for physical fitness and should not be done in patients.

EQUIPMENT REQUIRED

Step or platform 20 inches or 50 cm high (16 inches for women), stop watch, metronome (a metronome, is a device that produces an audible click or other sound at a regular interval that can be set by the user, typically in beats per minute).

PRINCIPLE

During exercise, there is a progressive increase in the heart rate and blood pressure. However, after the exercise is over, these values return to the pre-exercise levels during the next few minutes. The fact that, compared to a trained person, there is a greater increase in the heart rate and BP in an untrained individual during exercise, and that these values take a longer time to return to basal level, forms the basis of exercise tolerance tests. The response to physical exercise depends on the cardiac reserve, i.e., efficiency of the heart, muscle power, training, motivation and the state of nutrition. Therefore, the cardiac efficiency tests can also be used to test physical fitness in an individual.

PROCEDURE

- Explain the test procedures to the subject. Perform screening of health risks and obtain informed consent.
- Record basic information such as age, height, body weight and gender. Check step height and set metronome.
- Record the basal pulse rate.
- The subject, has to take steps up and down on a platform in a cycle of two seconds with four distinct foot movements (1) the right foot on (2) both feet on (3) right foot off (4) left foot off. The rate of 30 steps per minute must be sustained for 5 minutes or until exhaustion. To ensure the right speed, a metronome is used. Exhaustion is the point at which the subject cannot maintain the stepping rate for 15 seconds. The subject immediately sits down on completion of the test, and the heartbeats are counted for 1–1.5, 2–2.5, and 3–3.5 minutes.
- Start a stop watch at the beginning of the exercise and measure the duration of the exercise.
- Ideally, the exercise should be performed for 5 minutes. Stop the test if the subject feels breathless and exhausted and is unable to continue the test.
- Count the pulse rate 1 minute after the end of exercise.
- The pulse rate is inversely proportional to the degree of cardiac efficiency.

❖ To obtain an approximate idea of the cardiac efficiency index, count the pulse rate at the following intervals:
- Between 1 and one and a half minutes = a
- Between two and two and a half minutes = b
- Between three and three and a half minutes = c

The results are written down as *time until exhaustion in seconds* and *total heartbeats counted in the recovery period*.

Time after which the pulse rate returns to basal level = ……minutes

Fitness index equation is derived from the above data.

Cardiac efficiency index =
$$\frac{\text{Duration of exercise in seconds} \times 100}{(a + b + c) \times 2}$$

For example, if the total test time was 300 seconds (if completed the whole 5 minutes), and the number of heart beats between 1–1.5 minutes was 90, between 2–2.5 it was 80 and between 3–3.5 it was 70, then the long form fitness index score would be: $(100 \times 300)/(240 \times 2) = 62.5$. (The denominator is multiplied by 2 because we are using the total number of heartbeats in the 30 second period, not the rate (beats per minute) during that time.)

In normal individuals, the cardiac efficiency index is nearly 100%, but is more in sports persons.

Efficiency/Fitness Index

❖ Over 90%—efficiency is excellent
❖ 81–90%—efficiency is good
❖ 55–80%—efficiency is average
❖ Below 55%—efficiency is poor

DISCUSSION

The Harvard step test also known as aerobic fitness test was first developed by Lucien Brouha and associates in 1943. It is simple to conduct and requires minimal equipment. Now several modified versions exist such as the Kasch step test and Sharkey step test.

Uses

❖ The Harvard step test is a type of cardiac stress test for detecting and diagnosing cardiovascular diseases.
❖ It is also a good measurement of fitness and a person's ability to recover after a strenuous exercise by checking the recovery rate.

Grading of Exercise

The WHO grading of muscular exercise, according to the heart rate and relative load index (RLI), i.e., percentage of maximum oxygen utilization, is as follows:

Grade	Heart rate per minute	Relative load index (% of maximum O_2 consumption)
Light (mild)	<100	<25
Moderate	100–125	25–50
Heavy	125–150	51–75
Severe	>150	>75

Purpose of Exercise Tolerance Tests

The exercise tolerance tests are the best tests for determining the efficiency of the heart as a pumping organ. These tests take the place of cardiac output measurements which cannot be done with ease in most clinical settings.

Cardiac Reserve

Cardiac reserve refers to the maximum increase in cardiac output above normal and is expressed in percentage. In a healthy adult it is 4–5 times the resting value and in athletes it is 7–8 times.

For example, if the basal cardiac output = 5 L/min

Maximum achievable output = 25 L/min

Then, cardiac reserve percentage = $\frac{25 - 5}{25} \times 100 = 80\%$

A measure of the cardiac reserve can help predict the likelihood of heart failure if suspected. In persons with severe cardiac failure there will be no cardiac reserve. Any factor that prevents the heart from pumping blood effectively will decrease the cardiac reserve. The factors can be myocardial infarction, cardiomyopathy, vitamin B deficiency, valvular heart disease, etc. A diagnosis of low cardiac reserve can be made by asking the subject to exercise on a treadmill or by walking up and down the steps. Exercise tolerance is assessed by measuring the maximum heart rate attained after a standard exercise test, and the time required for the heart rate to return to normal. ECG and blood pressure will be monitored continuously during the test. Exercise tolerance is an excellent indicator of cardiac reserve.

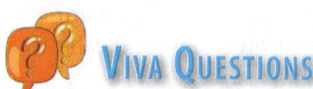

VIVA QUESTIONS

1. **How is muscular exercise graded?**
   Refer page 272.

2. **How will you calculate cardiac efficiency index?**
   Refer page 272.

3. **Define cardiac reserve. How will you calculate it?**
   Refer page 272.
4. **What does Harward step test measure?**
   It measures a person's aerobic fitness and can be used as a predictive test for their $VO_{2\,max}$. It also tests the cardiovascular system to cope up with increased muscular activity.
5. **Discuss the advantages of Harward step test.**
   » This test requires minimal equipment and cost
   » It can be performed without anybody's help
   » The person himself can assess his fitness level based on how quickly his heart rate recovers to the basal level after exercise.

57

Cardiovascular Autonomic Function Tests

LEARNING OBJECTIVES

- Discuss the tests employed to assess parasympathetic and sympathetic function tests
- Explain the immediate cardiovascular responses to standing from lying down
- Determine Valsalva ratio

PY5.14: CVS autonomic function tests in a normal volunteer.

AIM

To test the efficiency of the autonomic nervous system the following tests are done:
- Heart rate and blood pressure response to standing
- Heart rate response to tilting
- Heart rate variation with respiration
- Valsalva ratio
- Hand grip test (HGT)—blood pressure response to isometric exercise
- Cold pressor response test

CARDIOVASCULAR RESPONSE TO STANDING (30:15 R-R RATIO)

Aim

To determine the effect of standing from supine position on heart rate and blood pressure.

Apparatus

Four channel data acquisition system.

Principle

On standing from supine position, immediately the blood pressure falls by 20 mm Hg and heart rate increases by 10–20 beats within 5–15 seconds.

Procedure

- Connect the limb leads to record ECG in lead II. Connect the sphygmomanometer to record blood pressure.
- Ask the subject to lie down in the supine position with the sphygmomanometer and the ECG leads attached.
- He is asked to relax completely for a minimum of 10 minutes. Record the basal heart rate and blood pressure. Heart rate is measured from the continuous running ECG record using the formula
  Heart rate per minute = 60/R-R interval in second
- Ask the subject to stand up and note the change in heart rate and BP. Record BP serially at 1 and 2 minutes after standing. A continuous ECG is recorded during this period. Mark a point on the ECG to identify the time of standing from supine position.
- Note the heart rate at the 15th and 30th beat after standing.
- Determine the 30:15 R-R ratio from the ECG recording. Longest RR interval occurring about 30 beats after standing divided by shortest RR interval which occurs about 15 beats after standing gives the 30:15 RR ratio. Compare with the normal value.

Discussion

Blood pressure changes are studied to assess the integrity of the sympathetic functions and heart rate changes to study the integrity of parasympathetic functions of the autonomic nervous system.

- There will be changes in blood pressure and heart rate when the subject stands up from the lying down posture. On standing, there is pooling of blood in the lower extremities which leads to a decrease in venous return and cardiac output. This leads to a fall in systolic blood pressure by about 20 mm Hg. The sinoaortic reflex comes into play. There is decreased baroreceptor stimulation which results in increased sympathetic tone and decreased parasympathetic (vagal) tone. This produces reflex tachycardia and peripheral vasoconstriction. Thus the systolic blood pressure increases. The heart rate increases immediately upon standing and continues to rise for the next 10–15 beats. There after it slows to a maximum extent at the 30th beat.
- **30:15 R-R ratio** is the longest R-R interval where the heart rate is slowest occurring about 30 beats after standing divided by the shortest R-R interval where the heart rate is fastest which occurs about 15 beats after standing. Normal value is more than 1.04 and it is a measure of cardiac vagal function. RR ratio less than one indicate autonomic insufficiency.
- Patients with autonomic dysfunction have **orthostatic or postural hypotension,** where the systolic BP falls more than 20 mm Hg and the diastolic BP falls more than 10 mm Hg on standing up from lying down posture.
- In **orthostatic tachycardia**, the blood pressure on standing up will be normal or minimally decreased but there will be a sustained increase in heart rate by about 25 beats per minute.
- In vasovagal syncope, hypotension is accompanied by paradoxical bradycardia. In this condition there are overactive autonomic reflexes instead of autonomic insufficiency.

HEART RATE AND BLOOD PRESSURE RESPONSE TO PASSIVE TILTING

Principle

Cardiovascular response to change in position is tested using tilt table. A tilt-table test involves **changing a person's positioning quickly and seeing how their blood pressure and heart rate respond.**

Apparatus

Tilt table, ECG machine, sphygmomanometer and four channel data acquisition system.

Procedure

Ask the subject to lie down on a tilt table (**Fig. 57.1**). Connect ECG electrode to the four channel data acquisition system.

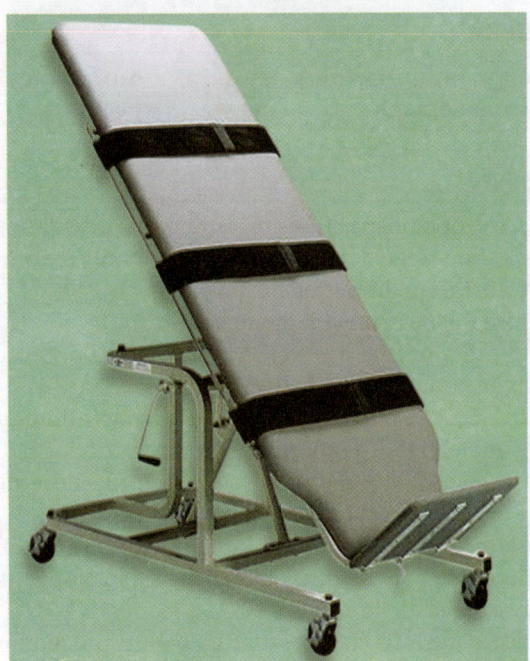

Fig. 57.1: Tilt table.

Tie the BP cuff to record blood pressure. Ask the subject to relax for 10–15 minutes. Record the baseline heart rate and blood pressure. Position the head side of the tilt table to an inclination of 80 degree from horizontal with the head up. Immediately record the blood pressure and heart rate and then record the BP at one minute interval for 3 minutes.

Discussion

This test is also known as **head up tilt table testing**. In this test the responses obtained are similar to that obtained in standing from the supine position. It is done for people who have symptoms like a rapid heartbeat or who often feel dizzy when they go from a lying down to standing position.

VALSALVA RATIO

Aim

To measure the change in heart rate and blood pressure during Valsalva maneuver.

Principle

Valsalva ratio is a measure of change of heart rate and blood pressure during a brief period of forced expiration against a closed glottis or mouthpiece connected to a mercury manometer. During and after Valsalva maneuver, there will be changes in cardiac vagal efferent activity and sympathetic vasomotor activity.

Apparatus

Mercury manometer, nose clip, mouth piece and electrocardiograph.

Procedure

- Give proper instructions regarding the procedure.
- Ask the subject to lie down in the semi recumbent posture or in the sitting posture.
- Close the nostrils with the nose clip.
- Put the mouth piece to the mouth of the subject and connect manometer to the mouth piece.
- Connect the electrodes of the electrocardiograph to record lead II ECG continuously.
- ECG recording 30 seconds before the procedure should be taken.
- Ask the subject to exhale forcefully into the mercury manometer and then ask him to maintain the expiratory pressure at 40 mm Hg for 10–15 seconds.
- Record the ECG changes throughout the procedure and up to 30 seconds after the procedure.
- Repeat the procedure three times and calculate the Valsalva ratio and select the largest ratio of the three.

The **Valsalva ratio** is the ratio of maximum heart rate during the Valsalva maneuver divided by the minimum heart rate occurring during phase 4, or the ratio can be calculated by dividing the longest R-R interval after the maneuver by the shortest R-R interval during the maneuver.

- Normal ratio: More than 1.45
- Borderline: 1.22–1.45
- Abnormal: Less than 1.22

Tachycardia ratio is defined as the ratio of shortest R-R interval during Valsalva maneuver to the longest R-R interval at rest. This is a better index of the functioning of the parasympathetic autonomic activity.

Precautions

- Subject should be instructed about the procedure properly.
- He should be allowed to practice the maneuver before actual performance.
- He should maintain the pressure constantly throughout the procedure.
- Procedure should be repeated three times.

Discussion

The Valsalva maneuver is done to assess the integrity of the baroreceptor mechanism. By monitoring the heart rate during the Valsalva maneuver, the Valsalva ratio can be measured. The Valsalva ratio is derived from the **maximum heart rate generated by the Valsalva maneuver divided by the lowest heart rate occurring within 30 seconds of the peak heart rate**. It possible, beat-to-beat BP recordings also should be recorded during the maneuver because the heart rate responses are baroreceptor reflex responses to changes in blood pressure. The normal cardiovascular response to a Valsalva maneuver has four phases.

The response is plotted with heart rate or systolic pressure in the Y axis and time in seconds in the X axis (**Fig. 57.2**).

Phase I (Initial Pressure Rise)

Phase I occurs at the onset of forced expiration or strain. There is a transient rise in blood pressure without any change in heart rate. The increase in blood pressure is due to increase in the intrathoracic pressure. When the pressure rises inside the chest, it forces blood out of the pulmonary vessels into the left atrium. This causes a mild increase in stroke volume during the first few seconds of the maneuver leading to a transient increase in systolic pressure.

Phase II (Reduced Venous Return and Compensation)

Phase II occurs during forced expiration. The venous return decreases due to increased pressure inside the chest leading to a fall in cardiac output and blood pressure. This initiates the baroreceptor reflex leading to reflex tachycardia and peripheral vasoconstriction. As a result of this compensation, the BP returns to normal or even above normal, but the cardiac output and blood flow to the body remains low. During this time the pulse rate increases (compensatory tachycardia). The heart rate increases throughout the phase due to vagal inhibition initially and sympathetic stimulation in the later stage.

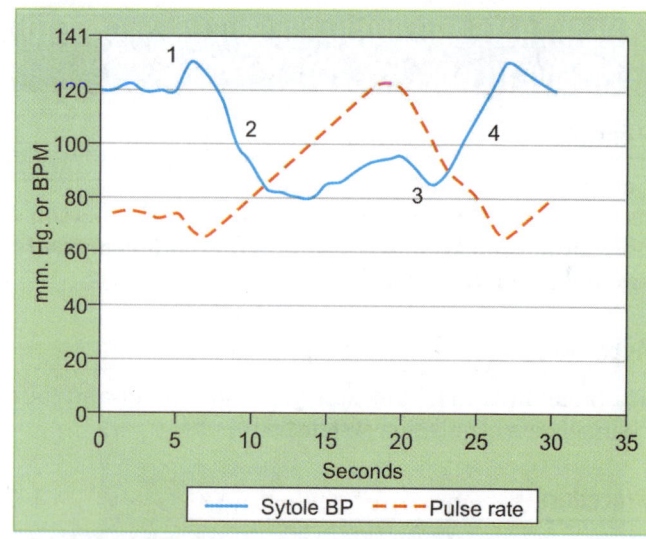

Fig. 57.2: Systolic blood pressure and pulse rate during a normal response to a Valsalva maneuver. Forty millimeter mercury pressure is applied at 5 seconds and relieved at 20 seconds.

Phase III (Pressure Release)

Phase III occurs when the pressure or strain is released. There will be a transient decrease in blood pressure without any change in heart rate. This is because when the intrathoracic pressure returns to normal the pulmonary vascular bed re-expand and gets filled with blood. This causes a further initial slight fall in stroke volume due to decreased left atrial return. Venous blood can once more enter the chest and the heart, and cardiac output begins to increase and BP returns to normal.

Phase IV (Return of Cardiac Output)

The intrathoracic pressure comes back to normal with complete cessation of strain. Venous return to the heart is increased by entry of blood which had been dammed back due to increase in intrathoracic pressure, causing a rapid increase in stroke volume and cardiac output. The blood pressure slowly rises above the normal level referred to as **overshoot phenomenon.** This rise in BP stimulates the baroreceptors leading to bradycardia and a fall in blood pressure to the normal level. With the fall of blood pressure, the pulse rate returns towards normal. In autonomic failure, the reflex bradycardia and blood pressure overshoot is typically absent.

Uses of Valsalva Maneuver

- Valsalva maneuver evaluates the sympathetic adrenergic functions using the blood pressure responses
- It evaluates parasympathetic (cardio-vagal) functions by assessing the heart rate responses
- Deviation from the normal response pattern signifies either abnormal heart function or abnormal autonomic nervous control of the heart.
- Valsalva method is also used by dentists following extraction of maxillary molar tooth. The maneuver is performed to determine if a perforation or antral communication exists.

HEART RATE VARIATION WITH DEEP BREATHING (SINUS ARRHYTHMIA)

Aim

To study the variation in heart rate with respiration.

Principle

Variation in heart rate with respiration is called sinus arrhythmia. Inspiration increases heart rate whereas expiration decreases heart rate. This change is mediated through vagus nerve and hence this test assesses the integrity of parasympathetic nervous system.

Procedure

- The subject lies in the supine position with the BP apparatus and ECG leads attached.
- Record the resting ECG and the heart rate.
- Ask the subject to breathe deeply at a rate of 6 breaths per minute with 5 seconds for inspiration and 5 seconds for expiration. Record the ECG during deep breathing.
- Determine the maximum and minimum heart rate with each respiratory cycle and find out the average heart rate in inspiration and expiration.
- Determine the expiratory to inspiratory ratio (E:I ratio) as the sum of 6 longest R-R intervals (slow heart rate), each of 6 repetitions divided by the sum of 6 shortest R-R intervals (fast heart rate).
- Normally, the fall in heart rate should be more than 15 beats per minute. In vagal insufficiency, the heart rate slows less than 10 beats/min.

ISOMETRIC EXERCISE (SUSTAINED HAND GRIP TEST)

Aim

To study the cardiovascular response to isometric exercise.

Principle

Sustained hand grip against resistance causes an increase in heart rate and blood pressure.

Apparatus

Sphygmomanometer, ECG machine, hand grip spring dynamometer **(Figs. 57.3 and 57.4).**

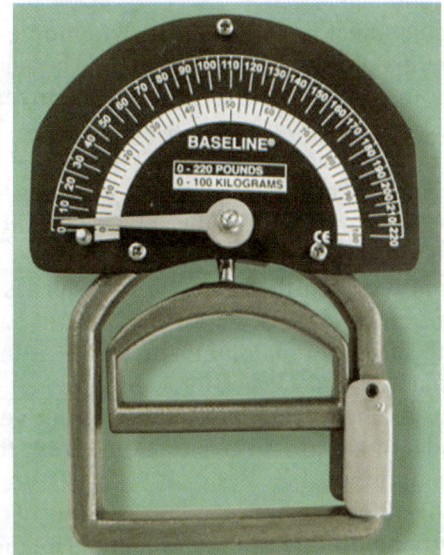

Fig. 57.3: Hand grip spring dynamometer.

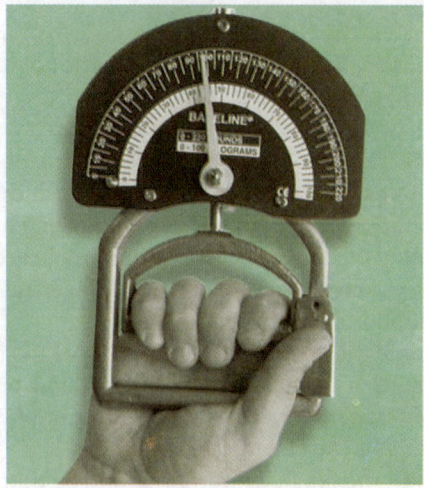

Fig. 57.4: Measurement of tension developed while squeezing the dynamometer.

Procedure

- Explain the test procedures and give proper instructions to the subject. Ask the subject to lie in a semi recumbent position.
- Connect the sphygmomanometer and the ECG electrodes for lead II recording.
- Record age, height, body weight, gender and hand dominance.
- Calibrate the dynamometer so as to suit the subject.
- Record the basal heart rate and blood pressure.
- Ask the subject to hold the dynamometer in the hand to be tested, with the arm at right angles and the elbow by the side of the body.
- The base of the dynamometer should rest on the first metacarpal, while the handle should rest on the middle of the four fingers.
- Ask the subject to squeeze the dynamometer with maximum isometric effort, which should be maintained for about 5 seconds. No other body movement is allowed. Measure the tension developed.
- Repeat the procedure twice and take second and the third reading. The forearm muscles are easily fatigued, so the best scores are usually achieved in the first or second trial.
- Select the highest of the three readings, which is referred to as maximal isometric tension.
- Ask the subject to maintain a pressure of 30% of the maximal isometric tension for 5 minutes.
- Record the heart rate and blood pressure every 30 seconds. Blood pressure is recorded from the non-exercising arm.
- Find the difference between the last value of diastolic pressure before the release of hand grip and mean value calculated by averaging the last three minute recording before commencing the exercise. The rise in diastolic blood pressure at the point just before the release of handgrip is taken as the index of response to the test.
- Normal response is a rise in diastolic pressure by about 15 mm Hg and rise in heart rate by 30%.

Precautions

- Proper instructions should be given to the subject.
- Basal diastolic blood pressure should be recorded.
- The subject should maintain the pressure of 30% of maximum isometric tension for 5 minutes.
- Diastolic blood pressure immediately before the release of hand grip should be recorded.

Discussion

- The purpose of the hand grip test is to measure the maximum isometric strength of the hand and forearm muscles. Handgrip strength is important for any sport in which the hands are used for catching, throwing or lifting. This test is often used as a general test of strength because people with strong hands tend to be strong elsewhere.
- **Determining the pulse rate and blood pressure responses to sustained hand grip test is an established technique to evaluate this autonomic balance**. A low variability in heart rate reflects an increase in sympathetic nervous system activity and reduced parasympathetic nervous system activity.
- This test is also useful to record whether the athlete is left or right handed, as this may help in the interpretation of results. The non-dominant hand usually scores about 10% lower.
- Results differ between male and females, between left and right (dominant and non-dominant) hands, and with age.
- The results can also be affected by the position of the wrist, elbow and shoulder, so these should be standardized.
- The blood pressure is increased due to increase in peripheral resistance and cardiac output. Peripheral vasoconstriction is due to stimulation of the alpha adrenergic receptors on the blood vessels. In sympathetic insufficiency the cardiovascular response to sustained hand grip is diminished or absent.
- If the diastolic BP is increased by more than 15 mm Hg, the response is normal. If it is between 11 to 15 mm Hg, then borderline and 10 or less than 10 mm Hg is an indicator of sympathetic insufficiency.

Section 5
Mammalian (Rabbit) Experiments

58. Perfusion of Isolated Rabbit's Heart and the Effects of Drugs and Ions
59. Recording of Rabbit's Normal Intestinal Movements and the Effects of Drugs

Chapter 58

Perfusion of Isolated Rabbit's Heart and the Effects of Drugs and Ions

LEARNING OBJECTIVES

- Discuss the composition of Ringer-Locke's fluid and its functions
- Effect of drugs and chemicals on rabbit's heart

PRINCIPLE

The isolated rabbit's heart will beat normally for some time if it is placed in Ringer-Locke's solution at a temperature of 37°C and pH between 7.4 and 7.6 and with adequate O_2 supply. The actions of drugs and ions on the activity of isolated heart can be studied.

REQUIREMENTS

Rabbit, Langendorff's apparatus, oxygen cylinder, freshly prepared Ringer-Locke's solution, kymograph and drum, scissors, thread and needle, drugs and electrolytes.

Composition of Ringer-Locke's Solution

- NaCl—0.9 g
- KCl—0.042 g
- $CaCl_2$—0.024 g
- $NaHCO_3$—0.015 g
- Glucose—0.1 g

The above ingredients are dissolved in distilled water and made up to 100 mL.

Glucose provides nutrition to the heart. The solution should be prepared on the same day because if glucose is added earlier, it gets fermented and alters the pH of the solution.

Langendorff's Apparatus

- A **reservoir bottle** fitted with a side glass tube with an opening at the bottom. The **glass tube** is connected to the reservoir bottle through a rubber tube. The reservoir bottle (Mariotte's bottle) is placed on a stand at a height of one meter. The bottle is filled with Ringer-Locke's solution. The tube connected to the oxygen cylinder is inserted into the side tube that contains the perfusion fluid (**Fig. 58.1**).
- The bottom of the side tube is connected to a **coiled glass tube** placed inside a rectangular perspex water bath.
- The **water bath** is provided with a heating element, a thermostat and an electric stirrer. These fittings help to maintain the temperature of water in the bath at 37°C.
- The other end of the coiled glass tube is connected through rubber tubing outside the water bath to a **cannula** having a central bulb, two side arms and a nozzle. One side arm is connected to a **mercury manometer** and the other side arm accommodates a **thermometer** to record the temperature of the fluid perfusing the heart. A manometer is used to record the perfusion pressure.
- The nozzle, which is directed downwards, is for introducing the aorta of the isolated heart.
- There is also a **lever** that that records the heart movements on the kymograph drum. The lever can be connected to the heart by means of a hooked pin tied to a thread.

PROCEDURE

- Fill the reservoir bottle with Ringer-Locke's solution.
- The side tube connected to the reservoir bottle will get filled with the Locke's fluid.

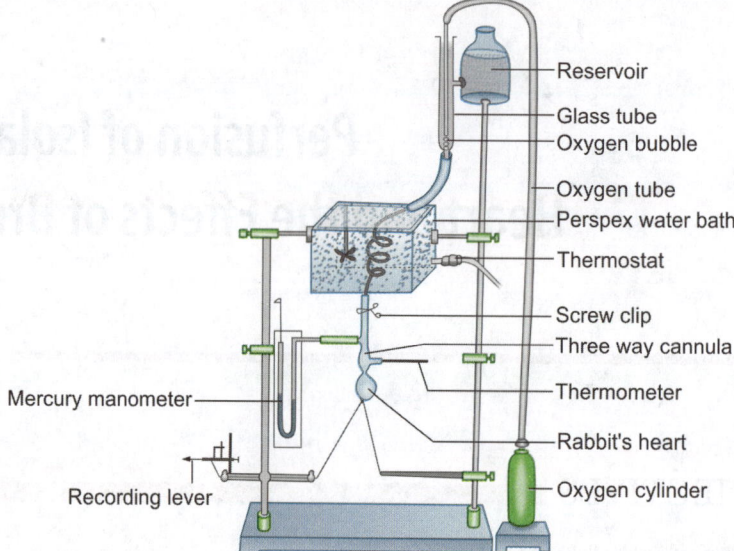

Fig. 58.1: Langendorff's apparatus.

Introduce the glass tube connected to the O_2 cylinder into the side tube and allow a good stream of O_2 bubbles to pass through it continuously **(Fig. 58.1)**.

- Fill the rectangular water bath with water. Connect it to the mains and adjust the thermostat in such a way that the perfusion fluid coming out of the cannula is maintained at 37°C.
- The rabbit is stunned by giving a hard blow on its head. The chest wall is quickly opened and the pericardium is removed from the heart.
- Hold the heart up and cut through the roots of the lungs and vena cavae. The heart is separated with sufficient length of aorta (at least 1–2 cm) attached to it.
- It is immediately transferred into the oxygenated chilled Ringer-Locke's solution. It is further washed in a series of bowls containing Ringer-Locke fluid (which is being continuously oxygenated) to remove all the blood from the heart before it clots. Air bubbles should not enter the vessels or heart chambers.
- Identify the aorta and pass a thread using a needle at its upper part. Carefully slide the aorta into the nozzle of the dripping heart cannula and the ligature is tied securely around it.
  Take care that the tip of the cannula does not penetrate the aortic valve. The temperature of the perfusing fluid should be maintained at 37°C.
- The perfusion pressure should be fixed around 60–80 mm Hg.
- When the warm oxygenated Ringer-Locke's solution flows through the coronaries, the heart starts beating. The outflow of fluid from the heart occurs through the pulmonary artery, which remains open.
- Now pass the hooked pin attached to the thread through the apex of the left ventricle. The other end of the thread is connected to the recording lever.
- Record a normal cardiogram on a slow-moving drum (speed 2.5 mm/s) of the kymograph
- After taking the normal cardiogram introduce the following agents by injecting through the side rubber tube just above the cannula with the help of a syringe and a hypodermic needle.
  - Adrenaline 1:100,000 (10 µg/mL)—1 mL
  - Acetylcholine 1:100,000 (10 µg/mL)—0.5 mL
  - 1% $CaCl_2$ solution—1 mL
  - 1% KCl solution—1 mL
- Wash out each agent with the perfusing fluid and wait for some time till the beats becomes normal. Take a normal cardiogram and then introduce the other agent and record the effect.

PRECAUTIONS

- The temperature of the perfusing fluid should be maintained at 37°C.
- Air bubbles should not enter the coronaries.
- Oxygen cylinder should be used for supplying O_2 at a regulated rate.
- The height of the fluid column should be sufficient to maintain a pressure of at least 60–80 mm Hg.
- Ringer-Locke's fluid should not contain any impurity
- The pH of the fluid should be in the range of 7.4–7.6.
- While introducing the nozzle into the aorta take care that it does not penetrate the aortic valve.
- Normal cardiogram should be taken before and after recording the effect of each agent.

OBSERVATION

- Each cardiac recording shows two types of waves; the small wave is the recording of atrial activity and bigger wave is the recording of ventricular activity.

Chapter 58: Perfusion of Isolated Rabbit's Heart and the Effects of Drugs and Ions

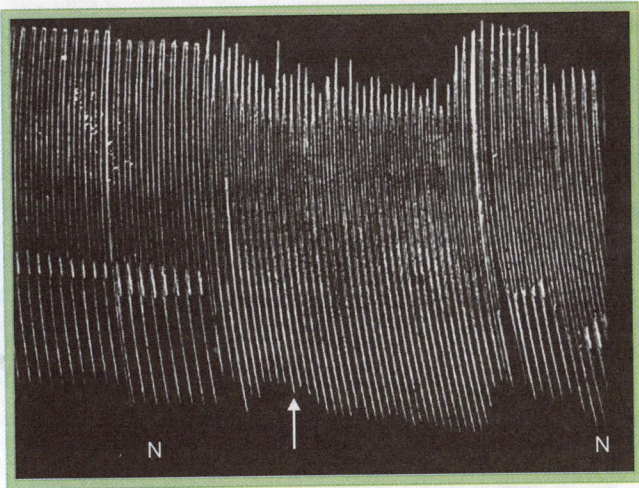

Fig. 58.2: Effect of adrenaline on rabbits isolated heart.

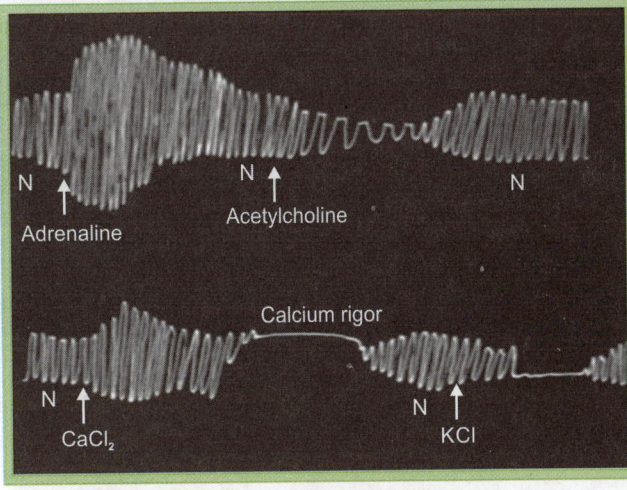

Fig. 58.3: Effect of drugs and ions on rabbit's heart.

- When adrenaline is introduced, there is marked increase in the heart rate and force of contraction (Fig. 58.2).
  - Adrenaline acts through β_1-adrenergic receptors in the nodal tissue. Adrenaline increases intracellular cAMP that facilitates the opening of long-lasting calcium channels. This increases heart rate by increasing the rapidity of the depolarization phase of the pacemaker action potential.
  - Adrenaline also acts on β_1-adrenergic receptors in the cardiac muscle cells and increases the intracellular Ca^{2+} concentration, which increases the force of contraction of heart.
- Acetylcholine decreases heart rate and force of contraction by acting through M_2 muscarinic receptors. Ach decreases the intracellular cAMP concentration in the nodal tissue and ventricular muscle cells and decreases heart rate and force of contraction. There is an increase in K^+ efflux leading to hyperpolarization of nodal tissues. There is also decrease in Ca^{2+} influx in the myocardium (Fig. 58.3).
- $CaCl_2$ increases force of contraction without allowing the relaxation of heart to complete. Finally, the heart may stop in systole. This is called **calcium rigor**. $CaCl_2$ may not significantly increase the heart rate.
- KCl decreases heart rate and force of contraction and finally the heart stops in diastole.

Effect of drugs and ions on rabbit's heart	
Agent	**Effect**
Adrenaline 1:100,000 (10 µg/mL)—1 mL	Marked increase in heart rate and force of contraction (Fig. 58.2)
Acetylcholine 1:100,000 (10 µg/mL)—1 mL	Decrease in the heart rate and force of contraction (Fig. 58.3)
$CaCl_2$ (1%)—1 mL	Increases heart rate and force of contraction and finally heart stops in systole (calcium rigor)
KCl (1%)—1 mL	Decreases heart rate and force of contraction and finally heart stops in diastole (Fig. 58.3)

VIVA QUESTIONS

1. **What is the composition and function of Ringer-Locke's fluid?**
   NaCl, $CaCl_2$ and KCl make the solution isotonic with plasma. $NaHCO_3$ maintains the pH between 7.4 and 7.6. Glucose provides nutrition to the heart.

2. **There should be no clots or air bubbles in the isolated heart while mounting it. Give the reason.**
   The perfusing fluid flows through the coronary vessels and not through the chambers. A clot in the coronary causes occlusion of the vessel. If the air bubbles enter the coronaries it will block the vessel leading to death of the heart.

3. **What happens if the nozzle pierces the aortic valve?**
   In this condition the perfusing fluid directly enters the left ventricle and the left ventricle enlarges leading to overstretching of the ventricle, which makes the heart nonfunctional. The mammalian heart depends on coronary circulation for nutrition and O_2. The coronaries arise from the root of aorta. So, there will be no coronary perfusion if the nozzle enters the ventricle.

4. **What is the mechanism of action of adrenaline, acetylcholine, CaCl$_2$ and KCl on heart?**
   - **Adrenaline** acts by stimulating β$_1$-receptors of heart. The effect is activation of adenylyl cyclase and increase in cAMP. This causes increased influx of Ca^{2+} into the myocardial cells leading to increase in the force of contraction. It increases Na$^+$ influx and decreases K$^+$ efflux from the nodal tissue leading to increase in heart rate.
   - **Acetylcholine** acts through M$_2$ muscarinic Ach receptors. It increases K$^+$ efflux leading to hyperpolarization. It also decreases cAMP levels and decrease Ca^{2+} influx into the myocardial cells. The effect is decrease in heart rate and force of contraction.
   - **CaCl$_2$** increases the force of contraction and in high doses the heart remains contracted and it stops in systole.
   - **KCl** decreases the magnitude of action potential and the heart finally stops in diastole.

5. **What are receptor blockers?**
   Substances that block the receptor site can prevent the combination of the transmitter with the receptor. They are called blocking agents. Thus atropine blocks the muscarinic receptors; hexamethonium block the nicotinic receptor on the peripheral ganglion cells; dihydroergotamine blocks the alpha adrenergic sites; DCI (dichloroisoproterenol) blocks the beta adrenergic sites and curare blocks the neuromuscular transmission.

59 Recording of Rabbit's Normal Intestinal Movements and the Effects of Drugs

Chapter

LEARNING OBJECTIVES

- Discuss the effect of adrenaline and acetylcholine on intestinal movements
- Explain the mechanism of action of acetylcholine on intestine
- Discuss receptor blockers and their mechanism of action

PRINCIPLE

Isolated pieces of small intestine continue to contract for some time if it is kept in a suitable solution at optimum temperature and adequate O_2 supply. The effect of various stimuli like drugs and ions on smooth muscles can be studied.

REQUIREMENTS

Dale's apparatus, Tyrode solution, petri dishes, thread and needle, oxygen cylinder, frontal lever, kymograph and smoked drum, 10 mL pipette, rabbit, drugs and chemicals.

Composition of Tyrode Solution

NaCl, KCl, NaH_2PO_4, $MgCl_2$, $CaCl_2$, $NaHCO_3$ and glucose (refer page 292).

Dale's Apparatus (Fig. 59.1)

It consists of a perspex rectangular water bath provided with a heating element and thermostat. There is a central organ bath of 20 mL capacity, which is provided with an outlet. There is a hollow bend glass tube curved at its lower end for fixing the intestine. This tube can be inserted in the center of the organ bath and is also used for supplying oxygen through the solution. The movements of the tissue are recorded on a moving kymograph with the help of a frontal lever attached to the assembly **(Fig. 59.1)**. The responses are very sluggish and the extent of movements of intestine is very small. Long levers can magnify the movements.

PROCEDURE

- Since the intestine of a fasting rabbit shows more movements, the rabbit is kept fasting overnight.
- Fill the organ bath with Tyrode solution and the water bath with water.
- Heat the water in the water bath and adjust the temperature to about 37°C.
- Take cold Tyrode solution in three petri dishes.
- The speed of the drum is adjusted for slow speed (2.5 mm/s).
- The rabbit is stunned and the abdomen opened.
- A midline incision is made on the abdomen quickly after stunning the rabbit and the upper piece of intestine (duodenum or jejunum) measuring about 15–20 cm should be cut and separated from the mesentery with the help of a pair of small sharp scissors. The separated piece is placed in the first petri dish containing cold Tyrode solution (cold solution prevents the activity of enzymes). The piece is then cut further into 4–5 pieces of approximately equal size. The contents are emptied carefully by allowing Tyrode solution taken in a 10 mL pipette to pass through the lumen of the intestine slowly without applying force.
- Transfer the pieces into the second and third petri dish containing Tyrode solution. Allow oxygen to bubble through it.
- Pass a long thin thread through the wall of one piece of intestine with the help of suture needle and tie a knot using a long piece of thread.

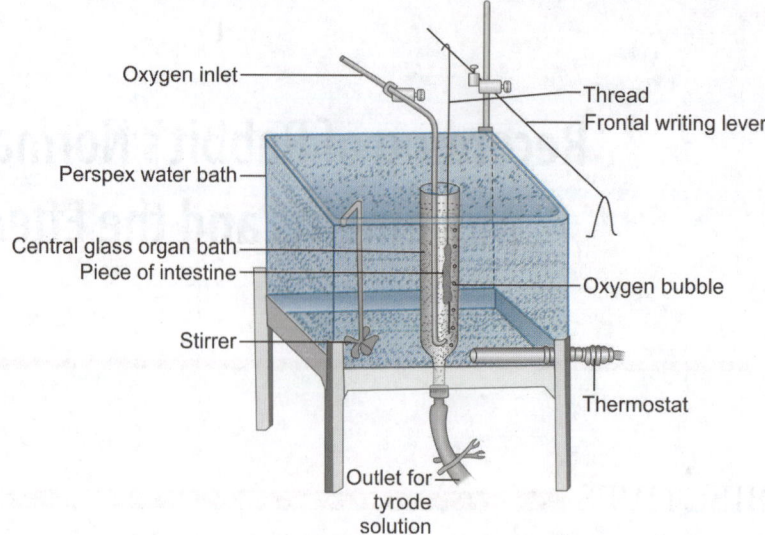

Fig. 59.1: Dale's apparatus.

- Pass a thread similarly on the opposite side of the piece, tie a knot and make a small loop that should be fixed into the curved end of the glass tube that provides an inlet for oxygen. These procedures should be completed as quickly as possible.
- Lift up the muscle with the glass tube and fix it in muscle bath as shown in the diagram. Allow oxygen to pass through the Tyrode solution immediately at a rate of 2–3 bubbles per second.
- The opposite end of the intestine is tied to the frontal lever with the help of the long thread attached to the intestine.
- Adjust the level of the lever so that it remains horizontal. For this purpose counterweight in the form of plasticine can be attached to the short arm of the lever in order to avoid undue stretch on the intestinal smooth muscle.
- If the pH of the fluid, temperature and the concentrations of ions in the Tyrode solution are correct and if the oxygen supply is adequate the intestine is seen to exhibit tonic and phasic contractions.
- Record a few normal contractions.
- The effects of drugs are studied by introducing a known quantity of the drug with help of tuberculin syringe into the central bath. After recording the effects of the drug, the preparation is washed by removing the fluid from the bath quickly through the outlet. An equal quantity of the fresh Tyrode solution should be introduced through the inlet. The effect of the next agent should be recorded only after the intestine shows a normal movement. Put arrow marks below the recording immediately after adding a particular agent to indicate the agents used for the recordings.

Observations (Fig. 59.2)

- Observe the rate and amplitude of intestinal movements recorded after the application of each agent and compare it with the normal recording.
- The responses given by the plain muscle are different from those given by the striated and the cardiac muscle.
- Smooth muscle is stimulated by acetylcholine and is inhibited by adrenaline.
- When acetylcholine is added to the preparation following the application of atropine, the effect of acetylcholine will be abolished (**Fig. 59.2**).

Effect of drugs and ions on isolated rabbit's intestine	
Agent	**Effect**
Acetylcholine 1:100,000 (10 µg/mL)—1 mL	Increase in the tone and frequency of intestinal movements (**Fig. 59.2**)
Adrenaline 1:10,000 (10 µg/mL)—1 mL	Decreases tone, frequency and amplitude of contraction
Atropine (0.01%)—1 mL	Decreases amplitude of contraction
Acetylcholine after atropinization	No effect
1% $CaCl_2$—1 mL	Increases height of contraction
1% $BaCl_2$—few drops	Marked increase in frequency and force of contraction
Histamine (50 µg/mL)—1 mL	Increases the frequency of contraction

- Histamine increases the tone of smooth muscle. It increases the amplitude of contraction. It acts by activating H_1 and H_2 histamine receptors. H_1 receptor stimulation activates phospholipase C, which in turn increases intracellular calcium ion concentration. By acting on H_2 receptors, it increases cAMP in the cells.

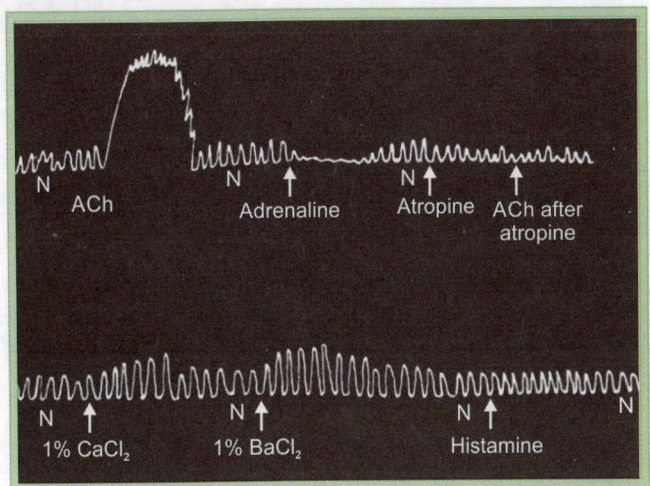

Fig. 59.2: Effect of drugs and ions on isolated rabbit's intestine.

- When barium chloride is added, the intestine contracts strongly due to the direct action of barium ions on the smooth muscles of the intestine. Potassium chloride has a similar action.
- $CaCl_2$ when added leads to tonic contraction of the intestinal muscle. This is due to increased entry of Ca^{2+} into the cells.

Precautions

- The animal should be kept fasting overnight to get good contractions.
- Removal of intestine into the cold Tyrode solution should be done immediately after killing the rabbit.
- The temperature of the water bath should be maintained at 37°C throughout the experiment.
- Oxygen should be supplied to the intestine throughout the experiment.
- Separate syringes should be used for adding chemicals into the organ bath.
- Normal recordings should be taken before and after adding the drugs.

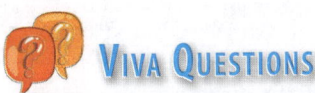

Viva Questions

1. **What are the types of smooth muscles? Give examples.**
   » Visceral smooth muscle, e.g., stomach, intestine, uterus, urinary bladder, walls of small arteries and veins.
   » Multiunit smooth muscle, e.g., walls of bronchioles, erector pili muscles, radial and circular muscles of iris.

2. **Classify receptors on the cell membrane of smooth muscle.**
   » Cholinergic muscarinic receptors and cholinergic nicotinic receptors
   » Adrenergic-alpha and adrenergic-beta receptors
   » Histaminergic receptors
   » Serotonergic receptors

3. **What is plasticity of smooth muscles?**
   Smooth muscles can undergo great changes in length without much increase in tension. As a result, organs like urinary bladder, stomach, etc., can increase their volume *within physiological limits* without much increase in intraluminal pressure. Thus, these organs can act as reservoirs.

4. **What is the effect of adrenaline in the intestinal movements? What is the mechanism of action?**
   Frequency and amplitude of contraction of the intestine is decreased when adrenaline is added. Adrenaline exerts its inhibitory effect by acting on both ∞ and β-receptors present on the smooth muscle. β-receptor stimulation decreases cAMP in the cells and there is increased intracellular binding of calcium. So, less Ca^{2+} is available in the cell. α-receptor stimulation causes increased calcium efflux from the cells so that less calcium is available in the cell. Thus, the frequency and amplitude of contraction decrease.

5. **What is the mechanism of action of acetylcholine in intestinal movements?**
   The smooth muscle becomes more active when acetylcholine is added. The rate and amplitude of contraction increase. There is an increase in tone of the muscle. Acetylcholine exerts its action by activating phospholipase C, which in turn forms inositol triphosphate (IP3). IP3 increases intracellular calcium ion concentration by mobilizing calcium from the intracellular stores and by facilitating calcium entry into the cell. Thus, there is an increase in the rate and magnitude of contraction.

6. **What is the effect of acetylcholine on smooth muscles after adding atropine?**
   Atropine is a muscarinic receptor blocker. It prevents the action of acetylcholine on the smooth muscle of intestine. It decreases muscle activity. If acetylcholine is added to the preparation following the application of atropine, the effect of acetylcholine will be abolished.

7. **What are the types of intestinal movements?**
   The movements of the intestinal muscle are slow and irregular. They are of two types: (1) Rhythmic or phasic movements, (2) Tonic movements. During a tonic contraction the rate and magnitude of rhythmic contractions are reduced.

Section 6

Normal Values

60. Hematologic Values and Fluids Used in the Laboratory

Chapter 60

Hematologic Values and Fluids Used in the Laboratory

NORMAL VALUES

Hematologic Values

RBC count:
- Men: 4.5–6 million/mm³ of blood
- Female: 4–5.5 million/mm³ hemoglobin content
- Male: 14–18 g/dL of blood
- Female: 12–15 g/dL PCV (hematocrit)
- Male: 40–50%
- Female: 35–45% blood indices
- MCV: 87 ± 6 fL
- MCH: 29 ± 4 pg
- MCHC: 30–35 g/dL or %

Total leukocyte count: 4,000–11,000 cells/mm³ of blood

Differential count
- Neutrophils: 45–70%
- Eosinophils: 1–5%
- Basophils: 0–1%
- Monocyte: 2–6%
- Lymphocyte: 20–40%

Platelet count: 1.5–4.5 lakhs/mm³ of blood
Reticulocyte count: 0.5–1% of erythrocyte count
Absolute eosinophil count: 40–400 eosinophils/mm³ of blood ESR
- Male: 3–5 mm at the end of first hour
- Female: 5–10 mm in the first hour

Osmotic fragility
Hemolysis begins in 0.45–0.38% NaCl
Hemolysis completed in 0.33–0.30% NaCl

Coagulation—Normal Values

- Bleeding time (Duke): 1–5 minutes
- Clotting time: 5–15 minutes
- Clot retraction time: 60 min

Prothrombin time: 11–14 seconds
Activated partial thromboplastin time (APTT): 25–40 seconds

Biochemical values
- Blood pH: 7.4
- Fasting blood sugar (FBS): 70–110 mg/dL
- Postprandial blood sugar (PPBS): 140–200 mg/dL
- Plasma proteins:
- Total protein: 6–8 g/dL
- Albumin: 3.5–5 g/dL
- Globulin: 2.5–3.5 g/dL
- Urea: 20–40 mg/dL

Uric acid:
- Male: 3–9 mg/dL
- Female: 2–8 mg/dL
- Creatinine: 0.5–1.5 mg/dL
- Sodium: 136–145 mEq/L
- Potassium: 3.5–5.4 mEq/L
- Calcium: 9–11 mg/dL
- Iron: 100–150 µg/dL

Serum
- Total bilirubin: 0.2–1.2 mg/dL
- Bilirubin direct: 0–0.4 mg/dL
- SGOT: 5–40 IU/L
- SGPT (ALT): 5–30 IU/L
- Alkaline phosphatase: 40–125 IU/L
- Total cholesterol: 150–200 mg/dL
- HDL: 40–60 mg/dL
- LDL: <100 mg/dL
- Triglyceride (40–50 years): 20–160 mg/dL
- Serum sodium: 135–145 mEq/L
- Serum potassium: 3.5–5.2 mEq/L

COMPOSITION OF DIFFERENT FLUIDS USED IN THE LABORATORY

Composition of Ringer, Ringer-Locke's and Tyrode solutions in 100 mL

	Ringer solution	Ringer-Locke	Tyrode solution
NaCl	0.65 g	0.9 g	0.8 g
KCl	0.014 g	0.042 g	0.02 g
$CaCl_2$	0.012 g	0.024 g	0.02 g
$NaHCO_3$	0.02 g	0.02 g	0.01 g
$MgCl_2$	–	–	0.01 g
NaH_2PO_4	–	–	0.005 g
Glucose	–	0.1 g	0.1 g
Distilled water	Made up to 100 mL	Up to 100 mL	Up to 100 mL

Hayem's fluid (RBC count):
- NaCl: 0.5 g
- Na_2SO_4: 2.5 g
- Mercuric perchloride: 0.25 g
- Distilled water: To make up the volume to 100 mL

Turk's fluid (total leukocyte count):
- Glacial acetic acid: 0.2 mL
- Gentian violet 1% solution: 0.1 mL
- Distilled water: To make the volume up to 100 mL

Rees-Ecker fluid (platelet count):
- Sodium citrate: 3.8 g
- Formalin (1% solution): 0.2 mL
- Brilliant cresyl blue: 50 mg
- Distilled water up to 100 mL

Dunger's fluid (absolute eosinophil count):
- Eosin (200 g/L): 10 mL
- 10% acetone: 10 mL
- Distilled water: 80 mL

Section 7: Model of Practical Examination

61. Sample Questions

Chapter 61: Sample Questions

PATTERN OF PRACTICAL EXAMINATION

	Total marks: 100
Practical I:	**40 marks**
Minor hematology:	10 marks
Human experiments:	10 marks
OSPE 4 Stations	20 marks
1. Amphibian graph (draw/interpret):	5 marks
2. Interpreting clinical conditions:	5 mark
3. Hematology: Skill assessment and calculation/interpret test results:	5 marks
4. Clinical and communication skill assessment:	5 marks
Practical II:	**40 marks**
Clinical examination:	20 marks
Major hematology:	20 marks
Viva voce:	20 marks

Four stations of 5 marks each
1. Laboratory data interpretation
2. Clinical scenario discussion
3. Instruments discussion
4. Common investigative data interpretation (ECG, spirometry, etc.)

Spotters

Identify the cell focused under the microscope—1 number
Neutrophil, eosinophil, lymphocyte or monocyte (basophil is usually not kept for the spotting examination)

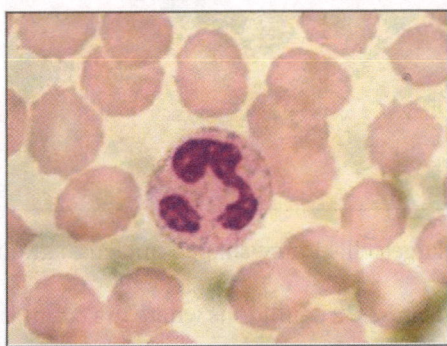

Neutrophil (multilobed nucleus, fine lilac-colored cytoplasmic granules)

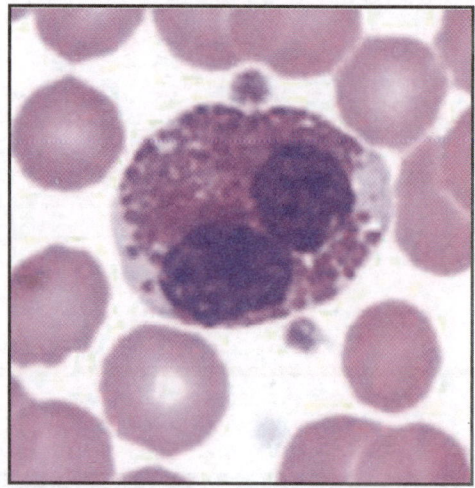

Eosinophil (bilobed nucleus, coarse orange red granules in cytoplasm)

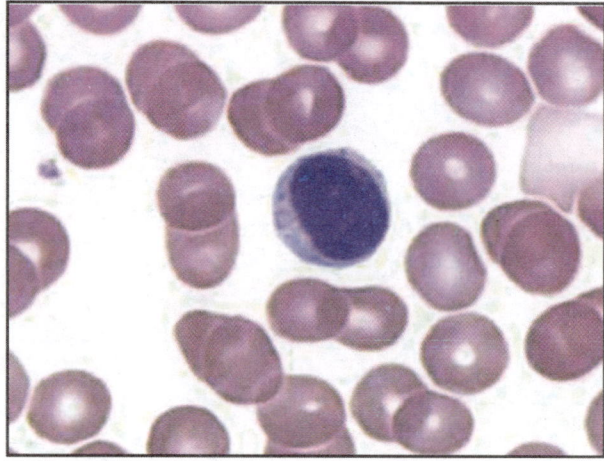

Lymphocyte (round nucleus, bluish gray cytoplasm)

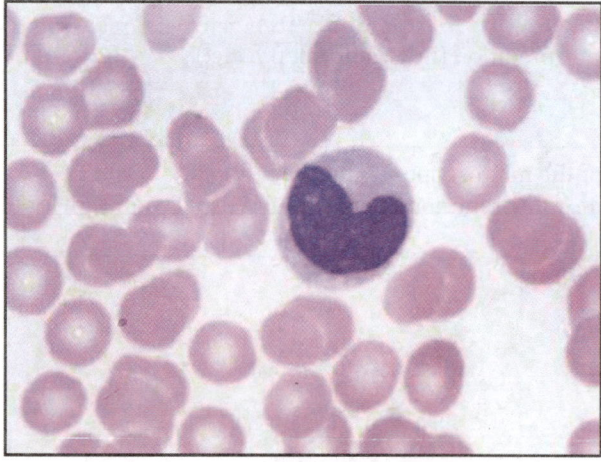

Monocyte (very large cell, kidney-shaped nucleus, agranular cytoplasm)

Subquestions: Give two identifying features, 2 conditions where the count is increased/decreased, two functions of the cell, etc.

Chapter 61: Sample Questions

Graphs of Amphibian Experiments

I.

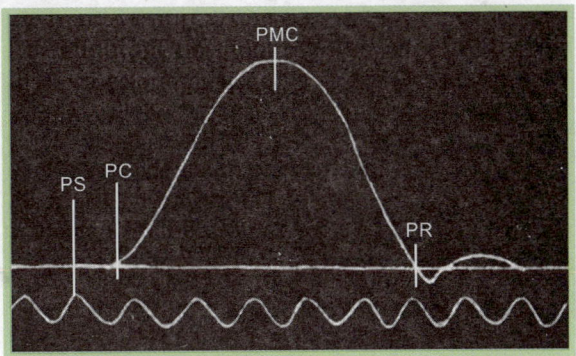

- Identify the graph (simple muscle twitch)
- Calculate the twitch duration (0.07 sec)
- What are the causes of latent period? (refer page 201 Q. 5)
- Find out the contraction period (0.03 sec)
- Calculate the relaxation period (0.04 sec)
- Give one condition where the relaxation period is increased (muscle fatigue)

II.

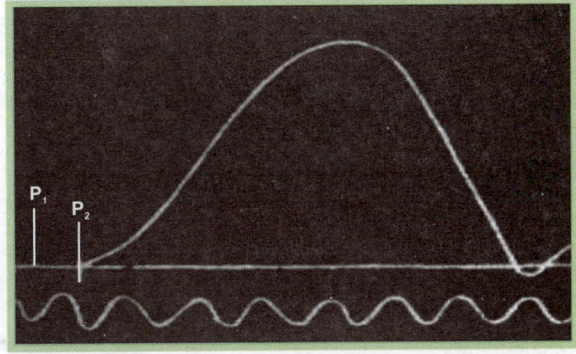

- Identify the graph (second stimulus falling in the latent period of first contraction).
- What is its difference from simple muscle twitch?
- What is the effect of second stimulus on this curve?
- Give the reason.
- What are the causes of latent period?

III.

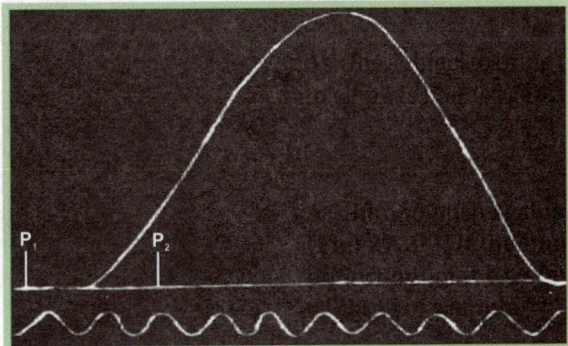

- Identify the graph (summation curve when second stimulus falls in the contraction period).
- What is the difference of this graph from simple muscle twitch?
- What is the reason for the change?
- Is this effect possible in cardiac muscle? Why?

IV.

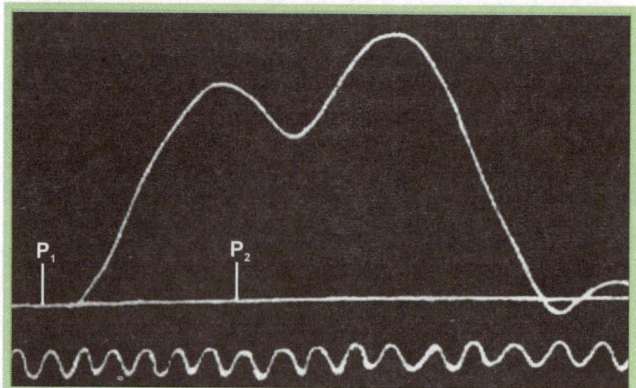

- Identify the graph (superposition).
- Why the second curve is taller?
- Is this effect possible in cardiac muscle?
- Why?

V.

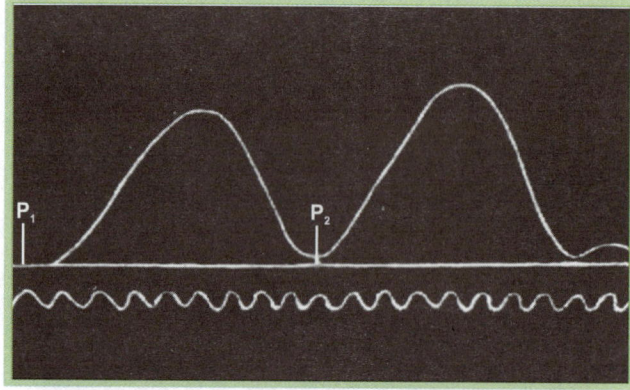

- Identify the graph (beneficial effect when the second stimulus falls immediately after relaxation).
- Why the second curve is taller? (Write the causes of beneficial effect, refer page 204 Q. 1)

VI.

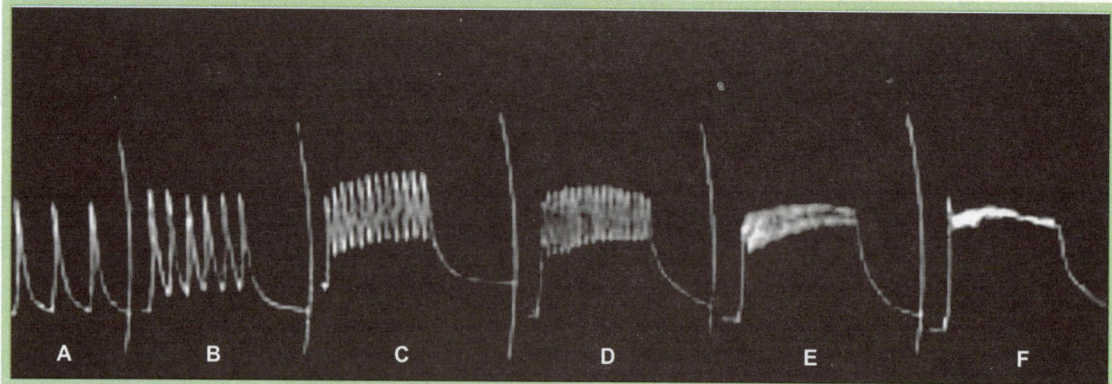

- Identify the graph (genesis of tetanus).
- Identify graph C (clonus).
- What is the reason for the effect?

VII.

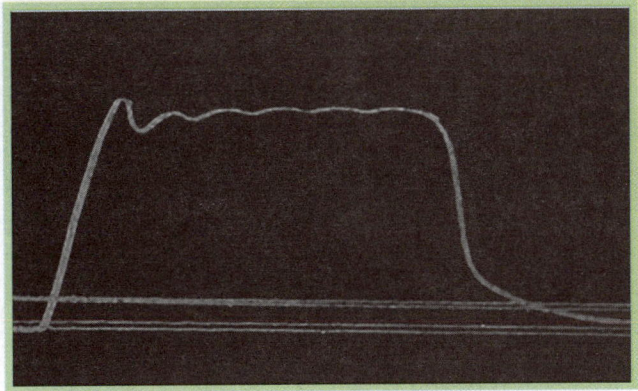

- Identify graph (tetanus).
- Is this effect seen normally in the body?
- What is critical fusion frequency?

VIII.

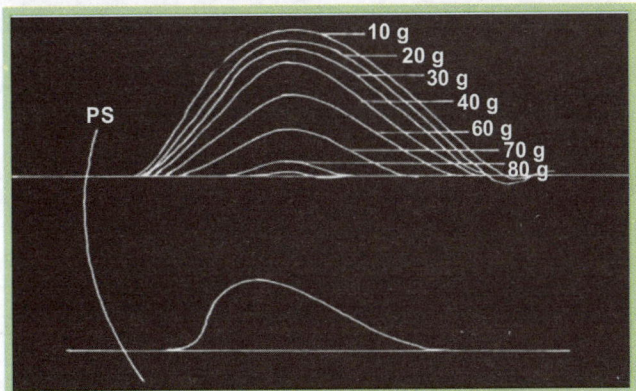

- Identify the graph (effect of load and afterload on muscle contraction).
- What is the reason for the lower curve?

IX.

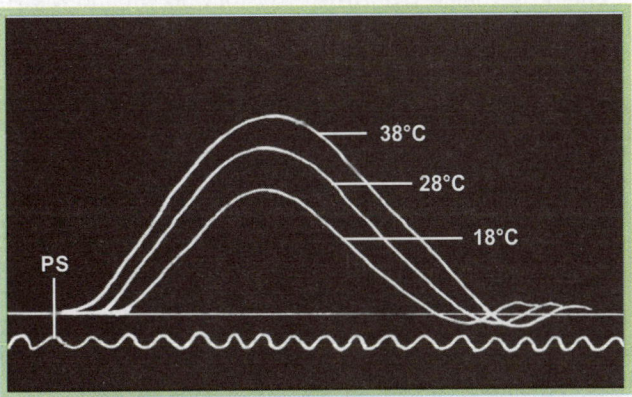

- Identify the graph.
- Why is the graph larger for hot water?
- What is its difference from the ideal curve that should be obtained?

X.

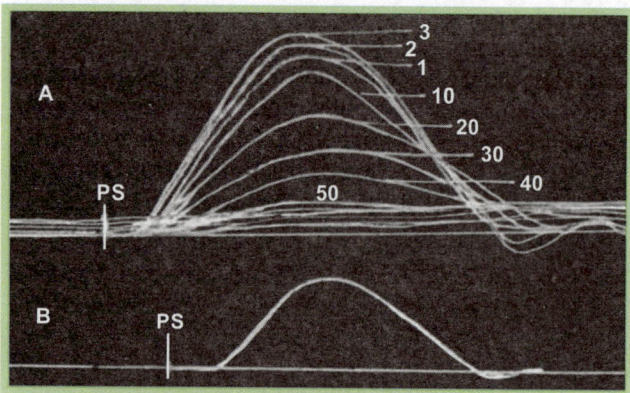

- Identify the graphs A and B.
- What are the reasons for the second graph marked B?
- Mention two causes for muscle fatigue.

XI.

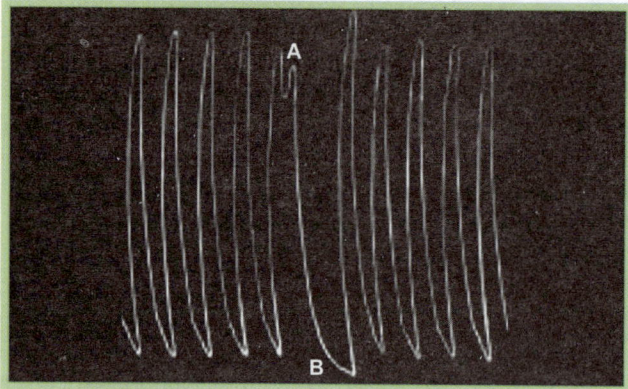

- Identify the part marked A (extrasystole).
- What is the reason for B? (Compensatory pause; when the next normal sinus impulse reaches the ventricle, it will be in the absolute refractory period of extrasystole and will not respond)
- Why is the graph following part marked B taller? (Due to extrasystolic potentiation as a result of increased availability of calcium ions in the cardiac muscle cell)

XII.

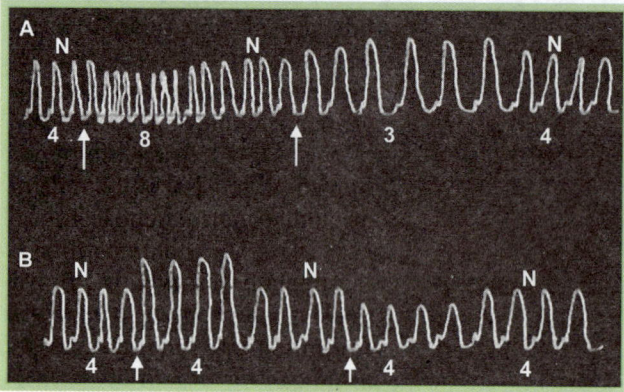

- Identify graph A (effect of heat and cold on sinus venosus).
- Give your reason (there is change in the heart rate when heat or cold are applied since sinus venosus is the pace maker of frog's heart)
- Identify graph marked B (effect of heat and cold on ventricle).
- Give the reason (there is no change in the heat rate, only the amplitude of contraction changes).

XIII.

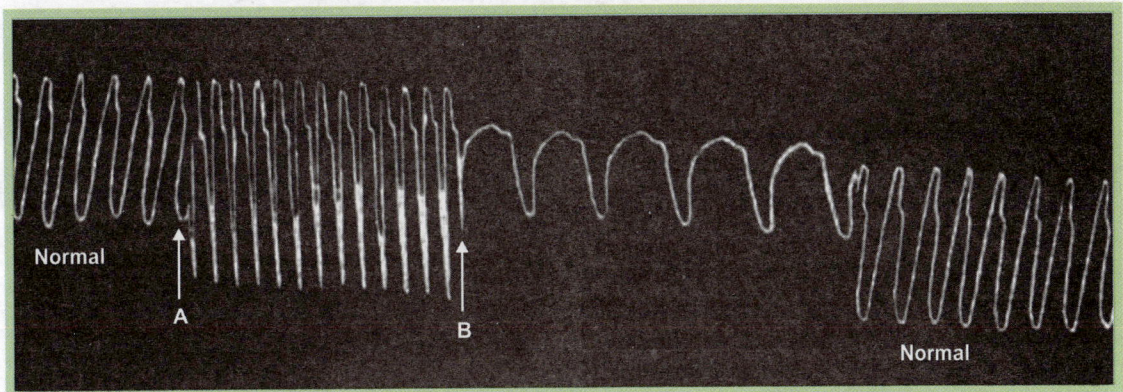

- Identify the drug applied at A and at B (A: adrenaline; B: acetyl choline on frog's heart).
- Give reasons (A: there is increase in heart rate and force of contraction; B: there is decrease in heart rate and force of contraction).

Calculations

1. Calculate the alveolar ventilation (AV) from the following data:
   Tidal volume = 600 mL
   Respiratory rate = 12/min
   Wasted ventilation = 2400 mL/min
   Ans: AV = (tidal volume – dead space volume) × RR
   Dead space air = 2,400/12 = 200
   AV = (600 – 200) × 12 = 4,800 mL/min
2. Calculate the dead space volume from the following data.
   Pulmonary ventilation (PV) = 6 L/min
   Alveolar ventilation (AV) = 4 L/min
   Respiratory rate (RR) = 10/min
   Ans: (PV – AV)/RR = 200 mL
3. Calculate the respiratory minute volume from the data given.
   Respiratory rate = 12/min
   Tidal volume = 500 mL
   Dead space volume = 150 mL
   Ans: 500 × 12 = 6,000 mL/min
4. Calculate the cardiac output from the following data
   Oxygen consumption = 300 mL/min
   Arterial oxygen content = 20 mL/dL
   Venous oxygen content = 15 mL/dL
   CO = amount of oxygen taken up by the body divided by arteriovenous concentration difference of oxygen

   $$CO = \frac{300 \text{ mL/min} \times 100 \text{ mL}}{5 \text{ mL}} = 6,000 \text{ mL/min}$$

5. Calculate the clearance value from the data given:
   Urine flow rate = 2 mL/min
   Urinary concentration of the substance = 150 mg/dL
   Plasma concentration = 15 mg/dL

   Ans: Clearance = UV/P = $\frac{150 \text{ mg/dL} \times 2 \text{ mL/min}}{15 \text{ mg/dL}}$ = 20 mL/min

   Name a substance that has a clearance value zero normally—glucose
   A substance whose clearance value is same as that of GFR—inulin
   Define clearance. Volume of plasma cleared of the substance in unit time is the clearance of that substance

6. Calculate the ventilation perfusion ratio from the given data
   Pulmonary blood flow = 5 L/min
   Respiratory rate =10/min
   Tidal volume = 500 mL
   Dead space volume = 100 mL
   V/P ratio = Alveolar ventilation/Pulmonary perfusion
   Alveolar ventilation = (500 – 100) × 12 = 400 mL × 10/min = 4,000 mL/min
   V/P = 4,000/5,000 = 0.8
7. Calculate the stroke volume from the following data
   Cardiac output = 24 L/min
   Heart rate = 120/min

   $$SV = CO/HR = \frac{24,000 \text{ mL/min}}{120/\text{min}} = 200 \text{ mL}$$

   One condition where cardiac output is increased—exercise
   Reason—increase in heart rate and increase in the force of contraction
8. Calculate the MCV.
   PCV = 45%
   RBC count = 5-million/mm^3
   MCV = PCV in mL per L of blood/RBC count in millions per mm^3 of blood = 45/5 × 10 = 90 fl
9. Calculate the MCH:
   RBC count = 5 million/mm^3
   Hemoglobin content = 15 g/dL
   PCV = 45%
   MCH = Hb in g per liter of blood/RBC count in millions per mm^3 of blood
   MCH = 15/5 × 10 = 30 pg
10. Calculate the MCHC from the following data and give the normal value:
    - Hemoglobin content = 7 g/dL
    - PCV = 24%
    - RBC count = 3 million/mm^3 of blood
    - MCV = 80 fl
    - MCH = 23 pg
    - MCHC = MCH/MCV × 100 = 28%
11. Calculate MCV and MCH from the following data:
    - Hemoglobin content = 7 g/dL
    - PCV = 24%
    - RBC count = 3 million/mm^3 of blood
    - MCV = 80 fl
    - MCH = 23 pg

Clinical Photographs

I. Acromegaly
- Identify the clinical condition. (Acromegaly)
- Give two identifying features. (Prognathism, prominent supraorbital ridge)

II. Cushing's syndrome
- Identify the condition. (Cushing syndrome)
- What is the reason for the purplish striae in the abdomen.

III. Gigantism
- Identify the condition. (Gigantism)
- What is the reason for hyperglycemia in this case?

IV. Myxedema
- Identify giving the cause. (Myxedema, hypothyroidism in adult)
- Mention two identifying features.

V. Tetany

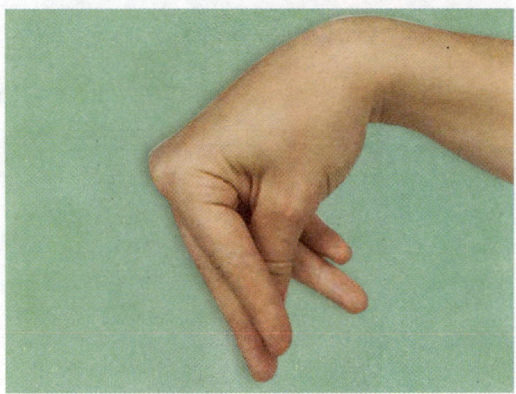

- Identify. (Tetany)
- What is the cause? (Hypocalcemia due to hypoparathyroidism)

VI. Cretinism
- Identify the condition mentioning two identifying features. (Cretinism; ugly looking, pendulous abdomen with umbilical hernia)
- What is the cause. (Hypothyroidism in infancy)
- Give two tests to confirm the diagnosis. (Estimation of thyroid hormones, serum cholesterol)

VII. Thyrotoxicosis
- Identify the condition (exophthalmic goiter or thyrotoxicosis)
- What is the cause for the exophthalmos in this case?
- Mention two tests to confirm the diagnosis.

VIII. Exophthalmos

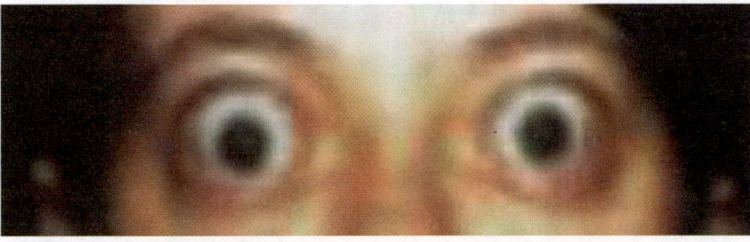

- Identify the condition. (Exophthalmos)
- Give a clinical condition where you get this finding. (Graves' disease or thyrotoxicosis)

IX. Pitting edema

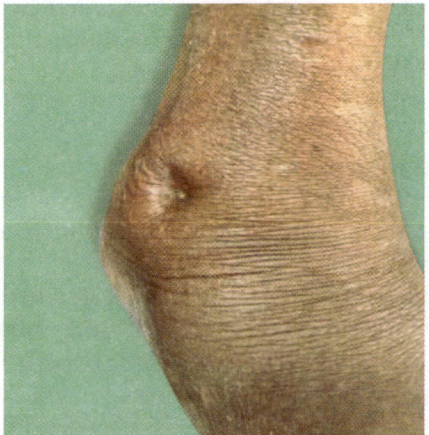

- Identify the sign seen over the lateral malleolus. (Pitting edema)
- Give two conditions producing it. (Hypoproteinemia, congestive cardiac failure)

X. LMN facial palsy

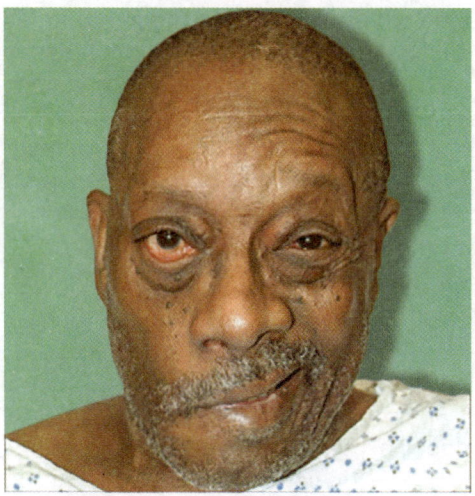

- Identify the condition.
- Where is the probable site of lesion?

Clinical History

1. A patient complains of polyuria, polydipsia and polyphagia. On investigation:
   - Fasting blood sugar = 300 mg/dL
   - Urine sugar = ++
   - Urine specific gravity = 1.080
     - Identify the condition. (Diabetes mellitus)
     - What is the reason for polyuria in this condition? (Osmotic diuresis)
2. A patient complains of polyuria and polydipsia. On investigation:
   - Fasting blood glucose = 80 mg/dL
   - Urine sugar = nil
   - Specific gravity of urine = 1010
     - Identify the condition. What is the underlying cause? (Diabetes insipidus; deficiency of ADH)
     - What is the reason for polyuria? (Decreased reabsorption of water in the distal nephron due to ADH deficiency)
3. Following an accident, a man was brought to the casualty with severe bleeding. On examination:
   - Cold, clammy skin
   - Pulse rate = 130/min
   - BP = 80/50 mm Hg
     - Identify the condition (Hemorrhagic shock)
     - What will be the RBC count and hemoglobin content in this patient? (Normal)
4. A 50-year-old lady complains of palpitation, increased sweating, intolerance to heat and tremor. On examination:
   - Skin was warm and moist; there was fine tremor of the hands
   - Pulse rate = 100/min
   - BP = 150/80 mm Hg
     - Identify the condition. (Hyperthyroidism)
     - What is the reason for the wide pulse pressure? (Systolic pressure is increased due to increase in cardiac output. Diastolic pressure is decreased due to peripheral vasodilatation as a result of increased metabolism and the resultant decrease in peripheral resistance)
     - Mention one test to confirm the diagnosis. (Estimation of TSH and thyroid hormones)
5. A 55-year-old lady complains of cold intolerance, hoarseness of voice, yellowish discoloration of skin and puffiness of face. On examination:
   Skin was thick and coarse; nonpitting edema was present
   - Pulse rate = 70/min
   - BP = 110/80 mm Hg
   - Serum bilirubin = 0.5 mg/dL

- Serum cholesterol = 300 mg/dL
  - Identify the condition. (Myxedema; hypothyroidism in adult)
  - What is the reason for generalized edema? (Accumulation of mucopolysaccharides in the subcutaneous tissue due to impaired metabolism of mucopolysaccharides).
  - What is the reason for yellowish discoloration of skin? (due to accumulation of β-carotene in the skin)
6. A 70-year-old man was brought to the casualty with weakness of right side of the body, deviation of angle of mouth to the right, and inability to speak. On examination:
   - BP = 160/110 mm Hg
   - Spastic paralysis of right upper and lower limbs
   - Babinski sign positive on the right side
     - What is the probable diagnosis? (Right sided hemiplegia)
     - Which is the probable site of lesion? (Left internal capsule)
7. A 10-year-old boy presented with uncontrolled bleeding following tooth extraction. Parents gave a history of episodes of uncontrolled bleeding following injuries for his grandfather. On examination:
   - Bleeding time = 3 minutes
   - Clotting time = 6 hours
   - Platelet count = 3 lakhs/mm^3 of blood
     - Identify the probable condition. (Hemophilia)
     - What is the defect here? [Deficiency of factor VIII (usually) or IX]
     - How will you treat him? (Fresh blood transfusion or injection of the cryoprecipitate of the factor which is deficient)
8. An 80-year-old man was brought to the OP with complaints of difficulty in walking, tremor of hands for the past one year. On examination:
   - Stooping gait
   - Disappearance of tremor when he is given water to drink
   - Rigidity of the muscles
   - Deep tendon reflexes—normal
     - Identify the probable condition. (Parkinson's disease)
     - What is the underlying defect? (Deficiency of dopamine due to lesion of nigrostriatal pathway in basal ganglia)
     - Which drug is given to treat him? (L-DOPA is given, since dopamine cannot cross the blood-brain barrier)
9. A 6-year-old child was brought with complaints of tiredness, difficulty in breathing, etc. Blood examination showed the following results.
   - Hemoglobin content = 7 g/dL
   - PCV = 24%
   - RBC count = 3 million/mm^3 of blood
   - MCV = 80 fl
   - MCH = 23 pg
   - MCHC = 28%
     - What is the probable diagnosis? (Hypochromic microcytic anemia or iron deficiency anemia)
     - What is the most common cause for this condition in children? (Worm infestation)
     - How will you treat it? (Deworming and administration of iron tablets or iron injection)

Diagrams

1. Lesions of optic pathway
   - Lesion of left optic nerve—anopia (complete blindness) of left eye
   - Lesion of optic chiasma central part showing a pituitary tumor—bitemporal hemianopia
   - Lesion of left optic tract—right homonymous hemianopia
   - Lesion of left optic radiation— right homonymous hemianopia
   - Lesion of left occipital cortex—right homonymous hemianopia with macular sparing
   - Lesion of pretectal nucleus—accommodation reflex present, pupillary reflex absent (Argyll-Robertson pupil)
2. Stretch reflex
   - Which is the receptor involved? (Muscle spindle)
   - Give one example. (Knee jerk)

3. Inverse stretch reflex
   - Which is the receptor involved? (Golgi tendon organ)
4. Renshaw cell inhibition
   - Identify the figure.
   - Name the interneuron marked. (Renshaw cell)
5. Diagram of ruptured Graafian follicle
   - Identify. (Ovulation)
   - Which is the hormone responsible? (LH)
6. Diagram of uterine cycle
   - Identify the phase marked. (5–14 days is proliferative phase due to the action of estrogen and 15–28 days is secretory phase due the action of progesterone mainly)
7. Diagram of juxtaglomerular apparatus
   - Identify the part marked. (Macula densa or juxtaglomerular cells)
   - Mention two functions.
8. Dark adaptation curve
   - Identify.
   - Normal period. (20 minutes)
9. Pyramidal tract lesions
   - What is the effect of lesion at A. (Left internal capsule—right sided hemiplegia or contralateral hemiplegia)
   - At B. (Left side of pons—right sided hemiplegia and left sided facial palsy, i.e., crossed hemiplegia)
10. Oxygen dissociation curve
    - Identify.
    - Factors that cause shift to right or left.
    - What is Bohr effect?
11. Cystometrogram
    - Identify.
    - What is plasticity of smooth muscle?
12. Diagram of a juxtamedullary nephron
    - Identify the type of nephron.
    - Name the ions reabsorbed and secreted in the segment marked.
13. JVP recording
    - Identify the wave marked. (a, c or v wave)
    - Give its cause and one abnormality.
14. Innervation of urinary bladder
    - What is the effect of stimulation of the nerve marked? (Hypogastric, pelvic or pudendal nerve)?
    - Mention the parasympathetic center. (S2,3,4)
15. Intrapleural/intrapulmonary pressure changes during respiration
    - Value at the end of normal expiration.
    - One cause for negative intrapleural pressure.

Interpretation

1. ECG
- Identify the lead. (aVR).

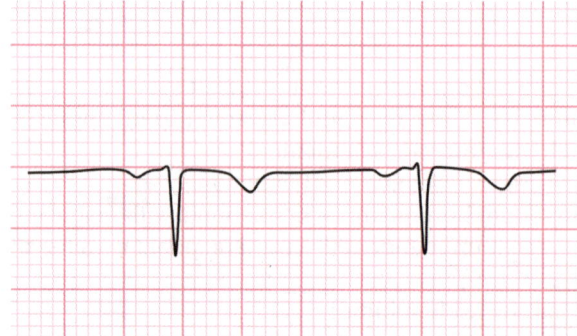

- Give the reason for the negative deflections. (In aVR, the deflections are negative because the depolarizing and the repolarizing waves travel away from the exploring electrode).

2. ECG

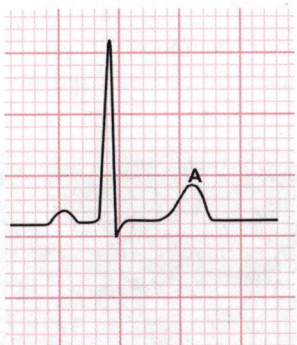

- Identify the part marked A. (T wave)
- Give its cause. (Ventricular repolarization)
- Calculate the duration and amplitude of the wave. (Duration = 0.04 sec × 3 = 0.12 sec; amplitude = 0.1 mV × 3 = 0.3 mV)

3. Perimeter chart

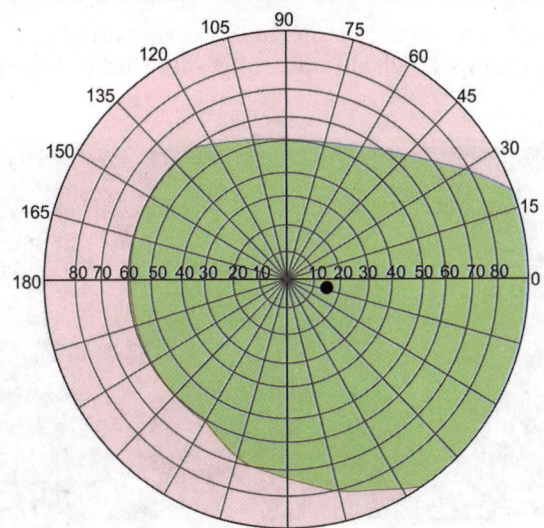

- Identify. (Perimeter chart showing field of vision of right eye)
- Why the field is not circular? (The field is limited by the nose medially, supraorbital ridge superiorly and maxilla inferiorly)
- Identify the black spot in the middle. What is the reason for it? (Blind spot; if the image falls in the region of optic disc since there are no photoreceptors the image is not seen)

4. Audiogram

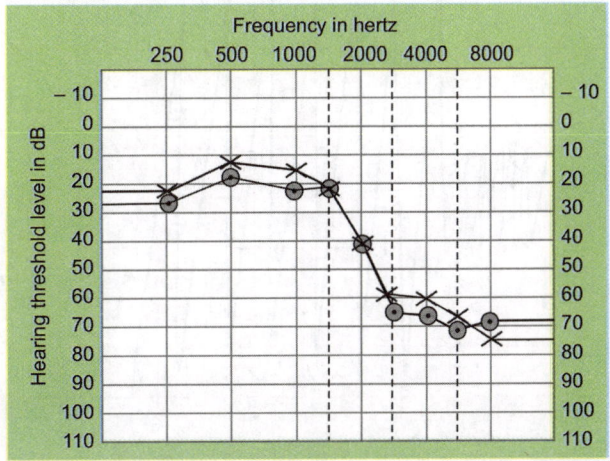

X = Bone conduction
O = Air conduction
- Identify. (Audiogram showing sensorineural deafness)
- Give your reason. (Both air and bone conduction are affected; hearing loss is more for higher frequencies)

5. Stethography

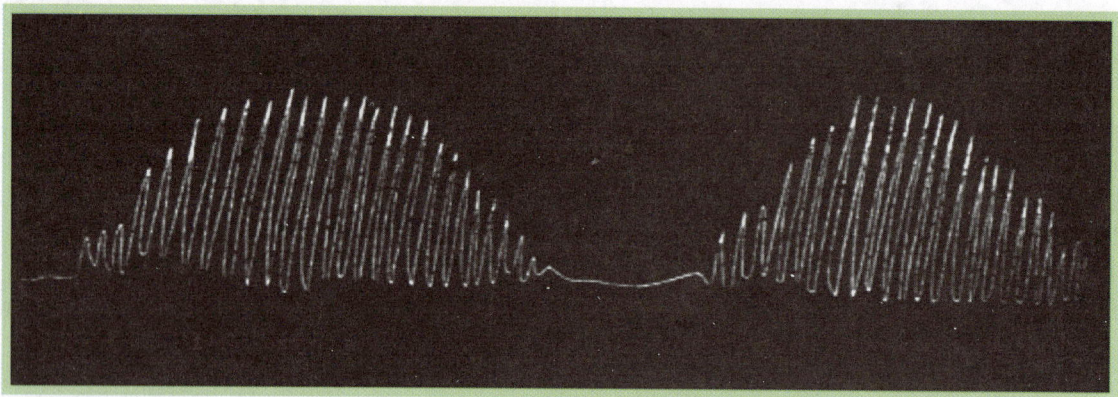

- Identify the graph. (Stethographic recording of Cheyne-Stokes breathing)
- Mention two conditions causing this. (High altitude, congestive cardiac failure)

6. Stethography

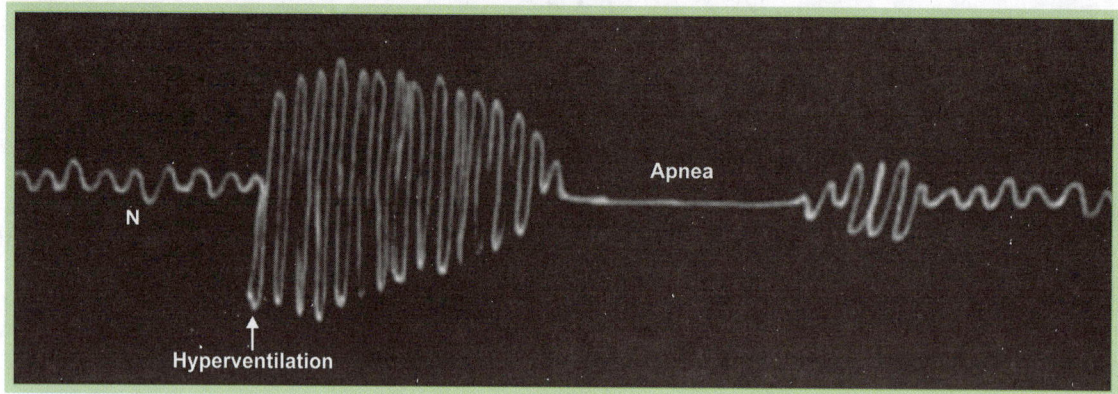

- Identify the part marked A. (Apnea following voluntary hyperventilation)
- What is its cause? (Washing off of CO_2 leads to decrease in arterial PCO_2. This causes depression of respiratory center and arrest of respiration for a brief period)

7. Spirometry

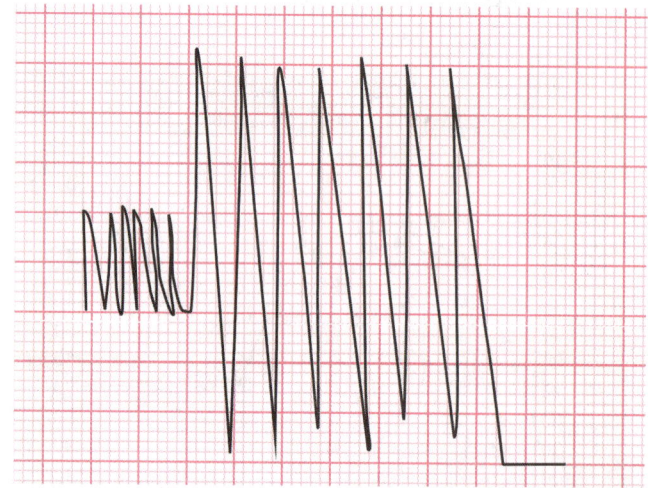

- Find out the maximum voluntary ventilation from the graph, which is recorded for 15 seconds. Smallest division in Y-axis = 30 mL
  Ans: (number of waves in 15 sec × volume of one wave) × 4 = (7 × 2100) × 4 = 58.8 L/min
- Give the normal value (125–170 L/min)

8. Hematocrit

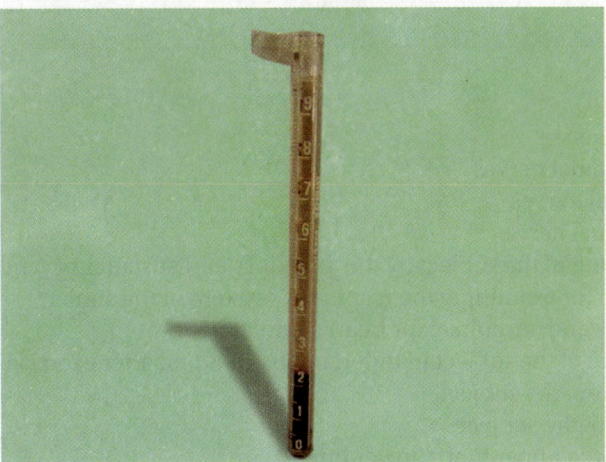

- Identify the condition giving reason. (Anemia; PCV is only 24%)
- Mention one cause. (Iron deficiency).

Skill

- Look for anemia, cyanosis, jaundice, and edema
- Demonstrate Rinne's/Weber's test
- Examine the radial pulse (rate, rhythm, character, volume and condition of vessel wall should be looked for and commented)
- Auscultate the aortic and pulmonary areas and comment
- Auscultate the mitral and tricuspid areas
- Demonstrate the power of right sternocleidomastoid
- Demonstrate accommodation reflex
- Pupillary light reflex of right eye (both direct and consensual reflexes should be elicited)
- Look for coordination of upper limb/lower limb
- Demonstrate any of the deep tendon reflexes (if side is not mentioned test both sides)
- Examine the cervical lymph nodes
- Elicit plantar reflex on the right side
- Test the power of biceps/triceps/supinator muscle and grade.

Short Experiments

One hematology experiment and one amphibian graph.

Hematology experiments (procedure and discussion together 5 marks). The procedure should be written briefly

- Hemoglobin estimation of your own blood
- PCV of the blood sample provided
- Demonstrate your blood group
- Find out your bleeding time and clotting time
- Determine the ESR of the blood sample provided.

Amphibian graph – 5 marks

- All graphs (muscle and heart) discussed in the laboratory can be asked
- Need not do the experiment
- Circuit diagram should be drawn if there are electrical connections
- A neatly labeled graph should be drawn
- Answer precisely to the questions asked.

Hematology Experiments

- Focus the counting chamber after charging for doing RBC count
- For doing WBC count
- Focus an eosinophil/neutrophil/monocyte or lymphocyte after Leishman's staining of your own blood smear.

Clinical Questions

- Elicit the deep tendon reflexes
- Elicit the superficial reflexes
- Examine the I and II cranial nerves
- Examine the III, IV and VI cranial nerves
- Examine the V and VII cranial nerves
- Examine the VIII and XI cranial nerve
- Examine the respiratory system of the subject by the palpatory and auscultatory method
- Do palpation and percussion for examining the respiratory system of the subject
- Percuss out the heart borders and auscultate for heart sounds
- Determine the blood pressure of the subject in different postures and after exercise
- Examine the higher functions of the subject
- Do the general examination of the subject
- Test the power of muscles of the upper limbs/lower limbs
- Test the kinesthetic sensations of the upper limbs of the subject
- Test the integrity of the motor system of the upper limbs of the subject
- Look for coordination of movements in the subject.

MARK DISTRIBUTION FOR I MBBS PHYSIOLOGY PRACTICAL EXAMINATION

MARKLIST FOR PRACTICAL / ORAL / VIVA VOCE
(Summer / Winter – 20…Exam (MBBS UG Courses)
(Applicable for batch admitted in M.B.B.S Course from Academic Year 2019-20 & onwards)

Course: FIRST MBBS   Subject : Physiology
CENTRE :   Marks : (Practical = Practical/Clinical + Viva) Min. 50 Max. 100
Date :   /   /20   Batch :

Practical									Oral/Viva	Total
Seat No.	C.V.C	R.S	C.N.S. & Special senses	Abdomen	Exercise (2) Hematology	Exercise (3) Short Exercise	Human Physiology Experiment	Practical (Total)	Oral/Viva Total	PR/Oral Total
	A	B	C	D	E	F	G	H	I	J
Max. Marks	10	10	10	10	10	15	15	80	20	100

Chapter 61: Sample Questions

MARKLIST FOR PRACTICAL / ORAL / VIVA VOCE
(Summer / Winter – 20…Exam (MBBS UG Courses)
(Applicable for batch admitted in M.B.B.S Course from Academic Year 2019-20 & onwards)

Course: FIRST MBBS
CENTRE :
Date :   /   /20

Subject : Physiology
Marks : (Practical = Practical/Clinical + Viva) Min. 50 Max. 100
Batch :

		Exercise 1				Exercise 2	Exercise 3*	Exercise 4**	Practical (Total)	Oral/Viva (Total)	PR/Oral Total
		Clinical Examination									
	C.V.C	R.S	C.N.S. & Special senses	General Exam & Abdomen		Hematology	Short Exercise	Human Physiology Experiment			
	A	B	C	D		E	F	G	H	I	J
Max. Marks	10.0	10.0	10.0	10.0		10.0	15.0	15.0	80	20.0	100

*Short exercises 3 marks each(3X5)
1. Case based scenarios/endocrine disorders photographs. 2. Interpretation of function tests. 3. One skeletal graph 4. One cardiac graph 5. Calculation

**Exercise 4: Human Physiology Experiment 1. Basic Life Support in a simulated environment 2. ECG 3. Spirometry 4. PEFR 5. EEG Interpretation 6. Ergography 7. Harward step test 8. Perimetry

* Suggested Methods of Assessment
Clinical exam & OSPE

(Please Note The above examination pattern will be applicable to the students admitted from Academic Year 2019-20 and onwards, which is informed to all Medical Colleges vide University letter No MUHS/X-1/UG/1692/2020 Date: 28/02/2020)

Index

Page numbers followed by *f* refer to figure.

A

Abdomen 130
    examination of 129
    muscles of 154, 157
    shape of 129
    stroking skin of 181*f*
    surface of 130
Abdominal cavity 134
Abdominal examination 129
Abdominal guarding 130
Abdominal organs, boundaries of 133
Abdominal reflex
    absence of 183
    eliciting 181*f*
Abdominal wall 131*f*
    movements of 130
Abductor digiti minimi 152
Abductor pollicis brevis 157
    testing 151*f*
ABO system 86
Absolute eosinophil count 71, 72, 291, 292
    by hemocytometry 71
    over indirect count 73
Accommodation reflex
    pathway for 175
    testing 164*f*
Acetylcholine 230, 231, 231*f*, 282, 284
    on heart, action of 231
Achilles tendon, squeezing 139*f*
Acid, superficial 29
Acid-citrate-dextrose 14
Activated partial thromboplastin time 82, 291
Adequate stimulus 142
Adrenaline 231, 282
    effect of 230, 231*f*, 283*f*
    mechanism of action of 284
Adventitious sounds 113
Agglutinogen 85
Agranulocytes 61
Agranulocytosis 68
Agraphia 137
Air conduction 169*f*, 262*f*
Alpha-antibodies 87*f*
Alzheimer's disease 136
Ammonium oxalate 77
Amphibian experiments 185
    graphs of 297
Amphibian heart 220
Amphibian nerve-muscle experiments, learning 216

Anacrotic limb 117*f*, 127
Analgesia 143
Anarthria 136
Anemia 19*f*, 39, 45, 94, 98
    mild 25*f*
    morphological classification of 42
    severe 25*f*
Anesthesia 143
    dissociated 143
Anhidrosis 163
Anisochromia 64
Anisopoikilocytosis 12*f*
Ankle
    clonus 179
    jerk 179, 179*f*
Anode, accelerating 235
Anopia 257
Anti-A
    antibodies 89
    sera 85*f*
    serum 87*f*
Anti-B antibodies 89
Antibody, warm 89
Anticoagulants 13
Anti-D
    antibodies 87*f*
    sera 85*f*
Antigens, types of 85
Aortic valve 283
Apex beat 110, 116
    locating 120*f*
Aphasia 136, 137
    nominal 137
Aplastic anemia 79
Apnea, reason for 254
Arc 255
Argyll-Robertson pupil 175
Arneth index 68
Arsenic poisoning 39
Arterial blood
    collection of 15
    pressure 103, 104*f*
        measurement of 118
Arterial obstruction 265
Arterial pulse 117*f*, 124
    abnormal 117*f*, 127*f*
    abnormalities of 127
    examination of 116
    recording of 126
    tracing 127*f*
Artery
    brachial 118

    carotid 118
    dorsalis pedis 118
    femoral 118
    popliteal 118
    pulmonary 218
    temporal 118
    tibial 118
Asbestos, inhalation of 93
Asbestosis 93
Asynergia 150
Ataxia 150
Ataxic gait 137
Athetosis 156
Atrial fibrillation 242*f*, 243
Atrioventricular nodal delay, causes of 246
Atropine, adding 287
Audibility curve 261
Audiogram 261, 307
    recorded, normal 262*f*
Audiometer 261
Auscultation, areas for 122*f*
Auscultatory gap 107
Auscultatory method 103, 105, 105*f*
Autologous transfusion 88
Automated analyzer 78
Automated electronic method 75
Autonomic balance 278
Autonomic function tests 274
Autonomic parasympathetic fibers 173
Axillary area 109

B

Babinski sign 183
Back 109, 188
    muscles of 154, 155, 157
Barany's test 169
Basopenia 67
Basophil 62, 62*f*, 66, 67
Basophilia 67
Behavior 135, 156
Biceps 153, 157
    jerk 178, 178*f*
    testing 153*f*
Bidder's ganglion 227
Bilirubin content 25
Biophysics experiments 233
Bipolar limb leads 237, 238
Bleeding time 80, 80*f*, 82
    determination of 80
Blind spot 257
Blinking 167

Blood
  accurately 17
  bank 87
  collection of 14
  components of 87
  elements of 66
  examination of 11
  film 61
  from anterior cubital vein, collection of 15f
  from heart chambers, collection of 15
  microscopic examination of 10
  specific gravity of 47
  to laboratory, transport of 15
  vessels, integrity of 84
Blood cell
  contain structures 58
  count 54
Blood contains
  diluted 72
  undiluted 72
Blood group
  determination 85, 87
    antibodies for 89
  O 89
  systems, inheritance of 89
Blood pressure 93, 97, 98, 103, 275
  after exercise 106
  changes 274
  measurement, principle of manual 103
  recording 103, 105, 105f, 106, 106f
  responses 278
  sitting posture 106
  standing posture 106
  supine position 106
  systolic 276f
Blood sample
  collection of 13
  methods of collection of 13
  overdilution of 30f
Blood smear 58, 59f, 65
  cover glass method of preparing 60
  good 66
  methods of making 59
  peripheral 58, 60f, 65, 69, 79
  preparing 58, 59, 59f
  stained 66
Blood transfusion 87, 88, 89
  complications of 88
Body
  left side of 142
  right side of 142
  temperature 83, 93, 98
  tube 4
Bombay group 89
Bone conduction 162, 169f, 263
Bowel sounds 133
Brachioradialis 157
  testing 153f
Breath holding, effect of 252
Breath sounds 113
  abnormal 113
  bronchial 115

Breathing
  bronchial 115
  deep 277
  type of 110
  using stethograph, movements of 251
Brecher-Cronkite method 77
Brilliant cresyl blue 74, 77
  stain 74
Bruit 124
Buccinator, testing power of 168f
Bulb, red bead in 34f

C

Calcium
  chloride 198
  deficiency 83
Calibrate dynamometer 278
Caloric tests 169, 170
Cannula 281
Capillary blood 14
  by finger prick, collection of 14f
Capillary space 37
Capillary tube method 81, 83
Carbon monoxide poisoning 39
Carboxyhemoglobin method 31
Cardiac efficiency index, calculate 272
Cardiac failure 97f
Cardiac impulse 119
Cardiac muscle 204, 206
Cardiac output, return of 277
Cardiac reserve 272, 273
Cardiogram
  normal 218
    recording of 219
Cardiorespiratory parameters 271
Cardiovascular autonomic function tests 274
Cardiovascular system examination 116, 123
Carotid pulsations 120
Catacrotic limb 117f, 127
Cathode ray oscilloscope 235, 235f, 238
  uses of 236
Cedar wood oil 58
Cell 52, 64
  counting 37
  distribution of 40
  identification of different 61
  mean, double population of 68
  nuclei of 55
  size 20
  swell 52
  types of 61
Central shaft with pulleys 190f
Centrifugal blood smear method 59, 60
Cerebellar
  disease 150
  lesion 158
Cervical
  group 96
  lymph nodes, examination of 96f
Charging counting chamber 37, 37f

Chest
  examination of 109
  expansion 111
  leads 237f
    normal ECG in 241f
    unipolar 238
  measurements 111
  movements 110
    during respiration 111
  palpation of 99f
  piece 101
  shape of 109
  wall, percussion over 113f
Cheyne-Stokes
  breathing recorded 254f
  respiration 253
Chin rest 255
Chorea 156
Citrate-phosphate-dextrose-adenine 14
Clavicular area 109
Clonus 183, 206
Clot retraction time 82
Clotting factors 82
  sources of 82
Clotting pathway 83
Clotting time 81, 82
  determination of 80
Cochlear function, tests for 173
Cochlear part, testing 168
Cog-wheel 157
Coiled glass tube 281
Cold pressor response test 274
Color blindness 174
Color vision 160, 162
  mechanisms of 173
  significance of testing 174
  testing 162f
Coma 136
Compensatory pause 225, 226, 226f
Compound microscope, parts of 3
Condenser, sub-stage 4
Conducting tubes 101
Conduction deafness 262, 263
  causes of 263
Confrontation test 161
Congenital cyanotic heart disease 39
Congestive cardiac failure 254
Conjunctiva 94f
Conjunctival reflex 180
  method of eliciting 180f
Connect limb leads 274
Consciousness, level of 135, 156, 182
Consensual light reflex 164
Copper sulfate 47
  advantages of 47
  method 47
Corrigan's pulse 117
Coumarin 14
Counting
  chamber, ruled area of 35f
  rules of 39
Cover slip preparation 74

Index

Cranial nerve 159, 163, 164, 173, 175, 180
    examination of 159, 172
    functions of 159
    integrity of 159
Cranial root 171
Cremasteric reflex 180, 181
    absence of 183
Cretinism 303
Critical fusion frequency 206
Cushing's syndrome 39, 131f, 302
Cyanmethemoglobin method 28, 31
Cyanosis 94, 98
Cyclopentolate drops 268
Cytoplasm 62f

D

Dacie's fluid 36
Dale's apparatus 285, 286f
Dancing movements 156
Deafness 137
    types of 263
Delusion 136, 137, 156, 172, 182
Dementia 135
Dense granules, contents of 79
Diabetic retinopathy 270f
Diadochokinesis 147, 148f
Diaphragm 101, 155, 157
Dicrotic notch 127
Distant vision 160
    testing 161f
Distension, symmetrical 130
Dorsalis pedis artery 118
Down-stroke catacrotic limb 127
Drowsiness 136
Drugs
    and ions, effects of 281, 287f
    effect of 283f, 285, 287
Dubois-Reymond inductorium 187, 187f
Duke's method 80, 81
Dunger's fluid 71, 292
    composition of 71
Dust particles 55
Dysarthria 136, 137
Dysdiadochokinesis 147
Dyskinesia 156
Dysmetria 150
Dysphasia 137, 136
Dysphonia 136

E

Ear piece 101
Edema 96, 96f, 98, 100
Elbow joint brachioradialis 153
Electric
    circuit, connections for 199
    connections 192, 197, 205, 211
    kymograph 190f
Electrical equipments 187
Electrical stimuli, advantages of 187
Electrically driven kymograph 190
Electrocardiogram 237
    normal 240
Electrocardiography, recording of 240f

Electrodes 237, 259
    stimulating 188
    types of 259
Electromagnet 188
Electromyogram 259
    uses of 260
Electron microscopy, scanning 7
Electronic recording device 235
Electronic stimulators 260
Elicit clonus, methods to 179
Embolus 84
Emotional behavior 135
Emotional state 156, 172, 182
Emphysema, severe 133
Endocrine disorders 39
Enophthalmos 163
Eosinopenia 67, 73
Eosinophil 62, 62f, 66, 67, 72f
    count, normal 73
    functions of 73
    granules 71, 73
Eosinophilia 67, 72, 73
Epitrochlear glands 96
Equipment required 271
Erector spinae 155, 157
Ergograph 264f
Erythroblastosis fetalis 88
Erythrocyte 11f, 65f
    sedimentation rate 17, 18
Erythropoiesis, stimulates 39
Esophageal lead 238
Esrite method 17, 18
Ethylenediaminetetraacetic acid 13
Exercise
    effect of 252
    grading of 272
    tolerance tests 272
Exophthalmos 163, 303
Expiratory reserve volume 249
Extensors of fingers, testing power of 152f
Extraocular muscles, examination of 165
Extrasystole 225, 226, 246
    pause 226f
Extremity, pendular movement of 147
Eye
    closure, forced 167
    icterus of 94f
    jaundice of 94f
    lens 5
    mean, conjugate movement of 174
    movements 164
    normal fundus of 163f, 269f, 270
Eyeball, movements of 165f
Eyepiece 5

F

Faradic current 187, 193, 193f
Fatigue
    causes of 212
    first site of 212
    phenomenon of 211
Feces 130
Femtolitres 44

Femur clamp 191
Festinant gait 137
Fetus 130
Fibrillation potentials 260f
Fibrin threads 81f
Fibrinogen 20
Field lens 5
Field of vision 160, 161
    binocular 258f
    test 162f, 255
Fine touch 138
    sensation 139f
Finger
    and wrist movements abductor pollicis
        brevis, muscles of 151
    clubbing of 95f
    extensors of 152
    flexors of 152, 157
    prick method 13, 80, 80f
Finger-nose test 147
    of right hand with eyes open 148f
    with eyes closed 148f
Finger-to-finger test 147
Fit 156
Flatus 130
Flexors of fingers, testing power of 152f
Fluid thrill, testing for 133
Foot
    dorsiflexors of 157
    dorsum of 96f
    drop 137
    plantar flexors of 157
Forced expiratory volume 249f
Forehead, wrinkling of 167
Formalin 77
Frank-Starling law 208, 222
Fresh blood under microscope 10f
    examination of 10
Frog
    board 191, 225
    heart rate 220
    muscle nerve preparation 199, 212f
    normal cardiogram of 218
    pithing of 194, 194f
    right side of 227
    sciatic nerve of 196f, 216, 217, 217f
    skeletal muscle graphs, recording 198f
    tissues 198
Frog's heart 218, 220, 223, 224f, 225, 226f,
        229, 230, 231, 231f
    anatomy of 218
    effect of
        drugs on 231f
        heat and cold on 221, 222f
        ions on 230
        temperature on 221
    isolated 230
    located, pacemaker of 220
    period in 225
    vagal stimulation on 227, 228f
Functional residual capacity 249
Fundus 269

G

Gait 136, 145, 156, 172, 182
   abnormalities of 135
   high stepping 137
   stamping 137
Gallbladder 132
Galvanic current 187, 193f
Gasometric method 28, 31
Gastrocnemius muscle 194
   separating tendon of 195f
Gear and pulley arrangement 191
Gentian violet 36
Ghost cell 11f
Gigantism 302
Glacial acetic acid 36, 54
Glass slide 10, 66
   method 58, 59
Glass tube 281
Globulin concentrations 20
Glossopharyngeal nerve 159, 170, 173
Gluteal nerve
   inferior 155
   superior 155
Granulocytes 61
Granulocytopenia 68
Graphesthesia 141

H

Hair 96
   esthesiometer 143
Haldane's method 28, 31
Hallucination 136, 137, 156, 172, 182
Hand grip
   spring dynamometer 277f
   test 274
Harvard step test 271
   advantages of 273
Hayem's fluid 36, 292
   composition of 36
Head's classification 137
Hearing by audiometry, test of 261
Heart 206, 222
   afterloading in 210
   borders of 116
   freeloading in 210
   level of 107
   lever 192, 192f, 225
   mean electrical axis of 243
   parasympathetic supply to 229
   rhythm of 242
   stimulation of nerves to 229
   vagal stimulation on 227
   while mounting 283
Heart block
   complete 243, 244f
   first-degree 243
   second degree 243f
   third-degree 243
Heart rate 275
   abnormalities in 246f
   generated, maximum 276
   lowest 276
   of frog 220
   per minute 272
   variation in 277
Heart sound
   first 122
   physiological split of second 124
   second 122
Heated stylus method 239
Heel-knee test 149, 149f
Heel-shin test 149
Hematocrit 17, 23, 309
   determination of 23
   findings 25f
   reading 24f, 25f
Hematologic values 291
Hematology 1
   experiments 310
Hemianopia 257
Hemiplegia 158
Hemiplegic gait 137
Hemocytometer 34
Hemocytometry 34, 54
Hemoglobin
   colorimetric estimation of 28
   concentration of 31
   estimate 28, 34, 44, 58, 80
   methods of estimation of 31
Hemoglobinometry 28
Hemolysis 52
Hemolytic disease of newborn, prevent 88
Hemophilia 82, 83
Hemorrhage, repeated small 39
Hemostasis 84
   steps in 83
Heparin 14
   act 71
Hepatojugular reflux 119. 125
Heteronymous hemianopia 257
Hip, extensors of 157
Histamine increases 286
Holmgren's colored wool test 162
Homeostasis 84
Homonymous hemianopia 257
Human heart, innervation of 229
Human sciatic nerve 217
Hyperalgesia 143
Hypersplenism, decreased in 79
Hypertension 107
Hyperthyroidism 39
Hypertonia 157
Hypertonic saline, blood in 11, 11f
Hypertonic solution 52
Hypochondriac, right 129
Hypochromia 45
Hypochromic anemia 64, 65f
Hypoesthesia 143
Hypotension, postural 275
Hypothermia 215
Hypotonia 158
Hypotonic saline, blood in 11, 11f
Hypotonic solution 50

I

Icterus 94
Ideal diluting fluid 40
Idiopathic thrombocytopenic purpura 79
Idioventricular rhythm 224f
Illumination system 5
Illusion 136
Immunity, types of 68
Impulse production, ectopic foci of 246
In vivo anticoagulants 14
Inductorium, parts of 187
Inflammatory conditions, acute 19
Infra-axillary area 109
Infraclavicular area 109
Inframammary area 109
Infraspinatus 153, 157
Ingredients, functions of 55
Inguinal lymph nodes, palpation of 133
Inspiratory reserve volume 249
Instruments used, study of 187
Intention tremor 147
Intercostal space, right second 113f
Interossei, testing of 151f
Intestinal movements 287
   types of 287
Intracardiac lead 238
Intravital staining 75
Iris diaphragm 5
Iron
   deficiency anemia 65, 65f
   estimation of 31
Ishihara's chart 162, 162f
Isolated muscle-nerve preparation 212
Isolated rabbit's
   heart 281
   intestine 287f
Isometric exercise 277
Isometric muscle lever 192
Iso-osmotic solution 51
Isotonic
   muscle lever 191, 192f
   saline 36, 208
   solution 11
Ivy's method 80, 81

J

Jaeger's test chart 160, 161f
Jaundice 94, 94f, 98
Jaw jerk 177
   eliciting 178f
Jendrassik's maneuver 177f, 183
Joint
   position of 146
   sense 138
Jugular pulse tracing 119
Jugular veins, external 120
Jugular venous pressure 93, 97, 118
   measurement of 119, 119f
   waveform of 124
Jugular venous pulse, waves of 119f

K

Kahn tubes 50
Kidney
   palpation of right 132f
   right 131

Index

K

Knee
- extensors of 155, 157
- flexors of 155, 157
- hammers, types of 177*f*
- jerk 179, 179*f*
  - elicit 177*f*

Korotkoff sounds 103, 107
Kymograph 214, 225, 253*f*, 281
- adjustments in 197, 199

Kyphotic posture 137

L

Langendorff's apparatus 281, 282*f*
Latent period
- causes of 199, 201
- decrease in 214

Latissimus dorsi 153, 157
Lead poisoning 93
Lead-pipe 157
Lee and White method 81
Left eye, testing pupillary light reflex of 163*f*
Left infraspinatus, testing 154*f*
Left kidney, palpation of 131
Leishman's stain 58, 61*f*, 65
- composition of 66
- preparation of 58
- smears 75

Lens, graded focal length 268
Lethargy 136
Leukemia 56
- types of 57

Leukemoid reaction 56
Leukocyte 61
- count, absolute 69
- different 66, 69
- differential counting of 44, 54, 58, 63
- distribution of 61
- functions of 56
- total count of 71

Leukocytosis 56
Leukopenia 56
- producing 56

Lid retraction 163
Light
- artificial 98
- natural 198

Light reflex 172
- abnormalities of 164
- testing indirect 164*f*

Limb
- active movements of 99
- leads, unipolar 238
- reflex movements of 99

Linen cuff, rubber bag with 103
Liver 131, 133
- lower border of 133*f*
- palpation of 132*f*

Low power adjustments 6
Low voltage
- terminal 193
- unit 187

Lower limb 149, 157
- muscles of 155, 157

Lower motor neuron facial palsy 304
Luca's trough 189
Lumbar, right 129
Lumbricals 151, 151*f*
Lung
- diseases, chronic 39
- volumes 247
  - and capacities, normal 248*f*

Lymphadenopathy 95
Lymphoblastic leukemia, acute 57
Lymphocyte 62, 63*f*, 65*f*, 67
Lymphocytic leukemia, chronic 57
Lymphocytosis 67
Lymphopenia 67

M

Macrocytes 44, 65
Malnutrition, severe 129
Mammalian
- experiments 279
- heart 220, 224

Mammary area 109
Mandibular division 165, 175
Marey's tambour 251, 252, 252*f*
Masseter of both sides, testing power of 166*f*
Mastication, muscles of 175
Maxillary division 165, 175
Mean arterial pressure 107
Mean corpuscular
- hemoglobin 39, 44
  - concentration 44, 45
- volume 44

Measles 67
Mechanical equipments 187, 190
Mechanical fragility 52
Mechanical kymograph 190*f*
Megaloblastic anemia 79
Memory 136
- and intelligence 156, 172, 182

Mental state 135, 156, 172, 182
Mercury
- commutator 189, 189*f*
- manometer 103, 276, 281

Metabolic flaps 156
Methylene blue stain 74, 75
Metronome 271
Microcytes 44, 65
Micro-erythrocyte sedimentation rate
- kit 19
- method 17

Microhematocrit method 23, 24, 25*f*
Microscope 7, 58
- adjustments of 6, 66
- binocular 3*f*
- care of 6
- compound 3, 4*f*, 10
- dark-field 7
- electron 3, 7
- fluorescence 7
- image formation by 5
- light 3
- magnification of 5
- phase contrast 7
- racking 6
- simple 3
- use of 3

Microscopic field, size of 76
Mini wright's peak flow meter 266, 266*f*
Miosis 163
Mitral area over apex beat 122*f*
Monocyte 62, 63*f*, 66, 68
Monocytopenia 68
Morphine poisoning 254
Mosso's ergograph 264
Motor
- aphasia 137
- component 165
- nucleus, main 170
- system examination 145, 156, 159
- unit 204

Motor cranial nerves 155
- purely 173

Mount counting chamber 55
Mounting cylinder 197
Mounting muscle nerve preparation 197
Movement 100
- abnormal 156
- coordination of 145, 147
- decomposition of 150

Murmur 124
- types of 124

Muscle
- acting 153
- bath 189
- bulk of 145, 156
- continuous stimulation of 211
- direct stimulation of 193*f*
- feel of 146
- grading of power of 155
- groups 150
- lever 191
- power of 145
- strength of 150, 157
- stretch reflexes 177
- summation 204
- temperature 214
- tone of 145, 146, 157
- twitch 201, 204
- type of 206

Muscle contraction 202, 203*f*, 206*f*, 208, 209*f*, 214
- amplitude of 208
- effect of temperature on 213, 214*f*, 215*f*
- strength of 204

Muscle nerve preparation 194
- dissection of 194

Muscle power 150
- abnormalities in 155

Muscular exercise graded 272
Mycobacterium tuberculosis 7
Myeloblastic leukemia, acute 57
Myeloid leukemia, chronic 57
Myocardial infarction 245, 245*f*
Myoclonus 156
Myograph
- and lever, adjustments of 198
- board 191, 225
- stand 191, 197, 225

Myxedema 302

N

Nails 96
Neck, muscles of 154
Needle electrode 259, 259f
Nerve
    abducent 159, 163, 172
    accessory 159, 171
    axillary 153
    facial 159, 166, 172
    femoral 155, 179
    hypoglossal 159, 172, 173
    in humans, conduction velocity of 217
    median 151, 152
    musculocutaneous 153, 178
    oculomotor 159, 163, 172
    olfactory 159, 172
    optic 159, 160, 172
    phrenic 155
    pudendal 182
    radial 152, 153, 178
    suprascapular 153
    thoracodorsal 153
    tibial 179
    trigeminal 159, 165, 172, 175, 177
    trochlear 159, 163
    ulnar 151, 152
    vagus 159, 170, 173
    vestibulocochlear 159, 168, 173
Nerve deafness 262
    causes of 263
Nerve impulse 217
    velocity of 216, 217
Nerve-muscle preparation, dissection of 195
Nervous system
    examination of 135
    functions of 135
Neubauer double counting chamber 35, 35f, 54, 77
Neural deafness 263
Neuromuscular junction 212
Neutropenia 67
Neutrophil 62, 62f, 65f, 67
    contain neutral substances 58
    functions of 66
Neutrophilia 67
Newbauer's counting chamber 40
Nose piece 5
    fixed 5
    revolving 5
Nozzle pierces 283
Nuclei 170
Numerical aperture 4
Nystagmus 174
    physiological 174

O

Obey 'rules of counting 37
Occipitofrontalis, anterior belly of 167f
Oil immersion, adjustments for 6
Olfaction 175
    abnormalities of 175
Olfactory nerve 159, 172
    examination of 160
Ophthalmic division 175
Ophthalmoscope 268-270
    direct 268, 268f
Ophthalmoscopy 270
    clinical significance of 270
    indirect 268
Opponens pollicis 151, 157
    testing 151f
Optic disc, cupping of 270f
Optic fundus 160
    examination of 162
Optical magnifying parts 5
Optical tube length 4
Opticokinetic nystagmus 174
Orbicularis oculi, testing power of 167f
Orthostatic hypotension 107
Orthostatic tachycardia 275
Oscillatory method 104
Osmotic fragility 17, 23, 50-52, 291
    determination of 50
    observation of 51f
    variation in 50
Oxygen
    carrying capacity determination 31
    cylinder 285

P

P wave 241
Packed cell volume 23, 24
    measurement of 23
Pain 138
    deep 138, 139
    pressure 138, 139
    sensation 139, 143
    superficial 139, 139f, 143
    visceral 143
Palmar interossei 151
Palpation 99, 110, 114, 120, 123, 130
Palpatory method 103, 104, 104f
    advantages of 103, 106
    disadvantages of 106
Pancytopenia 68
Paper recording 238, 239
Papilledema 269, 270f
Paradoxical cold fiber discharge 143
Parasternal heave
    elicitation of 116
    left 121f
Parasympathetic ganglia 219, 229
Parasympathetic nucleus 170
Paresthesia 143
Parkinson's disease 136, 156
Passive movement
    resistance to 146
    sense of 140
    testing sense of 141f
Pasteur pipette 23, 23f
Patellar clonus 179
Patellar jerk 179
Peak expiratory flow rate 266, 267
Peak flow meter chart 267f

Pectoral nerves
    lateral 153
    medial 153
Pectoralis 153, 157
Pendular knee jerk 183
Percussion
    correct technique of 100f
    rules of 100, 101, 115
Perfusion funnel 230f
Perimeter 255, 255f
    chart 256, 256f
    using 255
Perimetry 255
Peripheral cyanosis 95f
Peripheral smear 12f, 61, 62f, 63f, 66
    platelets 65f
Pernicious anemia 65
Petri dish 58, 285
Phillips and van Slyke's copper sulfate method 47, 48
Phloxin stains 71
Phosphorus 39
Physical examination 99
Physiograph 127f
Pilot's solution 71
Pipette 42
Pithing needle 194
Pitting edema 96f, 97f, 303
Plantar reflex 180, 181
    eliciting 181f
Plantar response, normal 181f
Plasma 20, 48
    column 23
    red color of 25
Platelet 64, 65, 78f, 79
    alpha granules of 79
    formation of 79
    function 79, 83
    life span of 79
Platelet count 77, 79, 82, 291, 292
    calculate 69
    normal 79
    variation in 78
Pleximeter 100
Plexor 100
Pneumothorax, large right 133
Poikilocytosis 65
Polycythemia 25, 39
    secondary 39
    types of 39
    vera 39
Popliteal nodes 96
Positive rebound phenomenon 147
Posture 136
    and gait, abnormalities in 137
Potassium chloride 198
Precordium 116
    examination of 119
    shape of 119
Preservation injury 88
Pressure 139
    pain, testing for 139f
    sensation, testing for 139f
Prick fingertip 77

Proptosis 163
Prothrombin time 82, 291
    one stage 81
Ptosis 163
Pulley driven kymograph 190
Pulse 93, 97
    abnormal 117
    alternans 118
    anacrotic 118
    biphasic 118
    bisferiens 118, 127
    character of 117
    dicrotic 118
    high volume 125
    paradoxus 118
    rate 124
    record 103
        normal 127*f*
    rhythm of 127
    three abnormal 125
    tracing, peripheral 127
    venous 124
    weak thready 128
Pulsus
    alternans 127
    bigeminus 127
    paradoxus 128
Pupillary light reflex 180
    pathway for 174
Pure tone audiometer 261, 261*f*
Purpura 79, 83, 84
Push spreader slide 59*f*
Pyramidal tract lesion 183

Q

QRS complex 241, 243*f*
    abnormalities in 244
QT interval abnormalities 244
Quadrantanopia 257

R

Rabbit's heart 283, 283*f*
    perfusion of isolated 281
Rabbit's intestine, isolated 286
Rabbit's normal intestinal movementsm,
    recording of 285
Rabbits isolated heart 283*f*
Radial pulse, palpation of 116*f*
Radiofemoral delay 118
Receptor 142
    adaptation of 143
    blockers 284
Record simple muscle twitch 201
Recording device 238
Red blood cell 20, 23, 34, 48, 64
    agglutination of 86*f*
    appearance of 10
    count 34, 36, 36*f*, 39, 44, 58, 80, 292
        normal 39
    determination of 50
    diluting fluid 36
    indices 44
    method of counting 38*f*
    osmotic fragility of 51*f*
    pipette 34, 34*f*, 41*f*, 42
        bulbs of 41*f*
Red bone marrow, malignant condition
    of 39
Red cell
    count, pathological variation in 39
    detect sickling of 10
    membrane 51
Red chilly powder appearance 86*f*
Reeling gait 137
Rees-Ecker diluting fluid
    composition of 77
    constituents of 79
Rees-Ecker fluid 292
Reflex 166, 182
    abdominal 180
    abnormal
        deep 183
        superficial 183
    accommodation 164, 180
    anal 180, 182
    arc, components of 183
    ciliospinal 180
    clinical examination of 176
    corneal 180
    deep 176, 177
    examination of 176, 182
    grade 183
    light 163
    organic 176, 182
    palatal 170, 180
    pharyngeal 171, 180
    properties of 183
    pupillary 163, 172, 180
    stretch 176, 183
    superficial 176, 180, 182
    types of 176
    visceral 176, 182
Refraction, errors of 173
Refractory period 204, 206
Remak's ganglia 219
Reservoir bottle 281
Residual volume 249
Resistance to passive movement, testing
    for 146*f*
Respiration
    breath-holding on 251
    mechanism of 251
    rhythm of 110
Respiratory movements 253*f*
    normal 252
    recording of 252*f*
Respiratory rate 93, 97, 98, 110, 111
Respiratory sinus arrhythmia 242
Respiratory system, examination of 109, 114
Resting tremor 156
Reticulocyte 75, 75*f*
    count 74-76, 291
        automated method of 76
    crisis 76
    span of 76
Reticulocytopenia 76
Reticulocytosis 76
Retina 256
    hypertensive changes in 270*f*
Rh system 86
Rh-negative
    baby 88
    mother 88
Rh-positive mother carries 88
Rhythm 117
Right axis deviation 243
Right eye 257*f*
    ptosis of 163*f*
Ringer's fluid, functions of 197
Ringer's solution 215, 223, 292
    composition of 198
Ringer-Locke's fluid 282, 292
    function of 283
Ringer-Locke's solution 281
    composition of 281
Rinne's test 168, 169*f*
Romberg's test 141, 149, 149*f*
Rotational tests 169
Rouleaux formation 10, 20
    degree of 61
    factors affecting 20
Rubber pump 104

S

Sahli's hemoglobinometer 29, 29*f*
Sahli's method 28
    disadvantages of 30
Saw-toothed voltage 235
Schwabach test 168
Sciatic nerve 155, 194
    gastrocnemius muscle preparation 196
Sclera 94*f*
Scotomas 257, 257*f*
Scotomata 257
Second-degree block 243
Seizure 156
Semantic aphasia 137
Semi-coma 136
Sensations 143
    deep 138
    superficial 138
Sense 143
    of position, testing for 141*f*
Sensibility 142
Sensorineural deafness 263*f*
Sensory
    ataxia 141, 150
    component 165
    cranial nerves, test 141
    functions 135
    general 167
    nerves, purely 173
    nucleus 170
    parts 141, 166
    receptors, classify 138
    system, examination of 138, 142
Serratus anterior 153, 157
    testing power of 154*f*
Serum 291

Shamroth's sign 95f
Sherrington-Starling recording drum 190
Shifting dullness, testing for 133
Shilling index 68
Shoulder, muscles of 153
Silent gap 107
Silicosis 93
Simple muscle twitch 199, 200f, 201, 203f, 211
   recorded 199
Simulated environment 159, 176, 237
Simultaneous stimulation, double 141
Sinus
   arrhythmia 246, 277
   bradycardia 246, 246f
   venosus increased 221
   venosus, effect of heat and cold on 221, 222, 222f
Sitting posture 108
Skeletal muscle
   contraction 203f, 208
   electrical events in 201f
   mechanical events in 201f
Skill 130, 309
Skin 96
   and hair, examination of 93
   clean 15
Sleep 135, 156, 172, 182
Small intestine, isolated pieces of 285
Smear
   fixing and staining of 60
   parts of 61
   preparation 74
Smoked drum 214, 219
Smoking 192
Smooth muscle
   cell membrane of 287
   plasticity of 287
   types of 287
Snellen's chart 160, 161f
Sodium
   bicarbonate 198
   chloride 74, 198
      solution 50
   citrate 74, 77
   fluoride 14
Somatic motor 167
Somatic pain, deep 143
Somnolence 136
Sounds heard, abnormal 122
Spastic gait 137
Special cover glass 36, 54
Special sensory 167
Specific gravity, normal values of 48
Spectrophotometry 31
Speech 136, 150, 156, 172, 182
   disorders, types of 136
   scanning 150
Sphygmomanometer 103, 104f, 129, 277
Sphygmomanometry, methods of 104
Spinal accessory nerve 173
Spinal root 171
Spinothalamic pathway 143
Spirometer 247, 247f
Spirometry, interpret 247

Spleen 131, 133
   deeper palpation of 132f
   palpable normally 134
   palpation of 132f
Spontaneous electrical activity, recording of 260
Spotters 295
Spreader slide 66
Squint 163, 174
ST segment, abnormalities in 244
Stain
   and water, mixture of 66
   peripheral smear 61f
Staining rack 58
Stannius ligature 223, 224f
   first 223
   second 223, 224
Starling's law 210
State Frank-Starling's law 210
State Landsteiner's laws 89
Stereognosis 140
   testing for 140f
Sternocleidomastoid, testing power of left 171f
Sternomastoid 171
Stethogram 251
Stethograph 251, 251f
Stethography 251, 308
   recording 253f
Stethoscope 101f, 129
   invented 101
   parts of 101
Stimuli
   successive 202
   types of 187, 193
Stokes-Adams syndrome 243
Straight-Line test 149
Striae gravidarum 131f
Stroke volume 127
Stupor 136
Suck blood 18
Summation 203
   types of 204
Supinator jerk 178, 178f
Supraclavicular area 109
Supraspinatus 153, 157
Surface disk electrode 259, 259f
Swallowing, effect of 252
Syme's cannula 230f
Syntactical aphasia 137
Systemic lupus erythematosus 20

▎T

T wave 241, 245f
   changes in 245
   inversion 245
   tall 245, 245f
Tachycardia 246
   ratio 276
Tactile localization 138
Tallquist's method 28, 31
Tandem walking 149, 150f
Tape recorder recording 239
Tape recording 238

Taste
   sensation 173
   sense of 167
Telemetry 238, 239
Temperature 97, 140
Temporal artery, superficial 118
Temporalis, power of 166f
Tenderness 100
Tendon
   jerks 177
   reflex, deep 176, 182, 183
Tension, measurement of 278f
Test tube 48
   method 89
Tetanic contractions 206
Tetanus 205
   affecting genesis of 206
   genesis of 205
Tetany 303
Thermometer 281
Thiazine eosinate 59
Thigh
   abductors of 155, 157
   adductors of 155, 157
   extensors of 155
   flexors of 155, 157
   rotators of 155, 157
Thoma glass pipette 34
Thoracic nerve, long 153
Thorn test 73
Thrombasthenic purpura 84
Thrombocytes 65
Thrombocytopenia 78
Thrombocytosis 78
Thromboplastin generation test 82
Thrombus 84
Thumb, adductors of 151, 151f
Thyrotoxicosis 303
Tibial artery, posterior 118
Tics 156
Tidal volume 249
Tilt table 275f
Tissue
   continuous stimulation of 193f
   staining 65
Toes
   extensors of 151, 155
   flexors of 151, 155
Tongue
   anterior 2/3 of 173
   posterior 1/3 of 173
Total bilirubin 291
Total leukocyte count 34, 44, 54, 55f, 58, 80, 291, 292
Touch sensation 138
Tourniquet 15
Trachea 109
   examining position of 111f
   position of 110
Transmission electron microscopy 7
Trapezius 155, 171
   lower part 157
   testing power of 171f
   upper part 157
Tremors 156

Index

Triceps 153, 157
    jerk 178, 178*f*
    testing 153*f*
Trisodium citrate 13
Tropicamide 268
Tube length 4
Tungsten filament 235
Turk's fluid 36, 54, 57, 292
    composition of 55
Tyrode solution 285, 292
    composition of 285

U

U wave 241
Umbilical hernia, normal 130*f*
Umbilicus 130
Upper limb 147, 157
    muscles of 151, 157
Upper respiratory tract 109
Uric acid 291
Urinary bladder 133

V

V wave, giant 124
Vagal escape, basis of 227
Vagal inhibition, basis of 227
Vagal tone 229
Vagosympathetic trunk 227
    stimulation of 228
Valsalva maneuver 275, 276, 276*f*
    uses of 277
Valsalva ratio 275, 276
Varnishing 192
Vascular defects 84
Vasculitis 84
Vector cardiography 243
Vein
    over abdomen, causes of prominent 134
    peripheral 13
Venous blood 48
    collection of 15
    sample 15

Venous pressure, assess 124
Venous pulsations 120
Ventilation, maximum voluntary 248*f*
Ventricle, effect of heat and cold on 222
Verbal aphasia 137
Vesicular breath 115
Vesicular breath sounds 115
Vessel wall, condition of 118
Vestibular function, tests of 173
Vibrating interrupter 188, 188*f*
Vibration sense 138, 139
    testing for 140*f*
Viral infections 67
Visible peristalsis 130
Vision
    acuity of 160
    binocular 258
    near 160, 161*f*
Visual field 255
    defects 162
Visual pathway 255
Vital capacity 247
Vocal fremitus 100, 111, 115
    testing for 112*f*
Vocal resonance 113-115
Voluntary hyperventilation 252, 254
von Willebrand disease 82

W

Waddling gait 137
Watch test 168
Water
    bath 281
    buffer 69
    distilled 30, 74
    hammer 117
        pulse 127
    tap 69
Waves 242
Weber's test 168, 169*f*
Wenckebach's phenomenon 243, 243*f*
Westergren's method 17, 18

Westergren's pipette 22, 23
    mounted 17*f*
Whispering pectoriloquy 115
White blood cells 10, 34, 61
    count 54
    diluting fluid 54
    pipette 35, 35*f*, 54, 56
        bulbs of 41*f*
    type of 11, 58
White coat hypertension 107
Whole blood 88
Willebrand disease 83
Wintrobe's hematocrit tube 23, 23*f*
Wintrobe's method 17, 18, 20, 23
Wintrobe's mixture 13
Wintrobe's tube 22, 23
Wright's method 81
Wright's peak flow meter 266, 266*f*
Wrist
    extensors of 152, 157
    flexors of 152, 157
    testing
        extensors of 152*f*
        flexors of 152*f*
Writing lever 191

X

X plates, set of 235
X-block 191

Y

Y plates 235
Yarn matching test 162

Z

Zero error' mercury manometer 106
Zeta potential 20